Current Advances in Drug Delivery Through Fast Dissolving/Disintegrating Dosage Forms

Edited by:

Vikas Anand Saharan

Department of Pharmaceutics, School of Pharmaceutical Sciences, Sardar Bhagwan Singh Post Graduate Institute of Biomedical Sciences & Research, Dehradun, India

Bentham Science Publishers Ltd.
Executive Suite Y - 2
PO Box 7917, Saif Zone
Sharjah, U.A.E.
Email: subscriptions@benthamscience.org

BENTHAM SCIENCE

CONTENTS

FOREWORD

The major challenge that I have experienced as a pharmaceutical science professional is to keep abreast of the ever-evolving developments in the field and translating the innovations to ensure better quality of life to human and animals. The history of pharmaceuticals is loaded with a concern for the development of new chemical entities. Only in recent years, the importance of dosage form design has been recognized as a vital component of safe and effective clinical outcomes.

Despite tremendous innovations in drug delivery, the oral drug delivery continues to be a step ahead as a preferred route of administration for therapeutic agents. Some obvious advantages include accurate dosage, low cost, self-medication, non-invasive and easy administration. At the same time, an important drawback with oral dosage forms is "dysphagia" or difficulty in swallowing in paediatric and geriatric populations, leading to noncompliance and ineffective therapy.

Recent advances in novel delivery systems aim to enhance the safety of drug molecules while maintaining the therapeutic efficacy with an overall aim of better patient compliance. To achieve this objective, the concept of Fast Dissolving/Disintegrating Dosage Forms (FDDF) was introduced. FDDF is a perfect example of patient-oriented pharmaceutical approach, which has emerged from the need to provide a convenient way to administer medicines. Solid dosage forms that disintegrate, dissolve, or get suspended in the saliva in the mouth rapidly (in seconds) without chewing or use of water, provide an excellent alternative to swallowing the solid dosage form. This technique facilitates easy swallowing providing significant benefits to the relevant patient population.

In addition to patient compliance, extending the pharmaceutical product life cycle is another reason for the increasing popularity of the FDDFs. As a drug entity reaches the end of its patent life, it is common for manufacturers to develop it in a new and improved dosage form that allows extension of market exclusivity, while offering its patient population a more convenient dosage form. It also leads to increased revenue for the company, while targeting underserved and undertreated patient populations. Generally, the additional cost of manufacturing these specialized dosage forms is only marginally higher, which is easily compensated by additional benefits to patients.

The book covers relevant topics in different chapters, *e.g.* basic introduction with advantages and key concepts, patented technologies, taste masking approaches, general ingredients for developing formulation, quality control parameters, and critical review of clinical trials, which will be useful for a wide range of readers. The book has also included application of FDDFs to achieve controlled and targeted release which is expected to be of considerable interest to experts as well as new researchers. I strongly feel that this addition to literature will be especially useful to undergraduate pharmacy and post-graduate pharmaceutical science students. The book will serve as a sound source of systematic information for FDDFs. Students and researchers who consider dysphagia or pharmaceutical marketing during innovative product development will find it as a welcoming tool. A single textbook that brings together inputs from experts in all of these subjects is certainly an invaluable asset to pharmaceutical industry.

I wish to congratulate the editor, team of authors and Bentham publisher for excellent work and contribution to the pharmaceutical sciences. It is especially pleasing to note that a small Master's project undertaken by Dr Vikas Anand in his early years motivated him to continue working in the field and led to this wonderful compilation.

Sanjay Garg
School of Pharmacy and Medical Sciences
University of South Australia, City East Campus
Adelaide, SA
Australia

PREFACE

The solid dosage forms that dissolve or disintegrate quickly in the oral cavity, resulting in solution or suspension, eliminating the need of water for swallowing, are known as fast dissolving/disintegrating dosage forms (FDDFs). Over the last 20 years, the field of FDDFs has expanded considerably to address not only concerns of immediate release dosage forms but additionally played an important role in controlled/modified release drug delivery. This is still an exciting and growing area of pharmaceutical research and education. Ironically, to date no single book provides detailed and specific information on FDDFs. Therefore, I decided to write a book comprising of chapters that collectively address this void and provide an insight into the various technologies and methodologies currently adopted to formulate, prepare and evaluate FDDFs. The idea for this book on the topic has been in mind since my first research project during M.S.(Pharm.) at NIPER, Mohali. Since, then it gradually strengthened when I was Assistant Professor at Seth GL Bihani SD College, Sri Ganganagar and Professor/Associate Professor at Sardar Bhagwan Singh Post Graduate Institute (SBSPGI) of Biomedical Sciences & Research, Dehradun. My teaching and research in relevant and related fields continuously helped me in understanding and developing deeper interests towards FDDFs.

The present book is an attempt to provide comprehensive information to the readers interested in FDDFs. The specific emphasis in this book has been given to various technologies of making FDDFs, formulation development, evaluation, clinical studies, and marketed FDDFs products. This book intends to serve as a source of reference work and some chapters may be used for classroom teaching in graduate/postgraduate programmes. The authors do feel that graduate/postgraduate programmes in pharmaceutical sciences often neglect to adequately address FDDFs as novel drug delivery systems. Research fellows and experience scientists also feel paucity to find few resources outside the primary literature for FDDFs.

Due to its organization into different chapters, the book can be read at different levels and a reader can start as per the sequence of chapters or may opt to go directly onto the desired chapter. Thus, this book could be useful for graduate, postgraduate and PhD students belonging to the pharmaceutical sciences. Nevertheless, we do hope that this book is also useful to expert as well as new researchers, who may find information and new ideas for novel advancements in the field of FDDFs.

I hope that all those who consult this book find it useful as an easy-to-understand text for FDDFs. Constructive comments/suggestions are also invited from readers for further refinements in this book.

CONFLICT OF INTEREST

The authors confirm that they have no conflict of interest to declare for this publication.

ACKNOWLEDGEMENTS

I am grateful and highly indebted to my M.S.(Pharm.) supervisor and teacher Prof.(Dr.) Sanjay Garg for teaching the concepts of research in pharmaceutics and extending his support to this book by writing a foreword to this book. I greatly acknowledge continuous motivation and support of my Ph.D. supervisor Prof.(Dr.) P.K. Choudhury for all my efforts to do the best in the field of pharmaceutical sciences.

I am extremely grateful to the management of SBSPGI, especially Sh. S. P. Singh (Chairman, SBSPGI) and Dr. Gauravdeep Singh (Managing Secretary, SBSPGI) for all round support during my entire tenure at SBSPGI. I am highly privileged to have some of my good teachers, like Dr. Luvkush (academic advisor, SBSPGI), Prof. Veerma Ram and Ms. Urmi Chaurasia, as a constant and continuous source of inspiration and motivation.

Without the support of my mother, father and wife, it was really impossible to complete this arduous task. They have sacrificed a lot of my personal time while I was working on this book. I also missed my son, Inesh, when I was working on this book and he was not beside me.

I would like to thank all the chapter authors for their hard work, valuable contributions and their patience in various phases of publication of this book. I am extremely thankful to Bentham for providing a platform from where this book can reach to it's readers.

Vikas A. Saharan
Department of Pharmaceutics
School of Pharmaceutical Sciences
Sardar Bhagwan Singh Post Graduate Institute
of Biomedical Sciences & Research (SBSPGI)
Balawala, Dehradun
India

List of Contributors

Anupama Singh	Department of Pharmacognosy, School of Pharmaceutical Sciences, Sardar Bhagwan Singh Post Graduate Institute of Biomedical Sciences & Research (SBSPGI), Balawala, Dehradun 248161, India
Arpita Jindal	Department of Clinical Pharmacy, Division of Pharmaceutical Sciences, Shri Guru Ram Rai Institute of Technology and Science, Dehradun 248001, Uttarakhand, India
D. N. Mishra	Department of Pharmaceutical Sciences, Guru Jambheshwar University of Science and Technology, Hisar 125001, Haryana, India
Hemant Jadhav	Department of Pharmacy, Birla Institute of Technology and Science, Pilani Campus, Vidya Vihar, Pilani 333031, Jhunjhunu, Rajasthan, India
Kalpana Nagpal	Amity Institute of Pharmacy, Amity University, Noida, Uttar Pradesh 201303, India
Mahaveer Singh	Department of Pharmacy, Birla Institute of Technology and Science, Pilani Campus, Vidya Vihar, Pilani 333031, Jhunjhunu, Rajasthan, India
Prashant Mathur	Department of Clinical Pharmacy, Division of Pharmaceutical Sciences, Shri Guru Ram Rai Institute of Technology and Science, Dehradun 248001, Uttarakhand, India
Shailendra K. Singh	Department of Pharmaceutical Sciences, Guru Jambheshwar University of Science and Technology, Hisar 125001, Haryana, India
Sokindra Kumar	RV Northland Institute of Pharmacy, Greater Noida 203207, Uttar Pradesh, India
Vandana Kharb	Sachdeva College of Pharmacy, Chandigarh-Ludhiana National Highway, Gharuan 140413, Punjab, India
Vikas A. Saharan	Department of Pharmaceutics, School of Pharmaceutical Sciences, Sardar Bhagwan Singh Post Graduate Institute of Biomedical Sciences & Research (SBSPGI), Balawala, Dehradun 248161, India

DEDICATION

Dedicated to
my Mother Mrs. Chanderpati

&

my Father Mr. Dayanand Saharan

Current Advances in Drug Delivery Through Fast Dissolving/Disintegrating Dosage Forms

Current Advances in Drug Delivery through Fast Dissolving/Disintegrating Dosage Forms

Editor: Vikas Anand Saharan

eISBN (Online): 978-1-68108-459-6

ISBN (Print): 978-1-68108-460-2

First published in 2017.

CHAPTER 1

Fast Dissolving/Disintegrating Dosage Forms: Introducing through Development, Market, Pharmacopoeial and Regulatory Status

Vikas A. Saharan[1,*], **Anupama Singh**[2] and **Vandana Kharb**[3]

[1] *Department of Pharmaceutics, School of Pharmaceutical Sciences, Sardar Bhagwan Singh Post Graduate Institute of Biomedical Sciences and Research, Balawala, Dehradun 248161, Uttarakhand, India*

[2] *Department of Pharmacognosy, School of Pharmaceutical Sciences, Sardar Bhagwan Singh Post Graduate Institute of Biomedical Sciences and Research, Balawala, Dehradun 248161, Uttarakhand, India*

[3] *Sachdeva College of Pharmacy, Chandigarh-Ludhiana National Highway, Gharuan 140413, Punjab, India*

Abstract: Fast Dissolving/Disintegrating Dosage Forms (FDDFs) have emerged as alternate dosage forms for patients who cannot swallow or who should not swallow or who refuse to swallow conventional tablets/capsules and liquid formulations. FDDFs include Fast Dissolving/Disintegrating Tablets (FDTs), Fast Dissolving/Disintegrating Oral Films (FDOFs), Fast Dissolving/Disintegrating Capsules (FDCs), Fast Dissolving/Disintegrating Pellets (FDPs), *etc*. These dosage forms dissolve/disintegrate quickly, when placed on tongue, resulting in solution/suspension, which can be swallowed easily and hence do not require water for their oral ingestion. This chapter introduces FDDFs rationale, their brief history, regulatory/pharmacopoeial aspects, advantages/disadvantages and their market potential.

Keywords: Absorption, Capsule, Dysphagia, FDT, Film, Freeze drying, Geriatric, Granule, Mini tablet, Nausea, ODT, Orodispersible, Paediatric, Parkinsonism, Pellet, Pharmacopoeia, Psychotic, Quality of life, Tablet, Travellers.

1. INTRODUCTION

Administering drug by oral route is simple, convenient and a first choice delivery

* **Corresponding author Vikas A. Saharan:** Department of Pharmaceutics, School of Pharmaceutical Sciences, Sardar Bhagwan Singh Post Graduate Institute of Biomedical Sciences and Research (www.sbspgi.edu.in), Balawala, Dehradun 248161, Uttarakhand, India; Tel: +91-135-2686246; Mobile: +91-8439820796; Fax: +91-135-2686286; E-mail: vikas.pharmaceutics@gmail.com

option among all other routes of delivering drug. Further, in orally administered dosage forms, the solid dosage forms, *i.e.* tablets and capsules, are mostly liked because of their ease of manufacture, low cost of production, and convenience in packaging and transportation. Conventionally, tablets can be manufactured by either direct compression or granulation methods. Although the basic mechanical compaction approaches for tablet manufacturing remains same. The tablet formulation technology has undergone great improvement and continuous efforts are still ongoing to improve the processes and techniques of tablet manufacturing and physical properties of the tablet *vis a vis* to the latest developments in science.

Sublingual tablets and buccal tablets are considered as precursors to FDDFs. Sublingual tablets have been developed for antianginal drugs like nitroglycerine, *etc.*, where sublingual and/or buccal absorption can provide faster onset of action in acute attacks and improve bioavailability. Buccal tablets are designed to dissolve on the buccal mucous membrane to improve bioavailability of drugs, which are inconvenient to administer parenterally, like steroids and narcotic analgesics. Absorption through buccal route bypasses the gastrointestinal tract for rapid systemic distribution. Not all FDDFs administered orally can offer buccal absorption and bioavailability/faster onset advantages. Most of the FDDFs have similar absorption, bioavailability, onset and similar pharmacokinetics to conventional solid unit dosage forms. However, a fast disintegration of dosage form, rapid dissolution of the drug in oral cavity, and a small tablet weight can enhance absorption in the oral cavity.

US Food and Drug Administration (FDA), in its guidance document *"Size, Shape, and Other Physical Attributes of Generic Tablets and Capsules"*, has emphasised on ability of disintegration to influence oesophageal transit time and the performance of the drug product for its intended use, especially in patients suffering from dysphagia [1]. In one estimate, it was reported that over 16 million people in the US are suffering from some sort of swallowing problems (dysphagia). Dysphagia is "subjective awareness of swallowing difficulty during the passage of a bolus from the mouth to the stomach or the perception of obstruction during swallowing" [2]. Depending on the location of this sensation, dysphagia is classified as oropharyngeal or substernal. Dysphagia may arise due to benign or malignant structural lesions, oesophageal motility abnormalities, oropharyngeal dysfunction (including aspiration), neuromuscular disorders, postsurgical changes and gastro-oesophageal reflux disease (GERD). Dysphagia is also a common consequence of many diseases like pneumonia, dehydration, and malnutrition [3]. Neurological disorders (*e.g.* Parkinson's disease, brain or spinal cord injury, muscular dystrophy, stroke multiple sclerosis) and gastrointestinal disorders (GERD, oesophagitis, cancer in oesophagus) are some of the major health problems, which may lead to dysphagia [4]. However, the problem of difficulties in swallowing tablets/capsules is more widespread to 40% of the patient population in US [1]. Paediatric, geriatric and neurologic patients often suffer more from the difficulty of swallowing tablets and capsules [5 - 7]. Tablet swallowing problems have also been observed in adults [3].

In one latest survey, frequent dysphagia was observed in 3% of the US population, uniformly across both gender and all adult ages, and GERD has been indicated as its main underlying cause [8].

FDDFs require less effort to swallow and do not results in increased levels of airway compromise, when swallowing of Orally Disintegrating Tablets (ODTs) is compared to conventional tablets in dysphagic patients [3]. FDDFs are, therefore, considered as an alternate drug delivery option for patients who are either suffering from some sort of dysphagia or patients where compliance is an issue related to size/shape of tablets/capsules or their swallowing ability. FDDFs are comparatively easier dosage form to administer in paediatrics, geriatrics, psychotic, and adult patients who experience dysphagia more often. FDDFs can be administered without water, which makes them more attractive for frequent travellers and situations where access to potable water is an issue. FDDFs improve quality of life in patients by alleviating problems of swallowing, compliance, medication administration without water (nocturea, frequent travellers, nausea) and improving quicker onset of action of medications for immediate action for pain, anxiety, cough-cold, sexual pleasure, anxiety, *etc.* [9 - 14].

2. PHARMACOPOEIAL AND REGULATORY STATUS

FDDFs were first introduced in late 1990s in the market. In the official pharmacopoeial point of view, these formulations are known as orodispersible tablets in European Pharmacopoeia [15] and Orally Disintegrating Tablets in USP [16] and Japanese Pharmacopoeia (JP 16) [17] uses both of these terms. USP, BP and JP have also included several monographs of ODT tablets (Table **1**).

Table 1. Monographs of ODTs in USP 35 NF 30 [16], BP 2010 [19] and JP 16 [17].

USP 35 NF 30	BP 2010	JP 16
Alprazolam Orally Disintegrating Tablet	Orodispersible Mirtazapine Tablets	Ebastine Orally Disintegrating Tablet [17]

(Table 1) contd.....

USP 35 NF 30	BP 2010	JP 16
Clonazipine Orally Disintegrating Tablet		Naftopidil Orally Disintegrating Tablets [20]
Donepezil Orally Disintegrating Tablet		Amlodipine besylate Orally Disintegrating Tablets [21]
Loratadine Orally Disintegrating Tablet		Taltirelin Orally Disintegrating Tablets [21]
Mirtazapine Orally Disintegrating Tablet		
Ondansetron Orally Disintegrating Tablet		
Risperidone Orally Disintegrating Tablet		
Carbidopa and Levodopa Orally Disintegrating Tablet (Second Supplement to USP 36 NF 31)		

USP 35 NF 30 defines ODTs as *"Orally Disintegrating Tablets are intended to disintegrate rapidly within the mouth to provide a fine dispersion before the patient swallow the resulting suspension where the active pharmaceutical ingredient is intended for gastrointestinal delivery and/or absorption. Some of these dosage forms have been formulated to facilitate rapid disintegration and are manufactured by conventional means or by using lyophilisation or molding process"* [18].

European Pharmacopoeia 7.4 and British Pharmacopoeia 2010 have defined orodispersible tablets as *"uncoated tablets intended to be placed in the mouth where they disperse rapidly before being swallowed"* [15, 19]. EP 7.4 and BP 2010 have specified a time limit of 3 minute for disintegration in pharmacopoeial apparatus for orodispersible tablets.

Japanese Pharmacopoeia specifies ODTs as "*tablets which are quickly dissolved or disintegrated in the oral cavity. Orally Disintegrating Tablets shows an appropriate disintegration*" [17].

US FDA defines ODT as "*solid dosage form containing medicinal substances which disintegrates rapidly, usually within a matter of seconds, when placed upon the tongue*" [22]. Disintegration time of 30s or less is specified, when disintegration is performed by USP disintegration test method or any other suitable disintegration test. An upper dose limit for ODT is 500 mg is considered appropriate, but a dose greater than 500 mg may be incorporated without affecting the performance, *i.e.* disintegration time. The idea of 500 mg weight limitation is, therefore, not appreciated by various research groups and pharmaceutical industries. Successful ODTs having more than 500 mg weight and disintegrating time less than a minute have been formulated.

In 2012, films for oral drug delivery became part of the European Pharmacopoeia, edition 7.4 [15]. Films were included in the monograph as 'oromucosal preparations' and described as fast-dissolving 'orodispersible films' or 'mucoadhesive/buccal films', which are intended to be attached to oromucosal sites. Unlike ODTs, pharmacopoeia does not specify any time limit for disintegration/dissolution of FDOFs (Fast Dissolving/Disintegrating Oral Films).

International Conference on Harmonisation (ICH) and drug regulating agencies like European Medicines Agency (EMA), US FDA, Pharmaceuticals and Medical Devices Agency (PMDA), *etc.* have issued several guidelines on developing age adapted dosage forms with an aim to improve health related quality of life of patients [23 - 27]. FDDFs, like Fast Dissolving/Disintegrating Pellets (FDPs), Orally Dissolving/Disintegrating Mini-Tablets (ODMTs), Fast Dissolving/ Disintegrating Granules (FDGs), provide dosing flexibility for paediatrics and thus their potential as dosage form is rising with the regulatory stringencies and requirements of special dosage forms for special populations. FDPs and ODMTs are currently under development and their entry in pharmacopoeia and market is expected soon.

3. SOME KEY CONCEPTS: RATIONALE, ADVANTAGES AND CHALLENGES

FDTs are also pronounced by various other names, which are presented in Box **1**. In this chapter and book, we have uniformly used Fast Disintegrating/Dissolving Tablets (FDTs) for ODTs and for all other similar tablet dosage forms, which disintegrate quickly in oral cavity or *in vitro*.

Box 1: Various synonyms of FDTs.

- Melt in mouth tablets
- Fast dissolving/disintegrating tablets
- Rapidly dissolving/disintegrating tablets
- Rapid melt tablets
- Fast melt tablets
- Fast dispersion tablets
- Mouth dissolving tablets
- Saliva soluble tablets
- Rapid suspension tablets

FDTs have been initially developed as immediate release dosage forms intended for faster and quicker onset and suited best, therefore, to drugs indicated for treatment of acute diseases. Fast acting, compliance critical and paediatric drugs are some good drug candidates for developing FDTs (Box **2**). However, FDTs have also been designed and developed for treatment of chronic diseases in patients who are dysphagic. Quick oral disintegration and administration without water have made FDTs popular as an alternative to conventional tablets in patients who are not dysphagic. Advantages of FDTs have significantly impacted the convenience, acceptability and compliance of delivering drugs in special populations. Persons, who often travel, also prefer FDTs over conventional tablets due to difficult access of water, sometimes.

Box 2: Therapeutic categories, which are considered as potential targets for developing FDDFs.

- Pain, fever, migraine drugs
- Cardiovascular drugs (angina, stroke, hypertension, *etc.*)
- Respiratory drugs (anti-asthmatics, systemic antihistamine, throat, cold and cough problems)
- Anticancer drugs
- Central nervous system drugs (sedatives, antiemetics, antipsychotic drugs, antimanic drugs, schizophrenia, Parkinson's disease, Alzheimer's disease, *etc.*)
- Over the counter drugs (multivitamin preparations, antacids, *etc.*).

3.1. Patient Specific Advantages of FDDFs

- Easy swallow by patients who have swallowing problems or patients who reject to swallow, *e.g.* geriatric, paediatric and psychotic patients.
- Easy swallow in dysphagia due to diseases, *e.g.* AIDS, parkinsonism, thyroidectomy, head and neck radiation therapy, neurological disorders, upper gastrointestinal surgery, diseases like injury in food-pipe, persistent nausea, *etc.*
- Bed-ridden patients can swallow FDT without water and without the need to rise or sit in the bed for swallowing.
- Situations when quick access of water is inconvenient, *e.g.* frequent travellers and busy persons.
- No water is required for dosing and hence beneficial for patients with renal failure, patients on anti-diuretic treatment and in places where access to water is a problem.

- Patient compliance due to convenience to carry and administration.
- Easy and discrete handling.
- Convenience and accurate dosage, when compared with liquids.
- Rapid pregastric absorption of drug from, mouth, pharynx and oesophagus. Hence, faster onset of action beneficial in stroke, migraine and pain therapy, and improved bioavailability for buccally absorbed drugs and drugs prone to first pass metabolism.
- Rapid drug therapy intervention.

3.2. Disadvantages/Challenges to FDDFs

- Undesirable taste of drug and excipients (bitter, sour, metallic and chalkiness).
- Friability problems due to Compression-less method of manufacturing or use of low to very low compression forces.
- Drugs sensitive to humidity and temperature.
- Need for special packaging and embossing of identification marks.
- Requirements of special equipments for production and packaging (freeze drying, cotton candy spinning apparatus, 3-D printing, *etc.*).
- High cost involved in production and packaging.
- Drug dose and limitation on the final size of the tablet.

4. THE DEVELOPMENT PATH

For the first time, FDDFs were developed and studied in 1970's by Wyeth Laboratories in the United Kingdom [28]. Patents covering these novel dosage forms were issued to Wyeth around the world [29, 30]. Later this technology was registered and trademarked by the name of Zydis®. Zydis® technology utilise a patented freeze drying process for removing water from an aqueous solution or suspension of active ingredient(s) and excipients kept in blister packs. The cost of making these novel dosage units were significantly higher and thus Wyeth associated with R. P. Scherer (now Catalent), from 1981 onwards, for sharing the costs of development and to bring specific expertise in developing these novel dosage forms. In that joint venture, Wyeth concentrated on the formulation technology and R.P. Scherer on the development of an efficient and economical freeze drying process. Wyeth marketed FDDF sunder Expidet™ trademark in some of the European countries such as Switzerland, Belgium and Germany [28]. A lorazepam fast dissolving formulation (Tavor Expidet™) was launched in 1992. Expidet™ was a trademark of American Home Products Corp. At that time, in 1990's, there was only one manufacturing plant at Scherer's Swindon site. Now, Catalent has four different facilities located at Somerset (New Jersey, US), Swindon (UK), Kakegawa (Japan) and Schorndorf (Germany) for the development and production of Zydis® FDDFs [31].

First generation FDTs were manufactured by freeze drying technologies. The dosage form was formulated with a water soluble carrier material and a unit dose of drug was dissolved in an aqueous solution. The composition was frozen and water was sublimed by freeze drying process to yield FDDFs described as Zydis® FDDFs. Simultaneously or later other companies like Farmalyoc (Lyoc®), Janssen Pharmaceutica (QuickSolv®), and Elan's (currently Perrigo) (NanoCrystal® Nanomelt™) developed their own freeze drying technologies for manufacturing FDTs. All these freeze drying technologies for manufacturing FDTs are discussed in ***Chapter 2***.

First generation FDTs, prepared by freeze drying technologies, have disadvantages of a low hardness, high friability, costly manufacturing process and special packaging leading to crumble and not so robust tablets. These disadvantages were tried to overcome by developing FDTs by modifying conventional tablet compaction methods to increase disintegration/dissolution time of tablets. Advent of faster and high functionality disintegrants had made this task easy. Tablets get enough hardness when compressed by conventional wet/dry granulation or direction compression, while faster disintegration/dissolution was achieved by adding high amounts of superdisintegrants in the formulation. Direct compression, granulation methods, compaction and subsequent treatments, and effervescent tableting methods evolved for preparing FDTs are described in Chapter 3. New compaction based technologies emerged to produce stronger FDTs. Ziplets®, Flashtab®, Easy Tec®, Advatab®, Frosta®, RACTAB® and other proprietary technologies have also been explored in ***Chapter 3***.

Through three decades, FDT technologies have advanced significantly with their rapid market growth across various countries and numerous therapeutic segments. New and novel methodologies like moulding, extrusion, floss, three dimensional printing have emerged in manufacturing FDTs. These novel methodologies and trademark technologies like EMP® tablet, FlashDose® and others are presented in ***Chapter 4***.

Technologies for manufacturing FDTs are extensively patented across the globe. Patents provide exclusive benefits to recover industry costs on developing a technology. Inventions in the field of FDDFs have led to several patents. Technologies based on the patents have been either registered or trademarked for their commercial exploitation. ***Chapter 5*** explores various inventions related to manufacturing, packaging and other aspects of FDTs through published patents and patent applications.

Formulating an FDT is a difficult challenge due to the expectation of striking a balance between hardness and quicker disintegration/dissolution. Excipients play important roles in striking a balance between mechanical strength and disintegration//dissolution time of tablets. ***Chapter 6*** deals with various excipients used in designing and developing FDTs. Superdisintegrants, diluents and taste masking excipients have been described with their dedicated roles, key properties and their importance in formulation development of FDTs.

Chapter *7* is a comprehensive coverage on various taste masking approaches used in formulating pleasantly flavoured and palatable FDDFs. Taste masking is essential required in FDDFs due to their quick disintegration/dissolution in oral cavity leading to fast access of bitter drug to taste buds. Various proprietary and technological advancements in controlling bitterness and improving taste in FDDF formulations are explained with the help of published research reports and patents.

Evaluation and quality control of novel FDTs require new set of equipments and methodologies for estimation of attributes like disintegration, dissolution, mechanical strength, *etc*. Various in house disintegration test apparatuses have been reported in literature for estimating quick disintegration/dissolution/water sorption. Some of these disintegration test equipments are available commercially. Special methodologies have been used for estimating drug release from such dosage forms. These evaluation methodologies have been refined and some of these have been accepted by pharmacopoeia/industry/drug regulatory agencies. ***Chapter 8*** provides a comprehensive review on latest quality control tests, quality control equipments and evaluation parameters of FDTs. Disintegration equipments and methodologies for measuring disintegration time are emphasised with due diligence to their development.

Clinical tests on FDDFs have established several pharmacokinetic and compliance/preference benefits of FDDFs over other conventional dosage forms. ***Chapter 9*** is authors' effort to describe clinical advantages through reported clinical studies on FDDFs.

FDOF or oral drug strip, when placed on the tongue, disintegrates/dissolves within seconds resulting in release of drug, which is swallowed with the saliva. FDOF utilises hydrophilic polymers, which dissolve/disintegrate in oral cavity and thus enable to deliver drug by dissolution followed by quick absorption to the systemic circulation. Absorption of the drug occurs *via* mouth, buccally or sublingually and/or *via* small intestine. FDOFs are also considered as advanced alternative to conventional tablets, capsules and liquid dosage forms. Some of these FDOFs are also regarded as good alternatives to FDTs/ODTs. The most popular and straightforward approach to manufacture oral films is the solvent casting method. Other alternative methods include wet and melt extrusion, and drug printing methodologies like flexography and ink-jet printing. Due to small dose incorporation, challenges of bitter taste and other complexities associated with FDOFs, not many products have reached in the market. ***Chapter 10*** describes various formulation factors, manufacturing technologies and evaluation of FDOFs.

FDCs, ODMTs, FDPs and sustained/controlled release FDTs are some latest entry to the family of FDDFs. ***Chapter 11*** gives a latest view on these new FDDF entrants. Perforation and vacuum drying are used to prepare fast disintegrating capsules (FDCs) from conventional hard capsules [32]. Low bloom strength gelatin and various other additives have been used to develop Fastcaps (hard capsules) characterised with rapid disintegration in saliva and adequate mechanical strength [33]. Fast disintegrating capsules are able to overcome disadvantages of other FDDFs especially low pay-load, unsatisfactory taste masking, and time consuming and expensive manufacturing process. Mini-tablet and the FDDF technologies have been combined to develop novel ODMTs with multifunctional excipients. ODMTs, of diameter 3 mm or less, provides easy measuring abilities coupled with rapid disintegration of tablets in small amount of saliva, making them most appropriate dosage form for not only children but also for infants and toddlers [34]. Pectinic acid and MCC Sanaq burst have been used in preparing FDPs by extrusion/spheronisation [35, 36]. These pellets can offer advantages of faster disintegration/dissolution as with other FDDFs and may provide easy measuring abilities in case of paediatric dosing. For reducing dosing frequencies, controlling/sustaining drug release, novel FDDFs utilises FDDF technologies coupled with various other controlled/sustained drug release technologies like ion-exchange resins [37], coating [38], microparticulate beads [39, 40], *etc.* ***Chapter 11*** also discusses such research reports where technologies have been used in combination to achieve the objectives of modified/controlled release *via* FDDFs.

5. FDDF MARKET

FDDFs offer various commercial advantages (Box **3**) for boosting significant profits to both brand and generic pharmaceutical companies. FDDF products are regarded as novel drug delivery systems by drug regulatory agencies and this viewpoint makes them eligible for patent protection and market exclusivity. The brand value of an established drug increases with patent life extension and market exclusivities by protecting the drug product from generic substitution, which in turn increases revenues. Availability of more oral drug products, based on a single drug, widens the preference/acceptance among special patient populations leading to increase in market demands. FDDFs are considered ideal for drugs that are off patent. Generic manufactures can introduce drug products based on FDDFs for an off patent drug and broaden the range of drug products.

Box 3: Commercial advantages of FDDFs.

- New dosage form according to drug regulatory agencies
- Patent line extension
- Exclusivity of product
- Life cycle extension
- Product differentiation
- Protect product from generic substitution

FDDF technologies provide simple and safe option to deliver a drug orally, when compared to other delivery technologies based on other routes of drug administration. ODTs, FDOFs and other FDDFs provide the advantage of formulating drugs as either generic versions or bioequivalent extensions of approved drug products offering minimum clinical hurdles in getting regulatory approval.

Zydis® ODT formulation of loratadine (Claritin® Reditabs®) was the first FDDF drug product approved by US FDA in December 1996 [41]. Zydis® ODT formulation of clonazepam (Klonopin®) and a Zydis® ODT formulation of rizatriptan (Maxalt®) entered in market in December 1997 and June 1998, respectively. Lyophilised FDTs were the first FDTs, which were marketed and achieved high success in sales, expanding market size and increasing number of worldwide product launches [42]. Market growth and successful entry of Lyophilised FDTs were possible due to their versatile applications like buccal absorption, stable formulation environment and bioequivalence.

Revenue of above $2 billion was generated by ODT products sales, which was a hike of 20% over revenues of 2003 [43]. ODT market, in regions of US, EU, and Japan, grew more than $8.4 billion in 2011 with an increase of 24 percent from the past two years [44]. Generic competition and approvals in FDT segment were main driving forces to increase the number of FDT products in the market. However, generic competition has eroded the US and EU ODT market faster than the Japan ODT market where minimum impact is observed. FDT market is expected to reach $12 billion globally by 2018 with the popularity and growth of FDTs in various developing countries [44].

In 2004, as an estimate about 92% of the ODT world market share was distributed among three different therapeutic segments, *viz.* central nervous system, gastrointestinal, and oncology [45]. It has led to conclude that most successful ODTs belong to therapeutic segments like nausea, pain, migraine, insomnia, GERD, Parkinson's disease and other CNS disorders.

Two commercially successful FDDF products are GlaxoSmithKline's Zofran® ODT (ondansetron) and Lilly's Zyprexa® Zydis® (olanzapine) [45]. Zofran® ODT (ondansetron) is used for treatment of nausea and emesis induced by chemotherapy, surgery and radiation. After its approval in Jan 1999 by US FDA, Zofran® ODT reached a worldwide sales of more than $300 million in 2004, which represented about 20% of total Zofran sales with an average annual growth rate of approximately 50% [45]. Motivated by such high growth eight different generic ODT versions for ondansetron appeared in June 2007 to February 2011 [46]. Zyprexa® Zydis® (olanzapine) ODT, for treating schizophrenia and bipolar disorder and approved in April 2000 by US FDA, achieved a worldwide sale greater than $400 million at the end of 2004 [45]. This growth in US market had led to entry of olanzapine ODT by 9 different pharmaceutical companies in Oct 2011 to May 2014 [46]. However, Zyprexa® Zydis® formulation still enjoys marketing exclusivity till 26 July 2016 [46].

FDOF market started with products in mouthwash, OTC and nutraceutical segments. Later the focus of the market was shifted to prescription FDOF. FDOF were first introduced as strips in early 2000 and the first product was Listerine pocket strips, in the mouthwash range [47]. As a pharmaceutical product in OTC section, Zentrip® was launched in US by Sato Pharmaceuticals in August 2009 for prevention of motion sickness. This was followed by approval of Novarits' Nexcede® (12.5 mg ketoprofen) by the US FDA in November 2009. In July 2010, US FDA approved Zuplenz® (Ondansetron HCl, 4 mg, 8 mg), which was first prescription oral film product. Suboxone® thin film (buprenorphine and naloxone), FDOF product of Reckitt Benckiser's, was successful commercially with sales of $513 million in 2011 [44]. FDOF products for treatment of CNS disorders, allergies and diabetes are continuously expanding. FDOF market is expected to reach $1 billion in 2015 [44].

Currently, 10 FDOF products are available in the market and 29 FDOF products are in the development pipeline out of which 6 are expected to be launched in

2015/2016 [48]. These FDOF drug products provide rapid onset of action when administered by oromucosal, buccal or sublingual route. PharmFilm® (MonoSol Rx) and RapidFilm® (Applied Pharma Research/teas Labtec) technologies dominate the FDOF market with their use in about 30% of the products. A total of 10 different FDOF technologies have entered in the market. FFT Medical, Cynapsus Therapeutics, IntelGenx are some new entrants in developing FDOF products. Some successful marketed FDOF products are Suboxone®, Breakyl®, Onsolis® and Zuplenz®.

Many FDDF drug products have entered in the market after proving their patient preference/compliance and/or clinical/pharmacokinetic benefits in clinical studies. Market success of these novel FDDF drug products has led to the development and commercial entry of numerous FDDF products. Exhaustive and comprehensive lists of approved and marketed FDDF drug products can be found in ***Chapter 12***.

CONCLUSIONS

Development of FDDFs offers considerable commercial advantages, like patent line extension, product exclusivity, life cycle extension and product differentiation, protect the drug product from generic substitution and market competition. Pharmacopoeial and regulatory acceptance of FDDFs have significantly attracted both big and small scale pharmaceutical manufacturers and specialty drug delivery companies to come up with more and more FDDF products. Market outlook for FDDFs is also potential and promising to both brand pharmaceutical companies and generic pharmaceutical manufacturers. Patient acceptance by all age groups for FDDFs has increased their market potential and outreach. Novel FDDFs, like ODMTs, sustained/controlled release FDTs, FDPs, FDCs, are in development pipeline, which may soon be commercialised.

REFERENCES

[1] FDA Guidance for industry Size, shape, and other physical attributes of generic tablets and capsules. Silver Spring, MD: U.S. Department of Health and Human Services, Food and Drug Administration, Center for Drug Evaluation and Research (CDER) 2013.

[2] Carucci LR, Turner MA. Dysphagia revisited: common and unusual causes. Radiographics 2015; 35(1): 105-22.
[http://dx.doi.org/10.1148/rg.351130150] [PMID: 25590391]

[3] Carnaby-Mann G, Crary M. Pill swallowing by adults with dysphagia. Arch Otolaryngol Head Neck Surg 2005; 131(11): 970-5.
[http://dx.doi.org/10.1001/archotol.131.11.970] [PMID: 16301368]

[4] Birmachu W. Orally disintegrating extended release (ODT-ER) dosage forms. Drug Deliv 2010; (April): 33-4.

[5] Llorca P-M. Discussion of prevalence and management of discomfort when swallowing pills: orodispersible tablets expand treatment options in patients with depression. Ther Deliv 2011; 2(5): 611-22.
[http://dx.doi.org/10.4155/tde.11.32] [PMID: 22833978]

[6] Lefton-Greif MA. Pediatric dysphagia. Phys Med Rehabil Clin N Am 2008; 19(4): 837-851, ix.
[http://dx.doi.org/10.1016/j.pmr.2008.05.007] [PMID: 18940644]

[7] Sura L, Madhavan A, Carnaby G, Crary MA. Dysphagia in the elderly: management and nutritional considerations. Clin Interv Aging 2012; 7: 287-98.
[PMID: 22956864]

[8] Cho SY, Choung RS, Saito YA, *et al.* Prevalence and risk factors for dysphagia: a USA community study. Neurogastroenterol Motil 2015; 27(2): 212-9.
[http://dx.doi.org/10.1111/nmo.12467] [PMID: 25376877]

[9] Überall MA, Müller-Schwefe GH. Sublingual fentanyl orally disintegrating tablet in daily practice: efficacy, safety and tolerability in patients with breakthrough cancer pain. Curr Med Res Opin 2011; 27(7): 1385-94.
[http://dx.doi.org/10.1185/03007995.2011.583231] [PMID: 21561313]

[10] Weiss JP, Herschorn S, Albei CD, van der Meulen EA. Efficacy and safety of low dose desmopressin orally disintegrating tablet in men with nocturia: results of a multicenter, randomised, double-blind, placebo controlled, parallel group study. J Urol 2013; 190(3): 965-72.
[http://dx.doi.org/10.1016/j.juro.2012.12.112] [PMID: 23454402]

[11] Shankar G, Nate C. Positive and Negative Syndrome Scale as a long-term outcome measurement tool in patients receiving clozapine ODT- A Pilot Study. Pharm Pract (Granada) 2007; 5(1): 42-5.
[http://dx.doi.org/10.4321/S1886-36552007000100007] [PMID: 25214917]

[12] Sand PK, Dmochowski RR, Reddy J, van der Meulen EA. Efficacy and safety of low dose desmopressin orally disintegrating tablet in women with nocturia: results of a multicenter, randomised, double-blind, placebo controlled, parallel group study. J Urol 2013; 190(3): 958-64.
[http://dx.doi.org/10.1016/j.juro.2013.02.037] [PMID: 23454404]

[13] Nalamachu S, Hassman D, Wallace MS, Dumble S, Derrick R, Howell J. Long-term effectiveness and tolerability of sublingual fentanyl orally disintegrating tablet for the treatment of breakthrough cancer pain. Curr Med Res Opin 2011; 27(3): 519-30.
[http://dx.doi.org/10.1185/03007995.2010.545380] [PMID: 21208151]

[14] Martin-Morales A, Gutiérrez-Hernández P, Romero-Otero J, Romero-Martín JA. Duration of erection: does it really matter? A randomised, double-blind clinical trial to assess the impact of vardenafil ODT on duration of erection and its correlation with patients and partners sexual quality of life and duration of intercourse: the VADEOPEN study. J Sex Med 2014; 11(6): 1527-38.
[http://dx.doi.org/10.1111/jsm.12496] [PMID: 24628736]

[15] European Pharmacopoeia – edition 74. Strasbourg, France: European Directorate for the Quality of Medicines (EDQM) 2012.

[16] USP 30 NF 25. Rockville, Md., USA: The United States Pharmacopeial Convention Inc 2007.

[17] The Japanese Pharmacopoeia. 16th ed., Japan: Society of Japanese Pharmacopoeia, Ministry of Health, Labour and Welfare 2011.

[18] USP 35 NF 30. Rockville, Md., USA: The United States Pharmacopeial Convention Inc 2012.

[19] British Pharmacopoeia. London, UK: TSO (The Stationery Office) 2010.

[20] Supplement II to JP XVI (Japanese Pharmacopoeia, Sixteenth edition): Society of Japanese Pharmacopoeia, Ministry of Health, Labour and Welfare. Japan 2014.

[21] Supplement I to JP XVI (Japanese Pharmacopoeia, Sixteenth Edition): Society of Japanese Pharmacopoeia, Ministry of Health, Labour and Welfare. Japan 2012.

[22] FDA Guidance for Industry Orally Disintegrating Tablets. Silver Spring, MD: U.S. Department of Health and Human Services, Food and Drug Administration, Center for Drug Evaluation and Research (CDER) 2008.

[23] Breitkreutz J, Tuleu C. Pediatric and Geriatric Pharmaceutics and Formulation. Modern Pharmaceutics. 5th ed. 2009; pp. 221-58.

[24] Shah RR. Drug development and use in the elderly: search for the right dose and dosing regimen (Parts I and II). Br J Clin Pharmacol 2004; 58(5): 452-69. [http://dx.doi.org/10.1111/j.1365-2125.2004.02228.x] [PMID: 15521892]

[25] Guideline on pharmaceutical development of medicines for paediatric use. Committee for Medicinal Products for Human Use (CHMP) Paediatric Committee (PDCO). London, UK: European Medicines Agency 2013.

[26] Reflection Paper EM. Formulations of choice for the paediatric population. London, UK: European Medicines Agency 2006.

[27] Zisowsky J, Krause A, Dingemanse J. Drug development for pediatric populations: regulatory aspects. Pharmaceutics 2010; 2(4): 364-88. [http://dx.doi.org/10.3390/pharmaceutics2040364] [PMID: 27721363]

[28] Virley P, Yarwood R. Zydis-a novel, fast dissolving dosage form. Manuf Chemist. 1990; 61: pp. 36-7.

[29] Gregory GK, Peach JM, Du Mayne JD. Articles for carrying chemicals. United States Patent 4371516, 1983.

[30] Gregory GK, Ho DS. Pharmaceutical dosage form packages. United States Patent 4305502, 1981.

[31] Zydis Fast Dissolve , 2014 [Accessed on 2 Jan 2015]; Accessed from http://www.catalent.com /index.php/offerings /A-Z-Offerings/zydis

[32] Ciper M, Bodmeier R. Modified conventional hard gelatin capsules as fast disintegrating dosage form in the oral cavity. Eur J Pharm Biopharm 2006; 62(2): 178-84. [http://dx.doi.org/10.1016/j.ejpb.2005.08.014] [PMID: 16260126]

[33] Ciper M, Bodmeier R. Preparation and characterisation of novel fast disintegrating capsules (Fastcaps) for administration in the oral cavity. Int J Pharm 2005; 303(1-2): 62-71. [http://dx.doi.org/10.1016/j.ijpharm.2005.07.004] [PMID: 16111845]

[34] Stoltenberg I, Breitkreutz J. Orally disintegrating mini-tablets (ODMTs)a novel solid oral dosage form for paediatric use. Eur J Pharm Biopharm 2011; 78(3): 462-9. [http://dx.doi.org/10.1016/j.ejpb.2011.02.005] [PMID: 21324357]

[35] Leuenberger H, Leuenberger MN, Puchkov M. Right First Time: Computer-Aided Scale-up for manufacturing solid dosage forms with a shorter time to market. Swiss Pharma 2010; 32: 3-13.

[36] Tho I, Sande SA, Kleinebudde P. Disintegrating pellets from a water-insoluble pectin derivative produced by extrusion/spheronisation. Eur J Pharm Biopharm 2003; 56(3): 371-80. [http://dx.doi.org/10.1016/S0939-6411(03)00071-7] [PMID: 14602179]

[37] Jeong SH, Park K. Development of sustained release fast-disintegrating tablets using various polymer-coated ion-exchange resin complexes. Int J Pharm 2008; 353(1-2): 195-204. [http://dx.doi.org/10.1016/j.ijpharm.2007.11.033] [PMID: 18164882]

[38] Fini A, Bergamante V, Ceschel GC, Ronchi C, de Moraes CA. Fast dispersible/slow releasing ibuprofen tablets. Eur J Pharm Biopharm 2008; 69(1): 335-41. [http://dx.doi.org/10.1016/j.ejpb.2007.11.011] [PMID: 18182280]

[39] Venkatesh GM, Stevens PJ, Lai J-W. Development of orally disintegrating tablets comprising controlled-release multiparticulate beads. Drug Dev Ind Pharm 2012; 38(12): 1428-40. [http://dx.doi.org/10.3109/03639045.2011.653365] [PMID: 22356215]

[40] Venkatesh GM, Swaminathan V, Lai J-W, *et al.* Rapidly dispersing granules, orally disintegrating tablets and methods. United States Patent 20120282335, 2012.

[41] Allamneni Y, Allamneni N, Amarnath R, *et al.* A review on new innovations and technologies in the formulation of orally disintegrating tablets , 2015 [Accessed on 3rd March 2015]; Accessed from http://www.pharmatutor.org/articles/review-on-new-innovations-technologies-in-formulation-of-orally-disintegrating-tablets

[42] McLaughlin R, Banbury S, Crowley K. Orally disintegrating tablets: the effect of recent FDA guidance on ODT technologies and applications , 2009 [Accessed on 3rd March 2015]; Accessed from http://www.pharmtech.com/orally-disintegrating-tablets-effect-recent-fda-guidance-odt-technologies-and-applications

[43] Oral fast- dissolving drug delivery: technologies, market analysis, business opportunities. Technology Catalysts International 2003.

[44] Tablet OD, Technologies F. Orally Disintegrating Tablet and Film Technologies. Technologies, Products, & Market Analysis. 7th ed., 2013. [Accessed on 3rd March 2015]; Accessed from http://www.technology-catalysts.com/pdf/ODT7_brochure.pdf

[45] Harmon TM. Orally disintegrating tablets: a valuable life cycle management strategy , 2007 [Accessed on 3rd March 2015]; Accessed from www.pharmaceuticalcommerce.com

[46] Approved Drug Products with Therapeutic Equivalence Evaluations (Orange Book). 34th edn., U.S. Department of Health and Human Services, Food and Drug Administration, Center for Drug Evaluation and Research, Office of Medical Products and Tobacco Office of Generic Drugs 2014.

[47] Dixit RP, Puthli SP. Oral strip technology: overview and future potential. J Control Release 2009; 139(2): 94-107. [http://dx.doi.org/10.1016/j.jconrel.2009.06.014] [PMID: 19559740]

[48] Oral Thin Films Market, 2015-2025 , 2015 [Accessed on 3rd March 2015]; Accessed from https://www.reportbuyer.com /product/2634536/ oral-thin -films-market- 2015-2025.html

CHAPTER 2

Freeze Drying Technologies for Developing Fast Dissolving/Disintegrating Tablets

Vikas A. Saharan*

Department of Pharmaceutics, School of Pharmaceutical Sciences, Sardar Bhagwan Singh Post Graduate Institute of Biomedical Sciences and Research, Balawala, Dehradun 248161, Uttarakhand, India

Abstract: Highly porous nature of freeze dried materials and their ability to retain shape and volume have motivated pharmaceutical scientists to explore application of freeze drying in manufacturing fast dissolving/disintegrating tablets (FDTs). The process of manufacturing lyophilised tablets as FDTs is extensively proprietary and patented. Zydis®, Lyoc®, QuickSolv® and NanoCrystal® Nanomelt™ technologies have been successful in developing drug products and obtaining regulatory clearances from drug regulatory agencies for their marketing authorisations. This chapter aims to discuss formulation, processing and manufacturing aspects of FDTs prepared by freeze drying and also provides an overview on some of these patented FDT technologies.

Keywords: Disintegration, Dissolution, Formulation, Freeze casting, Freeze drying, Gels, Granules, Lyoc®, Lyophilisation, Manufacturing, Matrix, NanoCrystal®, Nanomelt™, Nanoparticles, Patent, Proprietary, QuickSolv®, Tablet, Wafer, Zydis®.

1. INTRODUCTION

Freeze drying is widely used in fabricating amorphous, porous and compact structures that dissolve rapidly. Active ingredient can be entrapped in this water soluble compact structure to prepare a unit dosage form, which can dissolve/disintegrate quickly, either *in vitro* when placed in water or *in vivo* when placed in the oral cavity. The freeze dried matrix of such tablets comprises a water soluble mixture of saccharides and polymers, the proportions of which are optimised to rapid dispersion characteristics and sufficient mechanical strength

* **Corresponding author Vikas A. Saharan:** Department of Pharmaceutics, School of Pharmaceutical Sciences, Sardar Bhagwan Singh Post Graduate Institute of Biomedical Sciences and Research (www.sbspgi.edu.in), Balawala, Dehradun 248161, Uttarakhand, India; Tel: +91-135-2686246; Mobile: +91-8439820796; Fax: +91-135-2686286; E-mail: vikas.pharmaceutics@gmail.com

to withstand handling and transportation stresses. The tablet formulations essentially contain excipients like suspending agents or emulsifiers, viscosity modifiers, wetting agents, preservatives, antioxidants, colours, taste masking agents and flavours, which can either enhance the processing capabilities or improve the quality of the resulting tablets.

2. FREEZE DRYING

Freeze drying or lyophilisation may be defined as the process of removing water from solutions/suspensions/emulsions by sublimation under the influence of high vacuum at temperatures below freezing point of water. The resulting final product is dry and extremely porous. Lyophilisation, as a drying process, was developed in 1940s and till then it has advanced as an important manufacturing step in improving stability of pharmaceutical and biological products [1]. The process is helpful in inhibiting chemical, microbiological and physical degradation pathways that has been otherwise evidenced with the presence of water or residual moisture. Drying at a low temperature has made lyophilisation a safe and extensively applied process for thermolabile actives, pharmaceutical ingredients and biological drugs. Since its inception, lyophilisation has been widely applied in formulating long term stable vaccines, preservation of nucleic acid based pharmaceuticals, preserving red blood cells, and development of micro and nanoparticulate delivery of small molecules, proteins and peptides [2]. Novel lyophilisates have found their applications as FDTs, 3D scaffolds, respirable powders after milling, respirable powders from direct dispersion of lyophilisates and respirable powders from spray-freeze drying.

The freeze drying process essentially involves three steps: an initial freezing of the formulation followed by primary drying and subsequently secondary drying to remove residual moisture from the final product [3]. Liquid drug formulation, solution/suspension/emulsion, filled in vials/tubes/blisters is placed on temperature controlled shelves within a sterile chamber and cooled to low temperatures until solvent freezes. One of the most important targets in freezing step is to achieve uniform freezing of the entire batch. Apart from conventional shelf freezing protocols, other approaches like flash freezing with nitrogen [4, 5] and freezing with annealing [5, 6] are also used for freezing the liquid formulations and optimising the formulation characteristics. Annealing is the process of heating an amorphous substance at a temperature lower than T_g (glass transition temperature) for such a duration that can asymptotically transform it to equilibrium glassy state, resulting in changes in some physical properties like volume, entropy and enthalpy [2]. Primary drying involves reduction of chamber pressure and raising temperature to sublime the frozen solvent. This drying step may extend from several hours to few days to complete. Primary drying time can be reduced up to 10-30% with controlled nucleation of ice crystals during the initial freezing step [3]. Even after primary drying, some solvent still remains as chemically bound to the solid product, which is finally removed by a desorption process referred to as secondary drying. The drying process is concluded under sub-ambient pressure. Sometimes, primary and secondary drying are coupled in a freeze drier with gradual increase in the temperature for a longer duration (*e.g.* for overnight) [7]. The final dry product retains the shape and volume (fill level) of the container (vial, tube or blister) leading to the formation of a highly porous product.

Freeze drying is a reversible process and addition of water to a freeze dried product readily reconstitutes to its original liquid form, if desired. Freeze drying is frequently used to produce amorphous materials. The use of very low temperatures in the process limits molecular mobility and thereby prevent nucleation of the drug and the excipients resulting in reduction of crystallinity in the final formulation [8]. Optimising the conditions of the freeze drying process may offer a control on the solid state properties of the dried product.

2.1. Lyophilised FDTs: Formulation, Packaging, Advantages and Challenges

FDTs prepared by lyophilisation are highly porous tablets capable of quick oral disintegration/dissolution in the saliva eliminating the need of water for swallowing. However, highly porous tablets may fail due to low hardness and high friability issues, which require a careful optimisation of mechanical strength and quick disintegration time.

The desired attributes of a drug to be incorporated in a lyophilised FDT formulation are low dose, poor water solubility, sufficient chemical stability, fine particle size and tasteless [9, 10]. Ideally, the drug should be poorly water soluble, dose shall be less and a fine particle size range is required to allow formation of a stable aqueous suspension with the matrix components. Problems may arise with soluble drugs due to the formation of eutectic mixtures lowering the freezing point of the formulation, resulting in incomplete freezing or melting during drying. Materials having large particle size may lead to sedimentation problems. High dose actives can be accommodated but with higher dose it becomes difficult to achieve a rapidly dispersing unit. Sufficient aqueous stability is also required to prevent undue degradation of the drug during suspension formation. Very few drugs meet all the essential criteria of an ideal compound. However, certain problems can be resolved by incorporating suspending agents or by adding a milling process to reduce sedimentation. For water soluble drugs with high dose, the use of ion-exchange resins may be appropriate to render the soluble compound insoluble [11].

The matrix of lyophilised tablets essentially consists of two components, *viz.* a gum or water soluble polymer and a matrix supporting agent. These two components work simultaneously for successful development of lyophilised tablets [12]. Water soluble gums like gelatin, xanthan gum, dextran, arabic gum [12], alginate [11], maltodextrin [13], and water soluble polymers as the first component performs as binding agents. First component provides mechanical strength and shape to tablets. The second component acts as matrix supporting and disintegration enhancing agent. Saccharides and polyols, such as mannitol, sorbitol, sucrose, amino acids *etc.*, are prominently used as matrix supporting/disintegration enhancing agents for providing crystallinity, hardness and elegance [12, 14]. Viscosity modifying agents like Pluronic F127, Carbopol 974P-NF are used to improve mouth-feel and aid pre-gastric retention [15]. Water is used as a medium to provide porous structure, since water sublimes during the process of lyophilisation. Suspending agents, emulsifiers, pH adjusting substances and preservatives are required for physically stabilising the suspension/emulsion formulations prior to freeze drying. Lyophilised FDT formulations also contain sweeteners and flavours to improve the taste and palatability profile.

Physicochemical properties of active ingredient play a guiding role in the successful development of FDTs by freeze drying. Freeze drying process and technologies for making lyophilised tablet are not amenable to large doses of highly water soluble active ingredients [11]. Dose up to 400 mg of water insoluble drug can be incorporated in lyophilised FDTs, while water soluble drug has a highest limit of 60 mg [16]. The formation of easy to collapse glassy solids upon freezing and the formation of eutectic mixtures leading to depression of freezing point are two critical issues with the use of water soluble drugs [16]. High dose of active ingredient (500-1000 mg) and/or drug combinations resulting in such high dose make extreme challenge to develop FDT using a freeze drying process [11]. Some FDTs of bitter drugs have been prepared by freeze drying [17], but the challenge is quite obvious with the increase in dose of bitter drug as the taste masking process may additionally lead to an increase in the amount of total solids. Water quality is also a crucial concern for FDTs to be prepared by freeze drying method. The purified water as per compendial specifications is essential for such manufacturing [18].

Freeze drying process is a lengthy and relatively costly manufacturing process.

Highly porous nature of lyophilised FDTs make them unfit to conventional packaging and poor stability concerns frequently arise with storage under stress conditions like high moisture and high temperature. Friable nature of FDTs required the need for special packaging to protect the contents from environmental and physical stresses. Additionally, the package also play an important role in shaping (moulding) and stability. The package comprises a sheet of a thermoplastic film material having depressions thereon. The film is made up of polyvinylchloride or a laminate such as polyvinylchloride/polyvinylidene chloride, polyvinyl chloride (PVC)/polyvinylidene chloride/polyethylene chloride) [19]. Alternatively, the manufacturing may be performed in aluminium foil-foil or aclar laminates [16]. The active ingredient in the form of a suspension formulation is closed and frozen within the plastic sheet and then freeze dried. Stepped edge blister pack and child resistant blister pack having limited entry points are also available for packaging of FDTs [20].

Direct pressing technique to emboss identification mark may cause deformation, reduce porosity, increase dispersion and could lead to cracking the FDTs due to their inherent fragility, moisture sensitivity and chemical make-up. A desired logo or other product information is first embossed or framed into the base of the dosage packed or blister and later an appropriate dose of the medicament of liquid suspension is deposited into the embossed pockets [21].

2.2. Lyophilised FDTs: Some Literature Reports

The ability of a lyophilised formulation to retain the structure and volume on drying results in highly porous units. This shape and volume retaining property has attracted pharmaceutical formulation scientists in exploring lyophilisation in developing FDDFs using different methods and techniques. Table **1** represents some of the lyophilised tablets with their important excipients and freeze drying conditions.

Table 1. Lyophilised FDTs, their excipients and freeze drying conditions.

Drug	Excipients	Freeze Drying Conditions			Ref.
		Freezing	Primary Drying	Secondary Drying	
–	L-proline, L-serine and gelatin	-80°C for 2 h	48 h at -40°C shelf temperature	20°C shelf temperature and vacuum of 50 mTorr for 10 h	[22]

(Table 1) contd.....

Drug	Excipients	Freeze Drying Conditions			Ref.
		Freezing	Primary Drying	Secondary Drying	
–	Gelatin, D-sorbitol, D-mannitol, sucrose, Pluronic F127 and Carbopol 974 P-NF	-80°C for about 60 min	48 h at -40°C shelf temperature	20°C shelf temperature and vacuum of 50 mTorr for 10 h	[15]
–	L-form of alanine, serine, proline and gelatin	-80°C for 2 h	-35°C and vacuum of 0.1 mbar for 86 h	20 °C and vacuum of 0.1 mbar for 15 h	[23]
–	Gelatin and L-amino acids	-80°C for about 60 minutes	48 h at -40°C shelf temperature	20°C shelf temperature and vacuum of 50 mTorr for 10 h	[24]
ACE527: A trivalent live attenuated vaccine	Sucrose, trehalose, potassium phosphate, potassium glutamate, potassium citrate, Mannitol, M-500, Natrosol 250H, Natrosol 250L, polyvinyl pyrrolidone (PVP) K85-95 and CeraVacx	-40°C for 4 h;,frozen at a rate of -25°C per minute to -80°C for 1 h, fast freezing in a dimpled steel plate that had liquid nitrogen misting onto the bottom	-30°C to 30°C over an 8 h period	30°C for 12 hour	[5]
Clonidine HCl	Gelatin and saccharides	-80°C for about 60 minutes	-40°C shelf temperature for 48 h	20°C shelf temperature and vacuum of 50 mTorr for 10 h	[14]
Griseofulvin	Gelatin, glycine, sorbitol, fractionated coconut oil, sesame oil, Tween 80 and Span 80 and hydroxypropyl methylcellulose (HPMC)	-22°C for 24 h	-45°C and vacuum of 7×10^{-2} mbar for 48 h	Room temperature, over calcium chloride at a relative humidity of 0% in a desiccator	[25]
Hydrochlorthiazide	Maltodextrin, xanthan gum, PEG 6000, Miglyol 812 and Methocel A15LV	45°C for 1.5 h, frozen at the rate of 0.5°C/min	-10°C shelf temperature, 60°C condenser temperature and vacuum of 1 mbar for 8 h	25°C shelf temperature and a vacuum of 0.1 mbar for 6 h	[13]

(Table 1) contd.....

Drug	Excipients	Freeze Drying Conditions			Ref.
		Freezing	Primary Drying	Secondary Drying	
Meloxicam	Gelatin, mannitol, glycine, PVP K90, PVP K25, polyethylene glycol (PEG) 6000, PEG 4000, PEG 400, Tween 80 and Tween 20		-22°C for 24 h		[26]
Nimesulide	Gelatin, sorbitol, mannitol, glycine, Tween (20, 80), sodium chloride, potassium chloride, sodium lauryl sulphate, PEG (400, 4000, 6000) and PVP (K25, K30, K90)	-22°C for 24 h	24 h at -45°C condenser temperature and pressure of 7×10^{-2} mbar		[27]
Omeprazole enteric coated pellets	Gelatin, carrageenan and alanine	-80°C for 60 min, annealing in a pre-cooled freezer at -20°C for 12 h and later shifted to freezer maintained at −80°C	-40°C shelf temperature and a vacuum of 50 mTorr for 48 h	10 h at a shelf temperature of 20°C at a pressure of 50 mTorr	[6]
Phenobarbitol sodium	Gelatin and mannitol	-40°C for 60 minutes	40 h at a vacuum of 0.08 mbar with a gradual increase of shelf temperature up to 20°C	35°C shelf temperature for 2 h	[7]
Piroxicam nanocrystal	PEG 4000, maltodextrins, xanthan gum, gelatin and croscarmellose	-20°C	-10°C rising to 20°C at a vacuum of 0.5 mbar, overnight		[28]

(Table 1) contd.....

Drug	Excipients	Freeze Drying Conditions			Ref.
		Freezing	Primary Drying	Secondary Drying	
Ranitidine HCl, loperamide HCl, ibuprofen, 5-5 diphenylhydantoin	Gum arabic, alanine, sodium-octansulphonate, triethylamine, ammonium hydroxide, sodium-octansulphonate, triethylamine and sodium lauryl sulphate	Freezing at -80°C for 60 minutes, annealing in a pre-cooled (-20°C) freezer for 12 h and then shifted to the freezer maintained at –80°C	-35°C shelf temperature for 16 h	10°C shelf temperature and pressure of 50 mTorr for 1 h	[12]
Sildenafil citrate	Maltodextrin, Xanthan gum, xylitol, PEG 8000, gelatin, mannitol and glycine	-28°C for 24 h	24 hours at -45°C for 24 h and a pressure of 7×10^{-2} mbar	In a desiccator at room temperature	[29]
Sumatriptan succinate	Gelatin, Plasdone K90D, mannitol, glycine, sorbitol, sucralose, camphor, menthol, xanthan gum, disodium EDTA and magnesium stearate	-40°C for 12 h	-15 °C for 12 h at vacuum of 0.250 mbar	-15°C for 20 h at vacuum of 0.250 mbar	[30]

Ahmed *et al.* (2007) prepared FDTs of griseofulvin from a lyophilised dry emulsion [25]. An o/w emulsion was prepared with a gelatin solution as aqueous phase, sesame oil or medium chain glyceride (Miglyol) as oil phase and Tween 80/Span 80 and HPMC as emulsifiers. An increase in the rate of absorption (C_{max} reduced by 4 h) and 85% higher AUC were achieved with FDTs when compared to conventional tablets of griseofulvin.

Sildenafil solid dispersions, prepared from different grades of PEG and Poloxamer 188, were incorporated in sublingual tablets prepared by lyophilisation [29]. Instantaneous dissolution (100% in 1 minute) and relative bioavailability of 159.81% was obtained with lyophilised tablets of sildenafil.

Meloxicam aqueous dispersion, containing gelatin as matrix former, mannitol or glycine as a collapse protectant and different disintegration accelerators (1% w/v), *viz.* PVP K25, PVP K90, PEG 6000, PEG 4000, PEG 400, Tween 80 and Tween 20, was lyophilised to prepare FDTs [26]. All FDTs disintegrated in less than 46 s in pharmacopoeial disintegration apparatus. FDT formulation containing 1% w/w PEG 400 was found best in terms of *in vitro* disintegration and dissolution.

In one study, FDTs prepared by lyophilisation were used in delivering vaccine by oral route. FDTs of ACAM2027 strain (the most labile component of the trivalent ACE527 vaccine) were prepared by lyophilisation for their use in the prevention of *Escherichia coli* induced diarrhoea [5]. FDT formulation utilised cryoprotectants (sucrose and trehalose), buffers and stabilisers (salts of phosphate and glutamate) and binders (Natrosol®, PVP and mannitol). Optimised lyophilisation method resulted in a viability loss of less than 0.3 log10 (50% recovery). On the other hand, a viability loss of 0.4 log10 (40% recovery) was reported after storage for 12 months. Optimised FDTs were strong with disintegration time <10 s and found capable to preserve the bacteria for 12 months at 2–8°C.

Terahertz pulsed spectroscopy (TPS) was used as an important analytical off-line and in-line tool for evaluating the degree of crystallinity in FDTs, co-freeze dried mixtures, conventional tablets and spray dried microparticles [23]. In co-freeze dried amino acid (l-alanine, serine and proline) and gelatin mixtures, crystallinity was studied by TPS. Crystallinity of ~62±1% (n=3) and 72±0.5% (n=3) was observed in the co-freeze dried alanine and gelatin mixtures (50% w/w and 70% w/w, respectively), while no crystallinity was found in proline and gelatin mixtures. Crystallinity of ~41±0.5% (n=3) and ~80±0.5% (n=3) was observed in the serine and gelatin matrix in compositions of 30% w/w and 50% w/w, respectively. TPS has the potential to be used for in-line measurements, during the process of freeze-drying, to study and optimise and/or maximise the crystallisation of the excipients by annealing prior to initiating the primary drying stage.

FDTs of sumatriptan succinate were prepared by lyophilisation [30]. FDT formulations employed gelatin–mannitol (3.75% w/v and 3.5% w/v, respectively) as a matrix and camphor as a volatilising pore forming agent. Optimised FDTs disintegrated in less than 10 s and exhibited a rapid dissolution of 90% within 10 min.

FDTs of hydrochlorthiazide were prepared by lyophilising oil-in-water emulsion comprising maltodextrin, Miglyol 812 and Methocel A15LV or a suspension comprising maltodextrin, xanthan and PEG 6000 [13]. *In vitro* drug release from reference hydrochlorthiazide tablet and lyophilised emulsion FDT was found similar. In a pharmacokinetic study, FDTs prepared from suspension were found superior, with a higher C_{max} and $AUC_{0\text{-}24h}$ and lower T_{max} when compared to reference formulation and FDTs prepared by lyophilising emulsion. It was anticipated that a solid dispersion of hydrochlorthiazide with PEG 6000 might be formed during lyophilisation leading to faster *in vitro* drug release and improvements in bioavailability.

FDTs of phenobarital and phenobarbital sodium were prepared by lyophilisation [7]. Mannitol:gelatin in ratio of 5:1 was found optimum as matrix former composition in lyophilised tablets. Chemical form, drug concentration and physical properties of suspension/solution were found to affect the mechanical strength of FDTs. FDTs were characterised porous and minimum water absorption was observed after monthly storage at 60% relative humidity (RH). Tablets were regarded as non-hygroscopic, as there was only 1-3% increase of tablet mass after storage at 40% and 60% RH for 4 weeks. All FDT formulations disintegrated quickly within few seconds, when tested in water at 37°C.

Piroxicam nanocrystals, prepared by high pressure homogenisation using Poloxamer 188 as stabiliser, were incorporated with other excipients into FDTs [28]. Drug dissolution rate of piroxicam from nanocrystals based FDT formulations was significantly higher than from coarse piroxicam. Particle size reduction of piroxicam increased surface-to-volume ratio leading to improvement in the dissolution rate. Piroxicam nanocrystals based FDTs, prepared with gelatin or croscarmellose as excipients, showed a higher drug dissolution rate in comparison to the commercial formulation and FDTs prepared using xanthan gum.

In vitro dissolution and *in vivo* rate of absorption increased when nimesulide was formulated as FDTs by lyophilisation [27]. Sugar alcohol (sorbitol or mannitol) and gelatin were used as matrix formers and glycine as collapse protectant. Role of different disintegration accelerators [sodium lauryl sulphate (SLS), PEG, PVP and Tween] was also studied. Lyophilised FDTs disintegrated within few seconds and drug dissolution was considerably faster than plain powder drug and commercial tablets. A significant increase in C_{max}, an increase of 62% in AUC and T_{max} decrease by 1 h were achieved in comparison to reference commercial tablets.

Saccharides and polyols are extensively used as matrix forming agents in lyophilised FDTs, but their use has been restricted in paediatrics, diabetic and obese patients while treating chronic conditions. Alanine, glycine, threonine and proline were evaluated as alternate matrix forming agents for preparing zero saccharide lyophilised FDTs and compared for thermal, mechanical, wettability and moisture uptake properties [31]. Alanine and glycine were found potential matrix forming agents due to similar thermal and mechanical profiles and advantages of better wettability and low hygroscopic profiles, when compared to mannitol.

Several L-amino acids were evaluated for their possible use as matrix supporting/disintegration enhancing agents at 10-70% w/w concentration with an aqueous solution (5% w/w) of gelatin (60 bloom strength) as binder [24]. Lyophilised tablet index (LTI) values [using formula LTI=(H/DT)÷(H*/DT*) where, H= hardness of the test tablet, DT=disintegration time of the test tablet, H*=hardness of the control tablets, DT*=disintegration time of the control tablets] were calculated to estimate the effect of amino acids on mechanical strength and disintegration of tablets. LTI values > 1 indicated advantages over the gelatin formulations and LTI values <1 suggested deterioration in the desired tablet properties (disintegration time and hardness). Highest LTI value of 4.99 was achieved with 30% w/w of alanine. LTI value of 3.39 was obtained with 30% w/w glutamine and 10% w/w glycine. It was observed that alanine, serine, glutamine, histidine, glycine, threonine and arginine improved the overall tablet properties to different extents at different concentrations.

In another study, zero saccharide lyophilised FDTs were prepared with optimised combinations of proline and serine to achieve higher wettability and stability over that of individual amino acids [22]. Proline enhanced the disintegration by increasing the wettability of FDTs and high concentrations of serine increased the mechanical properties of FDTs. Large average pore diameter and a narrow pore size distribution was observed in annealed tablets leading to faster sublimation rate and quick disintegration time in comparison to the tablets prepared by freezing at pre-cooled shelves (without annealing) and by flash freezing with nitrogen.

A novel enteric coated multiparticulate formulation of omeprazole was incorporated in lyophilised FDTs [6]. Gelatin, used as a matrix in FDTs, provided a smooth and pleasant mouthfeel upon disintegration of tablets. Carrageenan, employed as viscosity modifier in gelatin solutions, increased the viscosity of gelatin solutions by forming complex coacervates. An increase of 100 times in viscosity of 5% w/w gelatin solution was achieved by adding 0.2% w/w carrageenan. Alanine was employed as matrix support/disintegration promoter. The optimised FDT formulation, as determined by central composite face centred design, contained gelatin (4.7% w/v), carrageenan (0.02% w/v) and alanine (3% w/v).

In an FDT optimisation study, gelatin (5% w/w, in combination consisting of a 1:1 ratio of 75:225 bloom strength gelatin) was found superior for preparing FDTs having hardness of 13.7±0.9 N and disintegration time of 24.1±0.6 s [15]. Increase in gelatin concentration further resulted in increase of both disintegration time and mechanical strength of FDTs. Hardness of FDTs remained unaffected with increase in the ratio of 225 bloom strength gelatin, but it significantly affected disintegration time. Saccharides like mannitol, sorbitol, sucrose, *etc*. were used as diluents and cryoprotectants. With 20-50% mannitol, the tablet properties like mechanical strength and disintegration time were found optimum. An amount of 50% w/w mannitol in FDTs resulted in hardness of 30.9 N and disintegration time 13.3 s. Addition of Pluronic F127 and Carbopol 974P-NF in the formulation improved mouth-feel and bioadhesion by increasing the viscosity of resulting suspension in saliva. However, addition of viscosity modifying polymers (2-10% w/w) was worsening to both disintegration time and mechanical strength of the FDTs.

Lyophilised FDTs of Clonidine HCl with highest LTI were prepared from 30% w/w mannitol in 5% gelatin stock solution [14]. A decrease in disintegration time of FDTs was observed with decreasing bloom strength and concentration of gelatin in the stock solutions. On the other hand, mechanical strength of the FDTs was found sensitive to concentration of gelatin rather than the bloom strength of gelatin. Stock solution concentrations of 2-5% w/w of low bloom strength gelatin were found most appropriate for the development of lyophilised FDTs. Crystallisation of mannitol during the freeze drying process resulted in superior FDTs. However, glucose, xylitol, maltotriose and trehalose resisted to greater extents during crystallisation. Parabolic relationship between disintegration time and gelatin/saccharide compositions was obtained. An optimum balance between the hardness and disintegration time was achieved at 30-40% w/w of mannitol.

Gum arabic and alanine based lyophilised FDTs of ranitidine HCl, loperamide HCl, ibuprofen and 5-5 diphenylhydantoin were prepared and optimised for a balance of disintegration time and hardness [12, 32]. Gum arabic (15% w/w) was used as an alternative to gelatin in lyophilised tablets. Alanine functioned as matrix supporter/disintegration enhancer. A 3^2 factorial design (three replicates) study was performed to identify the effect of selected formulation factors individually and simultaneously on the quality of FDTs. Surprisingly, for all the selected drugs alanine concentration of 40% w/w was found optimum.

3. FREEZE CASTING

The freeze casting process is a fluid-solid phase transition process [33]. An aqueous solution of drug, matrix former and suspending agent is subjected to frozen conditions. Freezing of water to ice crystals results in volume expansion of suspended solid particles, an effect which is referred as '*cold compression*'. A vertical temperature gradient is maintained during freezing to support growth of ice crystals only in vertical direction. This vertical temperature gradient is achieved by cooling the lower surface and top surface is kept exposed to ambient conditions. Evaporation of the ice crystals results in formation of a porous solid structure. Solid load, concentration of active ingredient(s), freezing temperature and drying temperature are critical process parameters, which controls the porosity of the resulting dosage form.

Szepes *et al.* (2007) prepared theophylline FDTs by freeze casting method [33]. A suspension of potato starch and theophylline was prepared in water. Citric acid or saccharose was used as suspending agent. These suspensions were poured in a cylindrical plastic moulds (13 mm) and maintained at 20°C in a cooling cell linked to a thermostat. Only the bottom surface of the moulds was in contact with cooling surface. The upper surface of the moulds was open to the surrounding ambient conditions. The vertical temperature gradient in the moulds supported the growth of ice crystals vertically in the moulds. An air drier was used to evaporate ice crystals by forced-air drying at 30°C.

4. PROPRIETARY AND PATENTED TABLET TECHNOLOGIES BASED ON FREEZE DRYING

Several proprietary, patented and trademark technologies for preparing FDTs using different lyophilisation protocols are Zydis®, Lyoc®, QuickSolv® and Nanocrystal® Nanomelt®.

4.1. Zydis®

Catalent Pharma Solutions' (www.catalent.com) Zydis® technology is a pioneer lyophilised oral dosage form platform for manufacturing FDDFs. FDDFs based on Zydis® technology disperses almost instantly in the mouth and does not require water for swallowing. Zydis® FDDF technology enhances investment value and accelerates a drug product's potential by attracting customers due to their advance pharmacokinetics through pre-gastric absorption and improvements in patient compliance.

Zydis® technology was jointly developed by R. P. Scherer and Wyeth. Most of the initial patents of Zydis® technology were assigned to John Wyeth and Brother's Ltd. (Maidenhead, Berks, UK) [19, 34] and R.P. Scherer [10, 35]. Wyeth concentrated on the formulation development, while R.P. Scherer worked on development of an efficient and economical lyophilisation process. Expidet™ formulations were first marketed formulations of Zydis® in some regions of Europe. Tavor™ Expidet™ was launched in 1992 by Wyeth (Italy) as a line extension to company's lorazepam products [36]. In 1998, R.P. Scherer was acquired by Cardinal Health, which was later renamed as Catalent Pharma Solutions. Principle of Zydis® technology consists of freeze drying of an aqueous solution or suspension of drug and excipients in blister packs, resulting in a friable and quick dissolving formulation, which is seal packed in peel-off blisters to offer long term physical stability and protection from adverse environmental conditions. A four step manufacturing process of Zydis® units is presented in Fig. (**1**). First step involve mixing of drug and excipients to prepare an aqueous solution or suspension. In step 2, prepared aqueous solution or suspension is transferred to preformed blisters for freezing by an optimised cryogenic freezing process, where a careful control on growing of ice crystals is kept. Step 3 utilises lyophilisation process to sublime water from the frozen units to obtain Zydis® units. Fourth and last step employs a hot seal process to seal and pack Zydis® units. Presently, Catalent has four different facilities for development and production of Zydis® FDDFs, which are located at Somerset (New Jersey, US), Swindon (UK), Kakegawa (Japan) and Schorndorf (Germany) [37].

Catalent has developed a bouquet of FDDFs under registered name of Zydis®. Zydis®*Fast Dissolve* dose forms are lyophilised FDTs, which disintegrate and disperse almost instantaneously (normally in 3 to 5 seconds) in saliva and does not require water for administration. Bitter tasting active ingredient may be incorporated into the tablet after masking the taste. Zydis® fast dissolve tablet and granules family includes *Zydis® Ultra, Zydis® Nano, Zydis® Bio and Zydis® Granules and Gels* [37].

STEP 1: MIXING
Drug + Excipient(s) + Solvents
STEP 2: FILLING AND FREEZING
Filling in Preformed Blisters + Cryogenic Freezing Process to Control Size of Ice Crystals
STEP 3: LYOPHILIZATION
Transfer of Frozen Preformed Blisters in Large Scale Freeze Dryer Followed by Lyophilization to Obtain Zydis® Units
STEP 4: SEALING
Heat Seal Process of Zydis ® Units for Long Term Stability and Protection from Environmental Conditions

Fig. (1). Four step process of preparing Zydis® units.

Zydis® Ultra offers enhanced fast dissolve formulations, greater taste masking abilities, increased dose and coating for controlled/sustained release profile.

Zydis® Nano is a nanoparticulate formulation, prepared by Zydis® technology, for delivering poorly soluble drugs in the form of an FDT. Nanoparticles have been found extremely useful in improving rate and extent of drug dissolution with a subsequent improvement in bioavailability and reduction in onset of action allowing, thereby, reduction in dose or dose frequency and improving patient safety by exposing less amount of total drug to the patient. Drug nanoparticles are formed by wet milling or other established methods and used in making suspension in the Zydis® process. This allows a rapid dispersion of the nanoparticles in the finished dose form (FDT) without breaking and fracturing of nanoparticles during the manufacturing process. To exemplify the application, nanosuspensions of indomethacin, fenofibrate, naproxen and phenacetin were prepared by wet milling with fish gelatin solutions, which also acted as an effective stabiliser to nanoparticles [38]. Prepared nanoparticles were incorporated into Zydis® tablets. Porous matrix of Zydis® tablets supported quick wetting and dissolution of nanoparticles. Ambient and accelerated stability conditions did not result in any significant changes in particle size of nanoparticles.

Zydis® Bio dose forms incorporate large biological molecules like allergens, peptides, proteins and viral vaccines. *Zydis® Bio* sublingual delivery overcomes various challenges of proteins and peptide drugs like harsh environment of gastrointestinal tract, use of absorption enhancers/bioadhesives, peptidases and proteolytic enzyme activity and potential interaction with gastrointestinal constituents. Sublingual delivery through *Zydis® Bio* formulations provides a relatively neutral salivary pH which improves bioavailability/onset of action of proteins and peptides drugs. Low temperature processing during manufacturing also prevents degradation of labile drugs. The advantage of solid dosage coupled with a protective packaging further aids long term stability. Liquid processing facilities helps in achieving good content uniformity of low dose/potent drugs.

Zydis® Granules and Gels are versatile and patient friendly single unit granule formulation as a stick pack with improved acceptance in patient care. These novel dosage forms share the same convenience of Zydis® Ultra products and allows high drug loading and broadest in applying taste masking methods. These granules can be sprinkled onto food and thereby provides high patient compliance and patient acceptance. Alternatively, *Zydis® Granules* can be dispersed or dissolved in water to prepare suspension or solution for dosing foods with drugs and thereby provides a novel means of administering drugs and patient care to special populations like paediatrics, geriatrics and psychiatric.

Uniformity of dose and horizontal splitting of the dosage units have been observed with sedimentation of coated particles in the blister pockets prior to freezing. Therefore, particle size of the drug in Zydis® suspension should be less than 100 μ to prevent settling of the coated particles in the preformed blister packs during holding time (freeze drying). However, taste masked microencapsulated paracetamol, pseudoephedrine HCl and ibuprofen (particle size >200 μ) were successfully incorporated in Zydis® units without any sedimentation of the drug particles in the Zydis® suspension and without any significant retardation on the disintegration of the final dosage unit [39]. Increase in viscosity of the Zydis® suspension (addition of xanthan gum, or CMC) and lowering of the temperature during dosing in the blister packs are two successful approaches in preventing settling of microencapsulated particles in the Zydis® suspension. Large holding time of the Zydis® suspension may lead to release of some amount of drug in the aqueous phase from coated particles, but the drug released in solution can be taste masked using sweetener and flavour.

Olanzapine Zydis® displayed improved disintegration and drug release profile among all generic ODTs (n=23) tested, regardless of their potency [40]. Disintegration test was conducted in a 30 mL of non-agitated simulated saliva at 37°C kept in a petri dish of 10 cm diameter. Olanzapine Zydis® disintegrated completely in less than 4 s for all tested strengths (5, 10, 15 and 20 mg). Prolanz ® Fast (5 mg) disintegrated in 12 s followed by risperidone ODT 4 mg, which disintegrated in 40 s. Generic olanzapine ODTs dissolve less than 10% w/w of olanzapine in 30 s. Slow dissolution of the olanzapine generics was due to one or more reasons like excipient nature and solubility, binder nature and strength, low drug load, particle size of drug/excipients, some of which may result in incomplete disintegration.

4.2. QuickSolv®

Janssen's (www.janssen.com, a subsidiary of Johnson & Johnson) proprietary QuickSolv® technology is based on a solid-state dissolution method for preparation of the matrix and a solvent exchange process for removing water from the frozen matrix. QuickSolv® technology of preparing porous units was initially developed by Mediventures and later sold to Janssen in 1991 [41]. Solid-state dissolution method involves preparation of a uniform high porosity matrix having sufficient resistance to disintegration or crumbling under normal manufacturing and handling conditions [42 - 45]. A matrix of gelatin, pectin and/or soy fibre protein, mannitol and one or more amino acid (*e.g.* glycine) is used in preparing the dosage unit [46]. A solution or suspension or emulsion of the drug and excipients is prepared in a solvent (generally water and referred to as the first solvent) and subsequently subjected to solidification by freezing. The frozen and solidified system is kept in contact with an another solvent (ethanol or menthol or acetone and referred to as second solvent) at a temperature greater than the freezing point of the first solvent. Drug and excipients are insoluble in the first solvent, while the second solvent is miscible in the first solvent. Hence, a solidified matrix free from the first solvent is obtained. However, the remaining second solvent in the matrix is evaporated at normal pressure or higher temperature by passing a stream of air or nitrogen or vacuum drying or by a microwave assisted drying process. The process of shaping tablets also involves dispersing gas (air, oxygen, nitrogen, argon) bubbles to generate foam in solution or suspension to prevent cracking and melting of the dosage form during lyophilisation [46].

Porous dosage forms developed from QuikSolv® technology disintegrates very rapidly. However, the use of this technology is limited to only low dose drugs and drugs which are insoluble in the second solvent. QuikSolv® technology offers more resistance towards cracking when compared to other freeze drying technologies and melt-back is less often observed as heat being applied during the drying process. These technological advantages of QuikSolv® have overcome the problems in packaging lyophilised tablets. High porosity of QuikSolv® FDTs is also attributed to the foaming process alongside the freeze drying process [46, 47]. Despite being highly porous, texture of FDTs is relatively thick.

4.3. Lyoc®

Lyoc® technology is currently owned by Cima Labs (www.cimalabs.com), which is a subsidiary of Cephalon. Lyoc® technology is regarded as the one of the pioneer and patent protected FDT technology, which entered very early in the commercial markets. Oral lyophilisates, also called oral Lyoc® are porous, crumbly solid preparations for oral administration disclosed for the first time in a U.S. Patent 3767807 [48]. In 1968, Lyoc® offered ODA Lyoc® (sodium saccharinate and flamenol) as world's first FDT [49]. Seven commercialised FDT products based on Lyoc® are Spasfon-lyoc® (phloroglucinol), Para-lyoc® (paracetamol), Loperamide-lyoc® (loperamide) and Proxa-lyoc® (piroxicam) [49]. This technology is suitable for drugs with different physicochemical properties and capable to incorporate drug particles with different functional coatings for taste masking, controlled /extended/modified release.

The process of making a Lyoc® involve preparation of a solution or suspension or o/w emulsion comprising filler, thickening agent, surfactant, non-volatile flavouring agents, sweetener and drug [50, 51]. Optimised homogenous formulation is filled into preformed blisters and subjected to freezing at a very low temperature at -40°C [51]. High amount of fillers (mannitol) or polymers are sometimes used to increase the viscosity of the formulation and to improve homogeneity of suspension or emulsion (paste). Water is removed from the frozen formulation by subjecting it to specific pressure conditions for direct ice to water vapour transformation. The process does not involve use of organic solvents and hence regarded as environment friendly and cost effective. The lyophilisation process is capable to produces highly porous tablets allowing disintegration of the resulting tablets in 2-20 s [51]. Bead or microparticles with suitable excipients may be incorporated to prepare paste, which is subjected to lyophilisation. Active ingredient amounts in range 500 µg to 500 mg can be incorporated in Lyoc® tablets.

4.4. NanoCrystal® Nanomelt™

Perrigo's (www.perrigo.com/) NanoCrystal® Nanomelt™ technology utilises orally administered nanoparticles of 2 µm or less in the form of FDT matrix. This technology was developed by Elan Pharma, later acquired by Perrigo in 2013. Nanocrystal™ particles are typically less than 1000 nm drug particles prepared by a proprietary wet milling technique and stabilised by surface adsorption onto selected stabilisers to prevent agglomeration in dispersion [52, 53]. NanoCrystal™ colloidal dispersions of poorly water soluble drug may be mixed with water soluble excipients, filled into preformed blisters and lyophilised to prepare Nanomelt™ dosage forms. Nanomelt™ dosage forms own characteristics of both a liquid formulation (easy to use) and a solid unit dosage form (convenience). The resulting FDTs dissolve/disintegrate in small amount of water or saliva in seconds. This technology is capable of improving compound activity by nano-sizing and improving characteristics of the final product by formulating as FDTs or conventional tablets. Decreasing particle size to nano ranges improves the dissolution rate and presentation of nanoparticles in FDTs improves patient compliance and acceptance. FDTs prepared with Nanocrystal™ additionally offer pharmacokinetic benefits by improving the bioavailability of orally administered nanoparticles.

This technology is quite promising and attractive for potent and hazardous materials as it can avoid operations like blending, granulation and tableting and thereby prevents liberation of large amounts of powder in air. Lyophilisation of nanoparticles enables incorporation of small quantities of drug into FDTs without negligible losses. Final product does not require special packaging and thus may be conventional blister or bottle packed. The technology utilises compendial

GRAS excipients, which are not moisture sensitive. Active ingredients in doses up to 200 mg per dosage unit can be accommodated.

NanoCrystal® technology has enabled an efficient delivery system of a poorly water-soluble drug Rapamune® (rapamycin) for preventing rejection of transplanted kidneys [54]. Rapamune® tablets are convenient to administer and easy to store than the Rapamune® oral solution. Some other marketed drug products based on NanoCrystal® technology are Emend® (Aprepitant), Tricor® (Fenofibrate), Megace ES® (Megestrol) and Theralux® (Theramycetin) [1]. All these drug products are conventional tablets with advantages of increase in dissolution rate leading to successful improvements in their pharmacokinetics.

5. CONCLUSIONS

With the advancements of science and technologies, the cost of freeze drying process has been considerably reduced and now it has become cost effective. Further technological advances are also required to make the process to be applied much more economically for the development of FDDFs. Quickest disintegration and faster dissolution characteristics can be achieved with lyophilised FDTs when compared to FDTs prepared by compression based methods. Lyophilised FDTs do possess technological limitations like low dose of active ingredient, low mechanical strength of FDTs and requirement of special packaging. For these reasons, the market of lyophilised FDTs is continuously shrinking and it has been slowly and steadily being captured by FDTs prepared by other methods. Introduction of Zydis® granules/gels, Zydis® Nano, Zydis® Bio and NanoCrystal® Nanomelt™ dosage forms in the market may attract new drug delivery opportunities and may possibly expand their market size with new drug products.

REFERENCES

[1] Junghanns J-U, Müller RH. Nanocrystal technology, drug delivery and clinical applications. Int J Nanomedicine 2008; 3(3): 295-309.
[PMID: 18990939]

[2] Kasper JC, Winter G, Friess W. Recent advances and further challenges in lyophilisation. Eur J Pharm Biopharm 2013; 85(2): 162-9.
[http://dx.doi.org/10.1016/j.ejpb.2013.05.019] [PMID: 23751601]

[3] Siew A. Controlling ice nucleation during the freezing step of lyophilization. Pharmaceut Technol 2013; 37: 36-40.

[4] Salazar J, Müller RH, Möschwitzer JP. Application of the combinative particle size reduction technology H 42 to produce fast dissolving glibenclamide tablets. Eur J Pharm Sci 2013; 49(4): 565-77.
[http://dx.doi.org/10.1016/j.ejps.2013.04.003] [PMID: 23587645]

[5] Lal M, Priddy S, Bourgeois L, *et al.* Development of a fast-dissolving tablet formulation of a live

attenuated enterotoxigenic *E. coli* vaccine candidate. Vaccine 2013; 31(42): 4759-64. [http://dx.doi.org/10.1016/j.vaccine.2013.08.010] [PMID: 23965220]

[6] Alhusban F, Perrie Y, Mohammed AR. Formulation of multiparticulate systems as lyophilised orally disintegrating tablets. Eur J Pharm Biopharm 2011; 79(3): 627-34. [http://dx.doi.org/10.1016/j.ejpb.2011.05.014] [PMID: 21693189]

[7] Sznitowska M, Płaczek M, Klunder M. The physical characteristics of lyophilised tablets containing a model drug in different chemical forms and concentrations. Acta Pol Pharm 2005; 62(1): 25-9. [PMID: 16022490]

[8] Zhang GG, Law D, Schmitt EA, Qiu Y. Phase transformation considerations during process development and manufacture of solid oral dosage forms. Adv Drug Deliv Rev 2004; 56(3): 371-90. [http://dx.doi.org/10.1016/j.addr.2003.10.009] [PMID: 14962587]

[9] Virley P, Yarwood RJ. Zydis-a novel, fast dissolving dosage form. Mfg Chemist. 1990; pp. 36-7.

[10] Grother L, Hall M, Bryans D, *et al.* Process for preparing solid pharmaceutical dosage forms. United States Patent US 6156339, 2000.

[11] Seager H. Drug-delivery products and the Zydis fast-dissolving dosage form. J Pharm Pharmacol 1998; 50(4): 375-82. [http://dx.doi.org/10.1111/j.2042-7158.1998.tb06876.x] [PMID: 9625481]

[12] AlHusban F. Novel formulation strategies for the fabrication of lyophilised orally disintegrating tablets. Birmingham, UK: Aston University 2010.

[13] Corveleyn S, Remon JP. Formulation of a lyophilised dry emulsion tablet for the delivery of poorly soluble drugs. Int J Pharm 1998; 166: 65-74. [http://dx.doi.org/10.1016/S0378-5173(98)00024-6]

[14] AlHusban F, Perrie Y, Mohammed AR. Preparation, optimisation and characterisation of lyophilised rapid disintegrating tablets based on gelatin and saccharide. Curr Drug Deliv 2010; 7(1): 65-75. [http://dx.doi.org/10.2174/156720110790396427] [PMID: 19863486]

[15] Chandrasekhar R, Hassan Z, Alhusban F, Smith AM, Mohammed AR. The role of formulation excipients in the development of lyophilised fast-disintegrating tablets. Eur J Pharm Biopharm 2009; 72(1): 119-29. [http://dx.doi.org/10.1016/j.ejpb.2008.11.011] [PMID: 19073253]

[16] Sastry SV, Nyshadham JR, Fix JA. Recent technological advances in oral drug delivery - a review. Pharm Sci Technol Today 2000; 3(4): 138-45. [http://dx.doi.org/10.1016/S1461-5347(00)00247-9] [PMID: 10754543]

[17] Green R, Kearney P. Process for preparing fast dispersing solid oral dosage form. Patent US 5976577, 1997.

[18] Anonymous . Pure water ensures the quality of fast dissolving dosage forms. Manufacturing Chemist 1997; p. 68.

[19] Gregory GK, Ho DS. Pharmaceutical dosage form packages. Patent US 4305502, 1981.

[20] Thompson AR, Marshall RW. Stepped edge blister pack. Patent US 5358118, 1994.

[21] Thompson AR, Yarwood RJ, Kearney P. Method of applying indicia to a fast-dissolving dosage form. Patent US 6212791, 2001.

[22] AlHusban F, ElShaer AM, Kansara JH, *et al.* Investigation of formulation and process of lyophilised orally disintegrating tablet (ODT) using novel amino acid combination. Pharmaceutics 2010; 2(1): 1-17.

[23] Darkwah J, Smith G, Ermolina I, Mueller-Holtz M. A THz spectroscopy method for quantifying the

degree of crystallinity in freeze-dried gelatin/amino acid mixtures: an application for the development of rapidly disintegrating tablets. Int J Pharm 2013; 455(1-2): 357-64.
[http://dx.doi.org/10.1016/j.ijpharm.2013.06.073] [PMID: 23850623]

[24] AlHusban F, Perrie Y, Mohammed AR. Formulation and characterisation of lyophilised rapid disintegrating tablets using amino acids as matrix forming agents. Eur J Pharm Biopharm 2010; 75(2): 254-62.
[http://dx.doi.org/10.1016/j.ejpb.2010.03.012] [PMID: 20332027]

[25] Ahmed IS, Aboul-Einien MH. *In vitro* and *in vivo* evaluation of a fast-disintegrating lyophilized dry emulsion tablet containing griseofulvin. Eur J Pharm Sci 2007; 32(1): 58-68.
[http://dx.doi.org/10.1016/j.ejps.2007.05.114] [PMID: 17628451]

[26] Abd Elbary A, Ali AA, Aboud HM. Enhanced dissolution of meloxicam from orodispersible tablets prepared by different methods. Bull Fac Pharm Cairo Univ 2012; 50: 89-97.
[http://dx.doi.org/10.1016/j.bfopcu.2012.07.001]

[27] Shoukri RA, Ahmed IS, Shamma RN. *In vitro* and *in vivo* evaluation of nimesulide lyophilized orally disintegrating tablets. Eur J Pharm Biopharm 2009; 73(1): 162-71.
[http://dx.doi.org/10.1016/j.ejpb.2009.04.005] [PMID: 19406232]

[28] Lai F, Pini E, Corrias F, *et al.* Formulation strategy and evaluation of nanocrystal piroxicam orally disintegrating tablets manufacturing by freeze-drying. Int J Pharm 2014; 467(1-2): 27-33.
[http://dx.doi.org/10.1016/j.ijpharm.2014.03.047] [PMID: 24680963]

[29] Zayed R, Kamel AO, Shukr M, El-Shamy Ael-H. An *in vitro* and *in vivo* comparative study of directly compressed solid dispersions and freeze dried sildenafil citrate sublingual tablets for management of pulmonary arterial hypertension. Acta Pharm 2012; 62(3): 411-32.
[http://dx.doi.org/10.2478/v10007-012-0027-9] [PMID: 23470352]

[30] Gugulothu D, Desai P, Pandharipande P, Patravale V. Freeze drying: exploring potential in development of orodispersible tablets of sumatriptan succinate. Drug Dev Ind Pharm 2015; 41(3): 398-405.
[http://dx.doi.org/10.3109/03639045.2013.871551] [PMID: 24384027]

[31] AlHusban F, Mohammed AR. Novel zero-saccharide orally disintegrating tablets. Eur Ind Pharm 2011; 9: 15-7.

[32] AlHusban F, Mohammed AR, Perrie Y. Tablet comprising gum arabic. Patent WO 2011058336 A3, 2012.

[33] Szepes A, Ulrich J, Farkas Z, *et al.* Freeze-casting technique in the development of solid drug delivery systems. Chemical Engineering and Processing: Process Intensification 2007; 46: 230-8.
[http://dx.doi.org/10.1016/j.cep.2006.06.004]

[34] Gregory GK, Peach JM, Du Mayne JD. Articles for carrying chemicals. United States Patent 4371516, 1983.

[35] Yarwood RJ, Kearney P, Thompson AR. Process for preparing solid pharmaceutical dosage forms. United States Patent 5738875, 1998.

[36] Scherer announces Zydis product launch in Italy , 1992 [Accessed on 2 Jan 2015]; Accessed from http://www.thefreeli brary.com/SCHER ER+ANNOUNC ES+ZYDIS +PRODUCT+LAUN CH+IN+ITALY-a012 141406

[37] Zydis fast dissolve , 2014 [Accessed on 2 Jan 2015]; Accessed from http://www.catalent.com /index.php /offerin gs/A-Z-Off erings/zydis

[38] Bahl D, Vitez I, Crowley K. Manufacture of nanoparticulate Zydis® fast-dissolve tablets using fish gelatin. , 2010 [Accessed on 2 Jan 2015]; http://www.catalent.com /index.p hp/conte nt/download/ 768/10493/file /AAPS%202010%20 -%20Zydis%20 Poster%2029 44(Crowley ,%20Bahl,

%20Vitez).pdf

[39] Groather L, Green R, Hall M, *et al.* Taste masking a fast -dissolving,freeze dried tablet form. Pham Manf Rev. 1998; pp. 22-7.

[40] Hobbs D, Karagianis J, Treuer T, Raskin J. An *in vitro* analysis of disintegration times of different formulations of olanzapine orodispersible tablet: a preliminary report. Drugs R D 2013; 13(4): 281-8. [http://dx.doi.org/10.1007/s40268-013-0030-8] [PMID: 24170256]

[41] Janssen acquires Quicksolv 1991. Accessed from https://www.pharmamedtechbi.com /deals /199110295

[42] Gole DJ, Levinson RS, Wilkinson PK, *et al.* Pharmaceutical and other dosage forms. Patent US 5558880, 1996.

[43] Gole DJ, Levinson SR, Carbone J, *et al.* Delivery matrices prepared by solid-state dissolution. Patent US 5330763, 1994.

[44] Gole DJ, Levinson SR, Carbone J, *et al.* Preparation of pharmaceutical and other matrix systems by solid-state dissolution. Patent US 5215756, 1993.

[45] Gole DJ, Levinson RS, Davies JD, *et al.* Preparation of pharmaceutical and other matrix systems by solid-state dissolution. Canada Patent 1991.

[46] Gole DJ, Wilkinson PK, Davies DJ. Pharmaceutical and other dosage forms. Patent WO/1993/023017 1993.

[47] Sandri G, Bonferoni MC, Ferrari F, *et al.* Differentiating factors between oral fast-dissolving technologies. Am J Drug Deliv 2006; 4: 249-62. [http://dx.doi.org/10.2165/00137696-200604040-00007]

[48] Blonde P. Process for the production of lyophilized pharmaceutical compositions containing vitamin C. United States Patent 3767807, 1973.

[49] Fulzele S, Moe D, Hamed E. Lyoc (Lyophilized Wafer): an orally disintegrating tablet technology Drug Development and Delivery , 2012 [Accessed on 2 Jan 2015]; Accessed from http://www.drug-dev.com /Main/B ack-Issues /Lyoc-Lyop hilized-Wafer -An-Orally -Disinte grating-Ta-50. aspx#s thash. b4EEFdyt .dpuf

[50] Lafon L. Galenical form for oral administration and its method of preparation by lyophilisation of an oil-in-water emulsion. Patent EP0159237, 1985.

[51] Lyoc™ orally disintegrating tablet technology. , 2008 [Accessed on 2 Jan 2015]; Accessed from www.cimalabs.com /assets/ Lyocword. pdf

[52] Cunningham J, Liversidge EM. Nanoparticulate compositions having a peptide as a surface stabiliser. United States Patent 7879360, 2011.

[53] Liversidge GG, Engers DA, Roberts ME, *et al.* Nanocrystalline formulations of human immunodeficiency virus (HIV) protease inhibitors using cellulosic surface stabilisers. United States Patent 6045829, 2000.

[54] First US. approval for Elan's NanoCrystal formulation , 2000 [Accessed on 2 Jan 2015]; Accessed from http://www.pharmaceuticalonline.com/doc/first-us-approval-for-elans-nanocrystal-formu-0001

CHAPTER 3

Modifications in Conventional Tablet Compaction Technologies for Developing Fast Dissolving/ Disintegrating Tablets

Vikas A. Saharan*

Department of Pharmaceutics, School of Pharmaceutical Sciences, Sardar Bhagwan Singh Post Graduate Institute of Biomedical Sciences and Research, Balawala, Dehradun 248161, Uttarakhand, India

Abstract: Fast dissolving/disintegrating tablets (FDTs) can be manufactured by direct compression provided the challenge of fast disintegration with adequate mechanical strengths can be addressed. Superdisintegrants, directly compressible coprocessed excipients and water soluble excipients have opened up the flood gates of opportunities in designing and developing FDTs by direct compression. Unacceptable properties of active pharmaceutical ingredient (API), like poor solubility, bitter taste, low bioavailability, may be addressed by making granules, micro-particulates and/or using various coating methods. Such treated API can be used in preparing FDTs. Effervescent agents have also gained attention as disintegrating agents in tablets so as to fasten tablet disintegration time to achieve pharmacopoeial or regulatory compliance for disintegration time. This chapter describes various FDT technologies based on modifications of conventional tablet manufacturing methods. These techniques can be grouped into four categories, *viz.* direction compression, granulation methods, effervescent tablets and direct compression with subsequent treatments.

Keywords: Advatab™, Crystalline transition, Direct compression, DuraSolv®, Easy-tec™, Effervescence, Flashtab®, Frosta®, Granulation, Humidity treatment, OraQuick®, OraSolv®, Pharmaburst®, Phase transition, Ractab®, Sintering, Spray drying, Sublimation, Wowtab®, Ziplet®.

1. INTRODUCTION

The rapid disintegration of FDTs is a result of fast uptake of water within highly

* **Corresponding author Vikas A. Saharan:** Department of Pharmaceutics, School of Pharmaceutical Sciences, Sardar Bhagwan Singh Post Graduate Institute of Biomedical Sciences and Research (www.sbspgi.edu.in), Balawala, Dehradun 248161, Uttarakhand, India; Tel: +91-135-2686246; Mobile: +91-8439820796; Fax: +91-135-2686246; E-mail: vikas.pharmaceutics@gmail.com

porous matrix of FDTs. Manufacturing of FDTs has to face several challenges like mechanical strength, optimum disintegration time, good mouth feel, taste masking, *etc*. Most of the innovations in manufacturing of FDTs are based on two conceptually exclusive characteristics of FDTs. Firstly, disintegration/dissolution time for tablet should be less than one minute and secondly, there should be enough mechanical strength to handle the formulation. The tablet matrix is made highly porous by the addition of disintegrating agents and/or highly water-soluble excipients or by sublimation of water or other subliming materials in the tablet formulation. The use of conventional tablet manufacturing and packaging machinery and ease in technology transfer make them more attractive. Various methods of preparing FDTs by modifications in conventional tablet technologies are shown in Box **1**.

Box 1: Various methods, adapted from conventional tablet compaction methods, for preparing FDTs.

A. **Direct compression**
   Superdisintegrant addition
   Water soluble saccharides/excipients
   Coprocessed excipients
B. **Granulation methods**
   Wet granulation
   Dry granulation
   Melt granulation
   Spray drying
C. **Compaction and subsequent treatments**
   Sublimation
   Humidity treatment followed by drying
   Sintering
D. **Effervescent tablets**

2. DIRECT COMPRESSION

Direct compression is a straightforward, popular and extensively used approach of manufacturing FDTs. Active Pharmaceutical Ingredient (API) is added to directly compressible diluent(s) followed by mixing with lubricant/glidant and subsequent compression. Direct compression utilises conventional manufacturing equipments, commonly available excipients, and requires the least time and efforts. Disintegrants and water soluble excipients are responsible for faster disintegration/dissolution of the tablet. Some new coprocessed excipients have also been developed especially for FDTs for either providing two or more functionalities in a single excipient or improvements in functionality of excipient. Some of these coprocessed excipients are directly compressible and require, therefore, minimum processing steps in making FDTs and aid in achieving faster *in vivo/in vitro* disintegration/dissolution with sufficient hardness and friability.

Microcrystalline cellulose (MCC) is a diluent of choice for FDTs due to superior compatibility, drug carrying capacity and faster disintegration. Another important category of diluents is saccharides, which have been extensively used and explored in formulating FDTs, due to the availability of highly compressibility grades, low cost, aqueous solubility, and sweet and acceptable taste. Availability of MCC and saccharides in high compressibility grades has made direct compression as the method of first choice for manufacturing tablet. However, sometimes high compressibility of MCC or other excipient may adversely impact on disintegration of FDTs, but this problem can be solved with optimising the composition. It has been observed that most of the FDT formulations, meant for faster disintegration/dissolution, incorporate some saccharide as their necessary component.

2.1. Superdisintegrant Addition

Addition of large amounts of superdisintegrant(s) to a direct compressible tablet can fasten disintegration/dissolution of the tablet. In this approach, the type of disintegrant and its amount in the formulation are critically important. The most popular superdisintegrants used in formulating FDTs are croscarmellose sodium (CCS), sodium starch glycolate (SSG), crospovidone and low-substituted hydroxypropyl cellulose (L-HPC). Some less explored superdisintegrants are Indion 414, modified polysaccharides or gums, novel combinations like glycine-chitosan, chitosan alginate complex and *Plantago ovata* mucilage. MCC has been used in most of the formulations as multifunctional excipient, which act as diluent and disintegrant. Some of the literature reports on use of various disintegrants in directly compressed FDTs are provided in Table **1**.

Table 1. Use of superdisintegrants and various diluents in FDTs prepared by direct compression.

Drug	Diluent	Disintegrant	Ref.
Acetaminophen, ascorbic acid	MCC (Avicel PH-M series) and spherical sugar granules	L-HPC	[1]
Ascorbic acid and nifedipine	Mannitol	Crospovidone	[2]

(Table 1) contd.....

Drug	Diluent	Disintegrant	Ref.
Buspiron	MCC (Avicel PH 102) and Pearlitol SD 200	Crospovidone, CCS and SSG	[3]
Carvidilol solid dispersion with polyvinylpyrrolidone (PVP)	MCC and mannitol	Crospovidone, SSG, CCS and polacrilin potassium	[4]
Celecoxib solid dispersion with sorbitol		SSG	[5]
Chlorpromazine HCl	MCC and Mannitol	Crospovidone, CCS, SSG, L-HPC and pregelatinised starch	[6]
Cinnarizine	Avicel PH102 and mannitol	Crospovidone	[7]
Clonazepam	MCC and mannitol	Crospovidone, CCS and SSG	[8]
Clozapine	Avicel PH102 and mannitol	Kollidon CL, Explotab	[9]
Dicyclomine HCl, roxithromycin, montelukast sodium	Avicel PH102	Indion 414, CCS, SSG and crospovidone	[10]
Epinephrine	MCC (Avicel PH 301)	L-HPC	[11]
Ethenzamide	MCC	L-HPC	[12]
Famotidine	Spray dried lactose, mannitol and Avicel PH 101	SSG (Primojel), Ac-Di-Sol and L-HPC	[13]
Famotidine	Dibasic calcium phosphate (DCP)	Ac-Di-Sol, Crospovidone and SSG	[14]
Famotidine	MCC, xylitol and sucrose stearic acid esters	CCS	[15, 16]
Fexofenadine	Avicel PH102 and mannitol	Ac-Di-Sol, crospovidone, SSG	[17]
Flutamide	Ludipress, mannitol and Avicel PH102	SSG	[18]
Gliclazide	MCC and DCP	Crospovidone and CCS	[19]
Glipizide	MCC and DCP	Crosspovidone and CCS	[20]
Glyburide/PEG 6000/Surfactant ternary solid dispersion	MCC and lactose monohydrate	Maize starch, pregelatinised starch	[21]
Granisetron HCl	MCC and mannitol	CCS, SSG, crospovidone	[22]
Hydrochlorthiazide	MCC	CCS and crospovidone	[23]
Ibuprofen solid dispersion with PEG 4000	MCC (Avicel PH 102)	Primogel, Ac-Di-Sol	[24]
Lamotrigene	Mannitol and MCC (Avicel PH102)	SSG, crospovidone XL-10 and CCS	[25]
Losartan potassium	MCC and Mannitol	Polyplasdone XL 10, CCS and Explotab	[26]
Meclizine	MCC (Avicel PH102 and Avicel PH301)	L-HPC	[27]
Meclizine	Mannitol and maltodextrin	CCS	[28]
Melatonin	Mannitol	PVP	[29]

(Table 1) contd.....

Drug	Diluent	Disintegrant	Ref.
Meloxicam	Pearlitol SD 200 and MCC	Polyplasdone XL 10, CCS and Explotab	[30]
Meloxicam PEG solid dispersion	MCC (RanQ102)	Ac-Di-Sol	[31]
Meloxicam-β-cyclodextrin complex	Co-spray dried micro-crystalline cellulose and mannitol (Avicel HFE-102)	CCS, SSG and crospovidone	[32]
Omeprazole and domperidone	Mannitol	Kollidon CL, SSG, Ac-Di-Sol	[33]
Ondansetron HCl	Spray dried lactose	Glycine-Chitosan, CCS and crospovidone	[34]
Oxcarbazepine	Mannitol and DCP	Crospovidone and CCS	[35]
Oxycarbazepine	Avicel PH102	Polyplasdone XL10, Primojel and Ac-Di-Sol	[36]
Piroxicam	MCC and mannitol	Crospovidone and SSG	[37]
Rosiglitazone	MCC and lactose	SSG, Crospovidone and CCS	[38]
Roxithromycin	MCC and spray dried lactose	Co-grinded treated agar (C-TAG) and co grinded treated guar gum	[39]
Salbutamol sulphate	Avicel PH102	Primojel, Ac-Di-Sol and Polyplasdone R-XL	[14]
Salbutamol sulphate	MCC and mannitol	Sodium starch glycolate, CCS and Indion 414	[40]
Salbutamol sulphate	MCC and Mannitol	CCS, SSG and crospovidone	[41]
Salbutamol sulphate	Mannitol	SSG	[42]
Sildenafil citrate	MCC and starch	SSG and CCS	[43]
Tinidazole taste masked microspheres with Eudragit E100	MCC	SSG	[44]
Tizanidine HCl taste masked granules with Eudragit E100	MCC and mannitol	SSG, CCS and crospovidone	[45]
Valdecoxib and Metoclopramide	MCC, mannitol	SSG, Ac-Di-Sol and Kollidon CL	[46]
Valsartan	MCC	Crospovidone, Ac-Di-Sol and SSG	[47]
Zidovudine and Lumivudine FDC	Avicel PH102	Explotab	[48]

Directly compressible FDT formulation contains high level of superdisintegrants, which may range from 10-20% by weight or even higher than this amount or lower in some other cases when high amounts of water soluble diluents are used [49]. At high levels, superdisintegrant may affect mouthfeel, tablet hardness and friability of FDTs [13]. Hence, apart from disintegrant action, several other properties like compatibility, mouthfeel, flow, particle size and distribution, particle shape and morphology, flowability play significant role in selecting an appropriate superdisintegrant for FDTs [49]. On the other hand, the properties of drug, amount of drug and presence of other additives are also paramount importance in defining quality of FDTs.

Pharmaceutical disintegrants act mainly by following mechanism [50]:

i. Capillary/wicking action: Disintegrant absorbs water through pores in the tablet that enlarges the pores and reduces the binding forces between the tablets.
ii. High swellability: Disintegrant absorbs water, which results in increased swelling pressure that leading to disintegration of the tablet.
iii. Act by both capillary action and high swellability process.

A force equivalent concept, to explain efficiency of disintegration, is defined as the equivalent ability of disintegrating agents to absorb water to convert into a swelling force referred to as the disintegrating force [51]. A critical concentration of disintegrant is required, while optimising tablet for disintegration. Disintegration time of tablet increases with a decrease in disintegration concentration below critical value and disintegrant concentration higher than critical concentration leads to either a constant or greater disintegration time.

Following are the factors affecting the disintegration/dissolution of FDTs:

i. Type and amount of disintegrant
ii. Combination of disintegrants and their mechanism of action
iii. Water absorption capacity of the formulation
iv. Hardness and size of tablets
v. Nature of drug substance
vi. Nature of other tablet excipients
vii. Particle size distribution of diluents
viii. Porosity and pore size distribution

MCC and L-HPC have been widely employed as diluent and disintegrant combination used to prepare FDTs. MCC and L-HPC in the ratios of 8:2 to 9:1 resulted in FDTs with the fastest disintegrating time [1, 27, 52]. FDTs produced at a compression force of 300 kg rapidly disintegrated within 30 s *in vitro* and in the oral cavity [53]. Watanabe *et al.* (1995) formulated FDTs comprising crystalline cellulose and L-HPC and the tablets achieved disintegration time less than 30 s [27]. The crystalline cellulose and L-HPC combination increases the porosity of tablets promoting osmotic capillary action. Ishikawa *et al.* (1990) prepared oxybutynin and pirenzipine taste masked FDTs using MCC as a diluent and

L-HPC as disintegrant and the ratio was 8:2 [54]. FDTs of acetaminophen and ascorbic acid were prepared by direct compression method using special grade of MCC (Avicel PH-M series, particle size 7-32 μm) as diluent and L-HPC as disintegrant in the proportion of 9:1 [55]. Particle size of granules/API/formulation component is an important parameter influencing the acceptance of FDTs among patients. Sensory evaluation by volunteers has shown superiority of FDTs prepared from MCC having small particle size (Avicel PH-M), when compared with tablets with normal grade MCC (Avicel PH-102). Fluidity problem was solved with the addition of crystalline sugar granules made from sucrose and starch in ratio 7:3 (nonpareil spheres).

MCC particles are relatively smaller with large degree of circularity, when compared to L-HPC (larger particles, fibrous). Pure MCC tablet has higher number of contact points for a unit cross sectional area than in pure L-HPC tablet. Also, strong intermolecular hydrogen bonds are present at contact points in MCC tablet, when compared to the relatively weaker intermolecular forces between hydroxypropyl groups in L-HPC tablet. Water uptake in L-HPC is greater than MCC due to the presence of three hydroxypropyl ether groups in the amorphous region of L-HPC. An optimised MCC/L-HPC system is able to give the desired tensile strength and porosity and ultimately faster disintegration [53]. FDTs prepared by direct compression of diluent and different levels of disintegrants showed that FDTs are produced at low compression forces. Improving the robustness of such tablets by increasing compression force reduces the porosity [56]. Ethenzamide FDT consisting of excipients MCC, lactose, erythritol and sodium carboxymethyl cellulose were made by direct compression [57]. Optimum combination of tablet porosity and formulation was obtained by superimposing the contour diagrams of tablet tensile strength and disintegration time. Eythritol granules, prepared by fluidised bed granulation with water, and L-HPC blend were compressed to prepare FDTs. Granules of fine micronised grades (15 μm) gave tablets of greater hardness, when compared with the original larger size (40 μm) [58].

Co-grinding of mannitol and crospovidone, followed by the addition of crospovidone, D-mannitol and magnesium stearate, and subsequent compression improved hardness of FDTs [2].Vibration rod mill was used to perform co-grinding and crospovidone was employed to assist grinding of D-mannitol. The size reduction of D-mannitol increased specific surface area, resulting in increased contact area among powder particles leading to appreciable increase in hardness of tablets. The method was found effective with other saccharides and disintegrants. Dissolution rate of nifedipine improved remarkably from FDTs of nifedipine prepared by this method.

Disintegration and/or dissolution of FDTs, prepared by direct compression, are dependent on nature of disintegrants and water soluble excipients and the mechanism of action of one or more excipients in disintegrating/dissolving the dosage unit. L-HPC and mannitol was used in formulating superior famotidine FDTs characterised by faster dissolution and disintegration time of 11.4 s [13]. However, the combination of other diluents (Avicel PH101 and spray dried lactose) and disintegrants (Ac-Di-Sol and SSG) in FDTs of famotidine produced inferior tablets, as FDTs disintegrated and dissolved slowly.

Chitosan-glycine mixture was used as disintegrant-disintegrant accelerator combination in preparing FDTs of ondansetron HCl [34]. The formulations prepared with 5.5% w/w of chitosan and 43.3% w/w of glycine (43.3% w/w) were directly compressed to produce FDTs capable of oral disintegration in 29±2 s. An interpolymer complex of chitosan-alginate (1:1 ratio) and chitin was used as a novel combination of disintegrants in preparing FDTs of ondansetron HCl [59] and salbutamol sulphate [60]. The chitosan-alginate complex was prepared by coacervation phase separation method. A combination of chitin (10% w/w), glycine (40% w/w) and chitosan-alginate interpolymer complex (3% w/w) was found to contribute fastest disintegration in FDTs of ondansetron HCl. Disintegration time of salbutamol sulphate FDTs, containing 50% w/w of glycine, 10% w/w of chitosan-alginate complex and 15% w/w of chitin, were lower than FDTs containing some other concentrations/compositions. Faster disintegration of FDTs was achieved with faster movement of aqueous medium assisted by glycine leading to quick swelling of chitosan-alginate complex. Disintegration time of FDTs was correlated to tablet hardness, effective pore radius, water sorption time and swelling index by a mathematical model [61].

An FDT formulation of perchlorperazine maleate, containing *Plantago ovata* mucilage (8% w/w) and MCC (60% w/w), succeeded in achieving 11 s wetting time, *in vitro* disintegration time of 8 s and water absorption ratio of 86% [62]. FDTs were prepared by directly compressing combination of diluents (MCC and Pearlitol SD 200) and disintegrants (*Plantago ovata* mucilage or crospovidone). *Plantago ovata* mucilage was able to disintegrate FDTs slightly better than crospovidone.

2.2. Water Soluble Substances/Saccharides

Directly compressed sublingual tablet of aspirin, comprising aspirin, granulated sugar and mannitol as major components, dissolved rapidly in the oral cavity allowing faster sublingual absorption of aspirin and thereby prevented the gastric irritation [63]. Tablet formulations of aspirin containing glycerine, mineral oil and surfactants (two) had made the tablet more porous so that a small amount of saliva was able to form an emulsion ensuring faster disintegration/dissolution of tablets. A formulation containing an active ingredient, a lubricant and a water soluble sugar, such as sorbitol, and polyethylene glycols/glycerides (melting point 25° to 45° C) were combined and compressed at about 1000 psi pressure to FDTs [64].

2.3. Coprocessed Excipients

A tablet formulation is composed of various excipients having different functions like diluents, disintegrant, binder, glidant, lubricant, *etc*. Two or more than two functions of excipients can be combined by suitably processing them by one or combination of two or more methods like granulation, fluidised bed drying, coating, melt extrusion, solvent evaporation, milling, crystallisation, *etc*. Simultaneous processing of two or more excipients to develop a composite excipient is referred to as coprocessing and the resulting composite excipient is termed as coprocessed excipient. These excipients have synonyms like multifunctional, high functionality and performance excipients. Developing a coprocessed excipient does not involve any chemical reaction or change in their chemical structure/composition. Excipient(s) is/are only physically modified to achieve enhanced physical property (ies), which is generally not possible by simple mixing.

Faster disintegration and adequate mechanical strength are two important quality attributes of FDTs. Keeping this in view, diluents and superdisintegrants have been combined by subjecting them simultaneously to various processes leading to preparation of coprocessed excipient, thereby offering the advantage of minimising the use of other excipients in direct compression of FDTs. Use of several coprocessed excipients, in FDTs developments are provided in Table **2**.

Table 2. Use of coprocessed excipients in preparing FDTs by direct compression.

Drug	Coprocecessed Excipient	Other Excipients	Ref.
Amlodipine	F-melt®	Magnesium stearate	[65]
Baclofen	Ludiflash®	Calcium stearate, aspartame, Aerosil® and sodium lauryl sulphate (SLS)	[66]
Benzocaine	F-melt®, Pearlitol® Flash, Ludiflash® and Prosolv® ODT	Magnesium stearate	[67]

(Table 2) contd.....

Drug	Coprocecessed Excipient	Other Excipients	Ref.
Cefopodoxime proxetil complex with Kyron T	Pharmaburst®	MCC, Kyron T (various grades), talc, saccharin, orange flavour and disintegrant (crospovidone or CCS or SSG)	[68]
Cetirizine dihydrochloride	Ludiflash®	Avicel PH101, Aerosil® 200, magnesium stearate and sodium stearyl fumarate (SSF)	[69]
Gliclazide	Ludiflash®	MCC, sodium saccharine, magnesium stearate and talc	[70]
Hydrochlorthiazide	Parteck® ODT, Ludiflash®, Pearlitol® Flash, Prosolv® ODT and Pharmaburst® 500	SSF	[71]
Ibuprofen, diclofenac sodium and diltiazem HCl	F-melt® Type C and Type M	SSF	[72]
Mirtazapine and Kleptose HPB complex	Ludiflash® and Pearlitol®	Kyron T314, Avicel PH101 and magnesium stearate	[73]
Rifampin	F-melt®	Avicel PH102, Ac-Di-Sol, cherry flavour and magnesium stearate	[74]
Sildenafil citrate	Pharmaburst® 500	Magnesium stearate, sucralose, mango flavour and colloidal silicon dioxide	[75]
Sildenafil citrate and Poloxamer 188 solid dispersion	Pharmaburst® 500	Peppermint, xylitol and magnesium stearate	[76]
Tramadol HCl	Pharmaburst®	Colloidal anhydrous silica, magnesium stearate, aspartame and tutti frutti flavour	[77]
	Ludiflash®	Cocoa powder	[78]
	Ludiflash® and Parteck®	Magnesium stearate, Kollidon (several grades), Avicel PH102 and Ac-Di-Sol	[79]
	Ludiflash®	Magnesium stearate and SSF	[80]
	RxCipient® FM1000 and Parteck®	SSG and magnesium stearate	[81]

Some of these coprocessed excipient require only addition of drug and/or lubricant before compression of tablets. However, to address undesirable taste and palatability issues, sweetener and flavours are also added in the formulations of FDTs.

2.4. Trademark Technologies

2.4.1. Ziplets®

Ziplets® technology (Actavis; www.actavis.com, previously Aptalis Pharma and more previously Eurand International) is patented and proprietary technology for making FDTs. High weight tablets, containing high dose of drug, can be manufactured with acceptable hardness, friability and disintegration. In this technology, water soluble or water insoluble drug particles are coated to prepare microparticles, which are then mixed with water insoluble excipients (*e.g.* di or tri basic calcium phosphate), one or more disintegrants (*e.g.* cross-linked PVP) and optionally one or more substantially water soluble excipient (*e.g.* lactose) and subsequently compressed at low pressure to FDTs [82]. Water insoluble inorganic excipients in tablets are capable to disintegrate tablets faster than water soluble excipients like saccharides or sugar alcohols. Rather, tablets containing saccharides or sugar alcohols dissolve to form a highly viscous solution leading to a reduction in water diffusion at the core of the tablet resulting in prolonged disintegration [82]. Amount of insoluble inorganic excipient, amount of disintegrant, and proportion of water insoluble and water insoluble excipients govern the disintegration of the tablet. Enough compression can be applied to the formulations to obtain good tensile strength and less friable tablets. However, hardness of such tablets is critical in determining the disintegration and optimising rate of disintegration. FDTs prepared by Ziplets® disintegrate in less than 40 s. Ziplets® tablets were found stable at accelerated conditions (40°C, 75% Relative Humidity (RH)) up to 6 months and at room temperature (25°C, 60% RH) for 18 months [83]. No significant changes in disintegration time and physical properties of Ziplets® tablets were observed in accelerated stability studies.

Ziplets® entered in commercial market with a successfully launch of Cibalgina® DueFast (Novartis) in some countries of Europe [84]. This product combines the use of Ziplets® with Microcaps® technology in ibuprofen drug product.

2.4.2. Flashtab®

Flashtab® (Ethypharm, S.A., Paris, France; http://www.ethypharm.com/), a rapidly disintegrating multiparticulate tablet, is prepared by compression of excipient granules (dry- or wet-compression) along with coated microcrystals of drug or coated or uncoated granules of the drug [85, 86]. Coated microcrystals of the drug may be prepared by pan coating, micro-encapsulation, coacervation, or extrusion-spheronisation. Coated microcrystals provide taste masking effect without compromising the bioavailability. Starch and or modified starch or cross linked PVP, cross linked carboxymethyl cellulose or other superdisintegrants are used to achieve faster disintegration of tablets. High compressibility of MCC is utilised to provide good compressibility in the tablet formulation. Tablet properties can be further improved with the use of microparticles having intrinsic compression properties. The simultaneous use of a disintegrating agent and a swelling agent produce rapidly disintegration in mouth in less than 60 s. Disintegration and/or dissolution of a Flashtab® are governed by the action of one or more disintegrants. When two disintegrants are used in combination, they shall differ in their ability to generate swelling force. Disintegrant which provides high swelling (or disintegration) force is referred to as "disintegrating agent" and the second disintegrant which generate a low swelling force is called "swelling agent", offers satisfactory physical resistance to the tablet [86]. Good mechanical strength of tablets, faster disintegration and masking of undesirable taste are major advantages of Flashtab®. Pleasant taste in Flashtab® tablets can be achieved with Ethypharm's T-mask® flavour masking technology. Flashtab® tablet technology is also compatible to develop modified release tablets and bilayer tablets for two or more APIs.

2.4.3. Easy-Tec™ Technology

EasyTec™ (Antares Pharma's, www.antarespharma.com) technology uses a direct compression process and conventional rotary tablet machines for high speed manufacturing of FDTs. Disintegration of FDTs is made quicker by adding a specific excipient and disintegrants in the formulation. This technology has the advantage of using a low cost and robust manufacturing process and equipment, and use of compendial excipients in FDT formulations to eliminate the requirements of special manufacturing or packaging processes. FDTs weighing 200-1000 mg are designed to disintegrate in 10-30 s. This FDT technology is compatible to a large range of active ingredients of high to low doses, use of conventional and new excipients, masking undesirable taste and addition of flavours to improve palatability.

2.4.4. Advatab™ Technology

Advatab® is a proprietary technology of Actavis (Actavis, www.actavis.com, previously Aptalis Pharma and more previously Eurand International). FDTs, using this technology, are manufactured by dispersing uniformly coated API particles in a rapidly disintegrating matrix characterised by low water content, fine particle size and good organoleptics. Advatab™ brand was introduced in 2013 by Eurand International after acquiring rights of several patents of a Japanese Company Kyowa Hakko Co [84]. Advatab™ technology utilise Kyowa's external lubrication system (ExLub®) in which lubricant is sprayed onto punches and dies [87]. Hence, lubricant does not coat the particles to be compressed. Contrary to this, conventional tablets require internal lubrication, wherein lubricant is to be dispersed throughout the granules/powder and make it available on the inner surface of the tablet. Internal lubrication process requires a large amount of hydrophobic lubricant, which decreases the hardness of a tablet by reducing the binding action of particles and adversely impact disintegration as lubricant may impede the absorption of water or liquid into the tablet matrix. External lubrication requires 10-30 times less amount of lubricant for faster disintegration and good mechanical strength of tablets. The increase in dissolution and/or disintegration, without impacting negatively on tablet strength, makes external lubrication a good choice for FDT development. Tablets, prepared by Advatab™ technology, dissolve intra-orally in 15-30 s making tablets convenient to administer without water and without chewing. Microcaps™ taste masking technology (developed by Eurand International) is used in Advatab™ tablets to coat drug particles to achieve pleasant mouthfeel. Simultaneous use of Advatab™ and Microcaps™ technologies in a single product results in a patient preferred drug product with better taste and pleasant organoleptic sensation. Advtab™ can also be combined with Diffucap™ to develop highly differentiated taste masked and sustained release drug products [84]. Eurand NV and GSK co-developed pleasant tasting Lamictal® (lamotrigine) ODT, using AdvaTab™ ODTs and Microcaps™ [88].

2.4.5. Panacea-Biotech's Proprietary Technology

Panacea-Biotech (New Delhi, India) used a low cost direct compression method utilising water soluble sugar (mannitol, sorbitol, or xylitol, *etc.*) and superdisintegrants (SSG, *etc.*) for making FDTs [89]. Tablet disperses in solution or suspension within one minute. Taste of bitter drug is masked by using non sugar sweetener in two parts. One part gives immediate sweetness upon ingestion and another part of sweetener is granulated in mucoadhesive polymer to form a matrix, which slowly release the sweetener and gives prolonged sweet taste thereby effectively masking the bitter taste or aftertaste of API.

2.4.6. Technology Developed by Royal College of Surgeons, Ireland

The School of Pharmacy, Royal College of Surgeons, Ireland has developed a direct compression technology to produce mechanically strong tablets having low friability and ability to withstand stresses of conventional blister-packing. This technology is used to prepare a directly compressed FDT, comprising non-granulated API (0.1-50% w/w), directly compressible sugar alcohol (10-80%), directly compressible MCC (10-80%), by one step direct compression method using a compression force of at least 5 kN [90]. Sugar alcohol is directly compressible mannitol, MCC is a silicified MCC (Prosolv®) and API to be used is a hydrophobic substance. Optionally formulation may contain one or more lubricant, disintegrant, flavouring agent or glidant. These FDTs disintegrates in less than 40 s. The manufacturing process utilises a cost effective conventional tablet presses and avoids the use of liquids and hence the process is suitable where stability of API is a major concern. This technology allows incorporation of microparticulates, solid dispersions, *etc.* to produce extended release and taste masked FDTs.

Prosolv® and combination of Prosolv® and mannitol was used in preparing FDTs by direct compression to prepare characterised by high mechanical strength, rapid disintegration and dissolution [91]. Solid dispersions of crystalline simvastatin were prepared by spray drying. These solid dispersions were incorporated in FDTs which showed an improvement in dissolution rate, when compared to the FDTs containing corresponding physical mixture or the marketed simvastatin Zocor® tablets [92]. Evaluation in a phase I pharmacokinetic study in human volunteers (n=18) of simvastatin FDT formulation showed a 50% increase in bioavailability when administered sublingually compared to oral administration of the innovator product, Zocor®.

2.4.7. PharmaBurst™

PharmaBurst™ (SPI Pharma, Wilington, US) is proprietary and patented fast disintegrating coprocessed excipient system to prepare FDTs with quick disintegration and lesser adhesion to contact parts of the tablet punching machine. This excipient combines various useful properties of its constituent excipients, *viz.* mannitol, crospovidone, sorbitol and precipitated silicon dioxide [71]. This fast disintegrating excipient system was prepared by coprocessing of the composition in a fluidised bed apparatus [93]. Drug, lubricant and flavour(s) are dry mixed with PharmaBurst™ excipient system and compressed directly on a conventional tablet machine to produce FDTs. The entire manufacturing process is conducted at normal temperature and humidity conditions. FDTs made with PharmaBurst™, generally dissolve within 30-60 s depending on their size and hardness, does not require special packaging and, therefore, could be either packaged in blister packs or high density polyethylene bottles.

PharmaBurst™ is an "off the shelf" excipient, which allows to develop FDTs in-house quickly and much more cost effectively. While, other FDT technologies require a third party manufacturer and thus marketed under a license, which are expensive. When used at levels 50% w/w or higher, PharmaBurst™ gives an excellent creamy mouth feel as the tablet dissolves flushing down the taste masked granules of the drug without exhibiting grittiness. Quick Melt (80 mg) Children's Non-Asprin Pain Reliever/Fever Reducer (Marlex Pharmaceuticals,

New Castle, Delaware, USA) utilises SPI Pharma's PharmaBurst quick dissolve technology.

2.4.8. RubiODT

RubiODT® technology (Rubicon Research; http://www.rubicon.co.in/) is a direct compression technology, which uses PanExceaODT® and taste-masked drug particles. PanExceaODT® (Avantor Performance Materials) is a coprocessed excipient, which ensures quick disintegration of the tablet in the saliva and thereby provides better taste and texture. Special particle characteristics and the unique composition of RubiODT® enable drug loading capacity up to 650 mg. this technology is suitable for drugs having different solubility profiles and bitter taste. The technology can be coupled with RubiCoat® taste masking technology and can also deliver drug in a controlled or sustained or delayed release manner. It employs conventional equipment for manufacturing and packaging.

3. GRANULATION METHODS

3.1. Wet Granulation

Wet granulation involves preparation of granules from raw materials with the aid of a binder solution/slurry prior to compression of the tablet. Modification of materials' properties is easier in the wet granulation, when compared to dry granulation or direct compression. Control of compressibility and disintegration, essential in making FDTs, by altering the manufacturing conditions is feasible and rather easy in wet granulation. A binder solution or slurry helps with the formation of inter-particle bonds and growth of granules enhancing the hardness of the resulting tablets. Some of the literature reports on preparation of FDTs by wet granulation are shown as Table **3**.

Table 3. FDTs prepared by wet granulation methods.

Drug	Diluent	Disintegrant	Binder	Ref
Acetaminophen and codeine phosphate	Mannitol	Ac-Di-Sol	Gelucire 44/14-Kollidon VA64	[94]
Acetaminophen	Mannitol	CCS, sodium carboxy methyl cellulose	PEG-6-stearate	[95]
Acetylsalicylic acid		Carmellose, carmellose sodium, carmellose calcium, L-HPC	Acid treated yeast cell wall	[50]

(Table 3) contd.....

Drug	Diluent	Disintegrant	Binder	Ref
Buspiron	MCC (Avicel PH 102) and Pearlitol SD 200	Crospovidone, CCS and SSG		[3]
Carbamazepine	Monohydrate lactose	Crospovidone	PEG	[96]
Diazepam solid dispersion with PEG 4000/6000	MCC (Avicel PH 102) and lactose monohydrate	CCS	Starch paste	[97]
Glyburide/PEG 6000/Surfactant ternary solid dispersion	MCC and lactose monohydrate	Maize starch	Pregelatinised starch	[21]
Meclizine	Mannitol	CCS	Maltodextrin solution	[28]
Meloxicam	MCC, dextrose, β cyclodextrin	Crospovidone, CCS	Starch mucilage	[98]
Oxacarbazepine	Avicel PH102	Ac-Di-Sol	Starch	[99]
	D-mannitol, corn starch	Pregelatinised starch	D-sorbitol, macrogol 4000, hypromellose, hydroxylpropylcellulose, povidone	[100]
	Maltrin QD580 and Mannogem EZ Spray		Sucrose	[101]
	Corn starch	Amino acids (L-alanine, glycine, L-lysine HCl and L-tyrosine)	Hydroxypropylcellulose-L	[102]

Makooi-Merchead *et al.* (2001) used wet granulation method to prepare efavirenz FDT in which MCC was used as filler and SSG was incorporated as superdisintegrant. In general, a disintegrant level ranges from 5-20% w/w in the FDTs was used [103]. The method of addition of disintegrant is also important, particularly in moist granulation process. Dividing the disintegrant into extragranular and intragranular portion is more advantageous. Extragranular addition of disintegrant is responsible for disintegration of tablet into granules, which further disintegrate into fine particulates by the action of disintegrant added intragranularly [104]. Croscarmellose slurry was utilised for preparation of wet granules, which were dried and then mixed with MCC and a coprocessed excipient Avicel AC-815 and subsequently the blend was compressed to FDTs [105]. Disintegrants that propagate capillary effects and water uptake by capillary constitute major portion of such FDTs. Pore structure of the tablet is also important as any inherent hydrophobicity of the tablet mass will adversely affect disintegration/dissolution.

Ito *et al.* (1996) used treated agar powder (TAG) as disintegrant in preparing FDTs [106]. Agar powder was made to swell by water absorption followed by drying at room temperature. Final grinding results in TAG with high porosity. TAG powder quickly absorbs water and swells significantly, without being gelatinous at physiological pH, thereby making it a superior quality disintegrant.

Low dose sublingual aspirin tablet (80 mg), having ability for fast dissolution or disintegration in saliva, comprising of compressible soluble starch as a disintegrant and filler along with other excipients, inhibited cyclooxygenase and platelet aggregation very effectively [107]. The sublingual tablet was prepared by moistening the blend with 10% moisture followed by slugging. Slugs were grinded, passed through sieve number 14/16 and compressed with moderate pressure to obtain sublingual tablets.

Highly plastic granules were prepared by wet granulation and compressed into FDTs at low pressure [101]. The highly plastic granules comprised three ingredients: maltodextrin as a plastic material (Maltrin QD 580), mannitol (Mannogem EZ spray) for increasing penetration of water and sucrose solution as a wet binder. Highly plastic granules were able to maintain high porosity in compressed tablets leading to faster penetration of water and ultimately resulting in quicker disintegration/dissolution of tablets. Sufficient mechanical strength and friability enough for multi-tablet packaging was achieved with tablets prepared from high plastic granules. An API or nutritional ingredient can be incorporated intragraularly into highly plastic granules or may be added extragranularly. Simple processing steps and easy incorporation of microparticulates makes this technology amenable to produce taste masked and sustained/controlled release drug products.

Rapid disintegration granules (RDGs) were prepared by spray coating of a suspension in a fluidised bed processor [108]. Intra/suspension method and a suspension method were investigated for preparing RDGs. The intra/suspension method involved addition of disintegrants to saccharides followed by blending and granulating in a disintegrant/water suspension. The suspension method involved the addition of disintegrants to a suspension, which was used in granulating saccharides. RDGs were lubricated with magnesium stearate and compressed in a rotary tablet machine to prepare FDTs. Rapid *in vivo* oral disintegration and optimum hardness were achieved with FDTs prepared with RDGs in which mannitol was spray coated with a corn starch and crospovidone (in ratio 2.5:1) suspension.

3.2. Dry Granulation

FDTs were prepared from a powder mixture having a density 0.2 to 0.55 g/mL [109]. To achieve the required density alkali metal earth salts (calcium carbonate) or carbohydrates (sorbitol or mannitol), were processed by a pre-compaction (dry granulation). In particular, the pre-compacting or pre-compressing process for making the granules can be accomplished by applying a compression force. A compression force of 1-9 kN/cm was applied by a chilsonator or compactor to increase the density of powder mixture from 0.2-055 g/mL to 0.4-0.75 g/mL. The resulting granules were compressed into FDTs with disintegration time less than 40 s in oral cavity without chewing.

Dry granulation was used to prepare atenolol FDTs for studying the effect of three superdisintegrants, *viz.* CCS, crospovidone and SSG [110]. Atenolol, mannitol and dibasic calcium phosphate were mixed and the blend was compressed to prepare slugs of harness 4.5-5 kg/cm^2. Slugs were milled to prepare granules. Further, these granules were mixed with magnesium stearate and disintegrant. Croscarmellose sodium gave least disintegration time of 31±2 s at 8% w/w and drug release was 98% after 10 min.

3.3. Melt Granulation

When a solid that melts during granulation or a molten liquid is used as a binder to granulate pharmaceutical powders, the process is termed as melt granulation. This process requires high-shear mixers with heating jacket for preparing granules. Optionally, heat may be generated during mixing by impeller in a high-shear mixer. Melt granulation offers several advantages over wet granulation by omitting the use of water or organic solvents and reduces processing time and energy by eliminating the need of a drying step. Wecobee® M, Wecobee® M hydrogenated vegetable oil, PEG 900 and Gelucire® 33/01 were used as a binder (2.5-20% w/w) for granulating a water soluble excipient (saccharide) to prepare granules in a high shear/low shear mixer [111]. These granules were mixed with an API to prepare FDTs of hardness 3 kP or less [111].

An optimum melt granulation was achieved with PEG 400 and 6000 (4:6 ratio, melting point 37°C) as a binder at 0.25:4 ratio with granular mannitol [112]. Mannitol granules and other additives were used in preparing sublingual tablet of ketotifen fumarate. Used primarily as a binder, PEG also increased buccal permeation resulting in rapid absorption of the drug. Fast-release tablets of carbamazepine were developed from granules prepared by melt granulation in a high shear mixer [96]. In these granules, polyethylene glycol (PEG) 4000 was used as a binder and lactose monohydrate was employed as a hydrophilic diluent. Crospovidone was added as disintegrating agent in the granules by intragranular addition approach to enhance dissolution and disintegration.

PEG-6-stearate (Superpolystate®) was used as a binder in a melt/wet granulation method for preparing FDTs [95]. FDTs disintegrated quickly in 40±2 s and a hardness of 47.9±2.5 N was achieved. Superpolystate® is a hydrophilic waxy material having a melting point of 33–37°C and HLB of 9. A high-speed blade mixer was employed for conventional hot-melt procedure of preparing granules at 40–44°C. Superpolystate®, as a binder cum disintegrating agent, increased the physical strength of tablets and decreased disintegration time of the tablets.

A modified melt granulation technique was used to prepare FDTs of taste masked ambroxol HCl [113]. Xylitol and dextrose were dry-mixed and screened through sieve number 80 followed by blending with MCC and colloidal silicon dioxide. PEG 1000 melt at 50°C was gradually added to the prepared powder blend and mixed continuously at high speed to form granules. Granules were congealed and sifted through sieve number 60 and subjected to vacuum drying for 2 h. Ambroxol hydrochloride FDTs were prepared from dried fast disintegrating granules.

3.4. Spray Drying

Spray drying is used in processing of two or more excipients to alter their pre-compression and post-compression properties so as to produce efficient excipient system for making FDTs. Critical processing steps like making a suspension of API in appropriate solvent, followed by evaporation of the solvent, drying the coherent mass and sieving play important role in modulating excipient characteristics of prepared granules. Table **4** enlists various attempts of modifying properties of excipients.

Spray dried product is characterised by high porosity and fine particle size due to faster evaporation of solvent in drying process. Allen *et al.* used a spray-drying method to prepare FDTs [114 - 117]. In FDT formulation, mannitol was used as diluent, gelatin (hydrolysed and non-hydrolysed) acted as supporting agent, disintegrants were SSG or CCS, and citric acid and sodium bicarbonate were used to improve disintegration and dissolution. FDTs prepared from spray-dried powder disintegrated very quickly within 20 s in water [114, 117]. Low density granules, consisting of mixtures of alkali earth metal salts (density 0.3 g/ml to about 0.55 g/ml) and water soluble carbohydrates, were prepared by spray drying or pre-compacting process [109]. Such low-density granules were mixed and compressed into FDTs using conventional tablet machine. Sometimes, high amount of drug poses problems in manufacturing FDTs. Dijkgraft *et al.* (1998) prepared granulates by fluid bed granulation for preparing FDTs containing high amount of APIs like antimicrobial compounds (*e.g.* cefaclor, amoxicillin, *etc.*) [118]. FDTs by direct compression of galanthamine HCl and HBr and a spray dried carrier comprising a mixture of diluents (lactose monohydrate and MCC) and disintegrant (crospovidone or croscarmellose) [119].

Table 4. Coprocessing of excipients by spray drying and other drying processes for preparing superior excipient combinations for preparing FDTs.

Drug	Excipients	Apparatus Used	Coprocessing Conditions	Other Excipients Used in Tableting	Ref.
Glipizide	MCC and mannitol	JISL mini lab spray drier	Outer temp. 60°C, inner temp. 120°C and pressure of 2 kg/cm^2	SSG, corn starch, aspartame sodium, talc, strawberry flavour and magnesium stearate	[120]
Granisetron HCl	Crospovidone and CCS	Beaker with magnetic stirrer and hot air oven	Suspension in ethanol evaporated in beaker, wet mass sieving, drying at 60°C for 20 min	Mannitol, MCC, and sodium stearyl fumarate (SSF)	[121]
Losartan potassium	Coprocessing Ac-di-Sol and crospovidone	Beaker with magnetic stirrer and tray drier	Suspension in isopropyl alcohol evaporated at 50-60°C, wet mass sieving, drying at 60°C for 20 min	Lactose, dextrose, MCC, talc and magnesium stearate	[122]
Metoclopramide	MCC, mannitol, saccharin, superdisintegrants (Ac-Di-Sol, Kollidon and SSG) and an amino acid (glycine)	Buchi 190 Mini spray drier (Büchi Labortechnik AG, Germany)	Air flow rate of 4 lb/cm^2, Inlet air temp. 13°C and outlet air temp. of 70°C	SSF	[123]
Valedecoxib and metoclopramide	Disintegrant (Ac-D--Sol/Kollidon CL/SSF), MCC, mannitol and aspartame	SMST Scientech Spray Drier	Outer temp. 105-110°C, inner temp. 260-270°C and pressure of 2 lb/cm^2	Magnesium stearate	[46]

(Table 4) contd.....

Drug	Excipients	Apparatus Used	Coprocessing Conditions	Other Excipients Used in Tableting	Ref.
Zolmitriptan	Lactose and disintegrants (CCS/SSG/crospovidone/PVP)	Rotary evaporator (Heidolph, Germany)	Evaporation of solvent at 80°C at 150 rpm under vacuum	Magnesium stearate	[124]
	Binary and ternary mixtures of lactose monohydrate, MCC, mannitol and silicon dioxide	Buchi Spray Drier B-191	Inner temp. 130 °C		[125]

FDTs of valedecoxib and metoclopramide were prepared with a spray dried excipient base [46]. A suspension of mannitol, MCC, superdisintegrants and aspartame was spray dried to achieve a solid excipient mass which was passed through a sieve number 120 to obtain granules. Valedecoxib/metaclopramide was added to the spray dried granules followed by addition of magnesium stearate and compression of biconvex tablets in a single punch tablet machine. Prepared FDTs were superior to FDTs prepared by direct compression due to better flow property of spray dried granules and enhanced dissolution of the drug.

A dispersion of mannitol, MCC, disintegrant and saccharin in deionised water was spray dried to prepare excipient bases for preparing metoclopramide FDTs [123]. SSG, Kollidon® Ac-Di-Sol® and glycine were used as disintegrants. Disintegrants added to excipient bases before drying were more efficient when compared to their addition after completion of the drying process.

F-melt® is a spray-dried excipient used in FDTs containing inorganic excipients, saccharides, and disintegrating agents (http://www.fujichemical.co.jp /english/ medical/medicine /f-melt/ index.html). Addition of F-melt® and lubricant to API and thereafter direct compression was an easy and relatively straightforward method of manufacturing FDTs.

A suspension was obtained by dispersing superdisintegrants, MCC, aspartame in aqueous solution of mannitol. The resulting suspension was spray dried in a SMST Scientech Spray Drier at pressure 2 lb/cm^2, outer temperature 105-110°C, inner temperature 260-270°C to obtain wet mass of excipient base. The wet mass was sieved through sieve #120 and dried to obtain a directly compressible excipient base [46]. Quick disintegration time and good drug release characteristics were achieved with FDTs prepared from Kollidon® CL excipient base. Direct compression of spray dried excipient base resulted in superior FDTs, when compared to FDTs prepared through simple mixing of excipients followed by direct compression.

Mannitol and MCC in various ratios were spray dried to prepare a direct compression excipient base for FDTs [120]. Suspension of excipients in ethanol to a solid content of 10% was prepared and homogenous dispersion was fed to a spray dryer to prepare the coprocessed excipient. Fast disintegration (<15 s) and good compressibility was achieved with an optimised coprocessed formulation of mannitol and MCC (in ratio 1.25:1). FDTs of glipizide were prepared by blending with coprocessed excipients and other excipients followed by compression.

Lactose was processed with disintegrants (CCS/SSG/PVP/crospovidone) in a rotary evaporator to obtain a directly compressible excipient base [124]. The coprocessed mixture of lactose and SSG, having superior properties among all prepared coprocessed mixtures, was used to prepare FDTs of Zolmitriptan.

Coprocessesing of crospovidone and Ac-di-sol was performed using a isopropyl alcohol as a solvent [122]. Excipients were dispersed in the solvent and resulting dispersion was heated to evaporate the solvent. Coprocessed excipient particles were achieved through sieving of wet mass followed by drying. Wetting time and disintegration time of tablets prepared from coprocessed excipient decreased when compared with tablets formulated with non-coprocessed excipients. On the other hand, no appreciable change in hardness and friability was observed.

Coprocessing of MCC with SSL-hydroxypropylcellulose 1:1, 1:2 and 1:3 ratio was performed in a spray drier [9]. FDTs of tinidazole, prepared by direct compression of drug with coprocessed excipient base in ratio of 1:3, showed minimum disintegration time of 9.15±0.04 s and a superior drug release of 93.75% at 15 min. SEM studies confirmed that coprocessed particles were spherical, a factor that had improved flow properties.

Through a spray drying process different ratios of crospovidone and CCS (1:1, 1:2 and 1:3) were used in formulating FDTs of granisetron HCl [121]. The process involved preparation of a suspension of disintegrants in ethanol, followed by evaporation of the solvent from suspension, subsequent drying the coherent mass and thereafter sieving to obtain dried granules of desired size. These granules, drug, diluents, and other excipients were mixed and compressed to FDTs. Coprocessed superdisintegrants were superior in flow and compression characteristics. FDTs prepared with coprocessed superdisintegrants showed quick disintegration and faster drug dissolution when compared to the physical mixture of the superdisintegrants.

Binary and ternary mixtures of low cost and easily accessible excipients mannitol, lactose monohydrate, MCC and silicon dioxide (SiO_2) were dispersed/dissolved (10% solid concentration) in water and spray dried at same conditions in a Buchi Spray Drier B-191 [125]. The ternary mixture of mannitol:MCC:silicon dioxide in ratio 13:6:1 showed the better flow properties, superior tablet strength (>3 kg) and sufficient wetting times (of about 30 s) when tablets of 200 mg were compressed with a pressure of 0.3 ton.

3.5. Trademark Technologies

3.5.1. Frosta®

Frosta® technology (Akina Inc., http://www.akinainc.com/frosta.htm) uses conventional tablet machines and wet granulation methodology for economical production of FDTs. This technology is based on low pressure compression of highly plastic granules to manufacture FDTs [101]. Maltrin® QD 580 of suitable size (US Standard Testing Sieve no. 20 and no. 60 sieve) and Mannogem EZ spray (spray dried mannitol) particles are mixed into a high shear granulator for 30 s. Sucrose solution is added to the granulator followed by mixing to achieve a wet mass which is passed through a no. 8 sieve. Obtained wet granules are dried and blended with lubricants in a blender. Lubricated highly plastic granules are compressed into tablets by a rotary tablet press.

Thus, highly plastic granules are prepared with a plastic material, wet binder and water-penetration enhancer [126]. The plastic material may be water soluble or water dispersible or even may be porous. The plastic material, like maltodextrins, corn syrup, *etc.*, provides adequate mechanical strength to the tablets. Two forms of maltodextrin, Maltrin® QD M580 and Maltrin® M180, are mainly used to prepare FDTs by this technology. However, during compression, because of its porous structure, Maltrin QD M580 granules undergo more plastic deformation than Maltrin® M180 granules and leads to high mechanical strength of tablets [101]. Another important component of the plastic granules is water penetration enhancer. An optimum amount of water penetration enhancer (Mannozem® EZ spray) is required to be identified for achieving the desirable mechanical strength and disintegration time. Tablets prepared with a mixture of plastic materials and a penetration enhancer doesn't have enough mechanical strength. So a binder is needed to be added during granulation process. Commonly used binders are sucrose, PVP, HPMC, *etc.*

The key benefits of Frosta® techniques are simple processing (one step granulation), low manufacturing cost, faster disintegration (less than 40 s), good mechanical property (friability less than 1%) and no need for special packaging [101]. As the API can be added as microparticles, it provides the opportunity of taste masking and sustained release of drug.

3.5.2. RACTAB®

Ractab® technology was developed by Towa Pharmaceutical Co., Ltd., Japan (www.towayakuhin.co.jp). FDTs, prepared by this technology, are easy to handle, have high resistance against humidity, possess adequate hardness and rapidly dissolve in the oral cavity. FDTs by this technology are manufactured by compressing rapidly disintegrating granules (RDGs). RDGs are prepared by a suspension spray coating of a saccharide (mannitol) with crospovidone and corn starch in a fluidised bed granulator [108, 127]. RDGs are characterised by narrow particle size distribution, large surface area and micropores. Micronised ethylcellulose is blended in RDGs followed by compression at low force to prepare tablets. Micronised ethylcellulose, used as a dry binding agent, offers high physical strength coupled with improved resistance against humidity to prepared tablets. These robust FDTs can withstand stresses of handling and friability during their clinical use [127]. Optimised amount of micronised ethylcellulose in prepared FDTs was 5% w/w, which did not significantly alter oral disintegration time. Ractab® technology can be used for a wide range of APIs to achieve taste masking and to sustain or control release profiles [128].

Ractab® technology has been successfully applied in designing ODT formulations containing enteric-coated particles of tamsulosin hydrochloride [128]. Ractab® has also been successfully incorporated in various drug products marketed in Japan. Amlodipine Ractab® was found safe, effective and palatable in a post-marketing surveillance study in Japan [129]. Ractab® dissolves quickly in the mouth, tastes good, and particles are not rough on the tongue.

4. COMPACTION AND SUBSEQUENT TREATMENTS

4.1. Sublimation

FDTs can be prepared by direct compression of volatile materials with other suitable excipients. Alternatively, granules can be prepared with volatile ingredients with suitable excipients using a binder dissolved in a non-aqueous liquid. Tablets prepared by direct compression or granules are subjected to drying, which eventually leave pores at locations where particles of sublimable/volatile materials were initially present in the tablet matrix (Fig. **1**). Thus, the process of sublimation of volatile ingredients results in highly porous FDTs. These porous tablets may additionally contain superdisintegrants, which can further fasten the disintegration of the tablet. Pores in the tablets provide channels to the movement of water or saliva for quicker wicking/swelling action of superdisintegrant resulting in faster disintegration.

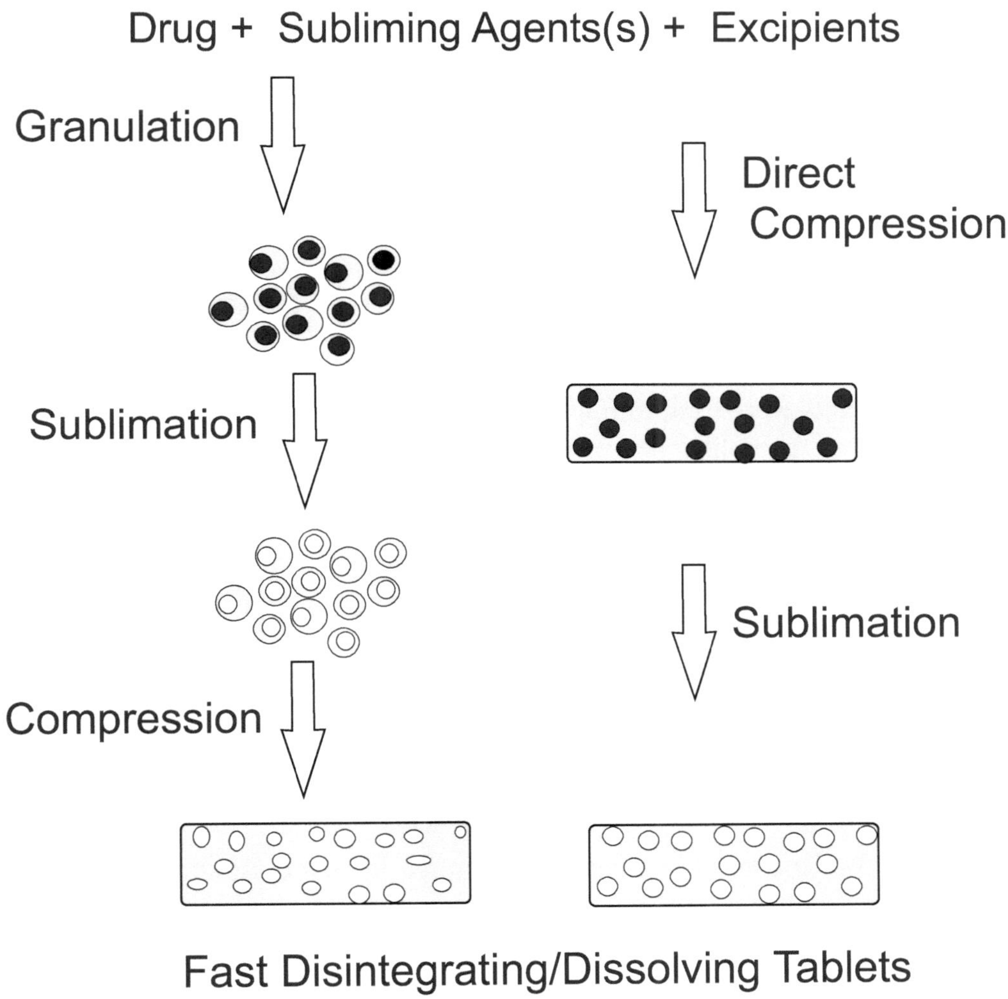

Fig. (1). Process of Preparing FDTs by Sublimation.

Heinemann and Rothe described urea, urethane, hexamethylenetetramine, ammonium bicarbonate, benzoic acid, naphthalene, phthalic anhydride, and camphor as subliming materials, which can be hard pressed with other excipients to produce porous tablets by sublimation [130]. Water, cyclohexane, benzene and tert-butanol were used as volatile agents to granulate mixture of drug and excipients to prepare porous FDTs [131]. The solvent (5-80% w/w) was solidified by liquid nitrogen, composition was pressed into tablets (temperature below the freezing point of the solvent) and the solvent was later evaporated by vacuum drying or lyophilisation. Volatile salts like ammonium bicarbonate, ammonium carbonate and ammonium acetate were used in preparing porous rapidly soluble tablets [132]. Diluent, volatile salt (30-50% w/w), and lubricant were used to formulate granules, which were compressed to tablets. The volatile salt was removed under a vacuum of for several hours to yield porous FDTs. A formulation containing menthol, a water-soluble, menthol-soluble polymer, and a drug at a temperature greater than the melting point of water was filled in a mould, solidified and the solvent menthol was removed by sublimation to prepare FDT [133]. The solidification was performed at a temperature sufficient to provide a substantially amorphous menthol structure.

FDTs of amlodipine besylate were prepared by direct compression followed by sublimation [134]. Camphor was used as subliming material and additionally superdisintegrants were used to improve disintegration and dissolution of tablets. The amount of camphor and crospovidone was significant in controlling disintegration time and friability of prepared FDTs, a full factorial design (3^2) study revealed. Rofecoxib solid dispersion was compressed to FDTs with subliming materials and superdisintegrant [135]. A full 3^2 randomised and reduced factorial designs were used to optimise tablet for best disintegration time and friability. Factorial designing helps in designing formulations and to achieve an optimised formulation with least efforts and minimum time [134, 135]. Vinpocetine:βCD:tartaric acid (1:2:2 molar ratios) kneaded solid system was incorporated in a sublingual tablet prepared by direct compression followed by sublimation [136].

A ratio of 7:3 of mannitol and camphor resulted in best dissolution time of few seconds, when tablets were prepared by direct compression and sublimation of camphor [137]. Addition of 10-30% camphor in mannitol resulted in reducing the dissolution time of tablet 45 s to 4 s. Incorporation of meclizine (10%) in the tablet containing mannitol and camphor (8:2 ratio) did not significantly affect dissolution time in saliva and tablets dissolved very rapidly in saliva within 18±3 s. Tablets prepared with camphor particles of size 105-149 μm were friable after sublimation of the camphor. On the other hand, camphor particles having size 355-500 μm were found optimum for preparing rapidly saliva soluble FDTs.

Camphor, menthol and urea were used in 10, 15, and 30% w/w with superdisintegrant Kyron® T-314 (5%) to prepare aceclofenac FDTs by direct compression followed by sublimation [138]. Tablets prepared with 5%

superdisintegrants and 20% camphor showed least disintegration time among all other formulations due to their high porosity and quicker uptake of water due to wicking action of Kyron® T-314. Faster dissolution of drug was also achieved in FDTs prepared with camphor due to their high porosity.

Vacuum-drying technique is an effective and alternative approach in preparing FDTs, when compared with the use of more expensive excipients or superdisintegrants [139]. Wet granulation using a non-aqueous granulating agent was used to prepare granules for making FDTs of salbutamol sulphate. Ammonium bicarbonate and camphor were used as subliming agents. MCC and mannitol were used as diluents. Formulations containing MCC disintegrated faster than formulations containing mannitol due to disintegration property of MCC and slow dissolution of mannitol. FDTs of haloperidol were prepared by wet non-aqueous granulation method using CCS and SSG as superdisintegrants and subliming material camphor [140]. Vacuum evaporation of camphor resulted in porous granules, which were compressed into tablets. Alternatively, tablets were also initially prepared and later subjected to vacuum evaporation of camphor from prepared tablets. Faster disintegration of tablets was achieved in tablets which were later exposed to vacuum evaporation. FDTs of norfloxacin were prepared by wet non-aqueous granulating method using camphor as subliming material [141]. Increasing the amount of camphor and superdisintegrant increased drug dissolution rate in FDTs of norfloxacin.

Some literature reports on preparation of FDTs by sublimation methods are provided in Table **5**. Sublimation technique for preparing FDTs is also compatible with taste masking [142] and incorporation of solid dispersions [135, 136]. Vacuum treatment for evaporation of subliming material is a cost adding and time taking process. However, use of other materials, which could be sublimed under/at room temperature and/or normal pressure is of great importance and utility and future scope on research on such tablets [143].

4.2. Humidity Treatment Followed by Drying

When tablets prepared by compression are conditioned to higher humidity, part of the moisture may dissolve water soluble components of the formulation, which can move around solid components. In this process, a layer of dissolved substance may spread over undissolved particles/granules, which can be dried to produce more contact points/bridges between the particles/granules in tablets. Thus, this process improves upon the hardness of the resulting tablet. When amorphous water soluble substances are used in the process and the conditioning process may convert them to crystalline, the process is referred as crystalline transition.

However, in all other cases it is simply referred as phase transition.

Table 5. Some literature reports on FDTs prepared by sublimation methods.

Drug	Subliming Agent	Sublimation conditions, drying apparatus	Tableting	Diluent	Disintegrant	Ref.
Aceclofenac	Camphor, menthol and urea	Tablets dried at 60°C until constant weight	DC	Lactose, MCC and mannitol	Kyron T-314	[138]
Amlodipine besylate	Camphor	Tablets dried for 5 h	WG	Mannitol and Avicel	SSG, Kollidon-CL and Ac-D--Sol	[134]
Cinnarizine	Camphor	Tablets dried at 60°C to constant weight, drying in oven	DC	Mannitol		[7]
Clonazepam	Camphor	Granules dried at 60°C, hot air oven, 6 h	DC	Mannitol	CCS	[144]
Clozapine	Camphor	Tablets dried at 60°C to constant weight, oven	DC	Mannitol		[9]
Domperidone	Camphor	Tablets dried at 60°C	DC	Mannitol, lactose	Crospovidone	[145]
Etoricoxib	Camphor, menthol and ammonium bicarbonate	Granules dried at 65°C, vacuum drying for 24 h	WG	Mannitol	Crospovidone	[146]
Flutamide	Camphor	Tablets dried at 60°C to constant weight	DC	Ludipress, mannitol and Avicel PH102	SSG	[18]
Haloperidol	Camphor	Granules dried at 60°C in tray dryer for 30 min	WG	Mannitol	SSG and CCS	[140]
Meclizine	Camphor	Granules dried at 80°C, vacuum drying for 30 min	DC	Mannitol		[137]
Meloxicam	Camphor	Granules dried at 60°C, vacuum drying for 24 h	WG	Lactose	Crospovidone	[147]
Meloxicam	Camphor, menthol and thymol	Tablets dried at 40°C, drying in oven till constant weight	DC		Ac-Di-Sol	[148]
Nimesulide	Camphor	Tablets dried at 60°C to constant weight	WG	Lactose	Crospovidone	[139]

(Table 5) contd.....

Drug	Subliming Agent	Sublimation conditions, drying apparatus	Tableting	Diluent	Disintegrant	Ref.
Norfloxacin	Camphor	Tablets dried at 80°C for 30 min	DC	MCC	Crospovidone and SSG	[141]
Rofecoxib solid dispersion	Thymol and camphor	Tablets dried at 60°C, vacuum drying for 24 h	DC	Dibasic potassium hydrogen phosphate and anhydrous lactose	CCS, crospovidone and SSG	[135]
Salbutamol sulphate	Camphor, ammonium bicarbonate	Tablets dried at 50°C	WG	MCC and mannitol		[149]
Sumatriptan succinate taste masked microspheres	Camphor, menthol and ammonium bicarbonate	Tablets dried at 40°C, drying in oven for 14-21 h	DC	Avicel PH112	Polyplasdone XL	[142]
Vinpocetine solid dispersion	Camphor and menthol	Tablets dried at 60°C, vacuum drying for 2 h	DC	Mannitol	Ac-Di-Sol	[136]

WG: wet granulation; DC: direct compression.

4.2.1. Crystalline Transition Method

Amorphous sugar in a formulation can be converted to crystalline sugar when it is exposed to humidity followed by drying. This crystalline transition improves the mechanical strength of the tablet resulting in optimum strong porous tablet. Hence, crystalline transition phenomenon is used to prepare FDTs of adequate mechanical strength.

A sugar, an amorphous sugar and API have been granulated and compressed to tablets, which are later subjected to humidification and drying to prepare tablets of hardness 3.7 kP [150]. Sugar includes lactose, glucose, trehalose, mannitol, erythritol or combinations of two or more thereof. Amorphous sugar, 2-20% w/w, can be glucose, fructose, lactose, sorbitol, trehalose, maltose, lactitol or a combination of two or more thereof. Freeze drying, spray drying or granulation methods are used to transform sugar into amorphous state. A solution of crystalline sugar in a suitable solvent is sprayed onto a drug and/or a sugar to granulate and/or coat. Granulate or coated particles are compressed to tablet and later humidified and dried. The preferred condition for humidity is 50-90% RH, and drying is 20-40°C. Humidification is performed at humidity greater than the apparent critical relative humidity required for the composition of the tablet. During the humidification process, amorphous sugar can absorb water at low moisture levels due to its low critical moisture content. The absorbed moisture is able to dissolve a part of surface of sugar particles. Later in the drying process, the strength of tablet increases due to the re-attachment and formation of fresh contact bridges between sugar particles. Crystalline transition of an amorphous sugar is an irreversible process. High critical relative humidity of the prepared tablets makes them less susceptible to moisture.

The mixture of freeze dried amorphous sucrose and mannitol was tableted at a low compression pressure and stored under defined humidity condition. The tensile strength of tablet increased with formation of contact bridges from crystallisation of amorphous sucrose [151 - 153]. An amount of 10-20% amorphous sucrose was found optimum for preparing FDTs [152, 154]. An industrial method based on fluid bed granulation of mannitol using sucrose solution as binder was developed. Thermal analysis and X-ray diffraction study confirmed the formation of amorphous sucrose in granules comprising mannitol (95% w/w) and sucrose (5% w/w), when granulated with water content of 4% w/w [151].

Some of the critical formulation factors for crystal transition methods are choice of amorphous sugar, diluents, nature of API as these can greatly affect disintegration time, tensile strength and porosity of tablets [154]. Selecting best amorphous sugar for a tablet formulation require a careful judgement on the basis of glass transition temperatures and hygroscopic nature. In one study, the tablets consisting of several diluents (erythritol, sorbitol, mannitol, glucose, xylitol) and amorphous sucrose (20% w/w) were stored for 5 days at 34% relative humidity and a temperature of 25°C [154]. Within the same porosity range, the extent of increase in tensile strength was found similar and independent of the diluent used. The increase in tensile strength seemed dependent on crystallisation of amorphous sucrose, rather than the diluent used.

In some other studies, diluents have been found considerably affecting the disintegration time even though the porosities were comparable. Shortest disintegration time was observed for tablets containing erythritol and decreases in order mannitol>xylitol>glucose>sorbitol [154]. Viscosity corresponding to diluent concentration of 100% was found to relate best with the disintegration time of tablets. High viscosity diluents resulted in longer disintegration time. Disintegration time in oral cavity was found within 10-30 s, when erythritol, xylitol or mannitol was used as the diluents. A higher oral disintegration time of 30 s or more was observed with sorbitol or glucose. Low viscosity diluents are considered more suitable for FDTs due to faster water penetration across tablet matrix and subsequent quick disintegration. High viscosity diluents retard water penetration into tablets by forming a highly viscous area inside the tablet leading to longer disintegration time of tablets.

Low drug loading in tablet, 20% or less, did not significantly affect tensile strength and disintegration time, but at higher loading, 60% and above, low water soluble drug resulted in a decrease in tensile strength and prolonging disintegration time in oral cavity [154]. Hence, high water solubility of the drug is considered more suitable in preparing FDTs by crystalline transition method.

On the basis of molding and dissolution rate, saccharides were classified into two types [155]. Type I Saccharides, *e.g.* lactose and mannitol, are characterised by low mouldability and high dissolution rate. Type II Saccharides, *e.g.* maltose and maltitol, possess high mouldability and low dissolution rate attributes.

High mouldability refers to a hardness of 2 kP or more for a 150 mg saccharide tablet of 8 mm diameter compressed at pressure 10-50 kg/cm$^{2.}$ [155]. High dissolution refers to the dissolution time less than 15 s in buccal cavity [155].

Granulating type I saccharides with type II saccharides improves the mouldability of type I saccharides. FDTs of desirable characteristics are thus prepared by compressing granules comprising type I and type II saccharides, and conditioning them later [156]. Coating or granulating type 1 saccharide with type II saccharide improves the compressibility of low mouldable type 1 saccharide particles, which are amenable for compression into FDTs. High-mouldability saccharide is used as a binder solution so that amorphous state of saccharide is maintained even after granulation. Prepared granules are compressed to FDTs, which are later subjected to a conditioning process, which enable conversion of amorphous state to crystalline state leading to increase in tablet hardness.

4.2.2. Phase Transition Method

In this approach of preparing FDTs, saccharides and/or sugar alcohols (dextrose, mannitol, sorbitol, fructose, maltose, maltitol, xylitol, *etc.*) are used as bulking agents in the tablet dosage form due to their good compatibility and a range of melting point 80-150°C. Saccharides and sugar alcohols can absorb moisture from surrounding atmosphere. This moisture can dissolve a part of saccharide or sugar alcohol, which can be dried later. During drying, the dissolved sugar or sugar alcohol can solidify resulting in formation of additional contact points/bridges among the particles/granules of tablet. Thus the process of humidification followed by drying can impart additional mechanical strength to tablet. High solubility of saccharides and sugar alcohols maintain their quick solubility and dissolution rate in oral cavity.

A drug and one or more saccharide may be granulated with water soluble polyvinylpyrrolidone and compressed into a tablets, which is humidified and dried to obtain a tablets of hardness 0.5-12.0 kP and oral disintegration time of 1-40 s [157]. The tablet formulation comprised one low mouldable saccharide (mannitol, xylitol, erythritol, lactose, lactitol, glucose, sucrose) or a mixture of two such saccharides or their derivatives of low mouldability, as diluents. In different tablet formulations, the saccharide of low mouldability ranged 25-98%. Additionally, the tablet formulation also contained 0.5-1% w/w of magnesium stearate or other insoluble lubricant and a disintegrant like PVP to further enhance the disintegration time of resulting tablets.

Humidification step involved the conditioning of prepared tablets at 50-100% RH for 5 minutes to about 12 hours at temperature between 20-50°C. For tablets compositions of mannitol (95% w/w) as diluent and maltose (5% w/w) as binder, humidification can be achieved at 85% RH and 25°C for 30 minutes, followed by drying for 30 minutes at 40°C and 30% RH. Similar treatment conditions are also recommended for tablet formulations using 0.5% w/w PVP or 4.5% w/w maltose solutions as binders.

An apparatus and method for manufacturing a highly porous (20-40% w/w) tablet capable of faster oral disintegration has been devised [158]. The apparatus comprises a punching section for compression between 0.20-0.01 t/cm^2, a transfer unit for transferring the punched tablets continuously, a humidification (or moisturising) section and a drying section at last.

Using this apparatus, API and one or more water-soluble saccharides, without using a water-soluble binding agent, can be compressed at 0.20-0.01 t/cm^2 and followed by humidification and drying. Lubricant, 0.5-2% w/w, may be added either internally or externally. Lubricant selection is based on compatibility, stability, sticking effect of drug and expected disintegration in oral cavity.

Maltodextrin (10-20% w/w) based tablets of meclizine, prepared by wet granulation and direct compression, were conditioned for 4 and 7 days respectively at 40°C and 75% RH [28]. X-ray diffraction confirmed the presence of maltodextrin in amorphous form from the beginning till the end of the operation and did not require any special treatment for amorphous form preparation. Direct compression followed by conditioning produced tablets with accepted hardness with a problem of long conditioning time and patch effect (aggregates of maltodextrin). Contrary to this wet granulation followed by conditioning alleviated the patch effect problem, while maintaining rapid disintegration. Maltodextrin hardening due to phase transition process manifested as glass-elastic deformation was proposed as mechanism for improving hardness of tablets.

4.2.3. Advantages and Disadvantages of Humidity Treatment Methods

FDTs prepared by humidity treatments are good in physical resistance towards transportation, handling and use. A pleasant mouthfeel and oral disintegration less than 60 s can be achieved. Several disadvantages of humidity treatment methods are lengthy process, use of extra equipments for humidification and drying and extra cost. Humidity has limitations of stability of API and thus this technique is considered unsuitable for moisture labile substances. Tablets prepared are extremely delicate before humidity treatment and require, therefore, careful handling during manufacturing process. Moisture proof packing and containers are essential for storage due to the hygroscopic nature of sugar alcohols/saccharides. Tablet hardness or oral disintegration time is susceptible to change due to solidification/crystallisation of low melting point sugar alcohol.

4.3. Sintering

When heat is applied to granules or a compact mass, some excipient or polymer may melt leading to movement across void spaces among particles. Upon cooling, the melted excipient or polymer solidify around the particles in the void space resulting a decrease in porosity of matrix and formation of bridges among particles. Sintering is the process of bonding surfaces of adjacent particles of powder or a compact upon heating. This process requires simple equipments like hot air oven or microwave oven and is, therefore, considered economic. Sintering has been used in retarding release of drug by reducing the porosity of the matrix in a tablet or granules. Many researchers have used sintering for the development of sustained/controlled release tablets [159 - 162].

Sintering action has also been explained as the process of subjecting a compact of powder to heating treatment around a melting point of a low melting-point material contained in the compact, cohesion between powder particles and contraction and densification of the compact are induced, resulting in solidification or densification of the compact [163]. Sintering has also been applied in preparing FDTs. Porous tablets of high tensile strengths have been achieved by subjecting the tablet components to high temperatures followed by solidification by cooling at lower temperatures [164].

The formulation components are drug, bulking agent, structural agent, binding agent and solvents. Bulking agents (10-95% w/w) include calcium carbonate, magnesium carbonate and carbohydrates like sucrose, fructose, mannitol, sorbitol, dextrose, xylose and mannose. The structural agents to be used are agar, albumin, gelatin and chondroitin. The most common structural agent is fish gelatin. Fish gelatin, bloom strength 0-25, allows the use of high concentration of the material on bead or the spray-dried matrix, making the spray drying process more efficient. Additionally, fish gelatin offers a highly porous matrix that quickly dissolves in saliva. Binding agent may be polyethylene glycol (PEG) or fatty acid alcohols or polypeptides. The binding agent of choice is PEG (1,000-1,000,000 mol. wt.), which has a melting point 50-90° C for easy sintering and thereafter re-solidification as temperature decreases during cooling. Additionally, PEG acts as a capillary attractant. The amount of 0.5-25% w/w of binding agent is considered sufficient for providing required sintering action and an optimum rigidity to the tablet. Water or ethyl alcohol or hydroalcoholic solutions are used as solvent, which provides desirable porosity to the granulated product or bead upon evaporation during drying. A suitable solvent is used to dissolve bulking agent and structural agent. The obtained solution was spray dried or dried to obtain granules, which are also referred as bead or a matrix. This is followed by dry blending of binding agent and drug with the matrix or bead. Optionally drug and/or binding agent may be added to the dissolved components before drying. This mixture was compressed to obtain a tablets. Prepared tablet is heated or sintered at a sufficient temperature for sufficient time to allow melting of the binding agent. Finally, the temperature reduction to ambient temperature allows binding agent to solidify.

The heating can be performed in an oven, convection oven or microwave. Industrial heating processes like radiant heat, UV and other short wave radiation, microwave heat, infrared heat and industrial equipments for such heating processes may be used in large scale production. A temperature of 50-100° C for about 3-45 minutes is sufficient to melt PEG. Cooling to ambient temperature solidifies binding agent resulting in bonding of particles in the tablet, which improves mechanical strength without drastically reducing porosity. Tablets prepared by sintering do not require special packaging and allows the tablet to remain intact during manufacturing, transportation, and handling during use.

PEG (particle size<100 μm, molecular weight between 3000-8000, 10-30% w/w of the powder blend) has been employed as a preferred radiofrequency meltable binder in preparing multilayered FDTs [165]. RF-meltable binder is a polar and solid binder that can be softened or melted upon exposure to radiofrequency (RF) energy and has the capability to re-harden or re-solidify upon cooling. The meltable binder has a melting point of about 30-140°C. The softening or melting of the meltable binder(s) results in the sintering of the tablet shape through the binding of the softened or melted binder with the API and/or other ingredients within the compacted powder blend. The tablet may be heated after it is removed from the tablet press or may be heated within the tablet press.

4.3.1. Sintering Action on Saccharides and/or Sugar Alcohols

FDTs can be prepared with mixture of sugar alcohol and/or saccharide, a sugar alcohol and/or saccharide, which differ appreciably (5°C or greater) in their melting points, and then subjecting the resulting powder to combined processing of compression and heating [163]. Heating followed by cooling (sintering) improves the inter-particle strength of FDTs. FDTs can be solidified or densified such that hardness can be imparted to an extent sufficient to withstand production, distribution and use. Using this method, FDTs having hardness of 2 kP or higher and disintegration in oral cavity within 30 s or less can be obtained.

Monosaccharides, disaccharides and sugar alcohols can be employed. Specific examples are erythritol, mannitol, lactitol, lactose, glucose, sucrose, maltitol, xylitol, sorbitol, trehalose and fructose. Any two or more of these saccharides and/or sugar alcohols may be used. Contents of these two or more sugar alcohols and/or saccharides may range between 75.0-99.95% w/w. Lowest melting point sugar alcohol and/or saccharide amount can be opted in range 0.3-50.0% w/w based on a total of respective content(s) of the remaining one(s) of the two or more sugar alcohols and/or saccharides. Any other suitable diluents or other excipient may be added. The powder mixture is dry blended together or wet granulated or fluid-bed granulated. The resulting mixture is compressed into compacts by a rotary or single punch tableting machine at 300-1,500 kgf. The resulting compacts are then heated at 80-140°C for 3-90 minutes and then allowed to cool down at room temperature to obtain FDTs.

Phase transition method has been used in preparing FDTs [166 - 168]. Saccharide or sugar alcohol with high melting point is granulated with low melting point sugar alcohol in a fluidised bed granulator. Granules are compressed to tablets and subjected to temperature between the low and high melting points of sugar alcohol/saccharide in an oven followed by cooling in a petri dish at 25°C/65% RH. The heating-cooling process results in an increase in hardness of tablets with melting, diffusion and solidification of low melting sugar alcohol. Phase transition of the lower melting point sugar alcohol induces an increase in inter particle bonds leading to a greater bonding surface area resulting in sufficient hardness of

FDTs and preserving high porosity. No special apparatus is required for preparing FDTs by this method.

Talc is recommended as best lubricant for FDT prepared by phase transition method as it provides a more hydrophilic surface upon heating [166] Use of magnesium stearate and sodium stearyl fumarate result in prolongation of *in vitro* disintegration time and oral disintegration time. Increase in amount of talc or heating do not adversely impact upon disintegration time of tablets. Water absorption rate in tablets and polarity on the surface of tablets increases with the use of talc, when compared with use of other lubricants.

FDTs can be prepared by direct compression method and later subjected to sintering action. In this process, sugar alcohols are mixed in a bottle for a few minutes. Low melting point sugar alcohol shall be kept at a low concentration (5% w/w). The resulting mixture is directly compressed to tablet [167]. Prepared tablets are dried in an oven at a temperature between melting points of sugar alcohols for 15-60 min. Later, tablets are exposed to room temperature for cooling.

In direct compression method, particle size of low melting point sugar alcohol play an important role in governing hardness of tablet. Use of sugar alcohol in small particle size results in harder tablets in comparison to tablets prepared with large particle size. For uniform distribution of a low melting sugar alcohol, wet granulation compression method is used, where solution of low melting point sugar alcohol is sprayed onto high melting point sugar alcohol to prepare granules in a fluidised bed granulator. Direct compression method requires more heating time to produce tablets of similar hardness, when compared with wet compression method.

Phase transition method was used to prepare Atenolol FDTs containing mannitol (Perlitol SD) as high melting point sugar alcohol and xylitol as low melting point sugar alcohol [169]. Sugar alcohols, drug, diluent and other excipients were mixed and compressed directly to tablets. Prepared tablets were placed in an oven at 93°C for 15 min for heating followed by cooling to room temperature for 4 h. Prepared FDTs were strong enough to get friability less than 1% and *in vitro* disintegration time of less than 60s was achieved in a pharmacopoeial disintegration tester.

FDTs prepared by phase transition method require moisture proof packing and container requirements due to hygroscopic nature of sugar alcohols/saccharides. Additionally, these tablets require careful handling under humid conditions and change in temperature during storage and usage as oral disintegration time and tablet hardness is susceptible to change due to phase transition of low melting point sugar alcohol.

4.4. Trademark Technologies

4.4.1. OraQuick®

Lumara Health's (http://www.lumarahealth.com, Earlier KV Pharmaceutical) proprietary OraQuick® technology uses sintering process in manufacturing robust FDTs. Tablets are sintered at temperature of about 50-100°C for several minutes to some hours or at 90°C for about 10 minute in an oven. During sintering step, PEG melts and binds particles to form stronger tablet. Taste masking technologies, FlavorTech® and MicroMask®, are used to suppress bitterness of the drug. MicroMask® provides taste masking by incorporating a drug into matrix microspheres. The matrix surrounding the drug particle is not disrupted during compression. The process does not utilise any kind of solvent leading to good mechanical strength tablets produced quickly and efficiently. When placed in mouth, the tablet disintegrates and dissolves within few seconds. The delivery system can hold a large payload of active drugs and produce a durable tablet that does not require special packaging requirements.

4.4.2. Wowtab® Technology

Wowtab® technology is a proprietary technology of Astellas Pharma, Inc. (www.astellas.com). This technology uses sugar and sugar based excipients to produce FDTs using conventional granulation and tableting techniques. Wowtab technology was initially developed and patented by Yamanochi Pharma Technologies, Inc. and the Wow in Wowtab® stands for 'to take Without Water. The Wowtab® products have adequate hardness so these are suitable for both conventional packaging, *i.e.* blister and bottle packaging.

Saccharides can be divided into two types, type I and type II based upon the dissolution rate and mouldability [155]. Type I saccharides (*e.g.* mannitol, lactose, glucose, sucrose, and xylitol) have low a high dissolution rate and low mouldability, whereas, type II saccharides (*e.g.* maltitol, maltose, sorbitol and an oligosaccharide) have low dissolution rate and high mouldability. Granulation with a solution of type II saccharides can improve the mouldability of type I saccharides. Granulated materials of type I with type II yields product have a high dissolution rate and high mouldability. In formulation of FDTs high mouldability and highly soluble granules are prepared by fluidised bed granulation of mixture of two types of saccharides listed above. Wowtab® FDTs utilise the same principle. Factors like nature of lubricant and particle size of drug have the most significant effect on quality of Wowtab®. In one study, micronisation of drug resulted in two-fold increase in disintegration [170].

FDTs consisting of active ingredient, a sugar and amorphous sugar were prepared by compression moulding followed by humidification and removal of solvent to make it dry and highly porous. Tablet strength was increased by humidification and drying steps. The process of granulation was performed in a fluid bed granulator. Drying of the tablet converted amorphous sugar to crystalline resulting in a high critical moisture point and high strength [171].

5. EFFERVESCENT TABLETS

Effervescence, a pleasant sensation, stimulates saliva secretion leading to the availability of some additional water for the effervescent action. Saliva stimulation occurs due to the presence of edible acids like tartaric acid, citric acid, ascorbic acid or malic acid as one of the components of the effervescent formulation [172]. One acid source and one carbonate source reacts with each other to produce effervescence. Mucus stripping properties of effervescence also enhances drug absorption [173]. Some of the effervescent tablets have demonstrated faster oral disintegration/dissolution (Table **6**).

Table 6. FDTs prepared by effervescent formulation approach.

Drug	Effervescent Couple	Diluent	Other Excipients	Ref.
Carbamazepine and SoluPlus® solid dispersion	Potassium bicarbonate and potassium carbonate	Avicel PH-102	Kollidon CL-F	[174]
Fexofenadine	Citric acid anhydrous and sodium bicarbonate	Pearlitol SD 2000	Crospovidone, CCS, SSG, aspartame, flavour, SSF and talc	[175]
Flutamide and PEG 6000 solid dispersion	Citric acid and sodium bicarbonate	Ludipress, mannitol and Avicel PH102	Sucralose and PEG 6000	[18]
Glibenclamide	Citric acid anhydrous, tartaric acid, sodium carbonate, sodium bicarbonate sodium hydrogen citrate, sodium glycine carbonate and potassium hydrogen phosphate	MCC and mannitol	PEG 1000	[176]
Lorazepam	Citric acid and sodium bicarbonate	Avicel PH102 and mannitol	Aspartame, talc and magnesium stearate	[7]

(Table 6) contd.....

Drug	Effervescent Couple	Diluent	Other Excipients	Ref.
Lorazepam	Citric acid, tartaric acid and sodium bicarbonate	Pearlitol SD 200	Crospovidone, aspartame, flavour, talc and SSF	[177]
Melatonin	Tartaric acid and sodium bicarbonate	Lactose	PVP and colloidal silica anhydrous	[29]
Prochlorperazine maleate	Citric acid and sodium bicarbonate	MCC and Pearlitol SD 200	Crospovidone, CCS, aspartame, SSF and pineapple flavour	[178]

Directly compressed effervescent dosage form, which completely and rapidly disintegrate, are described in various patents issued to Cima Inc [179, 180]. Rapid dissolving effervescent and robust tablets have been prepared from a matrix of powdered mannitol (a non-direct compression filler) and lubricant [181, 182]. Unpleasant gritty feeling increases in such dosage form due to non-direct compression filler and relatively large amount of lubricants. Hardness of such tablets also plays a significant role in disintegration time. Effervescent tablets are more susceptible to humidity conditions during the manufacturing process and storage, the strict controls of their carbon dioxide content becomes a guarantee for their physicochemical stability. Another disadvantage of using effervescent system in FDTs is their sensitivity to moisture. Manufacturing is required to be done in controlled environment and tablets should be packed in moisture-impermeable blisters. Cost of manufacturing increases for these tablets due to the above listed controls.

Michaelson *et al.* described the use of metal carbonic acid as disintegrant and alginic acid to prepare FDTs [183]. On placing in water, an acid-base reaction resulted in formation of a carbonic acid and alginic acid salt. Alginic acid salt caused the swelling of the tablet and carbonic acid generated carbon dioxide within the swelled tablet through which faster disintegration of the tablet was achieved. FDTs having starch as a bulking material and disintegrating agent are also described in patent literature [184, 185]. The tablet is formed of granules of a mixture of API, the effervescent base, starch, admixed to a blend of remaining ingredients, subsequently compressed to tablet form. Fast disintegration is achieved by using starch as a bulking and disintegrating agent and at the same time an effervescent couple as a supplement disintegrating agent. A starch degrading enzyme, which acts as a disintegration modulator, may also be added extragranularly to such formulation [184]. The enzyme (amylase, amyloglucosidase, glucose-fructose isomerase, *etc.*) upon contact with aqueous environment converts the starch to mono and polysaccharide, which quickly dissolves and improves the taste of the tablet and increases saliva secretions.

Effervescent tablets comprising microparticles, which rapidly disintegrates and forms a viscous slurry, have been prepared by common tableting processes [186]. API is coated over inert sugar beads followed by spray drying. Coated beads are blended with effervescent couple and other adjuvants and compressed to tablets. Sublingual buccal effervescent dosage form [187] have been prepared from effervescent granules by hot melt extrusion process [188] and fluidised bed granulation [189, 190].

Oral dissolving effervescent tablets of glibenclamide were developed by a modification of a wet granulation method involving absolute alcohol as a non-reactive liquid [176]. A solution containing PEG 1000 and effervescent couple (citric acid and sodium hydrogen citrate or tartaric acid) in absolute alcohol was used to granulate MCC. Effervescent granules were kept in oven for drying at 55°C for a duration of about 4 h. Dried granules were mixed with stoichiometric quantities of sodium glycine carbonate or sodium bicarbonate and mannitol. Various other excipients and glibenclamide were mixed with these highly plastic granules and compressed to FDTs. Citric acid was coated with PEG, which provided a physical barrier for effervescence reaction and thereby provided a stabilising effect. The effervescence reaction did not get any delay as PEG 1000 melts at body temperature.

FDTs of cinnarizine were prepared by effervescent method with other excipients like Avicel PH102, mannitol, talc, aspartame and magnesium stearate [7]. Citric acid and sodium bicarbonate were preheated at 70°C and all materials were mixed in a mortar and triturated. A single punch tablet machine fitted with 9 mm flat punches was used to compress homogenous powder mixture. Hardness of 2.5 kg/cm^2, friability 0.625% and disintegration time of 92 s was achieved with prepared cinnarizine FDTs.

FDTs of lorazepam were prepared by effervescent method [177]. Optimisation studies by 3^2 full factorial design were performed for finding optimum amount of CCS, sodium bicarbonate-citric acid and tartaric acid. Optimised formulation containing 18% w/w mixture of sodium bicarbonate-citric acid and tartaric acid and 8% w/w crospovidone was used in preparing FDTs characterised by *in vitro* disintegration time of 13s. Control FDTs, prepared without crospovidone, disintegrated in 180 s. Effervescent couple (anhydrous citric acid and sodium bicarbonate, in different ratios), superdisintegrants (CCS and crospovidone), MCC and mannitol containing formulations were used to prepare FDTs of prochlorperazine maleate [178]. FDTs containing 20% w/w sodium bicarbonate, 15% w/w anhydrous citric acid, 10% w/w crospovidone, and 20% w/w MCC were found optimum for *in vitro* disintegration time of 13 s. Prepared FDTs were found stable in a short term stability studies for 3 months.

Effervescent FDTs of fexofenadine HCl were prepared using crospovidone, SSG and CCS as superdisintegrants, different ratios of anhydrous citric acid and sodium bicarbonate and mannitol (directly compressible grade) [175]. The formulation containing 18% w/w anhydrous citric acid, 24% w/w sodium bicarbonate, 8% w/w crospovidone was optimised with best *in vitro* disintegration time of 20 s and achieved a four times faster release of drug ($t_{50\%}$ 4 min), when compared with the commercial conventional tablets of fexofenadine HCl ($t_{50\%}$=15 min). However, *in vitro* disintegration time and drug content remained same in a short term stability studies with the developed formulations.

Effervescent FDTs containing different dosages of melatonin were prepared for administration to paediatric patients. FDTs demonstrated disintegration times of less than 25 s and friability and hardness values that require no special storage or packaging conditions [29]. PVP was used an excellent binder as well as disintegrating agents in such effervescent tablets, resulting in acceptable friability and a lower disintegration time. The use of lactose as a diluent in these tablets did not offer sufficient resistance and therefore it was completely eliminated and PVP was used instead.

Combining effervescence and addition of superdisintegrant in a formulation was successful in achieving faster tablet disintegration but failed to achieve desired dissolution rate from flutamide FDTs [18]. Faster drug release, *i.e.* 73.12-96.99% after 15 min, was observed when flutamide was replaced with solid dispersion of flutamide with PEG 6000 in 1:5 ratio. Increase in the dissolution rate was an effect of the conversion of the crystalline drug into amorphous form while preparing solid dispersions.

Disintegration and dissolution of carbamazepine tablets containing Soluplus® improved with the use of potassium carbonate and potassium bicarbonate in tablet compositions. KinetiSol®, a proprietary methodology, was used in preparing solid dispersions of carbamazepine with Soluplus®. Soluplus® (BASF Corporation, Florham Park, NJ) is a hydrophilic graft copolymer of polyvinyl caprolactam–polyvinyl acetate–polyethylene. Addition of potassium bicarbonate and potassium carbonate allowed tablet hydration and effervescence. Effervescent reaction (Eq. 1 and 2) resulted in liberation of carbon dioxide, capable to destroy gel network and thereby accelerating drug release from tablets.

$$K_2CO_3 + 2HCl = 2KCl + H_2O + CO_2 \quad (1)$$

$$KHCO_3 + HCl = KCl + H_2O + CO_2 \quad (2)$$

Dissolution studies in 0.1 N HCl revealed that an amount of 1% w/w of potassium bicarbonate was effective as tablet disintegrant to achieve rapid disintegration of tablets. Dehydration of SoluPlus®, resulting in a weak hydrogel structure coupled with the liberation of carbon dioxide, was responsible for rapid disintegration and thereafter faster dissolution of the drug. Similar drug dissolution results were obtained in acetate buffer (pH 4.5) despite low polymer solubility.

5.1. Trademark Technologies

Effervescence or the liberation of carbon dioxide as a mechanism of disintegration in FDTs was described in several patents assigned to Cima labs (Table 7). Based on these patents, Cima labs developed trademark technologies, *viz.* OraSolv®, DuraSolv® and OraSolv$^{SR/LR}$. Due to softer and brittle nature OraSolv® tablets require special packaging system PakSolv®. However, DuraSolv® tablets are robust enough to pack in conventional packaging like bottles or foil pouches. Apparatus for handling and high speed packaging friable tablets like OraSolv® have also been designed and patented [191].

Table 7. Some of the patents relevant to proprietary technologies of FDDFs of Cima Lab, Inc.

Title	Inventive Step	Patent Issue Date	US Patent No.
Effervescent dosage form with microparticles	Microparticles and effervescent, which rapidly disintegrate in the mouth and provide adequate taste-masking	12 Jan 1993	5,178,878
Paediatric effervescent dosage form	ODT comprising effervescent disintegration agent, which is effective for rapid disintegration and positive organoleptic sensation to children	29 Jun 1993	5,223,264
Base coated acid particles and effervescent formulation incorporating same	Formulations include both an effervescent couple and an acid sensitive active agent. Formulations having an acid neutralisation capacity of 5.0 or less are also described.	2 Apr 1996	5,503,846
Taste masking microparticles for oral dosage forms	Taste masked microparticles made from sorbitol, mannitol, a mixture of an artificial sweetener and menthol, a mixture of a sugar and menthol, and methyl salicylate	4 Mar 1997	5,607,697
Rapidly dissolving robust dosage form	The tablet is made from an active ingredient mixed into a matrix of a non-direct compression diluent and a relatively high lubricant content.	15 Feb 2000	6,024,981

(Table 7) contd.....

Title	Inventive Step	Patent Issue Date	US Patent No.
Blister package and packaged tablet	A blister sheet defines one or more recesses in which fragile dosage forms are disposed and a peelable sheet of lidding material overlies the recesses to cover the dosage forms therein.	5 Dec 2000	6,155,423
Sublingual buccal effervescent	An additional pH adjusting substance is used in combination with the effervescent to promote the absorption of drugs	13 Mar 2001	6,200,604
Rapidly dissolving robust dosage form	ODTs consisting of an active ingredient and a matrix including a nondirect compression filler and a lubricant and having a friability of about 2% or less	24 Apr 2001	6,221,392
Apparatus for handling and packaging friable tablets	An assembly for handling and packaging pharmaceutical dosage forms includes an infeed structure, a laning structure, and a plenum structure extending from the infeed structure to the laning structure.	7 Aug 2001, 6 Nov 2001	6,269,615 and 6,311,462
Organoleptically pleasant in-mouth rapidly disintegrable potassium chloride tablet	ODT suitable for use in the delivery of potassium comprising 50-80% coated potassium chloride crystals for extended release	2 Apr 2002	6,365,182
Orally disintegrable tablet forming a viscous slurry	ODT for delivering coated/uncoated drug particles and/or microcapsules to achieve prompt/sustained/extended drug release	9 Apr 2002	6,368,625
Taste masking rapid release coating system	A core containing a drug encased in a spacing layer and a taste masking layer	25 May 2004	6,740,341

5.1.1. OraSolv®

OraSolv® technology utilises incorporation of taste masked microencapsulated drug in an effervescent composition to prepare FDTs [179, 180]. FDTs, prepared by OraSolv® technology, dissolve rapidly in saliva without the need of crushing/chewing, eliminate the need of administration of water, and allow for effective masking of taste of a large variety of prescription and non-prescription drugs. As the OraSolv® tablet dissolves in the mouth, it releases microparticles of the drug into the saliva forming a micro-suspension of the drug in the saliva. The microencapsulated drug suspension enters the stomach through normal swallowing process. Saliva triggers the effervescent action leading to generation of carbon dioxide, thereby assisting disintegration of tablets. Effervescence is perceived as pleasant sensations which also stimulate saliva production leading to availability of more water for further effervescence. OraSolv® effervescent composition makes use of an effervescent couple/pair, an acid source and a carbonate source, that release carbon dioxide when water is available as a medium to react. The acid sources are citric acid, malic acid, tartaric acid, fumaric acid, succinic acid, and adipic acids and the sources of carbonate comprise sodium bicarbonate, potassium bicarbonate, sodium carbonate and potassium carbonate [181]. Effervescent agent amount of about 20-25% w/w are employed in tablet compositions. Tablet compaction is performed at low pressure to achieve fast disintegration, high porosity and loading of large amount of taste masked API into the OraSolv® tablets. Normal blister packing of OraSolv® tablets is not feasible due to their highly friable nature and therefore requires special peel-off blister packing.

Apparatus for handling and high speed packaging friable tablets like OraSolv® have been developed [191]. The OraSolv® technology can be used to manufacture tablets with API dose range from 1-750 mg. OraSolv® tablets may be designed for hardness of 6–25 N and disintegration time of 10 to 40 seconds, which depends on formulation and tablet size. During manufacturing, OraSolv® requires controlled environment of low RH as effervescent excipient used in the formulation are hygroscopic and moisture sensitive. Taste of bitter drug may be masked by microencapsulation methods and effervescence. Saliva causes the OraSolv® tablet to quickly disintegrate in the mouth resulting in partial dissolution of constituents followed by swallowing of the resulting suspension with the saliva.

Low compression forces and disintegration in saliva without chewing reduces the potential for fracture of microparticles. Effervescent couple functions as disintegrating agent, aid taste masking and provide a pleasant fizzy sensation in the mouth. OraSolv® SR/CR tablets contain sustained/controlled release coated microparticulates in to a fast dissolving delivery system to combat the difficulty of swallowing controlled release/sustained release tablets.

The OraSolv® has a major disadvantage that it yields soft and fragile tablets in comparison to conventional tablets. So, it requires a special packaging system that protects the tablet during transport and shipment. PakSolv® is a proprietary blister unit package that resists tablets from breaking and additionally offers protection from moisture, light and child resistance. PakSolv®, “dome-shaped” blister package, is designed too narrow at its bottom to accommodate the tablet so as to restrict the vertical movement of tablet within the package to prevent breakage during transportation and handling.

The main disadvantage of using effervescent excipients is their anhydrous nature, which offers a challenge to protect the final dosage from absorption of moisture from surrounding atmosphere. Hence, manufacturing of effervescent units requires a controlled low humidity environment and packaging of tablets in moisture-impermeable blisters. As a result, the cost of effervescent FDTs is always higher than the cost of conventional tablets made by direct compression. However, the cost of effervescent FDTs is still lower than some other FDTs manufactured by more sophisticated technologies like freeze drying. Several FDT products based upon an effervescent formulation approach have been commercialised, *e.g.* Tempra® Quicklets 80 mg quick dissolving chewable tablet (Bristol Myers Squibb Co. NY), Zomig® Rapimelt Zolmitriptan fast dissolving tablets (Astra Zeneca PLC Wayne, PA).

The drawback of dissolving/disintegrating not quickly enough in saliva is common to many other technologies of manufacturing FDTs [179, 180]. OraSolv® SR/CR tablets contain sustained/controlled release coated microparticulates in to a fast dissolving delivery system to combat the difficulty of swallowing controlled release/sustained release tablets. Effervescent disintegrating agent rapidly disintegrate OraSolv® SR/CR tablets in saliva leading to the formation of a slurry or suspension of coated microparticulates in saliva, which is easy to swallow before the drug release starts from the coated microparticles.

5.1.2. DuraSolv®

DuraSolv® is an improved second generation FDT technology for manufacturing relatively hard and robust tablets which can withstand stresses of normal traditional packaging system such as foil pouches or bottles or blister packs. Use of high compaction pressure during compression makes DuraSolv® tablets stronger, durable, easy to handle and package in bottles/blisters, than OraSolv® tablets. Hence, DuraSolv® technology cost less to produce and package FDTs in comparison to OraSolv®. Similarities and differences in OraSolv® and DuraSolv® technologies are presented in Table **8**. The formulations of DuraSolv® tablets utilise large amounts of quickly dissolving excipients as fine particulates and wicking agents. Quick dissolution of the excipients and rapid ingress of saliva into the tablet matrix leads to faster dissolution of the tablet. This technology can also be utilised for sustained or controlled release quick dissolve system to improve compliance. Controlled release beads, pellets, microcapsules or microspheres or microparticulates can be incorporated in prepared FDTs.

Table 8. Similarities and differences in OraSolv® and DuraSolv® technologies.

Feature	OraSolv®	DuraSolv®
Route of Administration and Absorption	Oral, absorption from gastrointestinal tract	
Dose Range	1–750 mg	125 µg–500 mg

(Table 8) contd.....

Feature	OraSolv®	DuraSolv®
Disintegration Time	10–30 s	
Release Profile	Immediate, sustained, modified and enteric-coated	
Size of Tablet	1/4– 5/8 Inch	
Appeal	Can be coloured, flavoured as per requirement. De-bossing friendly	
Bitterness Control	Bitterness can be suppressed	
Packaging	Special blister packaging (including child-resistant options)	Bottle or blister packaging (including child-resistant options)
Tableting	Compression at low pressure in a tablet machine	Suitable automated tablet machine

Non-direct compression diluents and lubricant are two key components in a DuraSolv® formulation [181, 182]. Lactose, mannitol, sucrose, dextrose or sorbitol can be used as non-direct compression diluents responsible for quick dissolution without any gritty or sandy feeling in the mouth when used in particle size from 20-65 μm and their amount may range from 60% w/w to 95% w/w of the tablet composition. A significantly higher amount (1-2.5% w/w) of hydrophobic lubricants like magnesium stearate is required to be added in the tablet formulation when non-direct compression diluents are used. A considerably higher blending time, 10-25 minutes or longer, is also desired to achieve homogeneity of lubricant. When directly compressible diluents are added in the formulation, particle size greater than 100 μm is recommended for at least 85% of the particles. Gums (xanthan and gum arabic), Carbopol and hydroxyalkylcelluloses (HPMC and hydroxyethylcellulose) are employed as wicking agents to aid in the entry of water into the tablet matrix and thereby assisting in quick disintegration/dissolution of the tablet. Swelling disintegrants shall be used at its minimum. DuraSolv® FDTs can be manufactured for drug doses from 125 μg to 500 mg and disintegration times of 10-50 s can be achieved. Production cost of DuraSolv® tablets are significantly low due to the use of modest compaction forces for directly compressing the formulation in a conventional tablet machine followed by a conventional packing in a blister or bottle. Similar to OraSolv® technology, DuraSolv® technology is also compatible with PakSolv® proprietary packaging.

Use of high compaction pressure and low drug loading are two major limitations of DuraSolv® technology. Maintaining the structure of any coated microparticle is a great challenge with incorporation of high drug doses at a high compaction pressure. High pressure during compaction may fracture coating in DuraSolv® product leading to either quick exposure of bitter drug to taste buds or burst release from sustained/controlled release coated microparticulates. Therefore, the

DuraSolv® technology is best suited for drugs with relatively small doses.

CONCLUSIONS

In last two decades, FDTs have gained much attention because of their several advantages like patient acceptability, palatability and availability of numerous low cost manufacturing technologies. Various innovations surrounding FDTs primarily consider three basic parameters, *viz.* mechanical strength, disintegration time and mouth feel. FDTs have come up as a robust dosage form, which can be applied to achieve not only immediate drug release profile but also sustained/controlled release. Advancements in taste masking and flavour technologies have also increased the market demands of FDTs. The day seem not very far away when people may forget the swallowing of tablet with water. The developments of directly compressible excipients and availability of superdisintegrants have shifted the focus of pharmaceutical/nutraceutical industries towards direct compression for manufacturing FDTs. However, use of compression methods in manufacturing FDTs may fracture microparticulates leading to subsequent burst release of the drug. One another challenge of direct compression is to develop methods for loading drugs with very high doses, especially when the drug is also bitter in taste. Addressing issues of taste masking and poor solubility in the formulation further increases the drug loading level in FDTs.

REFERENCES

[1] Ishikawa T, Mukai B, Shiraishi S, *et al.* Preparation of rapidly disintegrating tablet using new types of microcrystalline cellulose (PH-M series) and low substituted-hydroxypropylcellulose or spherical sugar granules by direct compression method. Chem Pharm Bull (Tokyo) 2001; 49(2): 134-9. [http://dx.doi.org/10.1248/cpb.49.134] [PMID: 11217097]

[2] Shu T, Suzuki H, Hironaka K, Ito K. Studies of rapidly disintegrating tablets in the oral cavity using co-ground mixtures of mannitol with crospovidone. Chem Pharm Bull (Tokyo) 2002; 50(2): 193-8. [http://dx.doi.org/10.1248/cpb.50.193] [PMID: 11848208]

[3] Rajitha K, Shravan KY, Adhukondalu D, *et al.* Formulation and evaluation of orally disintegrating tablets of buspirone. Int J Pharm Sci Nanotechnol 2006; 1: 327-34.

[4] Singh H, Mishra SK, Varma R, *et al.* Formulation and evaluation of mouth dissolving tablets of carvedilol. Int J Pharma Bio Sci 2011; 2.

[5] Tiwari V, Kinikar DJ, Pillai K, *et al.* Preparation and evaluation of fast dissolving tablets of celecoxib. J Curr Pharm Res 2010; 4: 4-11.

[6] Gudas GK, Manasa B, Rajesham V, *et al.* Formulation and evaluation of fast dissolving tablets of Chlorpromazine HCl. J Pharm Sci Technol 2010; 2: 99-102.

[7] Patel BP, Patel JK, Rajput GC, Thakor RS. Formulation and evaluation of mouth dissolving tablets of cinnarizine. Indian J Pharm Sci 2010; 72(4): 522-5. [http://dx.doi.org/10.4103/0250-474X.73930] [PMID: 21218071]

[8] Shirsand SB, Suresh S, Swamy PV, Kumar DN, Rampure MV. Design and evaluation of fast dissolving tablets of clonazepam. Indian J Pharm Sci 2008; 70(6): 791-5. [http://dx.doi.org/10.4103/0250-474X.49125] [PMID: 21369444]

[9] Masareddy RS, Kadia RV, Manvi FV. Development of mouth dissolving tablets of clozapine using two different techniques. Indian J Pharm Sci 2008; 70(4): 526-8. [http://dx.doi.org/10.4103/0250-474X.44611] [PMID: 20046788]

[10] Amin P, Prabhu N, Wadhwani A. Indion 414 as superdisintegrant in formulation of mouth dissolve tablets. Indian J Pharm Sci 2006; 68: 117. [http://dx.doi.org/10.4103/0250-474X.22983]

[11] Rawas-Qalaji MM, Simons FE, Simons KJ. Fast-disintegrating sublingual tablets: effect of epinephrine load on tablet characteristics. AAPS PharmSciTech 2006; 7(2): E41. [http://dx.doi.org/10.1208/pt070241] [PMID: 16796358]

[12] Bi Y, Sunada H, Yonezawa Y, Danjo K, Otsuka A, Iida K. Preparation and evaluation of a compressed tablet rapidly disintegrating in the oral cavity. Chem Pharm Bull (Tokyo) 1996; 44(11): 2121-7. [http://dx.doi.org/10.1248/cpb.44.2121] [PMID: 8945778]

[13] Abdelbary A, Elshafeey A, Zidan G. Comparative effects of different cellulosic-based directly compressed orodispersable tablets on oral bioavailability of famotidine. Carbohydr Polym 2009; 77: 799-806. [http://dx.doi.org/10.1016/j.carbpol.2009.02.030]

[14] Khinchi MP, Gupta MK, Bhandari A, *et al.* Effect of various super disintegrants on drug release of orally disintegrating tablet. Int J Pharma Res and Dev 2010; 2.

[15] Koseki T, Onishi H, Takahashi Y, Uchida M, Machida Y. Development of novel fast-disintegrating tablets by direct compression using sucrose stearic acid ester as a disintegration-accelerating agent. Chem Pharm Bull (Tokyo) 2008; 56(10): 1384-8. [http://dx.doi.org/10.1248/cpb.56.1384] [PMID: 18827375]

[16] Koseki T, Onishi H, Takahashi Y, Uchida M, Machida Y. Preparation and evaluation of novel directly-compressed fast-disintegrating furosemide tablets with sucrose stearic acid ester. Biol Pharm Bull 2009; 32(6): 1126-30. [http://dx.doi.org/10.1248/bpb.32.1126] [PMID: 19483329]

[17] Solanki SS, Dahima R. Formulation and evaluation of fexofenadine mouth dissolving tablet. Dhaka Univ J Pharm Sci 2009; 8: 167-70.

[18] Elkhodairy KA, Hassan MA, Afifi SA. Formulation and optimization of orodispersible tablets of flutamide. Saudi Pharm J 2014; 22(1): 53-61. [http://dx.doi.org/10.1016/j.jsps.2013.01.009] [PMID: 24493974]

[19] Shinde AJ, Paithane MB, More HN. Development and in-vitro evaluation of fast dissolving tablets of gliclazide. Int J Drug Dev Res 2010; 2: 724-9.

[20] Patel B, Patel D, Parmar R, *et al.* Development and invitro evaluation of fast dissolving tablets of glipizide. Int J Pharm Pharm Sci 2009; 1: 145-50.

[21] Cirri M, Maestrelli F, Corti G, Mura P, Valleri M. Fast-dissolving tablets of glyburide based on ternary solid dispersions with PEG 6000 and surfactants. Drug Deliv 2007; 14(4): 247-55.

[22] Venkatalakshmi R, Sasikala C, Swathi R, *et al.* Formulation and evaluation of granisetron hydrochloride mouth dissolving tablet. Int J Pharm Sci 2009; 1: 336-41.

[23] Rangole US, Kawtikwar P, Sakarkar D. Formulation and *in vitro* evaluation of rapidly disintegrating tablets using hydrochlorothiazide as a model drug. Res J Pharm Tech 2008; 1: 349-52.

[24] Jain SK, Shukla M, Shrivastava V. Development and *in vitro* evaluation of ibuprofen mouth dissolving tablets using solid dispersion technique. Chem Pharm Bull (Tokyo) 2010; 58(8): 1037-42. [http://dx.doi.org/10.1248/cpb.58.1037] [PMID: 20686256]

[25] Patil C, Das S. Effect of various superdisintegrants on the drug release profile and disintegration time of Lamotrigine orally disintegrating tablets. Afr J Pharm Pharmacol 2011; 5: 76-82. [http://dx.doi.org/10.5897/AJPP10.279]

[26] Kakade SM, Mannur VS, Ramani KB, *et al.* Formulation and evaluation of mouth dissolving tablets of losartan potassium by direct compression techniques. Int J Res Pharm Sci 2010; 1: 290-5.

[27] Watanabe Y, Koizumi K, Zama Y, Kiriyama M, Matsumoto Y, Matsumoto M. New compressed tablet rapidly disintegrating in saliva in the mouth using crystalline cellulose and a disintegrant. Biol Pharm Bull 1995; 18(9): 1308-10. [http://dx.doi.org/10.1248/bpb.18.1308] [PMID: 8845832]

[28] Elnaggar YS, El-Massik MA, Abdallah OY, Ebian AE. Maltodextrin: a novel excipient used in sugar-based orally disintegrating tablets and phase transition process. AAPS PharmSciTech 2010; 11(2): 645-51. [http://dx.doi.org/10.1208/s12249-010-9423-y] [PMID: 20405257]

[29] Muñoz H, Castan H, Clares B, Ruiz MA. Obtaining fast dissolving disintegrating tablets with different doses of melatonin. Int J Pharm 2014; 467(1-2): 84-9. [http://dx.doi.org/10.1016/j.ijpharm.2014.03.054] [PMID: 24699354]

[30] Swamy P, Areefulla S, Shirsand S, *et al.* Orodispersible tablets of meloxicam using disintegrant blends for improved efficacy. Indian J Pharm Sci 2007; 69: 836. [http://dx.doi.org/10.4103/0250-474X.39448]

[31] Shenoy VS, Pandey S. Meloxicam-PEG6000 solid dispersions in rapidly disintegrating tablets: preparation, *in vitro* and *in vivo* characterization. Asian J Pharm Sci 2008; 3: 142-50.

[32] Obaidat AA, Obaidat RM. Development and evaluation of fast-dissolving tablets of meloxicam---cyclodextrin complex prepared by direct compression. Acta Pharm 2011; 61(1): 83-91. [http://dx.doi.org/10.2478/v10007-011-0005-7] [PMID: 21406346]

[33] Singh SK, Mishra DN, Jassal R, *et al.* Fast disintegrating combination tablets of omeprazole and domperidone. Asian J Pharm Clin Res 2009; 2: 74-82.

[34] Goel H, Vora N, Tiwary AK, Rana V. Formulation of orodispersible tablets of ondansetron HCl: investigations using glycine-chitosan mixture as superdisintegrant. Yakugaku Zasshi 2009; 129(5): 513-21. [http://dx.doi.org/10.1248/yakushi.129.513] [PMID: 19420882]

[35] Kalia A, Khurana S, Bedi N. Formulation and evaluation of mouth dissolving tablets of oxcarbazepine. Int J Pharm Pharm Sci 2009; 1: 12-23.

[36] Rizwanulla Madhubabu A. Preparation and evaluation of oxcarbazepine fast dissolving tablets. Int J Pharma Professional's Res 2011; 2: 201-5.

[37] Kiran NR, Palanichamy S, Rajesh M, *et al.* Formulation and evaluation of orodispersible piroxicam tablets. J Pharm Sci Res 2010; 10: 615-21.

[38] Arjun G, Prasad MS, Santhosha D, *et al.* Formulation and evaluation of rosiglitazone mouth dissolving tablet. Int J Pharma Bio Sci 2010; 1: 1-9.

[39] Sharma V, Philip AK, Pathak K. Modified polysaccharides as fast disintegrating excipients for orodispersible tablets of roxithromycin. AAPS PharmSciTech 2008; 9(1): 87-94. [http://dx.doi.org/10.1208/s12249-007-9026-4] [PMID: 18446466]

[40] Kumar A, Singh A, Saharan V. A comparative study of different proportions of superdisintegrants: formulation and evaluation of orally disintegrating tablets of salbutamol sulphate (In Communication) 2014.

[41] Thakur RR, Sardana V. Formulation optimization and evaluation of orally disintegrating tablets of salbutamol sulphate by cost-efficient direct compression method. IJPI's J Pharmaceut Cosmetol 2011; 1: 77-89.

[42] Sharma D. Formulation development and evaluation of fast disintegrating tablets of salbutamol sulphate for respiratory disorders. ISRN Pharmaceutics 2013; 2013 [http://dx.doi.org/10.1155/2013/674507]

[43] Kumar S, Sachdeva M, Bajpai M. Formulation and evaluation of mouth dissolving tablets sildenafil citrate. J Pharm Sci Technol 2010; 2: 202-6.

[44] Shishu KK, Rishi V. Development of taste-masked fast disintegrating tablets of tinidazole. Asian J Pharm Sci 2009; 4: 39-45.

[45] Zade P, Kawtikwar P, Sakarkar D. Formulation, evaluation and optimization of fast dissolving tablet containing tizanidine hydrochloride. Int J Pharm Tech Res 2009; 1: 34-42.

[46] Mishra DN, Bindal M, Singh SK, Vijaya Kumar SG. Spray dried excipient base: a novel technique for the formulation of orally disintegrating tablets. Chem Pharm Bull (Tokyo) 2006; 54(1): 99-102. [http://dx.doi.org/10.1248/cpb.54.99] [PMID: 16394558]

[47] Jain C, Naruka P. Formulation and evaluation of fast dissolving tablets of valdecoxib. Int J Pharm Pharmaceut Sci 2009; 1: 219-26.

[48] Kayitare E, Vervaet C, Ntawukulilyayo JD, Seminega B, Bortel V, Remon JP. Development of fixed dose combination tablets containing zidovudine and lamivudine for paediatric applications. Int J Pharm 2009; 370(1-2): 41-6. [http://dx.doi.org/10.1016/j.ijpharm.2008.11.005] [PMID: 19059324]

[49] Camarco W, Ray D, Druffner A. Selecting superdisintegrants for orally disintegrating tablet formulations. Pharm Technol 2006; 30: s28.

[50] Ozeki T, Yasuzawa Y, Katsuyama H, *et al.* Design of rapidly disintegrating oral tablets using acid-treated yeast cell wall: a technical note. AAPS PharmSciTech 2003; 4(4): E70. [http://dx.doi.org/10.1208/pt040470] [PMID: 15198565]

[51] Caramella C, Ferrari F, Bonferoni MC, *et al.* Disintegrants in solid dosage forms. Drug Dev Ind Pharm 1990; 16: 2561-77. [http://dx.doi.org/10.3109/03639049009058547]

[52] Ishikawa T, Watanabe Y, Utoguchi N, Matsumoto M. Preparation and evaluation of tablets rapidly disintegrating in saliva containing bitter-taste-masked granules by the compression method. Chem Pharm Bull (Tokyo) 1999; 47(10): 1451-4. [http://dx.doi.org/10.1248/cpb.47.1451] [PMID: 10553641]

[53] Bi Y, Sunada H, Yonezawa Y, Danjo K, Otsuka A, Iida K. Preparation and evaluation of a compressed tablet rapidly disintegrating in the oral cavity. Chem Pharm Bull (Tokyo) 1996; 44(11): 2121-7. [http://dx.doi.org/10.1248/cpb.44.2121] [PMID: 8945778]

[54] Ishikawa T, Watanabe Y, Utoguchi N, Matsumoto M. Preparation and evaluation of tablets rapidly disintegrating in saliva containing bitter-taste-masked granules by the compression method. Chem Pharm Bull (Tokyo) 1999; 47(10): 1451-4.

[55] Ishikawa T, Mukai B, Shiraishi S, *et al.* Preparation of rapidly disintegrating tablet using new types of microcrystalline cellulose (PH-M series) and low substituted-hydroxypropylcellulose or spherical sugar granules by direct compression method. Chem Pharm Bull (Tokyo) 2001; 49(2): 134-9. a

[http://dx.doi.org/10.1248/cpb.49.134] [PMID: 11217097]

[56] Gupte S, Kumbale R, Khankar R, *et al.* Evaluation of superdisintegrants in fast dissolve dosage form prepared by direct compression AAPS Annual Meeting and Exposition. Indianapolis, Indiana. 2000.

[57] Bi YX, Sunada H, Yonezawa Y, Danjo K. Evaluation of rapidly disintegrating tablets prepared by a direct compression method. Drug Dev Ind Pharm 1999; 25(5): 571-81. [http://dx.doi.org/10.1081/DDC-100102211] [PMID: 10219525]

[58] Obara S, Tanno F. Application of low-substituted hydroxypropylcellulose to tablets that rapidly disintegrate in oral cavity AAPS Annual Meeting and Exposition. Indianapolis, Indiana. 2000.

[59] Goel H, Tiwary AK, Rana V. Fabrication and optimization of fast disintegrating tablets employing interpolymeric chitosan-alginate complex and chitin as novel superdisintegrants. Acta Pol Pharm 2011; 68(4): 571-83. [PMID: 21796940]

[60] Kharade S, Bhutkar M. Novel superdisintegrants interpolymeric chitosan-alginate complex and chitin in the formulation of orodispersible tablets. IJPRD 2013; 5: 87-94.

[61] Goel H, Arora A, Tiwary AK, Rana V. Development and evaluation of mathematical model to predict disintegration time of fast disintegrating tablets using powder characteristics. Pharm Dev Technol 2011; 16(1): 57-64. [http://dx.doi.org/10.3109/10837450903479996] [PMID: 20028210]

[62] Shirsand SB, Suresh S, Para MS, Swamy PV, Kumar DN. Plantago ovata mucilage in the design of fast disintegrating tablets. Indian J Pharm Sci 2009; 71(1): 41-5. [http://dx.doi.org/10.4103/0250-474X.51952] [PMID: 20177454]

[63] Kracauer P, Gertrude G. Sublingual aspirin tablet. US Patent 4,206,209, 1980.

[64] McCarty JA. Fast dissolving buccal tablet. US Patent 5112616, 1992.

[65] Moghimi FJ, Asgharian R. S Mortazavi H. Formulation of amlodipine 5 mg oral disintegrating tablets and evaluation of its physicochemical properties. Res Pharm Sci 2012; 7: S352.

[66] Reza HM, Islam T, Shohel M, *et al.* Formulation design and evaluation of baclofen mouth dissolving tablets. Eur J App Sci 2012; 4: 110-6.

[67] Köllmer M, Popescu C, Manda P, Zhou L, Gemeinhart RA. Stability of benzocaine formulated in commercial oral disintegrating tablet platforms. AAPS PharmSciTech 2013; 14(4): 1333-40. [http://dx.doi.org/10.1208/s12249-013-0015-5] [PMID: 23990120]

[68] Raichur V, Khanum A, Pandit V, *et al.* Formulation and development of taste masked orally disintegrating tablets (ODTs) of cefpodoxime proxetil using ion exchange resins. Indo American J Pharmaceut Res 2014; 4: 151-65.

[69] Katewongsa P, Phaechamud T. Cetirizine dihydrochloride tablets comprising two different lubricants with highly loaded colloidal silicon dioxide. J Met Mat Min 2012; p. 22.

[70] Babu MK, Kumari SM, Sulthana MR, *et al.* Development and optimization of gliclazide sublingual tablets by using co-processed excipient to treat type II diabetes. World J Pharm Res 2014; 3: 3416-23.

[71] Stoltenberg I, Breitkreutz J. Orally disintegrating mini-tablets (ODMTs)a novel solid oral dosage form for paediatric use. Eur J Pharm Biopharm 2011; 78(3): 462-9. [http://dx.doi.org/10.1016/j.ejpb.2011.02.005] [PMID: 21324357]

[72] Krupa A, Jachowicz R, Pędzich Z, Wodnicka K. The influence of the API properties on the ODTs manufacturing from co-processed excipient systems. AAPS PharmSciTech 2012; 13(4): 1120-9. [http://dx.doi.org/10.1208/s12249-012-9831-2] [PMID: 22941425]

[73] Darwish MK. Application of quality by design principles to study the effect of coprocessed materials in the preparation of mirtazapine orodispersible tablets. Int J Drug Deliv 2013; 5: 309-22.

[74] Roth WJ, Kissinger CB, McCain RR, *et al.* Assessment of juvenile pigs to serve as human pediatric surrogates for preclinical formulation pharmacokinetic testing. AAPS J 2013; 15(3): 763-74. [http://dx.doi.org/10.1208/s12248-013-9482-6] [PMID: 23595360]

[75] Hiremath R, Mohanta GP. Orodispersible sildenafil citrate tablets: design and evaluation of formulation variables. World J Pharm Pharm Sci 2013; 2: 1298-308.

[76] Zayed R, Kamel AO, Shukr M, El-Shamy Ael-H. An *in vitro* and *in vivo* comparative study of directly compressed solid dispersions and freeze dried sildenafil citrate sublingual tablets for management of pulmonary arterial hypertension. Acta Pharm 2012; 62(3): 411-32. [http://dx.doi.org/10.2478/v10007-012-0027-9] [PMID: 23470352]

[77] Ponugoti RS, Gonugunta CR. Formulation and evaluation of mouth dissolving tablets of tramadol hydrochloride. Trop J Pharm Res 2014; 13: 669-75. [http://dx.doi.org/10.4314/tjpr.v13i5.3]

[78] Yoshita T, Uchida S, Namiki N. Clinical disintegration time of orally disintegrating tablets clinically available in Japan in healthy volunteers. Biol Pharm Bull 2013; 36(9): 1488-93. [http://dx.doi.org/10.1248/bpb.b13-00353] [PMID: 23995661]

[79] Amelian A, Winnicka K. Effect of the type of disintegrant on the characteristics of orally disintegrating tablets manufactured using new ready-to-use excipients (Ludiflash or Parteck) by direct compression method. Afr J Pharm Pharmacol 2012; 6: 2359-67. [http://dx.doi.org/10.5897/AJPP12.459]

[80] Kruse S, Gebert S, Meyer-Bohm K, *et al.* Compression characterization and lubricant sensitivity of orally disintegrating tablets based on Ludiflash APV World Meeting. Barcelona, Spain. 2008.

[81] Pabari RM, Ramtoola Z. Application of face centred central composite design to optimise compression force and tablet diameter for the formulation of mechanically strong and fast disintegrating orodispersible tablets. Int J Pharm 2012; 430(1-2): 18-25. [http://dx.doi.org/10.1016/j.ijpharm.2012.03.021] [PMID: 22465631]

[82] Dobetti L. Fast disintegrating tablet. Patent CA 2322315A1, 1999.

[83] Dobetti L. Fast-melting tablets: Developments and technologies. Pharm Technol Eur 2000; 12: 32-42.

[84] Fraher J. Eurand: creation of Advatab® - a new Technology for orally disintegrating tablets. Drug Deliv Technol 2007; 7: 62-5.

[85] Chauveau C, Gendrot E, Demichelis AG, *et al.* Multiparticulate tablet disintegrating in less than 40 seconds in the mouth. Patent US 6106861, 2000a.

[86] Cousin G, Bruna E, Gendrot E. Rapidly disintegratable multiparticular tablet. Patent US 5464632, 1995.

[87] Hayakawa E, Ishikawa Y, Goto T, *et al.* Tablet manufacturing method and tablet. United States Patent 6964779, 2005.

[88] FDA approves Lamictal ODT, co-developed by Eurand and GSK 2009. Accessed from http://www.manufacturingchemist.com/technical/article_page/FDA_approves_Lamictal_ODT_codeveloped_by_Eurand_and_GSK/42285#sthash.RIP34L6l.dpuf

[89] Singh A, Jain R. Fast dissolving composition with prolonged sweet taste. Patent WO 0139749A2, 2001.

[90] Ramtoola Z, Pabari R, Jamil A. Orodispersible tablets. Patent WO 2010/109019, 2010.

[91] Gowda V, Pabari RM, Kelly JG, *et al.* Influence of Prosolv and Prosolv:Mannitol 200 direct compression fillers on the physicomechanical properties of atorvastatin oral dispersible tablets. Pharm Dev Technol 2014.
[PMID: 24397821]

[92] Pabari RM, Jamil A, Kelly JG, Ramtoola Z. Fast disintegrating crystalline solid dispersions of simvastatin for incorporation into orodispersible tablets. Int J Pharm Investig 2014; 4(2): 51-9.
[http://dx.doi.org/10.4103/2230-973X.133029] [PMID: 25006549]

[93] Tillotson J, Propst C. Highly compactable and durable direct compression excipients and excipient systems. United States Patent 8617588, 2013.

[94] Popa G, Ochiuz L, Stoleriu I, *et al.* Binder and superdisintegrant influence on the properties of orally disintegrating high doses acetaminophen tablets. Farmacia 2010; 58: 303-7.

[95] Abdelbary G, Prinderre P, Eouani C, Joachim J, Reynier JP, Piccerelle P. The preparation of orally disintegrating tablets using a hydrophilic waxy binder. Int J Pharm 2004; 278(2): 423-33.
[http://dx.doi.org/10.1016/j.ijpharm.2004.03.023] [PMID: 15196646]

[96] Perissutti B, Rubessa F, Moneghini M, Voinovich D. Formulation design of carbamazepine fast-release tablets prepared by melt granulation technique. Int J Pharm 2003; 256(1-2): 53-63.
[http://dx.doi.org/10.1016/S0378-5173(03)00062-0] [PMID: 12695011]

[97] Giri TK, Sa B. Statistical evaluation of influence of polymers concentration on disintegration time and diazepam release from quick-disintegrating rapid release tablet. Yakugaku Zasshi 2009; 129(9): 1069-75.
[http://dx.doi.org/10.1248/yakushi.129.1069] [PMID: 19721383]

[98] Suresh VK, Ranjit K, Nikunj P, *et al.* Formulation and evaluation of fast disintegrating meloxicam tablets and its comparison with marketed product. Int J Pharm Pharmaceut Sci 2011; 3(1) http://www.ijppsjournal.com/Vol3Issue1/982.pdf

[99] Malke S, Shidhaye S, Kadam V. Formulation and evaluation of oxcarbazepine fast dissolve tablets. Indian J Pharm Sci 2007; 69: 211.
[http://dx.doi.org/10.4103/0250-474X.33145]

[100] Mimura K, Kanada K, Uchida S, Yamada M, Namiki N. Formulation study for orally disintegrating tablet using partly pregelatinised starch binder. Chem Pharm Bull (Tokyo) 2011; 59(8): 959-64.
[http://dx.doi.org/10.1248/cpb.59.959] [PMID: 21804239]

[101] Fu Y, Jeong SH, Park K. Fast-melting tablets based on highly plastic granules. J Control Release 2005; 109(1-3): 203-10.
[http://dx.doi.org/10.1016/j.jconrel.2005.09.021] [PMID: 16260059]

[102] Fukami J, Ozawa A, Yoshihashi Y, Yonemochi E, Terada K. Development of fast disintegrating compressed tablets using amino acid as disintegration accelerator: evaluation of wetting and disintegration of tablet on the basis of surface free energy. Chem Pharm Bull (Tokyo) 2005; 53(12): 1536-9.
[http://dx.doi.org/10.1248/cpb.53.1536] [PMID: 16327184]

[103] Makooi-Morehead WT, Buehler JD, Landmann BR. Formulation of fast-dissolving efavirenz capsules or tablets using super-disintegrants. Patent US 6238695, 2001.

[104] Shangraw R, Mitrevej A, Shah M. A new era of tablet disintegrants. Pharm Tech 1980; 4: 47-57.

[105] Augello M. Pharmaceutical suspension tablet compositions. Patent US 5995107, 1999.

[106] Ito A, Sugihara M. Development of oral dosage form for elderly patients: use of agar as base of rapidly disintegrating oral tablets. Chem Pharm Bull (Tokyo) 1996; 44(11): 2132-6.
[http://dx.doi.org/10.1248/cpb.44.2132] [PMID: 8945779]

[107] Amer MS. Low-dosage sublingual aspirin. Patent US 4866046, 1989.

[108] Okuda Y, Irisawa Y, Okimoto K, Osawa T, Yamashita S. A new formulation for orally disintegrating tablets using a suspension spray-coating method. Int J Pharm 2009; 382(1-2): 80-7. [http://dx.doi.org/10.1016/j.ijpharm.2009.08.010] [PMID: 19686825]

[109] Eoga AB, Valia KH. Method for making fast-melt tablets. Patent US 5939091, 1999.

[110] Shirwaikar AA, Ramesh A. Fast disintegrating tablets of atenolol by dry granulation method. Indian J Pharm Sci 2004; 66: 422-6.

[111] Abu-izza KA, Li VH, Look JL, *et al.* Fast dissolving tablet. United States Patent 6733781, 2004.

[112] Tayel SA, Soliman II, Louis D. Formulation of ketotifen fumarate fast-melt granulation sublingual tablet. AAPS PharmSciTech 2010; 11(2): 679-85. [LA - English.]. [http://dx.doi.org/10.1208/s12249-010-9425-9] [PMID: 20407934]

[113] Jacob S, Shirwaikar A. Preparation and evaluation of microencapsulated fast melt tablets of ambroxol hydrochloride. Indian J Pharm Sci 2009; 71(3): 276-84. [http://dx.doi.org/10.4103/0250-474X.56028] [PMID: 20490294]

[114] Allen LV Jr, Wang B. Process for making a particulate support matrix for making a rapidly dissolving tablet. Patent US 5587180, 1996.

[115] Allen LV Jr, Wang B, Davies JD. Method of making a rapidly dissolving tablet. Patent US 5635210, 1997.

[116] Allen LV Jr, Wang B. Particulate support matrix for making a rapidly dissolving tablet. Patent US 5595761, 1997.

[117] Allen LV Jr, Wang B, Davies JD. Rapidly dissolving dosage form. US Patent US 5776491, 1998.

[118] Dijkgraaf BL, Muhlenbruch A. Granulate for the preparation of fast-disintegrating and fast-dissolving compositions containing a high amount of drug. Patent US 5837292, 1998.

[119] Gilis PM, DeConde VF. Fast-dissolving galanthamine Hydrobromide tablet. Patent WO 9747304, 1997.

[120] Jacob S, Shirwaikar A, Joseph A, *et al.* Novel co-processed excipients of mannitol and microcrystalline cellulose for preparing fast dissolving tablets of glipizide. Indian J Pharm Sci 2007; 69: 633. [http://dx.doi.org/10.4103/0250-474X.38467]

[121] Nagendrakumar D, Raju S, Shirsand S, *et al.* Design of fast dissolving granisetron HCL tablets using novel co-processed superdisintegrants. Int J PharmaSci Rev Res 2010; 1: 58-62.

[122] Sharma S, Bhardwaj P, Gupta G. Formulation, evaluation and optimization of mouth dissolving tablets of losartan potassium: effect of coprocessed superdisintegrants. Int J Pharm and Biol Arch 2010; 1: 76-83.

[123] Alanazi FK. Evaluation of spray and freeze-dried excipient bases containing disintegration accelerators for the formulation of metoclopramide orally disintegrating tablets. Saudi Pharm J 2007; 15: 105.

[124] Gattani M, Singh V, Shukla M, *et al.* Development of directly compressible co-processed excipients for orally disintegrating tablets using rotary evaporation method. Int J Pharm PharmSci 2013; 5: 390-5.

[125] García MS, Gallo L, Palma S, *et al.* Coprocessed excipients production for direct compression of orally disintegrating tablets , 2014 [Accessed on July 7, 2014]; Accessed from www.fbioyf.unr.edu.ar/ricifa/.../GARCIA.pdf

[126] Fu Y, Pai CM, Park SY, *et al.* Highly plastic granules for making fast melting tablets. United States Patent 7749533, 2010.

[127] Okuda Y, Irisawa Y, Okimoto K, Osawa T, Yamashita S. Further improvement of orally disintegrating tablets using micronized ethylcellulose. Int J Pharm 2012; 423(2): 351-9. [http://dx.doi.org/10.1016/j.ijpharm.2011.10.050] [PMID: 22138608]

[128] Okuda Y, Okamoto Y, Irisawa Y, Okimoto K, Osawa T, Yamashita S. Formulation design for orally disintegrating tablets containing enteric-coated particles. Chem Pharm Bull (Tokyo) 2014; 62(5): 407-14. [http://dx.doi.org/10.1248/cpb.c13-00752] [PMID: 24789923]

[129] Fukui-Soubou M, Terashima H, Kawashima K, Utsunomiya O, Terada T. Efficacy, safety, and palatability of RACTAB(®) formulation amlodipine orally disintegrating tablets. Drugs R D 2011; 11(4): 327-36. [http://dx.doi.org/10.2165/11597650-000000000-00000] [PMID: 22133388]

[130] Heinemann H, Rothe W. Preparation of porous tablets. United States Patent US 3885026, 1975.

[131] Eberhard (Polling, DE1), Determann, Helmut (Starnberg, DE1), Production of porous tablets. United States Patent 4134943, 1979.

[132] Roser BJ. Rapidly soluble oral solid dosage forms, methods of making same, and compositions thereof. United States Patent 5762961, 1998.

[133] Lo JB. Method of producing porous delivery devices. Patent WO 1993018757 A1, 1993.

[134] Bhardwaj V, Bansal M, Sharma PK. Formulation and evaluation of fast dissolving tablets of amlodipine besylate using different super disintegrants and camphor as sublimating agent. American-Eurasian Journal of Scientific Research 2010; 5: 264-9.

[135] Sammour OA, Hammad MA, Megrab NA, Zidan AS. Formulation and optimization of mouth dissolve tablets containing rofecoxib solid dispersion. AAPS PharmSciTech 2006; 7(2): E55. [LA - English.]. [http://dx.doi.org/10.1208/pt070255] [PMID: 16796372]

[136] Aburahma MH, El-Laithy HM, Hamza YeS. Preparation and in vitro/in vivo characterization of porous sublingual tablets containing ternary kneaded solid system of vinpocetine with î-cyclodextrin and hydroxy Acid. Sci Pharm 2010; 78(2): 363-79. [http://dx.doi.org/10.3797/scipharm.0912-04] [PMID: 21179352]

[137] Koizumi K-i, Watanabe Y, Morita K, *et al.* New method of preparing high-porosity rapidly saliva soluble compressed tablets using mannitol with camphor, a subliming material. Int J Pharm 1997; 152: 127-31. [http://dx.doi.org/10.1016/S0378-5173(97)04924-7]

[138] Kulkarni U, Raghavendra NG, Hariprasanna RC, *et al.* Formulation and development of aceclofenac fast dissolving tablets: effect of functionality of subliming agents. J App Pharm 2011; 2: 179-90.

[139] Gohel M, Patel M, Amin A, Agrawal R, Dave R, Bariya N. Formulation design and optimization of mouth dissolve tablets of nimesulide using vacuum drying technique. AAPS PharmSciTech 2004; 5(3): e36. [http://dx.doi.org/10.1208/pt050336] [PMID: 15760070]

[140] Kumar R, Patil M, Patil SR, *et al.* Development and characterization of melt-in-mouth tablets of haloperidol by sublimation technique. Int J Pharm & Pharma Sci 2009; 1: 65-73.

[141] Pattanayak D, Das S, Pattanaik P. Formulation and evaluation of norfloxacin orodispersible tablets 2010; 1: 1-11.

[142] Sheshala R, Khan N, Darwis Y. Formulation and optimization of orally disintegrating tablets of sumatriptan succinate. Chem Pharm Bull (Tokyo) 2011; 59(8): 920-8. [http://dx.doi.org/10.1248/cpb.59.920] [PMID: 21804234]

[143] Jeong SH, Takaishi Y, Fu Y, *et al.* Material properties for making fast dissolving tablets by a compression method. J Mater Chem 2008; 18: 3527-35.
[http://dx.doi.org/10.1039/b800209f]

[144] Shirsand SB, Suresh S, Kusumdevi V, Swamy PV. Formulation design and optimization of fast dissolving clonazepam tablets by sublimation method. Indian J Pharm Sci 2011; 73(5): 491-6.
[http://dx.doi.org/10.4103/0250-474X.98984] [PMID: 22923860]

[145] Shailesh S, Gurjeet S, Gupta G. Formulation design and optimization of mouth dissolving tablets of domperidone using sublimation technique. Int J Pharm Sci 2010; 1: 128-36.

[146] Patel DM, Patel MM. Optimization of fast dissolving etoricoxib tablets prepared by sublimation technique. Indian J Pharm Sci 2008; 70(1): 71-6.
[http://dx.doi.org/10.4103/0250-474X.40335] [PMID: 20390084]

[147] Khemariya P, Gajbhiye KR, Vaidya VD, *et al.* Preparation and evaluation of mouth dissolving tablets of meloxicam. International Journal of Drug Delivery 2011; 2

[148] Abd Elbary A, Ali AA, Aboud HM. Enhanced dissolution of meloxicam from orodispersible tablets prepared by different methods. Bull Fac Pharm Cairo Univ 2012; 50: 89-97.
[http://dx.doi.org/10.1016/j.bfopcu.2012.07.001]

[149] Suresh S, Pandit V, Joshi H. Preparation and evaluation of mouth dissolving tablets of salbutamol sulphate. Indian J Pharm Sci 2007; 69: 467-9.
[http://dx.doi.org/10.4103/0250-474X.34568]

[150] Mizumoto TS. Tablets quickly disintegrating in the oral cavity and process for producing the same. United States Patent US 6589554, 2003.

[151] Sugimoto M, Narisawa S, Matsubara K, Yoshino H, Nakano M, Handa T. Development of manufacturing method for rapidly disintegrating oral tablets using the crystalline transition of amorphous sucrose. Int J Pharm 2006; 320(1-2): 71-8.
[http://dx.doi.org/10.1016/j.ijpharm.2006.04.004] [PMID: 16750604]

[152] Sugimoto M, Maejima T, Narisawa S, Matsubara K, Yoshino H. Factors affecting the characteristics of rapidly disintegrating tablets in the mouth prepared by the crystalline transition of amorphous sucrose. Int J Pharm 2005; 296(1-2): 64-72.
[http://dx.doi.org/10.1016/j.ijpharm.2005.02.031] [PMID: 15885456]

[153] Sugimoto M, Matsubara K, Koida Y, Kobayashi M. The preparation of rapidly disintegrating tablets in the mouth. Pharm Dev Technol 2001; 6(4): 487-93.
[http://dx.doi.org/10.1081/PDT-120000287] [PMID: 11775950]

[154] Sugimoto M, Narisawa S, Matsubara K, Yoshino H, Nakano M, Handa T. Effect of formulated ingredients on rapidly disintegrating oral tablets prepared by the crystalline transition method. Chem Pharm Bull (Tokyo) 2006; 54(2): 175-80.
[http://dx.doi.org/10.1248/cpb.54.175] [PMID: 16462059]

[155] Mizumoto T, Masuda Y, Fukui M. Intrabuccally dissolving compressed moldings and production process thereof. Patent US 5576014, 1996.

[156] Mizumoto T, Masuda Y, Yamamoto T, Yonemochi E, Terada K. Formulation design of a novel fast-disintegrating tablet. Int J Pharm 2005; 306(1-2): 83-90.
[http://dx.doi.org/10.1016/j.ijpharm.2005.09.009] [PMID: 16257154]

[157] Liu F-yF, He Min Michael, Nyshadham Janaki Ram, Sharma Kuldeepak, Chu James Shunnan, Fix Joseph A. Water soluble polymer-based rapidly dissolving tablets and production processes thereof. United States Patent 6465009, 2002.

[158] Tatara MT. Method and apparatus for manufacturing tablet capable of quick disintegration in oral cavity United States Patent 6316026, 2001.

[159] Patel D, Patel B, Patel H, Patel C. Design of controlled release non-erodible polymeric matrix tablet using microwave vven-assisted sintering technique. J Young Pharm 2011; 3(3): 176-80. [http://dx.doi.org/10.4103/0975-1483.83755] [PMID: 21897655]

[160] Rao MR, Ranpise AA, Thanki KC, Borate SG, Parikh GN. Effect of processing and sintering on controlled release wax matrix tablets of ketorolac tromethamine. Indian J Pharm Sci 2009; 71(5): 538-44. [http://dx.doi.org/10.4103/0250-474X.58188] [PMID: 20502573]

[161] Rao M, Ranpise A, Borate S, Thanki K. Mechanistic evaluation of the effect of sintering on Compritol 888 ATO matrices. AAPS PharmSciTech 2009; 10(2): 355-60. [http://dx.doi.org/10.1208/s12249-009-9211-8] [PMID: 19333763]

[162] Dave VS, Fahmy RM, Bensley D, Hoag SW. Eudragit(®) RS PO/RL PO as rate-controlling matrix-formers *via* roller compaction: Influence of formulation and process variables on functional attributes of granules and tablets. Drug Dev Ind Pharm 2012; 38(10): 1240-53. [http://dx.doi.org/10.3109/03639045.2011.645831] [PMID: 22257339]

[163] Nakagami H, Kuno Y. Medicinal compositions quickly disintegrating in the oral cavity and process for producing the same. United States Patent 20100080847, 2010.

[164] Lagoviyer Y, Levinson SR, Stotler D, *et al.* Means for creating a mass having structural integrity. United States Patent 6465010, 2002.

[165] Luber JR, Bunick FJ, Sowden HS, *et al.* Multi-layered orally disintegrating tablet and the manufacture thereof. Patent Patent Applicaton US 2011; 20110318411: A1.

[166] Kuno Y, Kojima M, Nakagami H, Yonemochi E, Terada K. Effect of the type of lubricant on the characteristics of orally disintegrating tablets manufactured using the phase transition of sugar alcohol. Eur J Pharm Biopharm 2008; 69(3): 986-92. [http://dx.doi.org/10.1016/j.ejpb.2008.02.016] [PMID: 18396020]

[167] Kuno Y, Kojima M, Ando S, Nakagami H. Effect of preparation method on properties of orally disintegrating tablets made by phase transition. Int J Pharm 2008; 355(1-2): 87-92. [http://dx.doi.org/10.1016/j.ijpharm.2007.11.046] [PMID: 18182258]

[168] Kuno Y, Kojima M, Ando S, Nakagami H. Evaluation of rapidly disintegrating tablets manufactured by phase transition of sugar alcohols. J Control Release 2005; 105(1-2): 16-22. [http://dx.doi.org/10.1016/j.jconrel.2005.01.018] [PMID: 15955365]

[169] Shahi SR, Kanzarkar MV, Khadabadi SS, *et al.* Formulation and evaluation of atenolol orodispersible tablets by phase transition technology. International Journal of Pharmacy and Pharmaceutical Sciences 2013; 5: 604-9.

[170] Rogers V, Dor PJ, Fix JA. Effect of formulation parameters on fast-disintegrating tablet performances AAPS Annual Meeting and Exposiotion. San Fransisco, CA. 1999.

[171] Mizumoto T, Mauda Y, Kajiyama A, *et al.* Tablets quickly disintegrating in the oral cavity and process for producing the same. Patent EP 1072256A1, 2001.

[172] Klienberg I, Sreehuy LM. Salivary stimulant. Patent US 4820506, 1989.

[173] Eichman JD, Robinson JR. Mechanistic studies on effervescent-induced permeability enhancement. Pharm Res 1998; 15(6): 925-30. [http://dx.doi.org/10.1023/A:1011936901638] [PMID: 9647360]

[174] Hughey JR, Keen JM, Miller DA, Kolter K, Langley N, McGinity JW. The use of inorganic salts to improve the dissolution characteristics of tablets containing Soluplus®-based solid dispersions. Eur J

Pharm Sci 2013; 48(4-5): 758-66.
[http://dx.doi.org/10.1016/j.ejps.2013.01.004] [PMID: 23348153]

[175] Nagendrakumar D, Raju SA, Shirsand SB, Para MS, Rampure MV. Fast dissolving tablets of fexofenadine HCl by effervescent method. Indian J Pharm Sci 2009; 71(2): 116-9.
[http://dx.doi.org/10.4103/0250-474X.54272] [PMID: 20336204]

[176] Jacob S, Shirwaikar A, Nair A. Preparation and evaluation of fast-disintegrating effervescent tablets of glibenclamide. Drug Dev Ind Pharm 2009; 35(3): 321-8.
[http://dx.doi.org/10.1080/03639040802337021] [PMID: 18821151]

[177] Shirsand SB, Suresh S, Jodhana LS, Swamy PV. Formulation design and optimization of fast disintegrating Lorazepam tablets by effervescent method. Indian J Pharm Sci 2010; 72(4): 431-6.
[http://dx.doi.org/10.4103/0250-474X.73911] [PMID: 21218052]

[178] Shirsand SB, Suresh S, Para MS, Swamy PV. Design of fast disintegrating tablets of prochlorperazine maleate by effervescence method. Indian J Pharm Sci 2009; 71(4): 447-51.
[http://dx.doi.org/10.4103/0250-474X.57298] [PMID: 20502555]

[179] Wehling F, Schuehle S, Madamala N. Effervescent dosage form with microparticles. Patent US 5178878, 1993.

[180] Wehling F, Schuehle S, Madamala N. Pediatric effervescent dosage form. Patent US 5223264, 1993.

[181] Khankari RK, Hontz J, Chastain SJ, *et al.* Rapidly dissolving robust dosage form. Patent US 6024981, 2000.

[182] Khankari RK, Hontz J, Chastain SJ, *et al.* Rapidly dissolving robust dosage form. Patent US 6221392, 2001.

[183] Michaelson J. Rapidly disintegrable tablet composition and method. Patent US 4414198, 1983.

[184] Acosta-Cuello TR, Ouali A. Fast-melt tablet and method of making same. Patent US 5807578, 1998.

[185] Ouali A. Fast-melt tablet and method of making same. Patent US 5807577, 1998.

[186] Siebert JM, Khankari RK, Kositprapa U, *et al.* Orally disintegrable tablet forming a viscous slurry. Patent WO 0009090, 2000.

[187] Pather SI, Khankari RK, Eichman JD, *et al.* Sublingual buccal effervescent. Patent US 6200604, 2001.

[188] Robinson JR, McGinity JW, Delmas P. Effervescent granules and methods of their preparation. Patent WO 0180822 A2, 2001.

[189] Bonadeo D, Ciccarilo F, Pagano A. A process for preparation of a granulate suitable to the preparation of rapidly disintegratinf mouth-soluble tablets. Patent WO 9904758, 1999.

[190] Bonadeo D, Ciccarello F, Pagano A. Process for the preparation of a granulate suitable to the preparation of rapidly disintegrable mouth-soluble tablets and compositions obtained thereby. Patent US 6149938, 2000.

[191] Amborn J, Tiger V. Apparatus for handling and packaging friable tablets. Patent US 6269615, 2001.

CHAPTER 4

Moulding, Extrusion, Floss and Three Dimensional Printing Technologies for Developing Fast Dissolving/Disintegrating Tablets

Vikas A. Saharan*

Department of Pharmaceutics, School of Pharmaceutical Sciences, Sardar Bhagwan Singh Post Graduate Institute of Biomedical Sciences and Research, Balawala, Dehradun 248161, Uttarakhand, India

Abstract: This chapter describes various developments in the designing, fabrication and manufacturing of FDTs using various technologies based on moulding, extrusion, floss, and three dimensional printing (3DP). Moulding has evolved from conventional moulding/tablet triturates to heat moulding, moulding methods involving use of compressed gases or low boiling point solvents, microwave drying, vacuum drying and compression of wet granules in especially designed moulding machine. Extrusion is not yet fully explored for developing FDTs. Floss techniques has moved ahead from Shearform® floss through liquiflash to creation of microparticulates. Rapid prototyping techniques, especially three dimensional printing (3DP), have enabled the use of computer aided designing (CAD) possibilities in manufacturing of highly porous dosage form offering immediate and complex drug release characteristics, tablets of any shape and dosage forms which can flash into a matter of seconds.

Keywords: 3DP™, Compaction, Compression, Computer aided design, Cotton candy, EMP®, FlashDose®, Floss, Formulation, Free form fabrication, Heat moulding, Microwave drying, Press through package, Rapid prototyping, Shearform®, Tablet, TheriFlash®, TheriForm®, Vacuum drying, Wet compression.

1. INTRODUCTION

The moulded tablet or tablet triturate was originally introduced by Fuller in 1781 as oral unit dosage form made from moistened powder, comprising drug and excipients, pressed in to a cavity, extruded and dried [1, 2]. Commercially, the use

* **Corresponding author Vikas A. Saharan:** Department of Pharmaceutics, School of Pharmaceutical Sciences, Sardar Bhagwan Singh Post Graduate Institute of Biomedical Sciences and Research (www.sbspgi.edu.in), Balawala, Dehradun 248161, Uttarakhand, India; Tel: +91-135-2686246; Mobile: +91-843-9820796; Fax: +91-135-2686286; E-mail: vikas.pharmaceutics@gmail.com

of moulding had started in 1990s with the successful market launches of lyophilised tablets. Lyophilisation is also a moulding technique in which solvent is removed by sublimation. However, this chapter deals with techniques other than lyophilisation for removal of solvent from moistened or wet powder. Several other methods for removing solvents are drying in an air-circulating oven, vacuum drying and microwave drying. Additionally, compressed gases/low boiling point solvents can also be used in the making of moulded tablets from which the solvent is removed at normal temperature and pressure. Wet compression methods have also been employed for manufacturing wet tablets, which are dried later.

Extrusion is a less explored approach in making FDTs. However, its use in creating taste masked particulates/granules is widespread. These taste masked granules of bitter drugs have found their immense use in manufacturing FDTs having wide acceptability among paediatric/geriatric patients.

Sugar floss is prepared from a cotton candy machine by melting the sugar inside and forcing it to extrude through small holes resulting in floss fibres. These floss fibres can be chopped, mixed with other excipients, conditioned and subsequently compressed to obtain FDTs. Special machines have also been designed for preparing microparticulates, which can be incorporated into FDTs.

Rapid Prototyping (RP) technology, exemplified by three-dimensional printing (3DP), uses powder processing method and liquid binders to bind powders in multiple layers leading to the generation of a layer-by-layer three dimensional structure *via* programming in a computer. Various literature reports have highlighted the usefulness of 3DP in developing FDDFs and controlled drug delivery systems.

2. MOULDED TABLETS

Conventionally, water soluble excipients like lactose, mannitol, sucrose, dextrose or other appropriate diluents are used as base in preparing moulded tablets [1, 2]. Lactose remains the most frequently used base. Mannitol is preferred for additional sweetness, cooling and pleasant sensation in the mouth. Drugs that are incompatible with sugar/sugar alcohol may require other diluents like precipitated calcium phosphate, precipitated calcium carbonate, bentonite or kaolin. In the process of moulding, the tablet components are mixed with water and/or with an organic solvent in which at least one of the components partially dissolve to give stiff slurry, which can be formed into tablets by filling in moulds or using special machines. Most frequently, hydroalcoholic mixtures containing 50-80% alcohol are used as solvent. Water content in solvent dissolves sugars and the resulting sugar solution acts as binder, while the alcohol speeds up the drying of the liquid. Water content can be reduced and sometimes completely eliminated, if tablet composition is water soluble. After shaping the tablet, the wet tablet is dried carefully. Evaporation of the solvent results in the binding of tablet components, whereby the tablets receive their strength. Fine hollow spaces remain after evaporation makes the tablet porous and penetrable to solvents for faster disintegration/dissolution. Conventional tablet triturates or moulded tablets provide satisfactory rate of dissolution but being too soft and brittle some difficulties may arise in packing and transporting due to practically pressure-less method of their production. The use of organic solvents may damage active ingredient, especially enzymes and indicators. Vapours of organic solvents require special provisions and safety measures in the production of the tablets. Water cannot be used as solvent for very readily water soluble drugs. When compared with conventional compressed tablets, moulded tablet suffers weight variation and content uniformity issues. Moulding methods have evolved with the development in science and technology to overcome some of these disadvantages. Moulded tablets have also gained great deal of attraction in recent years with the popularity and acceptability of FDTs among dysphagic, paediatric, geriatric, psychotic and frequently travelling patients. Compression moulding, heat moulding, moulding with the aid of compressed gas/low boiling point solvent, freezing with vacuum drying and microwave drying are some of the improvements which have been explored and employed for developing FDTs. Moulded tablets can be prepared by filling moulds with a dispersion of drug and excipients and subsequent drying of solvent by lyophilisation. However, this chapter deals with methods other than lyophilisation used in preparing moulded tablets.

2.1. Compression Moulding

Water soluble excipients are used in making moulded tablets because the resulting tablet is expected to dissolve rapidly and completely in mouth. Active ingredient is mixed with other water soluble excipients to obtain a uniform powder blend. Hydroalcoholic solvent is used to moist the powder blend followed by moulding of wet mass in moulding plates at a low compression pressure. Solvent from wet moulded tablet is removed by drying in air. Use of low compression pressure is helpful in maintaining desired porosity that is essential for quick disintegration/dissolution. Size of lactose (or other base material) particles, compression force, moisture content are some critical process parameters used for optimising tablets for quick disintegration/dissolution and adequate hardness. Poor mechanical strength of moulded tablets and masking undesirable bitter taste are two great challenges. Van Scoik disclosed a method of incorporating taste masked drug particles in lactose based moulded tablets [3]. Taste masking was achieved by spray congealing of bitter drug particles in a molten mixture of lecithin, hydrogenated cottonseed oil, sodium bicarbonate and polyethylene glycol (PEG). Taste masked drug particles were mixed with the carbohydrate and a hydroalcoholic solvent to form a wet mass. The wet mass was moulded into tablets at a low compression pressure. Wet tablets were dried to remove solvent resulting in a porous moulded tablet, also referred to as a tablet triturate. The tablet triturate contained a porous network of a water soluble but ethanol insoluble carbohydrate. However, the tablet triturate method is limited to active ingredient like estazolam that are not sensitive to the melting temperature of the glyceride. Furthermore, since the dosage form is formed into a damp mass and subsequently dried, conventional compression tableting machines cannot be used to manufacture this product. One major disadvantage of this technology is the poor mechanical strength of moulded tablets.

FDTs by moulding can be prepared by low pressure compression of wet lactose granules followed by drying of wet tablets in an air circulating oven [4]. The solvent (water) plays an important role in this wet compression method. Kneading of lactose with water dissolves a part of lactose and the resulting lactose solution forms a layer upon lactose particles. Drying of the tablets recrystallises lactose from lactose solution and form solid bridges (interparticle bonds) resulting in the rigid and highly porous tablets. This wet compression method is successful in preparing tablets having 0.5 MPa or more tensile strength and disintegration time of 15 s or less.

Takeda Chemical Industries (Osaka, Japan) has developed production methods wherein a mixture comprising drug, starches and sugars mixed with appropriate water is compressed at low pressure and then dried [5]. Highly porous FDTs weighing 1-2 g, disintegration time of 30-50 s in oral cavity and sufficient mechanical strength can be manufactured. However, such methods also require a special pharmaceutical technique/machine and adhesion of powder to the surface of a metal mould in compression process under moistening conditions. It may be, therefore, difficult to utilise this method for manufacturing purpose in a conventional plant. However, such moulded tablets require the use of either bitterless drug or necessitates taste masking of drug particles.

Using another technology developed by Novartis Consumer Health (Basel, Switzerland), moulded tablets are produced by filling a mould with a mixture solution containing a drug, a filler such as mannitol, a binder, and other auxiliary substances and subsequent drying the mixture solution [6]. Drying of moulded units can be performed by conventional drying at room temperature or at elevated temperature, pressure reduction or by microwave radiation. The process of drying is time consuming and depends upon the properties of API and the formulation components ability to sustain the conditions of drying.

2.2. Vacuum Drying of Frozen Wet Mass

A freezing process and subsequent vacuum drying has been used for preparing moulded tablets, which are considerably less porous than tablets prepared using freeze drying process [7]. A mixture of carbohydrate (*e.g.* lactose, dextrose, mannitol, maltose or maltodextrin), a gum (*e.g.* acacia, guar, xanthan, carrageenan or tragacanth) and a solvent is frozen in a tablet-shaped mould and dried in vacuum. Vacuum drying is performed at a temperature which is lower than the equilibrium freezing point and higher than the collapse temperature of the matrix. Unlike lyophilisation, solvent evaporate to gas *via* the liquid phase. Vacuum drying aids to dense the tablet matrix and thereby increases mechanical strength of tablets. Low pressures (*e.g.* 0.5-10 torr) during vacuum drying of unbound solvent are preferred, particularly if the primary drying temperature is near the collapse temperature (*e.g.* 1-5°C). Such low pressures retard the rate of phase change occurring at the collapse temperature results in producing a tablet having particularly good structural integrity.

A kneaded mixture of a drug and a rapidly water soluble pharmaceutical additive is subjected to compression in a wet state [8]. Optionally, a suitable binding agent may be added. The compression pressure for shaping tablets is relatively low, *e.g.* 50-1,000 kg. The resulting tablets are dried in a hot air circulating oven to yield FDTs. The tablet base component is a rapidly water soluble pharmaceutical additive, preferably xylitol, which is responsible for faster dissolution of the tablet. These tablets are different from conventional tablets in the sense that the compression and drying operations are reversed in order. Conventional tablets are produced by mixing starting materials, adding a binder, kneading and drying the mixture and subjecting the mixture to compression.

A compression moulded tablet process has been developed and patented by Eisai Co. Ltd. (Tokyo, Japan) [9]. In this process, a uniform blend of active ingredients and excipients is kneaded with solvent (alcohol or water) to a wet mass and filled in a mould. Upper and lower surfaces of the wet mass are lubricated to prevent sticking to the apparatus in a following compression step. A compression force of 5-100 kg for a 10 mm diameter tablet is applied onto the surface of wet mass. The compressed moulded tablets are taken out of the mould and dried. This method claims to prepare moulded tablets with both either water soluble or fat soluble active ingredient. However, conventional moulded tablet making process has been limited to water soluble active ingredient. Moulded tablets of a fat soluble active ingredient can be prepared by blending drug with water soluble excipients like D-glucose, mannitol, cane sugar or xylitol. Optionally, surfactant, wetting agent and favours may be added to the powder blend. Powder blend is kneaded with ethanol, and if required, a binder, to form a paste. Wet paste is charged in the mould and compressed at a suitable pressure resulting in shaping of the tablet. Wet tablets were removed from the mould and dried.

2.3. Microwave Drying of Moulded Tablets

Microwave drying has been used to improve hardness and disintegration properties of moulded tablets consisting of a polymeric disintegrant and mannitol [10]. Polyacetal punches are used to prevent sticking of wet mass. Pre-weighed wet granules are filled manually into a die followed by compression at 10 mm/min speed and the compression force is allowed to reach a limiting value of 0.3-0.7 kN. Obtained wet tablets are dried at 500 W in a microwave oven.

Using design of experiment approach, various factors like compression force, disintegrant ratio, amount of water and ratio of δ and β form of crystalline mannitol were studied for their possible impact on the properties of moulded tablets. Several disintegrants, *viz.* croscarmellose sodium (CCS), low substituted hydroxypropylcellulose (L-HPC) and crospovidone were assessed for their application in preparing FDTs [10]. NBD-020, L-HPC grade, gave best results for improved hardness and shorter disintegration time. An increase in disintegrant ratio leads to an increase of microwave induced swelling. Hardness of the tablet increased with microwave treatment and disintegration time reduced with increasing ratios of mannitol. Hardness and disintegration of tablets, upon microwave treatment, were significantly affected by change in crystalline forms of mannitol. Microwave treatment had increased β mannitol ratio in tablets leading to an increase in the hardness of the tablets and a decrease in the disintegration time. In an another study, water vapours generated during microwave drying caused either swelling or shrinking of tablets, a phenomenon, which depends on the manufacturing conditions and tablet compositions [11]. Transition of crystalline form of mannitol from δ to β, in the presence of water vapours, increased the tablet hardness. It was also observed that low volume of water and high ratio of silicon dioxide induced swelling of tablets upon microwave irradiation. The process of microwave drying of moulded tablets is limited to active ingredients having melting points higher than 110°C because higher temperatures can compromise chemical stability and dissolution rate of active ingredient [12].

2.4. Compressed Gas/Low Boiling Point Solvent for Moulding

Moulded tablets have also been prepared by a method that uses a compressed gas to prepare wet mass from homogenous mixtures of excipients and pulverised drug [13]. The wet mass is filled into moulds under pressure of between 101325 Pa (normal pressure or 1.01325 bar) and 107 Pa (100 bar) and decompressed to obtain highly porous moulded tablets. These porous moulded tablets can be of oral use with their characteristic fast disintegrating property. The pressurised liquefied gas has a boiling point below 0°C at normal atmospheric pressure and it may be selected among G 227 (1,1,1,2,3,3,3-heptafluoropropane), TG 134a (1,1,1,2-tetrafluoro-ethane), propane, n-butane, isobutane and dimethyl ether, and their mixture. Instead, a low-boiling solvent having a boiling point between 20-100°C at normal atmospheric pressure may be used.

2.5. Compression of Wet Granules

A wet compression method was used to prepare ethenzamide FDTs [14]. The process involved kneading of drug, a water soluble excipient and other excipients in a powder handling mill operated at a rotation speed of 2000 rpm. Distilled water was added to the powder mixture in small increments. With each addition of small amount of water, the powder was agitated for 60 s. Wet mass of powder was extruded through sieve of 710 μm into a container and prepared granules were covered with a wet paper to maintain moisture. Wet granules were compressed in a hydraulic press using flat punches. Wet tablets were dried through circulation of hot air in an oven. Dried tablets were kept in a desiccator until use/testing. This wet compression method successfully resolved the problem of weight variation in moulded tablets. Crystallisation of water soluble excipient during drying resulted in the formation of interparticulate bonds, which improved mechanical strength of tablets without compromising on high porosity of tablets. In wet compressed tablets, a logarithmic relationship between tensile strength and porosity was observed. Further, moisture content and decrease in particle size was found to decrease disintegration time of tablets, a trend analogous to the tensile strength of the tablets.

2.6. Moulding in Press Through Package (PTP) Moulds

FDTs containing *dl*-α-tocopheryl acetate, lactose and 2-hydroxypropyl-β-cyclodextrin as additives were prepared by moulding directly in its package [15]. Lactose, *dl* -α- tocopheryl acetate, 2- hydroxypropyl-β- cyclodextrin and water were agitated vigorously to prepare dispersion (without emulsification) for filling into PTP moulds. Filled PTP moulds were subjected to drying at 4°C for a day, 25°C for another day and a final drying at 40°C on the last day. Dispersion and filling at 25°C and 40°C caused cracking and chipping due to less crystallisation of lactose in the moulds. Drying of filled PTP sheets at 25°C or 40°C did not result in the formation of adequate number of tablets. Hence, a temperature of 4°C was found optimum for not only preparing and filling dispersion in PTP moulds but also for drying on first day. A subsequent drying at 25°C for the second day and a final third day drying at 40°C was able to produce tablets having sufficient hardness and faster disintegration.

2.7. Heat Moulding

Heat moulding involves preparation of a suspension, containing active ingredient, a sugar (*e.g.* lactose or mannitol) and agar, pouring this suspension into wells of blister packaging, forming a jelly of agar at room temperature and subsequent vacuum drying at 30°C [16].

Aqueous agar solution solidifies rapidly into a gel at room temperature within a short time, when it is filled in a mould. It provides the advantage of generating a uniform structural body with least chances of precipitation of solid components. Agar further improves the strength of the moulded tablet by forming a part of the structural body and during drying, especially under reduced pressure or with aeration, agar molecules move to the upper surface of the preparation with water molecules. Agar prevents reduction of hardness and formation of irregular shaped tablets by preventing expansion of the dried surface under reduced pressure conditions. Gelation of the preparation at room temperature prevents irregularity in shape and provides ease to various operations like transfer of the mould, drying *etc.*

2.8. Trademark Technology: EMP®Tablet

Eisai compression moulding machine (EMT 150) was designed by Eisai Co., Ltd. (Tokyo) and Sankyo Seisakusho Co. (Tokyo) for manufacturing moulded tablets [10, 17, 18]. Moulded tablets with small weight variation are easily prepared by a wet compression method performed in this machine. The tablets prepared by this machine have been marketed by Eisai Company as EMP® tablets.

Moulding tablets are manufactured by shaping wet powder in a mould followed by drying. This whole process can be accomplished at a single location by fitting a belt dryer to a compression moulding machine (EMT 150) [19, 20]. In actual practice, drug and water soluble excipient(s) are kneaded in a binder solution to prepare a wet mass, which is subsequently compressed in the compression moulding machine. Wet tablets are initially dried on a belt dryer attached to the compression moulding machine and final drying of tablets is performed in a tray dryer.

Wet powders are difficult to compress in a tableting machine due to adhesion/sticking of powder to machine parts and poor flowability leading to the problems of weight variation and low mechanical strength. The tablet moulding machine developed by Eisai Co. has considerably improved the handling of wet powder and subsequent compression. This machine uses a compression powder feeder to overcome the problem of weight variation. Compression powder feeder uses a two step process for transfer of wet powder from hopper to the die cavity. In the first step, oscillation of the feeding blade aids in the transfer of wet powder from hopper to a well on sub-table. The second step makes use of a plunger at a constant pressure for transferring wet powder from the wells to a die cavity set in the main table of the machine. A better control on weight variation is achieved through this two step process of transfer of wet powder. The problem of sticking of wet powder to punch can be resolved through a film compression system, which uses a 0.01 mm thick polyethylene film kept between the tableting punch and the wet powder. Wet tablets are dried on a belt dryer immediately after compression to provide sufficient mechanical strength. A secondary drying is essentially required to limit the moisture content to the desired level.

EMP® tabletis based on a formulation that is expected to make the swallowing of medicines easier for patients with mild dysphagia [21]. Eisai launched Aricept ODT in 2005, a line extension of donepezil in Japan in 2004 and in the US in 2005.

3. EXTRUSION METHODS

Steam extruded polymer (high maltose starch/hydrolysed gelatin/dextran/ dextrin/alginates) matrix can be shaped (cutting or moulding) in appropriate size tablets or other shapes [22]. Tablets produced by this method are non friable and claimed to dissolve in the mouth within 4 s. The polymer along with other excipients should have moisture content of 25% or less for desired expansion and structure formation. A part of the moisture is vaporised in the process leading to a low density matrix upon extrusion. The extruded matrix generally expands after processing. Drug and other excipients may be incorporated prior to extrusion.

PEG can be used as a vehicle for solvent based extrusion, both alone or in combination with the active ingredient [23]. PEGs (Carbowax 8000, Carbowax 3350, Carbowax 1450 and Carbowax 1000) are melted together at 45-65°C. Methanol and active ingredient are added and stirred continuously and the mixture is cooled to room temperature. When the materials are of semisolid consistency, they are transferred to the extruder and air pressure is applied to drive a regulator controlled extruder. The material is extruded on paper and dried at room temperature overnight (>12 h). A heated blade is used to cut the dried cylinders (extrudates) into equally sized tablets. Using mass extrusion approach, water soluble tablets with acceptable characteristics can be prepared on a small scale using a solvent based process. Extrudability is significantly affected by the composition of the mixture and addition of active ingredient. Extrudability is required to be optimised using a mixture design and application of ternary diagrams. It was observed that up to 30% of a soluble ingredient could be incorporated in the PEG vehicle. Tablets prepared by this method were found pharmaceutically elegant and passed content uniformity, friability and rapid disintegration/dissolution tests. Acetaminophen tablets prepared by mass extrusion were found to dissolve by erosion and the intrinsic dissolution rate was 0.86 mg/min/cm^2. It was proposed that currently available screw extruders may be adapted to extrude wide cylinders of the product and swig-blade cutting device could be used.

Hot melt extrusion/extrusion-precipitation/extrusion techniques have also been applied in preparation of taste masked granules, which can be incorporated into FDTs. Most of these studies have employed aminoalkyl methacrylate copolymer (Eudragit E100/Eudragit EPO) for masking bitter taste of drugs, *viz.* ibuprofen [24], hyoscine butylbromide [25], metoclopramide HCl [26], pirenzipine HCl [27], oxybutynin [27], chlorpheniramine maleate [28] and promethazine HCl [29]

4. FLOSS TECHNIQUES

Various patents have been assigned to Fuisz Technologies Ltd. for flash flow processing related to the spinning of one or more sugars with other substances in a cotton candy type machine [30 - 34]. APIs have been combined with sugar and spun into fibres to produce readily water soluble product [30]. Oleaginous substances can also be combined with sugar and the resulting mixture is subjected to melt spinning in a cotton candy type machine [35]. Heat sensitive active ingredient like protein can also be processed for flash flow, when a carrier material is selected from a maltodextrin and polydextrose. It includes the use of fructose as a processing aid in an amount sufficient to reduce the amount of heat required to create flash flow conditions in the carrier [36, 37].

Active ingredient [30] or a cosmetic [31] could also be added to fibres which are subsequently compressed to a sheet. However, adequate care shall be taken while compacting as it may break the fibrous mass. Wafer like structure containing medicament on or through spun fibres have been prepared and reduced in their size by chopping in a food grinder [34]. The process can reduce volume of floss as low as 15%. Compaction of spun fibres is described in some other patents also, but none of these patents disclose the formation of a compressed tablet [32, 38].

A compressed tablet for quick dispersion in the mouth has been prepared by compacting microparticles consisting of partially crystallised shearform matrix [39]. Shearform matrix is crystallised and mixed with additives to form compactible and flowable microparticulates. Alternatively, shearform matrix may be combined with additives and followed by crystallisation of shearform matrix to yield microparticles. Process of preparing FDTs from shearform matrix can be divided into following three steps [40].

First Step: This step involves preparation of a shearform matrix and mixing of active ingredient to it. Shearform matrix is formed by subjecting a carrier material to flash flow processing or flash-heat or flash shear.

Flash-heat process involve the heating of the carrier material to a point where an internal flow in carrier material results in movements at subparticle level, finally leading to the exit of carrier material from exit openings of a spinning head. Spinning at 3,000-5,000 rpm and a temperature of 150-250°C generates enough centrifugal force that can throw the carrier material out from the spinning head with simultaneous change in the structure of the carrier material. When drug and carrier material are present together, free form agglomerate of drug dispersed in carrier material are generated out off the spinning head. Cotton candy fabricating equipment is utilised for fabricating shearform matrices or floss. Cotton candy is a melt extrusion process in which the stock material is melted and forced through spinnerettes.

Flash-shear process involves raising the temperature of a non-solubilised carrier like a saccharide-based material that results in an internal flow, when a fluid shear force is applied. The carrier material moves ahead and ejects from spinning head in an internal flow condition leading to the formation of agglomerates. Agglomerates are cooled immediately after their contact with the shear force, allowed to continue in free flow condition and subsequently solidified. When drug is added to the carrier material, drug fuses as the composition undergoes an internal flow, followed by disruption and agglomerate formation. The process of flash shearing can be accomplished in a in a twin screw extruder having functionality of several heating zones. Nozzle is used as an ejector for casting out the carrier material at a very high pressure.

Second Step: The shearform matrix, obtained from first step processing, is chopped and combined with API, sweetener, binding/crystallisation inhibitor, flavour, colour, glidant, lubricant and any other excipient. Flavoured and compactible microparticulates are formed by combining shearform matrix and the additives. Substances like dextrose, surfactants (Tweens and Spans), polypropylene glycol and PEG act as binding/crystallisation modifiers and provide a control on the rate of crystallisation during binding of the matrix. Prepared microparticulates are agglomerates of relatively low density, which can withstand high compression force during tableting.

Third Step: Finally, the microparticulate mixture is subjected to compression (6-8 strong cob units) to yield FDTs characterised by good appearance, structural integrity and excellent drug release.

Improved processability, enhanced dissolution and taste masking properties can be combined in a drug product by using unifloss systems [41]. Shearform matrices or floss made from single sugar or sugar alcohol (*e.g.* xylitol) is referred to as single floss or unifloss. Flosses are shearform matrices containing a carrier and two or more sugar alcohols. The combination of two sugars or sugar alcohols like sorbitol and xylitol provides superior binding ability and flowability characteristics. FlashDose® tablets are prepared by mixing coated drug particles with unifloss, followed by blending with flavours, sweetener and lubricants and subsequent compressions in a rotary tablet press.

FDTs were prepared from amorphous shearform sugar masses, API and other excipients [42, 43]. The process includes fusion, mixing, filling and compression. Tablet ingredients were subjected to flash flow processing to obtain shearform matrices. Obtained shearform matrix masses were mixed with sweeteners, flavours, glidants and lubricants, and later filled into product wells (plastic blisters), where the composition is compressed at a low pressure (less than 250 psi and more preferably less than 80 psi), referred as tamping. Temperature and humidity were kept below the glass transition temperature for maintaining shearform matrix and API. Curing (binding and crystallisation) of the matrix material was achieved in a controlled humidity and temperature conditions for 1-4 days. Curing process transforms the product from amorphous to crystalline state, while the product remains in the bound state.

A friability of less than 1% and quick disintegration/dissolution of FDTs within 40 s was achieved, when liquiflash particles and excipients comprising a cellulose derivative and/or inorganic salt (directly compressible grade) were compressed to achieve hardness of 20-50 N [44]. In liquiflash conditions, a carrier material is quickly heated to achieve intraparticulate flow and partial deformation or liquefaction allows the composition to pass through small openings in a spinning device Liquiflash particles are expelled as discrete solid particles through the openings in the spinning head in response to centrifugal forces [45]. Drug or excipient can be fed to the spinning machine and microspheres can be obtained for drug alone or mixture of drug and excipient. There is no requirement of external shaping forces and thus expelled materials instantly reform into particles, which have different morphology from the feedstock. Thus liquiflash processing can result in a spheronise composition containing one or more drug(s) and/or excipient. Liquiflash conditions are dependent on the properties of the carrier material, API (if any) and other components.

4.1. Trademark Technology: FlashDose®

FlashDose® (Valeant Pharmaceuticals International, Inc.; Previously Biovail Corporation and more previously Fuisz Technologies) is a FDT containing a processed excipient called Shearform™. Various patents have been obtained for this Shearform™ technology [39, 42, 43, 46 - 49]. Shearform™ (Patented by Fuisz Technologies) is a floss of saccharides or polysaccharides processed into an amorphous fibre. Floss is generally made from dextrose, sucrose, lactose and fructose. A high shear mixer-granulator is used to reduce the size of fibres of floss by cutting or rotation. Appropriately sized floss fibres are mixed with API and other excipients like sweeteners, flavours, glidants and lubricants and the mixture is compressed to obtain tablets. The API may be either subjected to flash processing with the carrier material or may be added to the floss blend of the carrier material. FlashDose® tablets disperse rapidly in mouth, can house large amounts of API and have sufficient mechanical strength. However, the use of high temperature in melting the matrix may pose limitations for the application of the shearform matrix to thermolabile drugs. Proprietary Ceform® taste masking technology may be used for masking bitter taste in FlashDose® dosage forms of bitter drugs [50].

5. THREE-DIMENSIONAL PRINTING [3DP™ TECHNOLOGY]

Solid, free-form fabrication (SFF) methods offer some exclusive opportunities for the preparation of rapidly disintegrating/dissolving dosage units that can be constructed with a matrix having a three-dimensional architecture, which rapidly disperses, disrupts, disintegrates, or otherwise dissolves immediately. These novel dosage forms are built through an SFF process, such as 3DP. All process parameters and necessary instructions for fabricating these dosage forms are communicated *via* the computer that controls the operation of the 3DP machine. 3DP process ideally suits to prepare FDTs (disintegration in less than 90 s) dosage forms suitable for placement in a body cavity, on a body surface or exposed area such as an open wound [51].

3DP is a process of fabricating solid three dimensional objects by sequential addition of layers on layers in a laminated manner. This process is very similar to the inkjet printing process of creating a three dimensional object from two dimensional layers. This technique allows an excellent control over structure and composition of the fabricated dosage form. Computer-aided design (CAD) version of the object is used to calculate the intersection of planes required to form two dimensional segments of the objects and subsequently combined to form three dimensional structure of the object. In 3DP technology, both the macro and microstructure can be controlled since objects are built by addition of very small amounts of matter. 3DP can provide an excellent control at macroscopic shapes (cm level), intermediate features (about 100 μ level) and microscopic (about 10 μl level) features of the object. Thus, in other words, we can say that control can be exercised at size of the dosage form, size and orientation of pores or channels and the porosity in the structural walls of the dosage form. A computer controlled printing of microdrops of drugs, binders and other materials onto a very thin layer of powdered excipients, polymers and biomaterials results in fabrication of a dosage form [50]. Presence of binder in droplets is able to hold powders two-dimensionally in the form of a layer of the product. With the printing of each layer, the build platform descends for printing of another layer and this process repeats itself till printing process is complete and built of entire structure achieved. Thereby, 3-D printing process and production equipment precisely controls not only the surface composition but also the internal architecture of a product.

A 3DP tableting machine consists of a vertical piston, a spreading bar and a pair of horizontal X-Y axes motion controllers directed printing head [52]. Printing head is positioned above a platform, which holds a piston vertically and has a provision of spreading powder over piston plate *via* the spreading bar. The process of tablet fabrication starts with spreading a thin powder layer on a plate of the piston. A nozzle in the printing head directs the binder solution to powder bed leading to the formation of a layer. Thus, powder particles are attached to each other forming a two dimensional pattern. The piston is descended to a predetermined distance to form a new layer of powder over the existing layer. Repetition of this process results in formation of a defined three dimensional structure.

TheriForm®, a 3DP microfabrication technology, was used to make quickly dispersing dosage. Dispersion time of these dosage forms were as short as seconds in comparison to other FDTs and compressed tablets. A semi-automated technique for determination of dispersion time of such dosage forms was developed to generate accurate and reproducible measurements in a fast and simple way [53]. A formulation was optimised using Box Behnken design to develop rapid dispersing dosage forms by TheriForm® technology [54]. An amount of 97.5% w/w of mannitol and 2.5% w/w of maltitol, when used at 45% saturation level, was found optimum in a regression analysis for preparing FDTs.

3DP process has been used in designing internal structure and fabricating FDTs of acetaminophen [55]. A layer printing process was employed to deposit binder solutions onto chosen regions. Acceptable hardness (63.4 N/cm^2) was achieved by several binding mechanisms, but high friability (3.55%) was a critical disadvantage. FDTs disintegrated in 23.4 s and wetting time was 67.6 s. Acetaminophen release was 98.5% within 2 min. In another study with acetaminophen FDTs designed and fabricated by 3DP, friability was within the acceptable limit (0.92%) and hardness was 54.5 N/cm^2. Disintegration time and wetting time were 21.8 s and 51.7 s, respectively. Drug release of 97.7% was obtained after 2 min.

In one study, 3DP process was found efficient in fabricating dosage forms consisting of a very low drug content of 10 moles in a tablet [56]. Hardness and friability of prepared dosage forms were comparable to conventional dosage forms. 3DP is a novel technique used in the fabrication of complex oral delivery of pharmaceuticals. This technique has been used to attain zero order release of drug from acetaminophen tablets [57] and nearly zero order drug release from pseudoephedrine HCl formulations [58]. A doughnut shape multiple layered tablet has been fabricated and drug release was adjusted by optimising the design of the tablet [59]. Immediate-extended release tablet, a tablet for pulsed release followed by extended release, breakaway tablet and enteric dual pulsatory tablets were designed and fabricated by 3DP [60]. It was apprised that oral dosage form with two complex release profiles, erosion and diffusion, can be achieved through a single dosage unit composed of two different halves in a single unit. Pulsatory device capable of releasing drug in two pulses, one at stomach and another at intestine, was found efficient in attaining a time lag between drug release pulses by controlling device's geometry. Breakaway tablets consisting of three different sections, two drug releasing and one fast eroding, were also found feasible. Diclofenac was printed onto two different areas of a tablet constructed with one enteric excipient to obtain two drug release pulses in enteric tablets. In one study, a 3D printing process was used in adsorbing antibiotic onto a bioceramic powder [61]. Developed individualised implants were capable of treating different groups of patients or meeting the demands for individual drug delivery requirements.

3DP technology is flexible and can find numerous applications in various drug delivery systems like floating, colon targeted, oral fast disintegrating, controlled drug delivery, implantable and drug delivery systems with pulsed release and multiphase release characteristics [62]. Flexible and highly reproducible 3DP process can also be employed to address some of the challenging issues in drug delivery like delivery of peptides and proteins, poorly water-soluble drugs, highly potent and toxic drugs and controlled release of two or more drugs in a single dosage form. There are some critical challenges, which have limited the application of 3DP process. 3DP is still in pilot stage and commercial scale manufacturing machines are not yet available. The technique is too costly to be applied commercially at large scales, when compared to the conventional methods. Pharmaco-technical properties and selection of excipients are some critical challenges to formulation and dosage form development. More advancement in this technology is required to address these issues, especially for its commercial exploitation in pharmaceutical and healthcare industry.

CONCLUSIONS

The market of technologies for manufacturing FDTs seems much bigger than the expectations. These dosage forms have evolved from immediate release to controlled drug delivery and to more specialised drug delivery systems. FDTs have enormous potential for routes other than oral, *viz.* vaginal, topical, *etc. Vis--vis* to their advancements in therapeutic applications, technologies for manufacturing of FDTs are also upgrading. We have moved from adaptations of conventional methods to lyophilisation and more advanced RP/3DP technologies for designing and fabrication of FDTs. Some of these technologies have reached in the market, while some others are in pilot scale or even at the laboratory scale. The ongoing innovations in drug delivery systems and different unit operations are expected to bring together technological advancements and formulation knowledge to create newer technologies for developing FDTs.

REFERENCES

[1] Felton L. Pharmaceutical manufacturing. In: Troy DB, Beringer P, Eds. Remington: The Science and Practice of Pharmacy. 21 ed., Lippincott Williams & Wilkins 2006.

[2] Roberts M, Ford JL. Extrudable technologies of recontrolling drug release and absorption. In: Wilson CG, Crowley CJ, Eds. Controlled Release in Oral Drug Delivery. Springer 2011; pp. 239-56.

[3] Van Scoik KG. Solid pharmaceutical dosage in tablet triturate form and method of producing same. United States Patent 5082667, 1992.

[4] Bi Y, Yonezawa Y, Sunada H. Rapidly disintegrating tablets prepared by the wet compression method: mechanism and optimization. J Pharm Sci 1999; 88(10): 1004-10. [http://dx.doi.org/10.1021/js990061z] [PMID: 10514347]

[5] Makino T, Yamada M, Kikuta J-i. Fast dissolving tablet and its production. Patent EP0553777, 1994.

[6] Humbert–droz P, Seidel M, Martani R. Fast disintegrating oral dosage form. Patent WO/1997/038679, 1997.

[7] Pebley WS, Jager NE, Thompson SJ. Rapidly distintegrating tablet. United States Patent 5298261, 1994.

[8] Nakamichi K, Izumi S, Yasuura H. Fast soluble tablet. Patent EP0627218, 1994.

[9] Tsushima Y, Ashizawa K, Watanabe S. Method and apparatus for preparation of molded tablet and thereby prepared molded tablet. United States Patent 6036974, 2000.

[10] Sano S, Iwao Y, Noguchi S, Kimura S, Itai S. Design and evaluation of microwave-treated orally disintegrating tablets containing polymeric disintegrant and mannitol. Int J Pharm 2013; 448(1): 132-41. [http://dx.doi.org/10.1016/j.ijpharm.2013.03.023] [PMID: 23524122]

[11] Sano S, Iwao Y, Kimura S, Itai S. Preparation and evaluation of swelling induced-orally disintegrating tablets by microwave irradiation. Int J Pharm 2011; 416(1): 252-9. [PMID: 21763765]

[12] Sano S, Iwao Y, Kimura S, Noguchi S, Itai S. Impact of active ingredients on the swelling properties of orally disintegrating tablets prepared by microwave treatment. Int J Pharm 2014; 468(1-2): 234-42. [http://dx.doi.org/10.1016/j.ijpharm.2014.04.011] [PMID: 24709215]

[13] Bauer KH, Rohrer H-p. Fast–disintegrating tablets. Patent WO/2005/058284, 2005.

[14] Sunada H, Bi Y. Preparation, evaluation and optimization of rapidly disintegrating tablets. Powder Technol 2002; 122: 188-98. [http://dx.doi.org/10.1016/S0032-5910(01)00415-6]

[15] Motoyama K, Nagatomo K, Abd Elazim SO, Hirayama F, Uekama K, Arima H. Potential use of 2-hydroxypropyl-beta-cyclodextrin for preparation of orally disintegrating tablets containing dl-alph--tocopheryl acetate, an oily drug. Chem Pharm Bull (Tokyo) 2009; 57(11): 1206-12. [http://dx.doi.org/10.1248/cpb.57.1206] [PMID: 19881268]

[16] Masaki K, Ban K. Intrabuccally disintegrating preparation and production thereof. United States 5466464, 1995.

[17] Kato H, Tsushima Y, Ohwaki T, *et al.* Manufacture of tablet and device therefor. JP Patent 3179658, 2001.

[18] Kato H, Tsushima Y, Ohwaki T, *et al.* Method and apparatus for manufacturing tablets. United States Patent 5603880, 1997.

[19] Narazaki R, Harada T, Takami N, Kato Y, Ohwaki T. A new method for disintegration studies of rapid disintegrating tablet. Chem Pharm Bull (Tokyo) 2004; 52(6): 704-7.
[http://dx.doi.org/10.1248/cpb.52.704] [PMID: 15187391]

[20] Morita Y, Tsushima Y, Yasui M, Termoz R, Ajioka J, Takayama K. Evaluation of the disintegration time of rapidly disintegrating tablets *via* a novel method utilizing a CCD camera. Chem Pharm Bull (Tokyo) 2002; 50(9): 1181-6.
[http://dx.doi.org/10.1248/cpb.50.1181] [PMID: 12237533]

[21] Shoriken K, Yamaguchi M, Nakata H. Clinical evaluation of rapidly disintegrating tablets in patients with mild dysphagia. Iryo Yakugaku 2003; 29: 648-51. [Japanese Journal of Pharmaceutical Health Care and Sciences].

[22] Wigman LS, Thombre AG. Rapidly disintegratinf and fast dissolving dosage form. Patent CA 2331719, 2001.

[23] Murphy MP, Hollenbeck RG. A unique application of extrusion for the preparation of water–soluble tablets. Pharmaceutical Tehnology 1998 April; 94-102.

[24] Gryczke A, Schminke S, Maniruzzaman M, Beck J, Douroumis D. Development and evaluation of orally disintegrating tablets (ODTs) containing Ibuprofen granules prepared by hot melt extrusion. Colloids Surf B Biointerfaces 2011; 86(2): 275-84.
[http://dx.doi.org/10.1016/j.colsurfb.2011.04.007] [PMID: 21592751]

[25] Khattab IS, Zaghloul AA I, Afouna MI. Studies on the development of rapidly disintegrating hyoscine butylbromide tablets. Drug Discov Ther 2007; 1(1): 61-4.
[PMID: 22504365]

[26] Randale SA, Dabhi CS, Tekade AR, Belgamwar VS, Gattani SG, Surana SJ. Rapidly disintegrating tablets containing taste masked metoclopramide hydrochloride prepared by extrusion-precipitation method. Chem Pharm Bull (Tokyo) 2010; 58(4): 443-8.
[http://dx.doi.org/10.1248/cpb.58.443] [PMID: 20410620]

[27] Ishikawa T, Watanabe Y, Utoguchi N, Matsumoto M. Preparation and evaluation of tablets rapidly disintegrating in saliva containing bitter-taste-masked granules by the compression method. Chem Pharm Bull (Tokyo) 1999; 47(10): 1451-4.
[http://dx.doi.org/10.1248/cpb.47.1451] [PMID: 10553641]

[28] Shishu BA, Singh T. Preparation of tablets rapidly disintegrating in saliva containing bitter taste–masked granules by compression method. Indian J Pharm Sci 2007; 69: 80-4.
[http://dx.doi.org/10.4103/0250-474X.32113]

[29] Haware RV, Chaudhari PD, Parakh SR, Bauer-Brandl A. Development of a melting tablet containing promethazine HCl against motion sickness. AAPS PharmSciTech 2008; 9(3): 1006-15.
[http://dx.doi.org/10.1208/s12249-008-9133-x] [PMID: 18770049]

[30] Fuisz RC. Rapidly dissoluble medicinal dosage unit and method of manufacture. United States Patent 4855326, 1989.

[31] Fuisz RC. Spun fibrous cosmetic and method of use. United States Patent 4873085, 1989.

[32] Fuisz RC. Moderated spun fibrous system and method of manufacture. United States Patent 5034421, 1991.

[33] Fuisz RC. Taste masked medicated pharmaceutical. United States Patent 5028632, 1991.

[34] Fuisz RC. Method of producing compacted dispersible systems. United States Patent 4997856, 1991.

[35] Fuisz RC. Dispersed systems and method of manufacture. United States Patent 5011532, 1991.

[36] Fuisz RC, Cherukuri SR. Method of subjecting a protein–containing material to flash flow processing and product thereof. United States Patent 5503862, 1996.

[37] Fuisz RC, Cherukuri SR. Method of converting a feedstock to a shearform product and product thereof. United States Patent 5456932, 1995.

[38] Fuisz RC. Dispersed systems and method of manufacture. United States Patent 5096492, 1992.

[39] Cherukuri SR, Myers GL, Battist GE, *et al.* Process for forming quickly dispersing comestible unit and product therefrom. United States Patent 5587172, 1996.

[40] Cherukuri SR, Myers GL, Battist GE, *et al.* Process for forming quickly dispersing comestible unit and product therefrom. United States Patent 5895664, 1999.

[41] Mezaache D, Raiden MG, Sanghvi PP, *et al.* Dosage forms containing taste masked active agents. United States Patent 6165512, 2000.

[42] Myers GL, Battist GE, Fuisz RC. Apparatus for making rapidly–dissolving dosage units. United States Patent 5871781, 1999.

[43] Myers GL, Battist GE, Fuisz RC. Process and apparatus for making rapidly dissolving dosage units and product therefrom. United States Patent 5866163, 1999.

[44] Mezaache N, Frisbee SE, Woodall PB, *et al.* Quick dissolve compositions and tablets based thereon. United States Patent 7815937, 2010.

[45] Myers GL, Yang RK, Herman MR. Liquiflash particles and method of making same. United States Patent 5683720, 1997.

[46] Misra TK, Currington JW, Kamath SV, *et al.* Fast–dissolving comestible units formed under high–speed/high–pressure conditions. United States Patent 5869098, 1999.

[47] Myers GL, Battist GE, Fuisz RC. Process and apparatus for making rapidly dissolving dosage units and product therefrom. United States Patent 5851553, 1998.

[48] Myers GL, Battist GE, Fuisz RC. Process and apparatus for making rapidly dissolving dosage units and product therefrom. United States Patent 5622719, 1997.

[49] Myers GL, Battist GE, Fuisz RC. Delivery of controlled–release systems(s). United States Patent 5567439, 1996.

[50] Sastry SV, Nyshadham JR, Fix JA. Recent technological advances in oral drug delivery - a review. Pharm Sci Technol Today 2000; 3(4): 138-45. [http://dx.doi.org/10.1016/S1461-5347(00)00247-9] [PMID: 10754543]

[51] Yoo J, Kumar S, Monkhouse DC. Dosage form exhibiting rapid disperse properties, methods of use and process for the manufacture of same. United States Patent 6471992, 2002.

[52] Sherwood JK, Monkhouse D, Gaylo CM. Complex three–dimensional composite scaffold resistant to delimination. United States Patent 20030114936, 2003.

[53] Wang D, Nguygen CC, Bornancini ER, *et al.* The effect of media type, volume, and temperature on the dispersion time of quick–dispersing tablets made by the TheriFormTM process AAPS Annual Meeting.

[54] Lee K-J, Kang A, Delfino JJ, *et al.* Evaluation of critical formulation factors in the development of a rapidly dispersing captopril oral dosage form. Drug Dev Ind Pharm 2003; 29(9): 967-79. [http://dx.doi.org/10.1081/DDC-120025454] [PMID: 14606661]

[55] Yu DG, Shen XX, Branford-White C, Zhu LM, White K, Yang XL. Novel oral fast-disintegrating drug delivery devices with predefined inner structure fabricated by Three-Dimensional Printing. J Pharm Pharmacol 2009; 61(3): 323-9. [http://dx.doi.org/10.1211/jpp.61.03.0006] [PMID: 19222904]

[56] Katstra WE, Palazzolo RD, Rowe CW, Giritlioglu B, Teung P, Cima MJ. Oral dosage forms fabricated by three dimensional printing. J Control Release 2000; 66(1): 1-9. [http://dx.doi.org/10.1016/S0168-3659(99)00225-4] [PMID: 10708873]

[57] Yu DG, Yang XL, Huang WD, Liu J, Wang YG, Xu H. Tablets with material gradients fabricated by three-dimensional printing. J Pharm Sci 2007; 96(9): 2446-56. [http://dx.doi.org/10.1002/jps.20864] [PMID: 17497729]

[58] Wang C-C, Tejwani Motwani MR, Roach WJ, *et al.* Development of near zero-order release dosage forms using three-dimensional printing (3-DP) technology. Drug Dev Ind Pharm 2006; 32(3): 367-76. [http://dx.doi.org/10.1080/03639040500519300] [PMID: 16556541]

[59] Yu DG, Branford-White C, Ma ZH, Zhu LM, Li XY, Yang XL. Novel drug delivery devices for providing linear release profiles fabricated by 3DP. Int J Pharm 2009; 370(1-2): 160-6. [http://dx.doi.org/10.1016/j.ijpharm.2008.12.008] [PMID: 19118612]

[60] Rowe CW, Katstra WE, Palazzolo RD, Giritlioglu B, Teung P, Cima MJ. Multimechanism oral dosage forms fabricated by three dimensional printing. J Control Release 2000; 66(1): 11-7. [http://dx.doi.org/10.1016/S0168-3659(99)00224-2] [PMID: 10708874]

[61] Gbureck U, Vorndran E, Müller FA, Barralet JE. Low temperature direct 3D printed bioceramics and biocomposites as drug release matrices. J Control Release 2007; 122(2): 173-80. [http://dx.doi.org/10.1016/j.jconrel.2007.06.022] [PMID: 17655962]

[62] Yu DG, Zhu L-M, Branford-White CJ, Yang XL. Three-dimensional printing in pharmaceutics: promises and problems. J Pharm Sci 2008; 97(9): 3666-90. [http://dx.doi.org/10.1002/jps.21284] [PMID: 18257041]

CHAPTER 5

Patent Innovations in Fast Dissolving/ Disintegrating Dosage Forms

Kalpana Nagpal[1,*], **Shailendra K. Singh**[2] and **D. N. Mishra**[2]

[1] *Amity Institute of Pharmacy, Amity University, Noida, Uttar Pradesh 201303, India*

[2] *Department of Pharmaceutical Sciences, Guru Jambheshwar University of Science & Technology, Hisar125001, Haryana, India*

Abstract: The conventional oral drug delivery system, in spite of ease of administration and convenience of therapy, is associated with certain limitations especially for paediatrics, geriatrics, unconscious and travelling patients. To make the safe and effective usage of drugs, fast dissolving/disintegrating dosage forms (FDDFs) serves as an effective approach for rapid delivery of drugs. The present chapter is an effort to describe the various aspects of FDDFs including the different patented products and technologies, which are either commercially available in the market or in development pipeline. A systematic study of various patents related to formulation, packaging and evaluation of FDDFs is also provided. Thus, this chapter provides most comprehensive insights on different FDDFs technologies through their patents and innovative steps described therein.

Keywords: Advatab™, Disintegration, Dissolution, DuraSolv®, Dysphagia, Film, FlashDose®, Foamburst™, Frosta®, Lyoc™, Micap™, OraQuick®, OraSolv®, Proprietary, QuickSolv®, Soluleaves™, Superdisintegrant, Tablet, Technology, Trademark, Wafertab™, Wowtab®, Xgel™, Ziplets®, Zydis®.

1. INTRODUCTION

Drug delivery through oral route is a convenient and preferred route of administration. Solid dosage forms offer many advantages such as accurate dosing, stability, ease in manufacturing, small size of package and improved patient compliance [1], but they possess certain limitations like inconvenience or impracticability to be swallowed by paediatric (as their muscular and nervous systems are not fully developed), geriatric, dysphagic, psychiatric, travelling (no

* **Corresponding author Dr. Kalpana Nagpal:** Amity Institute of Pharmacy, Amity University, Noida, Uttar Pradesh 201303, India; Tel: +91-8447883427, E-mail: kalpananagpal@gmail.com, knchaswal@amity.edu

Vikas Anand Saharan (Ed.)

ready access to water), unconscious patients or nauseating and/or vomiting patients [1 - 7]. According to European Pharmacopoeia, "Orodispersible tablets are uncoated tablets intended to be placed in the mouth, where they disperse rapidly before being swallowed". The Center for Drug Evaluation and Research (CDER), US FDA defined Oral Disintegrating Tablets (ODT) as "A solid dosage form containing medicinal substances, which disintegrates rapidly, usually within a matter of seconds, when placed upon the tongue." FDDF offer certain advantages over effervescent tablets, dry syrups and chewing gums/tablets. The administration of effervescent tablets/granules requires water, whereas, the chewing gums/tablets cannot be chewed by elderly patients and for paediatrics unpleasant taste reduces their acceptability, if the taste masking coat get ruptured during mastication [4]. Moreover, FDDF offer more accurate dosing to patients as compared to liquid dosage forms. Thus, FDDF offers certain advantages [4, 5, 8 - 12] as well as certain limitations [1, 4, 5, 8 - 12], which are discussed in earlier chapters. FDDF is a solid unit dosage form usually in the form of tablets, although orodispersible films and modified hard gelatin capsules are also available. This type of dosage forms disintegrate and/or dissolve rapidly in the saliva without chewing or requiring water to swallow. The FDA uses the term '*Orally Disintegrating Tablets*' to describe them, whereas, European Pharmacopoeia enlisted them as '*Orodispersible Tablet*' [1]. Moreover, these are also referred in many literature as Melt-In-Mouth Tablets, Fast Dissolving, Oral Disintegrating, Mouth Dissolving, Porous Tablets, Quick Dissolving or Rapid Disintegrating Tablets [4, 5].

Patents provide legal protection to inventor(s) for their inventions, which includes new medicines also. The inventor(s) must satisfy the three conditions, *i.e.* novelty, inventiveness (non-obviousness) and usefulness. In patenting, the inventor(s) is given a limited period of time of exclusivity, generally 20 years, to make and sell a product incorporating his/her invention. In return, to the inventor(s) make the invention public, thereby encouraging the continuation of scientific discovery. In this way, the inventor(s) can easily regain their significant investment in research and development. Such an activity acts as a fundamental incentive to innovative activities. The individuals also get recognitions for their creative idea and profitable reward for their marketable inventions. Such incentives encourage innovations and assure continuous improvements in the quality of human life. In nut shell, patents provide not only protection to the intellectual rights of researchers but also serve as an source of inspiration to future researchers [13, 14].

FDDFs cater to the needs of patients, formulation scientist as well as the manufacturer [15]. An improved version of the existing drug may come in the market, especially for the drugs whose patent is about to expire. The market of the product will be extended exclusively, which in turn would benefit the manufacturer and has attracted lots of attention from the medium and large scale manufacturers of developing countries, who cannot afford heavy expenditure on search of new chemical entity.

2. PATENTED TECHNOLOGIES IN THE MARKET

2.1. Technologies in Fast Dissolving Tablets

The most common patented technologies used for formulating fast dissolving/ disintegrating tablets (FDTs) are briefly discussed hereunder [1, 4, 5, 16, 17]. The major advantages and the disadvantages associated with them are compared in Table **1**. Table **2** enlists some marketed products based on FDTs.

Table 1. A comparison of various patented technologies for FDTs.

Technology	Advantages	Disadvantages
Zydis®	• Light weight, eye pleasing, good to taste and touch product • Convenient and self preserving as final water content too low	• Expensive as freeze drying is involved and need special blister pack due to high fragile tablets • Poor stability • Maximum dose of water soluble drug is limited to approximately 60mg [27]
OraSolv®	• Two fold taste masking than Zydis® product • Low degree of compaction	• Appearance not too good like Zydis®; more brittle and weaker than conventional tablet
DuraSolv®	• Has durable product with higher mechanical strength than OraSolv® and can be packed in conventional blister pack • Faster and cost effective production • Structural integrity may be compromised with high dose of the drug Have fast disintegration time (<1 min) and hardness app.15-20 N	• Low drug loading capacity because the technology is not compatible with large dose of API • Not suitable for incorporation of taste masked coated pellets
Wowtab®	• Tablets so formed posses significant hardness and dissolution time; suitable for both conventional blister and bottle pack; more stable product than Zydis® or OraSolv® • Offers good taste as well as mouth feel and may incorporate various classes of drugs	• No significant change in bioavailability.
Flash Tab®	• Utilise most of the same excipients as in conventional tablets	-

(Table 1) contd.....

Technology	Advantages	Disadvantages
OraQuick®	• Faster and more efficient production as no solvent is used; appropriate for heat sensitive materials • Tablet compression do not disturb taste masking	-
FlashDose®	• Quick dissolution as product offer a very high surface area for dissolution • Tablets are highly porous and have pleasant mouth-feel	• Use of high temperature used may limit the use of drugs sensitive to heat, moisture and humidity • The dosage form can accommodate only up to 600 mg of drug.
Frosta®	• Disintegration within 5 and 50 s, depending on the tablet size • low manufacturing cost with one-step granulation processing • strong mechanical property with friability less than 1%, stable product offering multitablet packaging	• In general, the proportion of the two components (plastic material and water-penetration-enhancer) needs to be adjusted adequately so as to obtain the optimal properties in tablets
Advatab™	• Superior taste-masking offering controlled drug release capabilities • High dose capacity per dosage unit as the product is robust tablet-packaging choices include both standard bottles and push-through blister	-
Shearform®	• Tablets highly porous; offer pleasant mouth feel due to rapid solubilisation of sugars in presence of saliva	• Tablets are soft, friable and highly moisture sensitive
Lyoc™	• In contrast to OraSolv® and DuraSolv®, Lyoc™ technology is a lyophilised dosage form; offer greater porosity, shorter disintegration times (2-20 s)	• Yields a moisture sensitive product
Ziplets®	• Good mechanical strength of the tablets; handling problems may be avoided • Satisfactory features can be obtained at high dose (450 mg) and high weight (850 mg)	• As soluble component dissolves, rate of water diffusion in to tablet is decreased because of formation of viscous concentrated solution

2.1.1. Zydis®

FDTs in this method (www.catalent.com/zydis) are produced by freeze drying of the drug contained in the matrix (the matrix is usually made of gelatin). It utilises colours, sweeteners, ion-exchange resins and micro-encapsulation technique for taste masking. The processing involves the two main steps:

In Step 1, there is the formation of bulk preparation of an aqueous drug solution or suspension. It is followed by its subsequent precise dosing into pre-formed blisters. The tablet shape is formed by such blister and is an important component of product pack.

Table 2. List of US FDA approved products available in the market [17, 36].

Patented Technology	Products	Name of the Company	Composition/API
Zydis®	Claritin Reditab	R. P. Scherer/Schering Plough, Kenilworth, USA.	Micronised loratadine (10mg), citric acid, mannitol, gelatine and mint flavour
	Feldene Melt	Pfizer Inc, NY, USA.	Piroxicam (10 or 20 mg), mannitol, gelatin, aspartame and citric acid anhydrous
	Maxalt-MLT	R.P.Scherer/Merck & Co., NY, USA.	Rizatriptan (5 or 10 mg), mannitol, gelatin, aspartame and peppermint flavour
	Pepcid. RPD	Merck & CO., NY USA	Famotidine (20 or 40 mg), mannitol, gelatin and aspartame
	Zyprexa Zydis®	R.P.Scherer/Eli Lilly, Indianapolis, USA	Olanzapine (5, 10, 15 or 20 mg), mannitol, gelatin, aspartame, methylparaben sodium and propylparaben sodium
	Zofran ODT	R.P.Scherer/Glaxo Wellcome, Middlesex, UK.	Ondansetron (4 or 8 mg), mannitol, gelatin, aspartame, methylparaben sodium, propylparaben sodium and strawberry flavour
	Zelapar	Valeant Pharm	Selegiline HCl (1.25 mg),gelatin, mannitol, glycine, aspartame, citric acid, yellow iron oxide and grapefruit flavour
	Klonopin	Roche	Clonazepam (0.125 mg, 0.25 mg, 0.5 mg 1 mg, 2 mg) gelatin, mannitol, methylparaben sodium, propylparaben sodium and xanthum gum
	Dimetapp Quick Dissolve	Wyeth	Brompheniramine maleate and phenylpropanolamine HCl
	Feldene melt	Pfizer	Piroxicam, gelatin, mannitol, aspartame and citric acid
Zydis®	Maxalt-MLT	Merck	Rizatriptan benzoate, lactose monohydrate, microcrystalline cellulose, pregelatinised starch, ferric oxide red and magnesium stearate

(Table 2) contd.....

Patented Technology	Products	Name of the Company	Composition/API
OraSolv®	Remeron Soltab	CIMA/Organon, Glaxo Wellcome, Middlesex, UK	Mirtazepine (15, 30 or 45 mg), mannitol, aspartame, citric acid, crospovidone, Avicel, $NaHCO_3$, HPMC and magnesium stearate povidone, PMA, starch, sucrose, orange flavour
	Tempra First Tabs	CIMA/Mead Johnson, Bristol Myers Squibb, USA.	Acetaminophen (80 or 160 mg), mannitol (currently available in Canada)
	Nulev	CIMA/Schwarz Pharma.	Hyoscyamine sulphate (0.125 mg), aspartame, colloidal silicon dioxide crospovidone, mint flavour, magnesium stearate, mannitol and Avicel
	Zoming ZMT	CIMA/AstraZeneca, Wilmington, USA.	Zolmitriptan (2.5 mg), mannitol, aspartame, citric acid anhydrous, crospovidone, Avicel, sodium bicarbonate and magnesium stearate colloidal silicon dioxide and orange flavour
	Alavert	Wyeth CONS	Loratadine (10 mg) aspartame, citric acid, colloidal silicone dioxide, corn syrup solid, crospovidone, magnesium stearate, mannitol, microcrystalline cellulose, sodium bicarbonate, modified food starch and artificial flavours
	Kemstro	Schwarz Pharma	Baclofen (10 mg, 20 mg) aspartame, colloidal silicon dioxide and crospovidone, magnesium stearate, mannitol, microcrystalline cellulose, natural and artificial orange flavour and povidone
DuraSolv®	GasterD	Yamanouchi Pharma Tech., Inc.	Famotidine
	Fluxid	Schwarz Pharma	Famotidine, citric acid, colloidal silicone dioxide, corn starch, crospovidone, hypromellose, magnesium stearate, mannitol, MCC, methacrylic acid copolymer, natural and artificial cherry flavour, sodium bicarbonate, sucralose and sucrose
Wowtab®	Nurofen FlashTab	Ethypharm	Ibuprofen
	Relivia FlashDose®	Fuisz Technology Ltd.	Tramadol HCl
	Rybix ODT	Shionogi INC	Tramadol HCl, aspartame, copovidone, crospovidone, ethyl cellulose, magnesium stearate, mint flavour, mannitol and silicone dioxide
Advatab™	Lamictal *ODT*	Co-developed by Eurand and GSK	Lamotrigine, artificial Cherry flavour and crospovidone

(Table 2) contd.....

Patented Technology	Products	Name of the Company	Composition/API
Frosta® Technology	Propulsid Quicksolv	Janssen Pharmaceutica	Cisapride monohydrate (Formulation is withdrawn from US)
Advatab®	Risperdal-M-Tab	Janssen Pharmaceutica	Risperidone, Amberlite resin, gelatin, mannitol, glycine, simethicone, carbomer, sodium hydroxide, aspartame, red ferric oxide and peppermint oil
	Spasfon Lyoc	Farmalyoc	Phloroglucinol hydrate
	Cibalgina DueFast	Eurand International	Ibuprofen
QuickSolv®	Propulsid Quicksolv	Janssen Pharmaceutica	Cisapride monohydrate (Formulation is withdrawn from US)

In Step 2, the filled blisters are passed through specially designed cryogenic freezing process. This process controls the ultimate size of the ice crystals and ensures the porous matrix of tablets, which may facilitate their rapid disintegration. This is followed by transferring the frozen units to large-scale freeze dryers for the sublimation process to remove residual moisture from tablets [26, 27].

2.1.2. OraSolv®

This technique (CIMA Labs) utilises low compression force for making the tablets and is based on effervescence mechanism to release CO_2 when such a tablet comes in contact with saliva. The gas so released will help tablets to disintegrate with a pleasing sensation in the mouth of the patient. The organic acid crystals are coated using a stoichiometrically low quantity of base material as compared to the acid and comparatively greater particle size of base material in such a way that the base gets uniformly coated onto the acid crystals. The initiation of the coating process is done by the addition of a reaction initiator (such as purified water) and proceeded until the completion of base coating on organic acid crystals, which can be determined by measuring CO_2 evolution. This effervescent couple after mixing with polymer-coated drug particles and other required excipients, is utilised for the preparation of tablets [18].

Some workers have prepared the microparticles, using this technique, by dispersing the drug into a suitable polymer (such as ethyl cellulose, methyl cellulose, acrylate or methacrylic acid resins) along with other excipients called release promoters (like, mannitol and magnesium oxide). The drug and mannitol (as release promoter) are added to the polymeric dispersion under stirring; followed by the addition of magnesium oxide, drying for an hour at 50°C, de-lumping and drying for another hour at the same temperature. Further, the resulting mixture is screened (8 mesh) and dried for one hour at 60°C. Such microparticles are mixed with effervescent agents (the combination of organic acid like, citric, fumaric, tartaric, malic, adipic, succinic acids, *etc.* and carbonate source like sodium and potassium carbonate and bicarbonate salts) and other excipients and subsequently compressed to tablets [19, 20].

2.1.3. DuraSolv®

It is the second generation technology (Cima Labs) for preparing fast dissolving tablets. Here, higher compression pressure is utilised for compression of tablets. The ingredients used in the formulation is non-direct compression fillers (*e.g.* dextrose, mannitol, sorbitol, lactose, sucrose, *etc.* with particle size ranging from 20-65 μm) which show fast dissolution as well as minimises the gritty feeling of the direct compression fillers. The dry blend of non-compressible fillers, taste masking excipients and Active Pharmaceutical Ingredient (API) are then compressed into tablets using a conventional rotary tablet press.

2.1.4. Wowtab®

In this technique, two different types of saccharides are combined in a way so as to produce tablet with adequate hardness and fast dissolution rate (Yamanouchi Pharma Technologies, Norman, Oklahoma). Low mouldability sugar coated with highly mouldable sugar and exposed to a specific humidity condition. The high compressible saccharide used in the form of binder solution was present in amorphous form after granulation. The change from amorphous to crystalline by conditions involved in preparation of granules are obtained by spraying maltose solution and subsequent compression. The resulting tablets have higher hardness by increasing adhesion between particles. Maintaining a low disintegration, the conditioning process can be utilised to achieve sufficient hardness of a tablet.

2.1.5. Flashtab®

In this technique, microgranules (microcrystals) of the drug are used in tablet formulations (Ethypharm, http://www.ethypharm.com/drug-technologies/ proprietary-technologies.html). Microgranules of the drug may be prepared by coacervation, microencapsulation or extrusion spheronisation and subsequently compressed utilising conventional tableting methods to obtain FDTs. For producing quicker disintegration, an appropriate disintegrating agent and swelling agent are used in combination with the coated drug particles.

2.1.6. OraQuick®

The patented taste masking technology of KV pharmaceuticals (http://www.kvpharmaceutical.com) is OraQuick®. For taste masking process, this technique does not utilise solvents of any kind. Therefore, it leads to faster and efficient production of tablets with sufficient mechanical strength maintaining the taste masking property after tablet compression.

2.1.7. FlashDose®

FlashDose® (Fuisz Technologies, Ltd.) utilise a unique Shearform™ technology (Fuisz Technologies, Ltd.) and Ceform TI™ technology (Chantilly biopharm LLC; http://chantillybiopharma.com/patents.html) spinning mechanism to eliminate the bitter taste of the medicament and to prepare a matrix with a 'floss' like structure made of saccharides (such as sucrose, dextrose, lactose and fructose) at temperatures ranging between 180–266°F [21] and other polysaccharides such as polymaltodextrins and polydextrose. These polysaccharides should be used at 30–40% lower temperature than sucrose for thermolabile drugs [22].

The manufacturing process can be divided into the following four steps:

I. *Floss Blend:* The first step of this technique involves blending of 80% w/w sucrose is with mannitol/dextrose and 1% w/w surfactant so as to form the floss mixture. In this mixture, the surfactant helps to convert the sugar to crystalline state and also acts as a crystallisation enhancer to maintain the structural integrity of the floss fibres. This process helps in retaining the dispersed drug in the matrix and hence minimise migration of the drug out of the mixture [23].

II. *Floss Processing:* Flash heat and flash flow processes are utilised to produce matrix from the carrier material. The machine used is similar to a 'cotton-candy' formation machine, which consists of a spinning head and heating elements. The heat induces an internal flow condition of the carrier material which is then followed by its exit through the spinning head (2000–3600 rpm). The head flings the floss under centrifugal force and draws into long, amorphous and thin floss fibres, which are utilised in Step 3 [24 - 26].

III. *Floss Chopping and Conditioning:* The third step involves the conversion of fibres into smaller particles using a high shear mixer granulator. Thus is followed by their conditioning by partial crystallisation through an ethanol treatment (1%), which is sprayed onto the floss. This solution is subsequently evaporated to impart improved flow and cohesive properties to the floss [21].

IV. *Blending and Compression:* In the final step of the process, the chopped and conditioned floss fibres are blended with the drug along with other required excipients and compressed into tablets. A curing step is also carried out which involves the exposure of the dosage forms to elevated temperature and humidity conditions (40°C and 85% RH for 15 min). This is done to improve the mechanical strength of the tablets and is expected to cause crystallisation of the floss material resulting in binding and bridging to improve the structural strength of the dosage form [22].

2.1.8. Quicksolv®

Quicksolv® technology is owned by Janssen, a subsidiary of Johnson & Johnson, New Brunswick, NJ. This technology yields product by freezing an aqueous dispersion/solution of the drug containing matrix and then drying it by removing the water using excess of alcohol. With this, the final form obtained is very rapidly disintegrated but has low drug content and can be used for those drugs which are insoluble in the extraction solvent. For this technology to work better, the drug must have relatively low aqueous solubility, fine particle size <50 µm [27] and good aqueous stability in the suspension [9, 27]. The most common problem associated with water soluble drugs is the formation of eutectic mixtures resulting in freezing-point depression and the formation of a glassy solid on freezing, which might collapse on drying due to the loss of supporting structure during sublimation process [9, 10, 27].

2.1.9. Frosta®

The technique by Akina, Inc., (http:// www. akinainc.com /frosta. html), involves compressing highly plastic granules at low pressure for preparing them fast dissolving/disintegrating. All the components (the highly plastic granules, a water penetration enhancer and a wet binder) have their unique roles in the formulation of FDTs. The porous plastic material is mixed with water penetration enhancer and then they are granulated with suitable binder. It utilises the conventional wet granulation process and tablet press for cost effective production of tablets.

2.1.10. AdvaTab™

This technique by Adare Pharmaceuticals, (http://www.adarepharma.com/) is distinct from other FDTs technologies in that it can be combined with Microcaps® and Diffucaps® technology to achieve taste masking and customised release profiles [28]. The products created by the pairing of AdvaTab™ with Microcaps® offer the dual advantage of a patient preferred dosage form, together with a superior taste and smooth mouth feel. Traditional tablets are produced using an internal lubrication system in which lubricant is incorporated throughout the tablet blend to achieve lubrication of surfaces of tablet and contact parts of machine. With the use of internal lubricant, the tablet is made hydrophobic, which necessitates the use of higher tablet compression forces for a given tablet hardness. Due to low compression force required after applying lubricant, the tablets do not repel liquids such as saliva when ingested. Consequently, AdvaTab™ tablets are robust, disintegrate rapidly in the oral cavity and the tablet compression step does not lead to breakage of the drug particles.

2.1.11. Ziplets®

Ziplets® technology, owned by Eurand International S.P.A., (http: //www. eurand .com), utilise water insoluble drugs or coated microparticles of drugs. An excellent physical resistance to the tablet is provided by the addition of a suitable amount of a water insoluble inorganic excipients and an optimal disintegration is achieved with the use of disintegrants [29]. The use of water insoluble inorganic excipients offers a better enhancement of disintegration of tablets in comparison to the most commonly used water soluble sugars or salts which tend to dissolve rather disintegrate forming a concentrated viscous solution which reduces the rate of water diffusion into the tablet core [29, 30].

2.1.12. Lyoc®

Lyoc® is a lyophilised dosage form technique, which may be utilised for drug molecules having varying physicochemical properties (http://www.cimalabs.com/technology/lyoc). The components of the tablets produced by this technology include the drug, fillers, binders, flavours, sweeteners, surfactants, absorption enhancers and suspending agents. The use of additives and preservatives in the formulation is not necessary, as the conditions experienced by the drug formulation during the manufacturing process is lyophilisation. The process encompasses formation of an aqueous solution, suspension or emulsion of the drug compound and excipients, followed by the optimisation of liquid homogeneous formulation. The formulation is freeze-dried, after distributing them into preformed blisters by freezing at a very low temperature (below -40°C) Followed by exposure to specific pressure conditions that results in sublimation (direct ice to water vapour transformation). This will remove water from the formulation producing tablets with greater porosity, allowing for shorter disintegration times (in the range of 2 to 20 s). The process, being operated in absence of organic solvents, is environmentally friendly and cost effective. The usual drug product strengths range is 500 μg to 500 mg using this technology. In order to meet virtually any immediate or controlled release requirement, the release of the drug from the formulation can be tailored [31].

FDTs have also been successfully formulated and evaluated by phase transition of sugar alcohols [32]. Recently, multiparticulate systems [33] for tablet formation and swelling induced FDTs by microwave irradiation have been carried out for the formulation of fast dissolving tablets [34].

Beside this, ODTs of Ibuprofen have also been formulated by application of the new Sedem ODT Expert System [35]. A number of products based on these technologies are now available in the market and are revolutionising the tablets and pills domain in the healthcare system. The FDA approved products available in the market are summarised in Table **2**.

2.2. Technologies in FDFs

The second dosage form for fast release of API is fast dissolving films. Few of them are described hereunder:

2.2.1. Soluleaves™

Soluleaves™ technology is used to formulate a variety of oral delivery films that can incorporate API, colours and flavours (http://www.bioprogress.com/pages/content/index.asp? PageID=50). Such films can be designed to dissolve rapidly on contact with saliva, quickly releasing the API and flavours [37 - 39]. The quick release quality makes edible films an excellent delivery method for a large range of drug products, requiring fast release in the mouth, especially useful for paediatric or elderly patients' having difficulty swallowing conventional tablets or capsules. The conditions like cough/cold, gastrointestinal and pain nutritional deficiency can be treated using this delivery system. The films can also be tailored to adhere to mucous membranes for release of API over 15 minutes. This technology may also be applied to flavour-release products such as mouth fresheners, confectionery and vitamin products.

2.2.2. Wafertab™

The patented drug delivery system, Wafertab™ (http: //www.bioprogress.com /pages/ content/ index.asp? PageID=50), uses a unique process to prepare drug-loaded thin films for their topical or oral applications [37 - 39]. Ingestible filmstrip is prepared incorporating API pharmaceutical actives in a film prepared by casting and subsequent drying. The formulated film provides rapid dissolution and release of API when it comes into contact with saliva in the mouth. Films can be flavoured for improved taste masking. The API is precisely dosed and integrated into the body of a pre-manufactured XGEL™ film thus preventing exposure of API to unnecessary heat and moisture and thereby enhancing product stability. The Wafertab™ films offer many possibilities for innovative product design, enabling multiple films with different APIs to be bonded together such as a variety of shapes and sizes. This is a good method for delivery of medicines for fast release of APIs and for use by patients having difficulty in swallowing conventional tablets/capsules.

2.2.3. Foamburst™

The patent for Foamburst™ (http://www. uk-wire.com /cgi-bin/ articles/ 2004 112207 001146 35f.html, BioProgress PLC) was granted in September 2004 for capsules made of foamed film [37 - 39]. The product is a variant of the Soluleaves™ technology, where an inert gas is passed into the film during production resulting into a film with honeycomb like highly porous structure, which dissolves rapidly with a pleasant sensation. The voids created during the formation of the film may be gas-filled, empty or filled with other materials to produce specific taste-burst characteristics or to deliver APIs. The structure is light and the honeycomb shape results in capsules that dissolve rapidly, causing a melt-in-the mouth sensation. This technique has attracted a great deal of interest from food and confectionary manufacturers as a means of carrying and releasing flavours.

2.2.4. XGel™

XGel™ film technology was developed by BioProgress. It is at the heart of Meldex International's intellectual property, used in all its film systems and ingestible dosage delivery technologies [37 - 39]. The technology offers unique product benefits for healthcare and pharmaceuticals. It is approved on religious grounds as it is non animal-derived, suitable for vegetarians and GMO (Genetically Modified Organisms) free. Furthermore, continuous production and processing provides an economic and competitive manufacturing platform. The films, incorporating the API, can also be coloured, layered, taste masked and made capable of being enteric coated. The film systems can be made to encapsulate any oral dosage form and is soluble in either cold or hot water. The film is comprised of a range of different water-soluble polymers, specifically optimised for the intended use. The ingredients of the XGel™ are well known and generally regarded as safe (GRAS).

2.2.5. Micap™

Micap PLC signed an option agreement in 2004 to combine its expertise in microencapsulation technology with the BioProgress water-soluble films [37 - 39]. The aim of the agreement was providing new delivery mechanisms for the $1.4bn global market for smoking cessation products (SCPs) [37 - 39].

3. RECENT PATENTS IN FAST DISSOLVING DOSAGE FORMS

3.1. Patents in FDTs

Cary et al. (1991), through US patent 5073374, introduced a fast dissolving buccal tablet for administering a medicament that includes the API, a pharmaceutically acceptable lubricant (preferably sodium dodecyl sulphate, 1-3% w/w) and a water soluble sugar (directly compressible), such as sorbitol, combined such that the buccal tablet dissolves in about one minute [40]. The rapid delivery of the drug from the buccal tablets unexpectedly obviates the need for an adhesive, which would otherwise be required to prevent the patient from swallowing the dosage form. The preferred sugar is sorbitol, particularly sorbitol N.F. and /or spray dried sorbitol in an amount ranging from 90-99% w/w. The final formulation desirably have a diameter of about quarter a inch and a thickness of about 0.05 inches [40].

Wehling et al. (1993), in US patent 5178878, described a taste masking approach for tablets containing microparticles which rupture upon chewing and provide immediate release of API contained in the microparticles [41]. These microparticles release about 70% of API within 30 minutes, when tested using USP XXII apparatus 2, 900 ml water as dissolution medium at 50 rpm using. These microparticles are incorporated in a tablet along with an effervescent disintegration agent. When the tablet comes in contact with the saliva during chewing, the effervescent disintegration agent aids in rapid dissolution of the tablet and permitting quick release of the API from microparticles and also provides effervescence equivalent to about 20-60 cm^3 of gas for fizzing sensation and swallowing of the microparticles. Very effective taste masking is achieved by the combination of microencapsulation and effervescence mechanisms [41].

Wehling et al. (1993), in US patent 5223264, disclosed formation of an oral paediatric vitamin supplement tablets, comprising of at least one effervescent disintegrating agent (20-25% w/w) and at least one component comprising of vitamin or mineral effective as paediatric dose, having good organoleptic sensation and size and shape adapted for direct oral administration to children

[42]. Effervescences were achieved using the mixture of an organic acid and a base selected from carbonate, bicarbonate or their mixture. Such effervescence not only masks the taste of the tablet giving a pleasant oral organoleptic sensation but also improves the disintegration of the tablet [42].

Wehling et al. (1996), in US patent 5503846, described preparation of a base coated and a highly compressible acid formulation [18]. A stabilised effervescent dosage form comprises of an acid sensitive API and effervescent couple is intimately mixed therewith. Both an effervescent couple and an acid sensitive API are mixed in such a way that the in the effervescent couple (edible acid as core and base as its coating) the edible base remain slight less than the base required stoichiometrically. The coating of the base retards the reaction between acid and acid sensitive API to have an acid neutralisation capacity of less than about 5.0 meq. When the acid sensitive API is a gastro-intestinally active agent, the ratio of API to effervescent couple ranges from about 1:300 to about 1:0.25. The preparation method involves charging at least one particulate edible acid and at least one particulate edible base selected from the group consisting of sodium bicarbonate and potassium bicarbonate into a reactor keeping in mind that the edible base should have a particle size less than the particle size of the particulate edible acid, followed by mixing particulate, adding liquid to particulate in reactor with continuous mixing and allowing the particulate to react in the presence of liquid for a period of time so as to form a coating of edible base around the particulate edible acid. This reaction can be terminated by applying vacuum and heat to said reactor, while physically tilting said reactor, so as to provide for rapid and even liquid removal from particulate and so as to prevent a coating of edible base from being abraded from edible acid; and discharging particulate, whereby particulate edible acid is coated with edible base and has an acid neutralisation capacity of less than about 5.0 meq [18].

Allen et al. (1996), through European patent EP0743850, disclosed a support matrix, produced using standard spray-drying techniques (polymeric primary component, *e.g.* non-hydrolysed gelatin, a first polypeptide and a second solubilising component, *i.e.* hydrolysed gelatin), a solid dosage form and its process thereof, which disintegrate or dissolve in a few seconds on coming in contact with oral cavity fluid [43]. The hydrolysed gelatin helps the unmodified gelatin as a structural component of the matrix. It also increases the solubility of the matrix. In order to have a net positive charge on the protein and protein hydrolysate, their solution is made acidic and individual protein molecules become repellent to each other, when in solution. This will reduce the tendency for the protein molecule to cling to each other. Also, an effervescent agent (that will help in the disintegration of the dosage form), a binding agent and a flavouring agent may also be added for specific purposes. Firstly, a porous particulate powder is produced that will serve as tablet support. Then, API and other additives are combined with the powder and the mixture is formed into a tablet. In order to enhance the intactness and durability of the tablet, a coating may be applied to its outer surface. The tablets are formulated using very light compression pressure and such tablets have been reported to be of convenient size, stable, easy to dispense, easily transportable, easy to alter the dose and easy to administer. The tablets so formulated are suitable not only for the oral cavity but also for other moist areas of orifices of the body, such as rectum [43].

Alkire et al. (1997), in Patent 5607697, reported a solid pharmaceutical dosage form for direct oral administration which contains a core and a coating [44]. The core consists of many microparticles, comprising one API and a sweetening agent with negative heat of solution (0-80% w/w) selected from mannitol, sorbitol, a mixture of an artificial sweetener and menthol, a mixture of a sugar and menthol, and methyl salicylate that will provide sweetness as well as cooling sensation. The coating material, selected from ethyl cellulose, 5-75% w/w, either retards dissolution of said API in the mouth or masks the objectionable taste of API. The solid dosage form is sized, shaped and have a composition and hardness in such a way that is adapted for direct oral administration and is disintegrable in the mouth so as to release said microparticles [44].

Gergely et al. (1998), in patent 5792473, disclosed a technique for administrating acid sensitive API with hydrophobic properties which may influence the surface tension of water to the patient and result in pleasant-to-drink effervescent solutions [45] The resulting product will be an instant effervescent granular one with acid binding capacity of less than 5 meq. This will avoid the undesired antacids effects (especially advantageous for all H2 blockers. Such tablets dissolve rapidly in water at a temperature of about 15-20°C in less than 2 minutes. To achieve such a dosage form, the acid particles are coated with a small amount of one neutral substance (polymers soluble in water and/or alcohol), which causes a depression of the melting point of the acid grains at the surface, especially sorbitol solution. The melting point depression so caused may protract the re-crystallisation time of the citric acid or of the citrates that have formed, which signifies better compressibility of the effervescent granules over a longer period of time. The next step is anchoring by providing at least one second coating which contains an alkali and/or alkaline earth carbonate and /or bicarbonate, and optionally a partial reaction product of the carbonate or bicarbonate with the same or a different organic acid. The resulting product is claimed to have more shelf life, permits the preparation of substantially smaller tablets; offers a retarded reaction in terms of product preparation and better compressibility into tablets [45].

Acosta-Cuello et al. (1998), patent 5807578, introduce an improved fast melting solid dosage form for quick disintegration when placed in the mouth [46] The primary ingredients of such tablet are API (antacid in general, about 30-50% w/w), an effervescent couple (2-5% w/w of an effervescence base and about 2-5% w/w of an effervescence acid, generally sodium bicarbonate and malic acid), starch as a bulking and disintegrating agent (35-50% w/w, generally corn starch, modified starch or SSG or mixture thereof), a starch degrading enzyme (about 0.04-1% w/w, generally an equal mixture of amylo-glucosidase and alpha amylase) and tablet lubricant (about 2-5% w/w). The formulation is preferably intended to be manufactured in compressed tablet form. The formulation consists of an admixture and direct compression of a mixture of internal phase (consisting of granules) and a powderous external phase. The internal phase is prepared by mixing and sieving the dry ingredients and wet granulating them with purified water and sizing them with a sieve. The granules can then be admixed with powder blend of the external phase ingredients (effervescence acid, starch degrading enzyme, tableting lubricant, a sweetener and an aroma agent). The addition of starch contributes to the palatability, improved salivation and thus rapid ingestion of API and subsequent rapid disintegration of the tablet. The starch degrading enzyme will immediately begin to convert starch to mono and polysaccharides which quickly dissolve in the aqueous environment and further improve the taste of the tablet and increase salivation reducing the dryness in mouth [46].

Katzner et al. (2000), in patent 6155423, disclosed a blister package for containing frangible dosage forms while protecting the dosage forms from damage during transport and opening of the package [47] A blister sheet defines one or more recesses in which frangible dosage forms are disposed and a peel-able sheet of lidding material overlies the recesses to cover the dosage form packed inside. The indications on the pack direct the user for its safe use without damaging the dosage form. An empty space, between each dosage form and the bottom of recess, in which dosage form is disposed, cushions the dosage form from impact, when the package is dropped. Moreover, it offers plurality of unit packages [47].

Pather et al. (2001), in patent 6200604, described a pharmaceutical dosage form, for administering API to the oral cavity for buccal, sublingual or gingival absorption, which contains the orally administrable API along with an effervescent couple and a pH adjusting substance (any buffer system that is not harmful to the oral mucosa), both for promoting the absorption of API [48] The effervescent agent is added as penetration enhancer for influencing oral drug absorption. The effervescent agent acts by reducing the mucosal layer thickness and/or viscosity, tight junction alteration, inducing structural changes in the cell membrane and by inducing the hydrophobic environment within the cellular membrane [48].

Khankari et al. (2001), in patent 6221392, reported less friable (friability less than 2%), yet hard (15-50 Newton) tablets, which can rapidly dissolved in patients' mouth, can be stored, packaged and processed in bulk [49] Such tablets are created from mixture of API with matrix of non-direct compression filler, a wicking agent and a relatively high lubricant content. The tablet matrix comprised at least 60% w/w of the water soluble ingredients. Such tablets can be handled and packaged like other non rapidly dissolving dosage forms.

Makooi-Morehead et al. (2001), through patent 6238695, disclosed a formulation of a compressed tablet comprising a therapeutically effective amount of efavirenz (5-800 mg), a surfactant (preferably sodium lauryl sulphate, 0.1-5% w/w), a disintegrant or a superdisintegrants (1-10% w/w of croscarmellose, crospovidone or SSG), a binder (lactose starch or various sugars), a diluent (lactose or cellulose), a lubricant, a glidant (talc and colloidal silicon dioxide), and optionally additional pharmaceutically acceptable excipients [50]. The presence of one or more disintegrants enhances the dissolution rate of efavirenz in the gastrointestinal tract thereby improving the rate and extent of absorption of efavirenz in the body. To this kind of tablet, a superdisintegrant SSG (>10% w/w, swells 7-12 fold in less than 30 sec) is incorporated. The mixture of efavirenz and SSG is then wet granulated in the presence of an aqueous solution of sodium lauryl sulfate; dried; milled and blended with SSG and additional pharmaceutically acceptable excipients. This is then encapsulated or compressed into tablets of the resulting product [50].

Green et al. (2001), in US patent application 20010055611 A1, described a process for preparing taste masked fast dispersing solid dosage form, wherein prior to freeze drying, the suspension is treated for their delayed release that would at least be sufficient to mask the taste in mouth before swallowing [51] To reduce the sedimentation rate, particles are made coarser (size upto 1 mm) and viscosity was adjusted by reducing the temperature (from about 23-25°C to about 14-20°C) during the holding time in the suspension. This size range would allow the formulator to apply a uniform intact coating on the particles in order to achieve efficient freeze dried dosage forms with slow drug release rate [51].

Karali et al. (2002), in patent application WO/2002/015886, reported a new process for preparation of an oral, fast-melt tablet comprising a step of wet granulating the API (selective cyclooxygenase-2 inhibitory drug) with a binding agent (selected from gums, polypeptides, natural and modified starches, cellulosic materials, alginic acid and salts thereof, polyethylene glycol, poly-vinylpyrrolidone, polymethacrylates, silicate salts and bentonites). These are then blended with the saccharide of low mouldability (may be selected from lactose, mannitol, glucose, sucrose, xylitol, *etc.*) to result in formation of granules [52]. A preferred polypeptide is gelatin; the preferred starches include corn starch and pregelatinised starch; preferred cellulosic materials include MCC, methyl-cellulose, ethylcellulose, hydroxylpropyl cellulose, hydroxylpropylmethylellulose, carboxymethylcellulose and salts thereof, *e.g.* sodium carboxymethyl cellulose; preferred alginic acid salt is sodium alginate) referred silicate salt is magnesium aluminium silicate. One or more binding agents are present in a total amount of about 1-10% w/w, preferably about 1-7.5% w/w, and more preferably about 1-5% w/w of the composition. Moreover, the process may include a step of blending the granules with at least one of a lubricant, wetting agent, hydrophilic polymer, certain clays, a sweetening agent and a flavouring agent to form a tableting blend. This tableting blend is then subjected to compression to form oral fast-melt tablets.

Khankari et al. (2002), in patent 6365182, invented ODTs suitable for use in the delivery of potassium that contains potassium chloride crystals (about 50-80% coated by weight of the tablet, particle size 100-2,000 μm), an extended release coating (10-20% w/w may be selected from the group consisting of: cellulose ethers, cellulose esters, polymethacrylates and copolymers, polyvinylacetate copolymers and polyvinyl pyrrolidone), a rapidly dissolvable sugar or sugar alcohol filler (10-35% w/w, selected from the group consisting of mannitol, lactose, sucrose, maltose, dextrose, sorbitol, xylitol, maltitol, lactitol and maltodextrins), binder (0-15% w/w, selected from MCC, alginic acid, sodium alginate and starch), disintegrant (3-10% w/w selected from PVP, SSG, CCS, MCC and starch) and an effervescent couple (0-15% w/w, 5-25 meq of potassium) [53] The rapidly dissolving sugar or sugar alcohol filler should have complementary particle size to that of coated potassium chloride crystals and being between about 150 and about 1,500 microns. The tablet is claimed to dissolve in about 45 seconds or less [53].

Siebert et al. (2002), in US patent 6368625, disclosed an oral rapidly disintegrating dosage form which comprised of an API (as powder form or microcapsule), filler, and one in-mouth viscosity enhancing material (1-36% w/w, selected from the group consisting of methylcellulose, HPMC, hydroxyethyl cellulose, Carbopol and silicon dioxide). The microcapsule comprises an enteric, sustained release or extended release coating. Additionally, the tablet contains a filler (selected from sucrose, mannitol, xylitol, lactose and maltose), a binder (0-35% w/w selected from MCC and methyl cellulose), a disintegrant (0-40% w/w, selected from the group consisting of SSG and crospovidone); and optionally an effervescent couple (0-35% w/w).The dosage form is claimed to provide an organoleptically acceptable viscous slurry (viscosity 25,000-500,000 cps) upon the disintegration of the dosage form in a patient's mouth [54] The viscosity of the resulting slurry increases after disintegration of the dosage form in the mouth and this will form an organoleptically pleasant viscous material which retards the spread of insoluble materials including the drug [54].

Johnson et al. (2002), in US patent application 2002/0156056 A1, described a FDDF, which rapidly release the API in the oral cavity and promote pregastric absorption. The pregastric absorption can take place from buccal, sublingual, oropharyngeal and oesophageal absorption. The dosage form is made up of a carrier and an API (a dopamine agonist, an anti-emetic and/or an opioid antagonist for the treatment of Parkinson's disease) [55] Such dosage form may avoid first pass metabolism of the drug in the liver and reach directly into the systemic circulatory system, thereby increasing the bioavailability of dopamine agonists [55].

Aylward et al., (2002), in US patent application 2002/0194815 A1, introduced an assembly for handling and packaging pharmaceutical dosage forms [56]. It includes an infeed structure, a laning structure, and a plenum structure extending from the infeed structure to the laning structure. The infeed structure is for accepting a series of dosage forms including a surface movable in a downstream direction, a laning structure defining a plurality of lanes extending in said downstream direction and having a downstream end, and a plenum structure extending from said infeed structure to said laning structure including a guide portion for guiding dosage forms carried by said surface into said laning structure. The assembly also has a form handling device for receiving dosage forms and transporting dosage forms from said laning structure to a packaging device. There is also a dump gate having a closed position wherein said dump gate blocks said lanes at said downstream ends thereof, whereby dosage forms will accumulate in said lanes when said dump gate is in said closed position and an open position in which said dump gate does not block the lanes. Moreover, a timed controller is there for opening said dump gate after said handling device receives dosage forms whereby debris will be carried downstream out of said laning structure after said form handling device receives dosage forms from said laning structure. The said timed controller further comprises a computer communicating with said form handling device and said dump gate [56].

Furitsu et al. (2004), in US patent 6743443 B1, discussed an intraoral quickly disintegrating tablets of a phosphodiesterase inhibitor for treatment of erectile dysfunctions and a method of its manufacturing [57]. Such tablets can be easily taken up by the aged people, even without water, as this tablet have quick dissolving property and solubility in the mouth along with the strength in retaining the shape during preservation and manufacturing the tablet. The surfactant and/or the water soluble polymer plays an important role of improving the solubility, whereby wetting of the slightly API per se with water is improved. The method will improve the solubility of the slightly soluble API, provide quick disintegration in mouth and ensure a good touch to the tongue during the disintegration of tablet in mouth [57].

Ogasawara et al. (2005), in patent EP1552851 A1, describes formation of small-sized, intra-buccally rapidly disintegrating tablets comprising D-mannitol having an average particle diameter of 31-80 µm, an active ingredient, a disintegrant and stearic acid or a metallic stearate (0.01-0.5% w/w), which have sufficient hardness and able to withstand stresses of handling and transportation [58]. The tablets have a faster disintegration in the oral cavity and a pleasant feeling in a mouth. It further provides a method for producing an intra-buccally rapidly disintegrating tablet containing stearic acid or a metallic stearate by an external lubricating compression method, during which stearic acid or a metallic stearate as a lubricant is previously sprayed to adhere onto the punches and the dies of the tableting machine and the un-adherent surplus of stearic acid or a metallic stearate is recovered [58].

Suga et al. (2005), in patent EP1595533 A1, describes an intra-orally rapidly disintegrating tablets having hardness in the range of 35 N or more and disintegration within 1 minute. Such tablets can be produced easily with a usual tableting machine [59]. In this approach, the cores of the containing a medicament (water soluble API or a containing a API and a pharmaceutically acceptable sugar like mannitol, xylitol, lactose, sucrose, glucose, *etc.* alone or in combination) are coated with a pharmaceutical disintegrating agent (like crystalline cellulose, carmellose, carmellose sodium, crospovidone, starch, sodium carboxymethyl starch and partial gelatinised starch). The ratio of medicament to the sugar is 0.6-500 parts. The disintegrating agent is applied preferably in a form as thin as possible onto the whole of the core. The other ingredients of such tablets may include the fluidising agent, the lubricant, colouring agent and the aromatics.

Jeong et al. (2006), in US patent 20060115529, proposed to change the API into a complex with ion-exchange resins for preparing drug/ion-exchange resin complex [60]. The method being simple in preparation, and offer no uncontrolled burst effect in drug resin complex even at high drug loading. The disadvantage is exchanging capacity of the resin and an incomplete drug release, when tightly cross-linked gel-type resins are used [60]. The complexes of drug with ion-exchange resins may be incorporated into FDDFs.

Casey et al. (2006), US patent application 2006/0280788 A1, basically aimed to the deliver the mast cell stabilisers for their targeted delivery to the colon [61]. The different approaches such as FDT, powder or effervescent have been utilised in this direction. The use of a colon targeted formulation (through oral or rectal administration) allows the direct treatment of colon specific diseases and ailments. Such administration will lead to comparatively less degradation of API. The release of the API can be further delayed or slowed by increasing the amount of water insoluble polymer relative to the amount of water soluble polymer. The claimed invention may significantly enhance the patient ease of use, patient compliance and may also reduce drug misuse by the patient due to increased size of the product and requirement of reconstitution, without compromising pharmacokinetic/pharmacodynamic properties [61].

Monteith et al. (2007), in US patent application 2007/0031349 A1, invented a rapid release pharmaceutical formulation (which can be lingual strip, sublingual strip, oral mist, FDTs, lyophilised wafers, granulated particles and gum) [62]. The formulation consists of at least one PDE5 inhibitor and an orally disintegrating carrier, where the rapid release component results in a therapeutically effective blood concentration of the PDE5 inhibitor in about 1 minute to about 20 minutes. API combination therapy may be opted to address side effects of API. The said formulation is claimed to provide buccal and/or sublingual absorption in a manner that can rapidly achieve effective blood level at comparative lower dose. The approach is relatively non-invasive, easily administrable, well tolerable and has a faster onset of action. It may also avoid the disadvantages encountered with GIT absorption (such as slow absorption and degradation of API by fluid present in the GIT or first pass activation by the liver). Moreover, lower dosage also reduces the side effects associated with the API. Other ingredients of the formulation are pH buffering agents, disintegrants, suitable diluents, binders and conventional flavouring agents [62].

Tomoya Akutagawa et al. (2007), in US patent application US 2009/0117182 A1, have made an effort to overcome the limitations associated with the use of sugar alcohol, a major component in formulation of FDTs [63]. The tablet is composed of a granule that comprises a disintegrant (preferably crospovidone, 4-20% w/w of the whole tablet, average particle size 10-100 μm) inside thereof and coated with a disintegrant, an ordinary apparatus can be used to form a tablet using compression moulding, which has hardness with no practical problem and disintegrates rapidly with good mouthfeel. Drug is preferably kept only in the outside of granules to secure rapid disintegration. It may be added during the granule preparation and/or during the compression moulding. Coating with the disintegrant also contributes to improvement of compression mouldability [63].

Amborn et al. (2007), through patent EP1591360 B1, provides a transition between the infeed structure and the laning structure which is shaped to prevent jamming or a bottleneck effect in this transitional area which may result in damage to or destruction of the dosage forms [64]. It provides an assembly for guiding pharmaceutical dosage forms in a packaging assembly, comprising a surface movable in a downstream direction, a laning structure extending in a lateral direction transverse to the downstream direction and defining a plurality of laterally spaced lanes extending in the downstream direction. The assembly also comprises guide wall structures including a curved portion and a wall structure defining a plenum upstream of the laning structure. The curved portion guides the dosage forms carried by said surface so that dosage forms enter the plenum structure at a plenum entry adjacent a first side of the laning structure and travel laterally toward a second side of the laning structure before entering the lanes. The assembly preferably includes a form handling device for receiving dosage forms and transporting dosage forms from the laning structure to a packaging device. The packaging device may include a top plate and a bottom plate for engaging a packaging material and a lid stock there-between to seal the packaging material and lid stock together, forming packaged dosage forms. The assembly may include a top plate and bottom plate including a plurality of blocks and a base for floating support for the blocks. The lanes may have a downstream end and the assembly may further comprise a dump gate at the downstream end, having an open position and a closed position. A timed controller may be provided for opening the dump gate after the handling device receives dosage forms so that debris will be carried downstream out of the laning structure [64].

Hinrichs et al. (2009), in Patent EP1572157 B1, described that the lipophilic drugs (solubility below 33 g/l in gastric fluid of pH about 1-3) exhibit a low and irregular bioavailability upon oral administration [65]. Thus the objective was to provide adequately solubilised aqueous solution, a formulation comprising a crystallisable lipophilic compound. The sugar glass serves as a matrix for the lipophilic compound or compounds. In principle, the sugar glass can comprise any amorphous pharmaceutically acceptable sugar and/or derivative thereof (the term sugar includes oligo-sugars, poly-sugars and sugar alcohols or polyols, *e.g.* oligo and polysaccharides based upon glucose units (*e.g.* dextran, maltodextrin) fructose units (*e.g.* inulin, levan), mannose units (*e.g.* mannan) and oligo- and polysaccharides based upon galactose units (*e.g.* galactan)). Particularly suitable are non-reducing sugars. Preferred are fructans, such as those mainly containing β-1, 2 bonds as in inulin or mainly containing β-2,6 bonds as in levan. It has been found that the lipophilic compound in a pharmaceutical composition according to the invention is solubilised more effectively when the sugar dissolves relatively slow. Furthermore, thus the absorption of the lipophilic compound in the body can be improved. It has been found that the effective dissolution rate of a lipophilic compound is very well in an aqueous medium, in case the dissolving time of a matrix material is at least 2 min, preferably at least 5 min. Very good results have been achieved with a matrix material that has a dissolving time of 30 min of less. Further it has been found advantageous to provide a composition with a matrix that exhibits a high viscosity (least 60 mPas, at 37°C) both inside the tablet and/or in the boundary layer around the tablet during dissolving. The number average degree of polymerisation (DP) of the sugar molecules of the sugar glass is at least 10 (very good results with DP of 11-24) [65].

Fukushima et al. (2009), in patent Application WO/2009/151072, invented quickly disintegrating tablets containing a large amount of the API [66]. Such tablet is obtained by granulating a powder containing the API with the use of a binder solution containing mannitol and gelatinised starch originating in corn, mixing the obtained granules with at least one kind of a disintegrating agent selected from among corn starch, hydroxypropyl starch, carmellose and crospovidone and compression moulding the resultant mixture, characterised by containing the API in an amount of 25% w/w or, showing a disintegration time of 40 s or shorter and having an absolute hardness of 1.8 N/mm^2 or more [66].

Sugimoto et al. (2010), in patent application WO/2010/061846) disclosed an orally rapidly disintegrating tablet that can be produced in a conventional tablet manufacturing facility and has a satisfactory level of hardness for practical applications, and these changes in properties of the tablet are rarely caused by factors such as humidity [67]. The orally rapidly disintegrating tablet has hardness of 40N or more, can be disintegrated in the oral cavity within 60 seconds, and is produced by compressing of a mixture of an API, an excipient having good water wettability, a water insoluble polymer (can be 1 to 10 parts by weight, preferably 3-10 parts by weight, to 100 parts by weight of the tablet and are selected from the group consisting of HPMC acetate succinate, ethylcellulose, HPMC phthalate, CMC, methacrylic acid copolymer L, methacrylic acid copolymer S and amino methacrylate copolymer; one or more disintegrating agents) that is well compactible and does not substantially cause a decrease in the water wettability of the excipient and (d) a disintegrating agent (selected from the group consisting of carboxymethylcellulose calcium, L-HPC, carboxymethylcellulose, cross-linked carboxymethylcellulose sodium, crystalline cellulose, corn starch, pregelatinised starch, carboxymethyl starch sodium and cross-linked PVP) and the mixture can contain one or more additives selected from the group consisting of binders, plasticisers, coating agents, deflocculating agents, solubilisers, sweeteners, acidulants, flavouring substances, pH adjusters, solubilising agents, colorants and flavouring agents; and wherein a disintegration time in the oral cavity is within 60 s. The water-insoluble polymer that is well compactible and does not substantially cause a decrease in the water wettability of the excipient can be any polymers having said property without any limitation, and includes an enteric polymer such as HPMC acetate succinate, ethylcellulose (*e.g.* Ethocel®), methacrylic acid copolymer L (*e.g.* Eudragit L), methacrylic acid copolymer S (*e.g.* Eudragit S), HPMC phthalate (*e.g.* HP-50) or carboxymethylethylcellulose (*e.g.* CMEC), or amino methacrylate copolymer (*e.g.* Eudragit RS or RL). Among them, HPMC acetate succinate or HPMC phthalate is preferable. The average particle size of the water-insoluble polymer is usually 0.1-500 μm, preferably 0.5-300 μm, particularly preferably 1-100 μm of the water-insoluble polymer without any limitation. The lubricant includes magnesium stearate, calcium stearate, stearic acid, sucrose fatty acid ester, talc, polyethyleneglycol, *etc.* The contained amounts of the lubricant can be 0.01-3 parts by weight, preferably 0.01-2 parts by weight, more preferably 0.01-1 parts by weight, to 100 parts by weight of the tablet. The orally rapidly disintegrating tablet of the present invention can be prepared in accordance with conventional methods in the tablet production [67].

Fu et al. (2010), in US patent US7749533, disclosed fast dissolving easily swallowable tablet capable of melting rapidly in the buccal cavity and comprises a plurality of highly plastic granules [68]. These granules were comprised of a porous, plastic substance, a water penetration enhancer (1%-95% w/w) and a binder (1-90% w/w). The water penetration enhancer may be chosen from the group consisting of dextrates, dextrin, dextrose, fructose, lactitol, lactose, maltitol, maltose, mannitol, mannose, sorbitol, sucrose, erythritol, xylitol, MCC, silicified MCC, powdered cellulose, cellulose acetate, calcium sulfate, calcium carbonate, dibasic calcium phosphate, tribasic calcium phosphate, carboxymethylcellulose-calcium salt, and combinations thereof. The water penetration enhancer is characterised by exhibiting complete wetting of a 200 mg tablet (formed at 300 pounds in a 0.5 inch diameter die) within 60 s after contacting a 0.5 ml water drop provided on a flat surface on which the water drop does not spread. The role of the binder is to permit particles of the porous, plastic substance and the water penetration enhancer to adhere to each other sufficiently to prevent particle segregation and to increase granule adherence even at the low pressure used to form the tablet. The binder may be selected from the group consisting of dextrates, dextrin, dextrose, fructose, lactitol, lactose, maltitol, maltose, mannitol, mannose, sorbitol, sucrose, erythritol, xylitol, starch, gelatin, acacia, alginic acid, sodium alginate, cellulose, CMC, ethylcellulose, hydroxyethylcellulose, hydroxypropylcellulose, HPMC, methylcellulose, polydextrose, poly(acrylic acid), carbomer, poly(ethylene oxide), and povidone. The method of preparation of such a tablet involves combining a porous, plastic substance, and a water penetration enhancer to form an admixture. This admixture is treated with an effective amount of binder to form a mass of agglomerated particles. The agglomerates are then sieved and dried to isolate a plurality of highly plastic granules; and compressed the highly plastic granules under low pressure to afford the fast melting pharmaceutical tablet [68].

Szamosi et al. (2010), through US patent 7799342, relates to processes for the preparation of tablets having low hardness (about 1 kP or less) but good physical stability, acceptable degree of friability (withstands 20-50 rotations in the friability apparatus before any tablet break and friability less than 1% after 20 rotations), but dissolve rapidly in the mouth providing an excellent mouthfeel [69]. The tablets of the invention comprise a hydrophilic/hydrophobic compound which melts at about 37°C or lower (0.01-2.5% w/w; *e.g.* PEG mixtures, low melting triglycerides, monoglycerides and diglycerides, semi-synthetic glycerides, hydrogenated oil and its derivatives *etc.*), a water soluble excipients (40-80% w/w, *e.g.* saccharides, amino acids, *etc.*), one or more disintegrants, flavours, colorants, sweetners, souring agents, glidants or lubricants, and API. The tablet offer fast stable dissolution, good tablet mouthfeel and good physical stability (even the tablet contains a low melting ingredient; it is relatively stable to high temperatures). Degradation takes place by a combination of melting, disintegration of the tablet matrix and dissolution of water soluble excipients [69].

Ahmed et al. (2010), in US patent 7811604, described a non-effervescent, orally disintegrating solid pharmaceutical dosage form comprising a substantially homogeneous compressed dry mixture of free base clozapine (10-30% w/w), a non-polymeric, water-soluble carrier; a hydrophilic water-insoluble polymer (1-20% w/w of the dosage form), and a disintegrant (20-60% w/w), and is selected from the group consisting of crospovidone, CCS, SSG and combinations thereof) [70] The dry mixture and pharmaceutical dosage form are free of acids, water-soluble polymers, taste-masking polymers, and coatings. This dry mixture after mixing is directed for compression. The dosage foam thus obtained disintegrates in about 60 s or less [70].

Ahmed et al. (2011), in US patent 7867515, described a non-effervescent, orally disintegrating solid pharmaceutical dosage form comprising: a progestin equivalent to 0.5-2 mg of levonorgestrel, an ionic disintegrant (*e.g.* CCS, SSG, polacrilin potassium, carboxymethyl cellulose calcium and their combinations) and no non-ionic disintegrant and a hydrophilic water-insoluble non-ionic excipient (*e.g.* MCC, pregelatinised starch, cellulose compounds, starches, crospovidone and their combinations); wherein the ionic disintegrant is present in a concentration of greater than 8% to about 60% by weight of the dosage form and the hydrophilic water-insoluble non-ionic excipient is present in a concentration of about 1% to about 20% by weight of the dosage form [71]. The process involves mixing an ionic disintegrant and a progestin equivalent to about 0.5 mg to about 2 mg of levonorgestrel to form an initial mixture; adding to the initial mixture a hydrophilic water-insoluble non-ionic excipient to form a final mixture; and compressing the final mixture to produce the pharmaceutical dosage form [71].

Tanaka et al. (2011), in US patent application 20110091546, described a method for producing FDDFs having a high productivity by means of compression moulding and are prepared using a specific saccharide (40-90% w/w, mannitol and xylitol), a disintegrating agent (5-40% w/w, crospovidone, low substituted hydroxypropyl cellulose, CCS, crystalline cellulose, *etc.*) and an inorganic excipient (1-30% w/w, average pore diameter of 100 nm or smaller, *e.g.* magnesium aluminometasilicate, magnesium aluminosilicate, calcium hydrogen phosphate, *etc.*) in specific ratio show a significantly shortened disintegration time in the oral cavity and sufficient hardness for practical use [72]. The composition has such a structure that the disintegrating agent and the inorganic excipient are homogeneously dispersed in complex particles comprising mannitol and xyltiol. This will result in an improved disintegration property and an excellent moulding property as well. It is also believed that water-introducible pores of the specific inorganic excipient introduce small amount of water into the tablet and the water effectively act on the disintegrating agent which is also dispersed, thus a favourable rapid disintegration in oral cavity is obtained [72].

Hallgren et al. (2011), in patent application WO/2011/060290, provides an immediate release pharmaceutical formulation (tablet/capsule) comprising metformin, a sodium dependent glucose transporter inhibitor (SGLT2), and optionally a coating and the methods of preparing the formulations [73] The challenges for such formulation was the large drug-to-drug ratio between metformin and the SGLT2 inhibitor makes content uniformity, with respect to dapagliflozin or dapagliflozin (S) propylene glycol hydrate in the final formulation, an important issue. It is necessary to have this relatively small amount of dapagliflozin or dapagliflozin (S) propylene glycol hydrates evenly distributed throughout the final granules or tablet formulation and thus avoid any variation in content. In addition, the large difference in physical properties between dapagliflozin or dapagliflozin (S) propylene glycol hydrate and metformin, and especially the poor compaction properties of metformin, make it difficult to produce tablets having acceptable mechanical strength. After several unsuccessful attempts, including dry granulation by roller compaction and traditional wet granulation, it has now been found that both of the above requirements can be met by spraying a solution or a suspension comprising dapagliflozin or dapagliflozin (S) propylene glycol hydrate and a binder onto the metformin particles in a fluid bed equipment, thereby producing granules that have uniform dapagliflozin or dapagliflozin (S) propylene glycol hydrate content and good compaction properties. Good compaction properties of these granules are thought to result from the spray granulation process together with the fact that this process makes it possible to use larger amounts of a binder than was possible in the earlier tested granulation processes. The way in which the granules are built up during the spray granulation process gives them suitable density/porosity and a suitable particle size distribution with little variation between batches. The granules also have superior flow properties. It has further been found that these beneficial formulations can be achieved while maintaining the chemical stability of the dapagliflozin or dapagliflozin (S) propylene glycol hydrate despite using a process in which at least part of the dapagliflozin is dissolved in water. The composition of such tablet is 0.1-2% w/w dapagliflozin or dapagliflozin (S) propylene glycol hydrate; about 55-85% w/w metformin hydrochloride; about 1-15% w/w hydroxypropyl cellulose; about 2-25% w/w) microcrystalline cellulose; about 1-12% w/w SSG or about 3-10% w/w hydroxypropyl cellulose, low substituted; and about 0.25-5% w/w> magnesium stearate. The optional coating can be Opadry® II white, Opadry® II orange, Opadry® II brown, or Opadry® II yellow. The pharmaceutical formulation is in the form of a tablet, a stock granulation, or a capsule. In another aspect, the present invention provides immediate release pharmaceutical formulations that comprise about 0.1-1% dapagliflozin or dapagliflozin (S) propylene glycol hydrate; about 60-80%) metformin hydrochloride; about 1-10% w/w hydroxypropyl cellulose; about 2-25% w/w) microcrystalline cellulose; about 4-10% w/w SSG or about 3-10% w/w hydroxypropyl cellulose, low substituted; and about 0.25-2.5% w/w magnesium stearate. The optional coating can be Opadry® II white, Opadry® II orange, Opadry® II brown, or Opadry® II yellow. The pharmaceutical formulation is in the form of a tablet, a stock granulation, or a capsule [73].

Kashid et al. (2011), in US patent 8048449, disclosed a formulation of an orally disintegrating compressed tablet comprising of an API (may be water-soluble or water insoluble), an indirectly compressible filler (an average particle size of 150 μm or above, 42-72% w/w, selected from mannitol, dextrates, sorbitol, xylitol, sucrose, fructose, lactitol, erythritol or maltitol, should be in granulated, compacted or agglomerated form), silicon dioxide (10-30% w/w, covers the surface of filler used and optionally an effervescent couple) [74]. The effervescent couple used is citric acid (anhydrous)/sodium hydrogen carbonate and is used in an amount of about 5-20% w/w. The said formulation dissolves in the mouth in 60 s or less. Additionally it may contain a disintegrant (crosslinked polyvinylpyrrolidone or polacrilin potassium or a combination thereof and its used 10-30% w/w), surfactant (sodium lauryl sulphate, 1-4% w/w), lubricant (sodium stearyl fumarate, 1-5% w/w), antiadherant (colloidal silicon dioxide or amorphous silicon dioxide or a combination thereof, 0.5-2% w/w), glidant, sweetener (aspartame, 1-5% w/w) or flavouring agent (strawberry, cherry or orange or a combination thereof, 1-5% w/w). The process comprised of preparing granules of an active ingredient along with silicon dioxide and a conventional excipient, mixing the granules so obtained with a filler and a conventional excipient so that said silicon dioxide covers the surface of said filler and finally compressing this blend to form an orally disintegrating compressed tablet [74].

Motohiro Ohta et al. (2011), in US patent 8071128, described in the invention the method of producing an intrabuccally rapidly disintegrating tablet [75]. Such said intrabuccally rapidly disintegrating tablet comprised a sugar alcohol or saccharide in the form of primary particles having an average particle size of not more than 30 μm, an active ingredient and one or more disintegrants selected from the group consisting of crospovidone, CCS, low substituted hydroxypropylcellulose, and a mixture thereof. The method involves granulating a powder material comprising the sugar alcohol or saccharide and said one or more disintegrants, thereby producing granulated material having a predetermined size; mixing the said granulated material and said active ingredient; and compressing the mixture into an intrabuccally rapidly disintegrating tablet [75].

3.2. Patents for Fast Dissolving Oral Films (FDOFs)

Leung et al. (2003), in patent 6596298, introduced a mouth dissolving fast disintegrating single-layer water-soluble film. The film comprised of pullulan and an antimicrobial effective combination of at least two essential oils [76] The essential oils are selected from the group consisting of about 0.01-4% w/w of thymol, methyl salicylate or eucalyptol and/or about 0.01-15% w/w menthol. In the film, at least thymol and menthol should be present in the film. The other components are stabilising agent (0.01-5% w/w), colouring agent (0.001-0.1% w/w), water (0.1-8% w/w), sweetening agent (0.1-15% w/w), flavouring agent (0.1-15% w/w), cooling agent (0.1-4% w/w) and a surfactant (0.1-5% w/w).

Kulkarni et al. (2003), in a US patent application 2003/0206942 A1, described a mouth dissolving consumable film comprised of at least one water soluble polymer; at least one antitussive agent and a mucosa-coating effective amount of a mucosa-coating agent (selected from the group consisting of pectin, gelatin and their combinations, 0.01-5% w/w) [77]. The water soluble component can be selected among pullulan, HPMC, hydroxyethyl cellulose, hydroxypropyl cellulose, polyvinyl pyrrolidone, carboxymethyl cellulose, polyvinyl alcohol, sodium alginate, polyethylene glycol, tragacanth gum, guar gum, acacia gum, arabic gum, polyacrylic acid, methylmethacrylate copolymer, carboxyvinyl polymer, amylose, high amylose starch, hydroxypropylated high amylose starch, dextrin, chitin, chitosan, levan, elsinan, collagen, zein, gluten, soy protein isolate, whey protein isolate, casein and their combinations. The purpose of mucosa-coating agent is to soothen and coat the throat when released from the consumable film. An antimicrobial, up to about 30% w/w, may be selected from the group of effective amount of at least one essential oil (carvacrol, thymol, eucalyptol, menthol, methyl salicylate, eugenol, gerianol, verbenone and their combinations). The said formulation will provide extended throat coating and mucosa adherence properties [77].

Kulkarni et al. (2003), in US patent application 2003/0211136 A1, described a film which is adapted to adhere to and dissolve in the oral cavity of a warm-blooded animal including humans [78]. The film comprised at least one water soluble polymer, a taste masking agent; the API and optionally may incorporate saliva stimulating agent and suitable preservative. The water soluble polymer may be selected from the group consisting of pullulan, HPMC, hydroxyethyl cellulose, hydroxypropyl cellulose, polyvinyl pyrrolidone, CMC, polyvinyl alcohol, sodium alginate, polyethylene glycol, tragacanth gum, guar gum, acacia gum, arabic gum, polyacrylic acid, methylmethacrylate copolymers, carboxyvinyl polymers, amylose, high amylose starch, hydroxypropylated high amylose starch, dextrin, pectin, chitin, chitosan, levan, elsinan, collagen, gelatin, zein, gluten, soy protein isolate, whey protein isolate, casein and mixtures thereof). The effective amount of a sucralose and sweetener (0.1-10% w/w) selected from saccharin, aspartame, xylitol, acesulfame potassium and mixtures may be used ad sweetener. The addition of sucralose, a chlorinated sucrose, enhances the sweetness as well as masks the unpleasant taste [78].

Leung at (2008), in US patent 7407669, described an oral, rapidly dissolving film which comprised of a single layer of polymer including pullulan, a stabilising agent (0.1-2% w/w) comprising a mixture of xanthan gum, locust bean gum and carrageenan and at least one API (selected from the group consisting of non-steroidal anti-inflammatory agents, antitussives, decongestants, anti-histamines, expectorants, anti-diarrheal, H2-antagonists, proton pump inhibitors, central nervous system agents, analgesics and mixtures thereof) [79]. Such films contain an effective amount of the essential oils like thymol, methyl salicylate, eucalyptol and menthol. As the film is to be administered in oral cavity, it may also be used in dental plaque, gingivitis and bad breath as this is effective at killing the plaque-producing germs. The method of preparation is: mixing the film forming agent and stabilising agent (to provide a film forming mixture); preparing an aqueous solution using all water soluble ingredients; combining the above mentioned two mixtures (to form a hydrated polymer gel); formation of oil mixture by mixing oils to form oil mixture; addition of the oil mixture to hydrated polymer gel and mixing so as to form a uniform emulsified gel. The so formed emulsified gel is then casted onto a suitable substrate so as to obtain the requisite fast dissolving film [79].

Bess et al. (2010), through US patent 7648712, introduced a fast dissolving film that is adapted to adhere to and dissolve in the mouth of consumer. The claimed film comprises at least one water soluble polymer, an API, taste masking agent, water and additional ingredients such as antimicrobial agents, plasticising agents, flavouring agents, saliva stimulating agents, cooling agents, surfactants, stabilizing agents/preservatives, emulsifying agents, thickening agents, binding agents, colouring agents and sweeteners [80]. Ion exchange resins preferred for use in the films of the invention are water-insoluble. They consist of a pharmacologically inert organic or inorganic matrix containing covalently bound functional groups that are ionic or capable of being ionised under the appropriate conditions of pH. The organic matrix may be synthetic (*e.g.*, polymers or copolymers of acrylic acid, methacrylic acid, sulfonated styrene, sulfonated divinylbenzene), or partially synthetic (*e.g.*, modified cellulose and dextrans). The inorganic matrix can also be, *e.g.*, silica gel modified by the addition of ionic groups. The covalently bound ionic groups may be strongly acidic (*e.g.*, sulfonic acid), weakly acidic (*e.g.*, carboxylic acid), strongly basic (*e.g.*, quaternary ammonium), weakly basic (*e.g.*, primary amine), or a combination of acidic and basic groups. To prepare such film, the water-soluble ingredients are dissolved in water to provide an aqueous solution which is then mixed with at least one water soluble film former and at least one stabilising agent to provide a film-forming mixture. By combination of the film-forming mixture and the aqueous solution, a hydrated polymer gel will result, which is subsequently mixed with oil/oil mixture to provide a uniform gel. The uniform gel is then casted on a substrate and dried gel to provide the film [80].

Wrenn et al. (2011), in US patent 7946296, described formulation of a dissolvable tobacco film strip adapted to be consumed orally [81]. It comprised of a tobacco component, a binder and a humectant. The humectant is present in an amount (by weight) which exceeds a total amount of the at least one binder. The film strip comprises tobacco component (50-80% w/w), binder (3-12% w/w, pectin and/or a natural gum) and/or humectant (20-40% w/w, glycerine). The tobacco component may be ground or powdered, optionally agglomerated with binder (average particle size of between about 100 nm and 1 mm.). The tobacco component comprises a pattern on a free surface of the film strip. The other additives consist of flavours (up to 6% w/w), sweeteners, fragrances, colouring agents, filling agents and preservatives. The film strip comprises a laminate of two or more layers and the tobacco component is incorporated between at least two of the layers. The film strip has an average thickness of from about 50-500 μm. The steps for making a dissolvable tobacco film strip for oral tobacco enjoyment are: forming a mixture of at least one tobacco component in an amount of about 50-80% by w/w, at least one binder and at least one humectant in an amount of about 20-40% w/w, wherein the at least one humectant is present in an amount by weight which exceeds a total amount of the at least one binder; casting or extruding the mixture to form a film; drying the film; and forming the film into film strips [81].

The recent patents related to the fast dissolving dosage forms (FDDFs) are summarized in Table **3**.

Table 3. Recent patents related to FDDFs.

Patents in Fast Dissolving Tablets/Capsules				
Title	**Invention**	**Patent Issue Date**	**Patent No.**	**Citation**
Fast dissolving buccal tablet	Rapid delivery of the drug from the buccal tablets and obviates the need for an adhesive if a water soluble lubricant and a directly compressible sugar is used	17 Dec 91	5073374	[40]
Effervescent dosage form with microparticles	Effervescent microparticles rapidly disintegrate in the mouth and provide adequate taste-masking	12 Jan 93	5178878	[41]
Paediatric effervescent dosage form	Utilise effervescent disintegration agent, which is effective for rapid disintegration and good organoleptic sensation to children	29 Jun 93	5223264	[42]
Base coated acid particles and effervescent formulation incorporating same	Uses both an effervescent couple and an acid sensitive active agent. Formulations having an acid neutralisation capacity under 5.0 are used for making particulate base coated acid	2 Apr 96	5503846	[18]
Rapidly dissolving oral dosage form	A support matrix is produced using standard spray-drying techniques. It disintegrates or dissolves in a few seconds on coming in contact with oral cavity fluid	27-Nov-96	EP0743850 (A1)	[43]
Taste masking microparticles for oral dosage forms	Taste masked microparticles made from mannitol, sorbitol, a mixture of an artificial sweetener and menthol, a mixture of a sugar and menthol, and methyl salicylate	4 Mar 97	5607697	[44]
Granular product or tablet containing an effervescent system and API	Granular product of effervescent granules (made from carrier crystals of at least one solid, edible organic acid, and are coated with at least one layer of a neutral substance soluble in water and/or alcohol) for acid-sensitive API	11 Aug 98	5792473	[45]
Fast-melt tablet and method of making same patent	The effervescent fast melting tablet is created using the synergistic effect of effervescence couple, starch as bulking, disintegrating agent and starch disintegrating enzymes	15 Sep 98	5807578	[46]

(Table 3) contd.....

Patents in Fast Dissolving Tablets/Capsules				
Title	**Invention**	**Patent Issue Date**	**Patent No.**	**Citation**
Blister package and packaged tablet	A blister sheet defines one or more recesses in which fragile dosage forms are disposed and a peelable sheet of lidding material overlies the recesses to cover the dosage forms	5 Dec 00	6155423	[47]
Sublingual buccal effervescent system	The use of an additional pH adjusting substance in combination with the effervescent for promoting the absorption drugs is disclosed	13 Mar 01	6200604	[48]
Rapidly dissolving robust dosage form	The tablet is created from an active ingredient mixed into a matrix of non-direct compression filler and a relatively high lubricant content	24 Apr 01	6221392	[49]
Formulation of fast-dissolving efavirenz capsules or tablets using super-disintegrants	Using higher amount of sodium starch glycolate, as a superdisintegrants >10% amount/wt of tablet	29 May 01	6238695	[50]
Process for preparing Fast dispensing solid oral dosage form	At low temperature, the drug particles may be coated with a water insoluble polymer or lipid material to prevent release of drug during processing, mask the taste of the drug and permits controlled release of the drug	27 Dec 01	US2001/0055611 A1	[51]
Oral Fast-Melt Dosage Form of A Cyclooxygenase-2 Inhibitor	A process of the invention comprises wet granulation of a selective cyclooxygenase-2 inhibitory drug together with a saccharide of low mouldability and a specific binding agent	28 Feb 02	WO/2002/015886	[52]
Organoleptically pleasant in-mouth rapidly disintegrable potassium chloride tablet	ODT suitable for use in the delivery of potassium comprising: between about 50 and about 80% coated potassium chloride crystals for extended release	2 Apr 02	6365182	[53]
Orally disintegrable tablet forming a viscous slurry	ODT for the delivery of sustained or extended release microcapsules and/or prompt release coated or non-coated drug particles	9 Apr 02	6368625	[54]
Oral fast-dissolving compositions for dopamine agonists	A process for preparing fast dissolving tablets comprised of a carrier, a dopamine agonist, an anti-emetic and/or an opioid antagonist for the treatment of Parkinson's disease	24 Oct 02	US 2002/0156056 A1	[55]

(Table 3) contd.....

Patents in Fast Dissolving Tablets/Capsules				
Title	**Invention**	**Patent Issue Date**	**Patent No.**	**Citation**
Apparatus for handling and packaging friable tablets	An assembly for handling and packaging pharmaceutical dosage forms includes an infeed structure, a laning structure, and a plenum structure extending from the infeed structure to the laning structure	26 Dec 02	US 2002/0194815 A1	[56]
Tablets immediately disintegrating in the oral cavity	Dissolving slightly soluble API in organic solvent or an aqueous organic solvent together with a surfactant and/or a water soluble polymer, coating the solution on a filler or granulating it with a filler to obtain mixed products, mixing a saccharide, adding an organic solvent, water or an aqueous organic solvent, followed by kneading, and then compression moulding	01 Jun 04	US 6743443 B1	[57]
Rapidly disintegrating tablet and process for producing the same	Tablets formulated using a rotor type powder compressing machine equipped with an external lubricating system; suitable for applying lubricant on to the punches and the dies; affected by spraying the dispersion of lubricant in constant air flow onto the punches and the die	13 Jul 05	EP1552851 A1	[58]
Tablet quickly melting in oral cavity	Tableting machine yielded tablets with unproblematic hardness and rapid disintegration; tableting cores (containing a water-soluble API or API and a sugar) coated with a disintegrating agent	16 Nov 05	EP 1 595 533 A1	[59]
Fast melting tablets having taste masking and sustained release properties	Ion-exchange resin complex is used to mask the unpleasant taste of API and complex may further be coated to impart sustained release of API	28 Sep 06	US 2006,0115529	[60]
Delivery and formulations of mast cell stabilisers	API targeted to the colon using fast-dissolving tablet, powder or effervescent, the targeted release is upon ingestion which comprise of at least one mast cell stabiliser	16 Nov 06	US 2006/0280788 A1	[61]
Rapidly absorbing oral formulations of PDE5 inhibitor	The dosage form can be lingual strip, sublingual strip, oral mist, rapidly disintegrating tablets, lyophilised wafers, granulated particles and gum	4 Jan 07	US 2007/0031349 A1	[62]

(Table 3) contd.....

Patents in Fast Dissolving Tablets/Capsules				
Title	**Invention**	**Patent Issue Date**	**Patent No.**	**Citation**
Intraorally rapidly disintegrating tablet	Such tablet can be formed using an ordinary apparatus, having hardness with no practical problem and that disintegrates rapidly with good mouth feel	18 May 07	US 2009/0117182 A1	[63]
Apparatus for handling and packaging friable tablet	It provides an assembly for guiding pharmaceutical dosage forms in a packaging assembly, comprising a surface movable in a downstream direction, a laning structure and guide wall structure	22 Aug 07	EP 1591360 B1	[64]
Formulation for fast dissolution of lipophilic compounds	Comprising at least one lipophilic compound and one glass of a sugar, a sugar alcohol, a mixture of sugars, a mixture of sugar alcohols, or a mixture of at least one sugar and at least one sugar alcohol, wherein the lipophilic compound is incorporated in the sugar glass and the manufacturing method	06 May 09	EP 1572157 B1	[65]
Tablet quickly disintegrating in the oral cavity and method for producing the same	Such tablet contains a large amount of the API and obtained by granulating a powder containing API with the use of a binder solution, mixing the obtained granules with a disintegrating agent and compression molding	17 Dec 09	WO/2009/151072	[66]
Orally rapidly disintegrating tablet and process for producing same	Using the conventional tableting machine, these tablets with hardness >40 N, can be disintegrated in the oral cavity within 60 s, produced by compression molding of the mixture of API; excipient with good water wettability; water-insoluble polymer with good mouldability; and a disintegrating agent	3 Jun 10	WO/2010/061846	[67]
Highly plastic granules for making fast melting tablets patent	Such tablet comprises a porous, plastic substance, a water penetration enhancer and a binder; tablets dissolve rapidly in the mouth, have good hardness and low brittleness	6 Jul 10	US7749533	[68]

(Table 3) contd.....

Patents in Fast Dissolving Tablets/Capsules				
Title	**Invention**	**Patent Issue Date**	**Patent No.**	**Citation**
Fast dissolving tablet	The invention comprise of a compound which melts at about 37° C or lower, have a low hardness, high stability and comprise few insoluble disintegrants which may cause a gritty or chalky sensation in the mouth	21 Sep 10	US 7799342	[69]
Non-effervescent, orally disintegrating solid pharmaceutical dosage forms patent	Such non-effervescent FDDS comprise of free base clozapine substantially free of acids, water-soluble polymers, taste-masking polymers, and coatings, and methods of making and using the same	12 Oct 10.	7811604	[70]
Orally disintegrating solid dosage forms comprising progestin and methods of making and use thereof	A non-effervescent FDDS comprised of an ionic disintegrant and a hydrophilic water-insoluble non-ionic excipient	11 Jan 11	7867515	[71]
Composition for rapid disintegrating tablet in oral cavity	The composition of the tablet is: saccharides (40-90% w/w); inorganic excipients (1-30% w/w); and disintegrating agent (5-40% by wt)	21 Apr 11	20110091546	[72]
Immediate release tablet formulations	The invention involves the methods of preparing the formulations and of treating disorders associated with sodium dependent glucose transporter activity	19 May 11	WO/2011/060290	[73]
Mouth dissolving pharmaceutical composition and process for preparing the same patent	Formulation comprising one or more API, fillers with particle size of 100 microns or above, a high and desirable amount of silicon dioxide, one or more disintegrating agents, optionally effervescent couple	01 Nov 11	8048449	[77]
Intrabuccally rapidly disintegrating tablet and a production method of the tablets	Tablet prepared by growing a powder material into a granulated material with a fixed particle diameter, by mixing the obtained granulated material with API and a disintegrant, and compressing the mixture into a predetermined shape	06 Dec 11	8071128	[78]

For artificial taste simulation system using different approaches like developing electronic circuit [82 - 89]. Kuhlman *et al.*, 2004 [81] developed an electronic device which allowed simultaneous measurement of the presence of particular chemical species in a sample as well as the particular physical properties of the sample.

The developed device can monitor pH, the presence of inorganic species, organic species, gases, conductivity and oxidation-reduction potential (ORP) biological signatures of organisms or residual chemical mixtures characteristic of the presence of organisms.

In the very next year, Burgman *et al.*, 2005 [83] had taken patent on development of method and apparatus (tongue plate) for simulating taste sensations in a taste simulation system. The sensations like sweet, sour, salty and bitter were simulated in various regions of the tongue by fitting the plate over the human tongue keeping in view prevention of injury to the soft tissue of the human's tongue.

Another patent for taste recognition was granted to Harada *et al.*, 2006 [84]. For this, letting a solvent flow through a holding section which holds an object to be recognized and measuring the solvent which has flowed through the holding section by a taste sensor. If the flow rate of the solvent is set at about 1 ml/min, the solvent whose quantity is almost equal to that of saliva secreted in a mouth can be supplied to the object to be recognized, and hence the taste recognition can be performed by the taste sensor.

4. FORMULATION OF FAST DISSOLVING DRUG DELIVERY SYSTEMS

4.1. Challenges in Formulation of FDDF

In spite of certain limitations, ease of administration and convenience of therapy has stimulated the research which resulted in numerous dosage forms and technologies being patented in design and development of FDDF for improved therapy and patient compliance. However, these challenges must be taken care of during the formulation of FDDF [27, 36, 90 - 98]:

4.1.1. Palatability

Many drugs have unpleasant taste or are unpalatable because of their bitter taste. FDDF disintegrate and/or dissolve in the oral cavity of the patient and release the active ingredients which come in contact with the taste buds. Therefore, it is a prerequisite to mask the taste of drugs in FDDF for better patient compliance. FDDF usually contain the medicament in a taste-masked form.

4.1.2. Mechanical Strength

As the aim of the formulation is to make it fast dissolving or disintegrating in the oral cavity, it should be made of either porous or soft-moulded matrices. The other option is to compress into tablets with very low compression force. This makes the tablets friable, brittle and difficult to handle. Therefore, specialised peel-off blister packing is preferred for their packing.

4.1.3. Hygroscopicity

FDDF are generally hygroscopic (particularly the freeze dried products and modified brittle capsules) and thus cannot maintain physical integrity under humid conditions. Protection of formulated product from humidity also is a major challenge for the formulation scientist.

4.1.4. Amount of Drug

The limited amount of drug can actually be incorporated in the dosage form as for lyophilised dosage forms, the drug dose must be less than 400 mg for insoluble drugs and less than 60 mg for soluble drugs. Such criterion is quite challenging while formulating a fast-dissolving dosage forms.

4.1.5. Aqueous Solubility

The water soluble drugs pose various formulation challenges as they form eutectic mixtures, which may result in freezing-point depression. Therefore, there is formation of glassy solid that may collapse upon drying because of loss of supporting structure during the sublimation process.

4.1.6. Tablet Size

The size of the dosage form decides its degree of ease in administration. Reports say that the easiest size of tablet to swallow is 7-8 mm. The easiest size to handle is one larger than 8 mm.

4.2. FDTs: Composition and Role of Superdisintegrants

The excipients used in the formulation of a FDT play a crucial role in formulation development and affects its properties thereof [99]. Other than the API, a FDT contains an emulsifying agent (0.05-15% w/w, to aid in rapid disintegration without taking water or chewing; stabilising the immiscible blends and enhancing the bioavailability), binder (to maintain the integrity of tablet during compression), superdisintegrant, antistatic agent, lubricant (prevent the tablets from sticking to the die wall and punch faces), diluents, flavour, sweetener, filler and surface active agents. The examples of the excipients used thereof are summarised in Table **4**.

Table 4. The excipients used in fast dissolving tablets [15, 27].

Component	Examples
Emulsifying agent	Alkyl sulphates, propylene glycol esters, lecithin, sucrose esters
Binders	Cellulosic polymers (ethyl cellulose, hydroxypropyl cellulose, HPMC, alone or in combination), acrylic polymers (amino methacrylate copolymer *e.g.* Eudragit RL and RS), polyacrylate (Eudragit NE) and polymethacrylate (Eudragit E)
Antistatic agent	Colloidal silica (Aerosil), precipitated silica (Sylod FP244), micronised and non-micronised talc, maltodextrin and β-cyclodextrin
Lubricants	Magnesium stearate, stearic acid, sodium stearyl fumarate, micronised polyoxyethylene glycol (Macrogol 6000), leucine and sodium benzoate
Diluents	Cellulose derivatives, starches, lactose, polyols and mannitol

Superdisintegrants help in faster disintegration of the tablets into fine powder, when FDTs comes in contact with the saliva. The tablet should be compactable enough to produce less-friable tablets and able to produce good mouth feel to the patient. The FDTs should be of smaller size (8 mm) to achieve better patient compliance and the superdisintegrants should have good flow to improve the flowability of the blend [100]. A wide variety of superdisintegrants with varying physicochemical properties and their corresponding mechanism of disintegration are available which are summarised in Table **5**.

Table 5. List of superdisintegrants along with their mechanism of action.

Superdisintegrants (Brand Name)	Chemical Name	Mechanism of Action	Special Comment
Croscarmellose®, Ac-Di-Sol®, Nymcel ZSX®, Primellose®, Solutab® Vivasol®, L-HPC	Crosslinked Cellulose	Swells 4-8 folds in < 10 s; swelling and wicking both.	Swells in two dimensions; - Direct compression or Granulation; Starch free
Crospovidone, Crospovidone M®, Kollidon®, Polyplasdone®	Crosslinked PVP	Swells very little and returns to original size after compression but act by capillary action	Water insoluble and spongy in nature so get porous tablet
Sodium starch glycolate, Explotab®, Primogel®	Crosslinked Starch	Swells 7-12 folds In < 30 s	Swells in three dimensions and high level serve as sustain release matrix

(Table 5) contd.....

Superdisintegrants (Brand Name)	Chemical Name	Mechanism of Action	Special Comment
Alginic acid NF, Satialgine	Crosslinked alginic acid	Rapid swelling in aqueous medium or wicking action	Promote disintegration in both dry or wet granulation
Soy polysaccharides, Emcosoy®	Natural superdisintegrants		Does not contain any starch or sugar. Used in nutritional products.
Calcium silicate	Calcium silicate	Wicking action	Highly porous, Optimum concentration is between 20-40% w/w

There are four major mechanisms and the superdisintegrants utilise one or more of them for rapid disintegration of tablets which are as follows [101]:

1. *Swelling:* Generally, swelling is the most widely accepted general mechanism of tablet disintegration. Disintegration of tablet is poor with their high porosity resulting in lack of adequate swelling force in contrast to low porosity tablets. Also, fluid is unable to penetrate in the tablet and disintegration again slows down if the packing fraction is very high.
2. *Porosity and capillary action (Wicking):* As far as the mechanism is concerned, disintegration by capillary action is always the first step. When the tablet comes in contact with suitable aqueous medium, the medium penetrates into the tablet and replaces the adsorbed air on the particles. This weakens the intermolecular bond and breaks the tablet into fine particles. Hydrophilicity of drug/excipient governs water uptake capacity of the formulation. For fast disintegration, maintenance of porous structure and low interfacial tension towards aqueous fluid is necessary and creates a hydrophilic network around the drug particles.
3. *Disintegrating particle/particle repulsive forces:* The third mechanism of disintegration of the swelling of tablet made with 'non-swellable' disintegrants. It was proposed by Guyot-Hermann (particle repulsion theory) based on the observation that non-swelling particle also cause disintegration of tablets [102]. The mechanism is electric repulsive force between particles and water is required for it and repulsion is secondary to wicking.
4. *Deformation:* The disintegrated particles undergo some deformation during tablet compression, which on coming in contact with the aqueous media get normalised into their original structure. Occasionally, the swelling capacity of starch improves with deformation of granules during compression. The increase in size of the deformed particles results in breaking of the tablet.

Effect of powder characteristics on disintegration time of tablets [103]: The relation between powder characteristics and disintegration time of tablets revealed that a high bulk density results in a short disintegration time. The powder bulk density was greater than 0.5 g/mL may result in tablets with a disintegration time less than 60 s. Tablets with a short DT value tended to possess low hardness. However, the use of high-compressibility excipients in the formulation may increase the hardness to values greater than 3 kg.

Table **6** summarises the drugs and the method thereof that have been formulated as FDTs.

Table 6. Some example of recently prepared orodispersible tablets.

Drug	Method	Reference
Ofloxacin	Taste masked microspheres of ofloxacin were prepared using Eudragit and orodispersible tablets of the formulated microspheres were using natural superdisintegrant.	[110]
Nimesulide	Orodispersible tablets were prepared using locust bean gum as a natural superdisintegrant.	[111]
Cetirizine dihydrochloride	Tablets were prepared using cetirizine along with camphor and mannitol in different proportion.	[112]
Pheniramine maleate	Effervescent method	[113]
Diazepam	ODTs were prepared using different types of superdisintegrants at different concentration using wet granulation and direct compression methods.	[114]
Valsartan	Tablets were prepared by freeze-drying technique.	[115]
Ondansetron HCl	Direct compression method.	[116]
Roxithromycin	ODTs were prepared using modified polysaccharides as rapidly disintegrating excipients.	[117]
Indomethacin	The tablets were made by non-aqueous wet granulation technique with superdisintegrant incorporated both intragranularly and extragranularly.	[118]
Ibuprofen	To prevent bitter taste and side effects of the drug, the drug was associated with Phospholipon 80H, a saturated lecithin, by wet granulation. The granules were then coated using different film forming agents (Kollicoat SR 30, Amprac 01, Kollidon 90F, Eudragit RD 100) obtaining four lots. Coated granules were then formulated with a sweetener (Aspartame), a mannitol-based diluent (Pearlitol SD 200) and Kollidon CL or Explotab were added as superdisintegrants and compacted under low compression force.	[119]
Doxilamine	To prevent bitter taste and unacceptable odour of the drug, the drug was taste masked with weak cation exchange resins like Indion 234, Indion 204 and Indion 414	[120]
Omeprazole and Domperidone	The tablets were prepared by direct compression using mannitol as diluent and sodium saccharin as sweetening agent along with three different levels of disintegrant. The superdisintegrant used in this study were Kollidon CL, Ac-Di-Sol and SSG.	[121]

For the purpose of taste masking of the drugs, various techniques [104] have been utilised, so far, such as using flavours and sweeteners, such as aspirin by sodium phenolate [105]; chlorpheniramine and phenyl propanolamine by sodium bicarbonate, citric acid, and orange/cream flavour [106]; famotidine by sodium bicarbonate, citric acid and lemon flavour [18]; ibuprofen by sodium citrate dehydrate and sod. saccharin and refined sugar [107]; theophylline by d-sorbitol, sodium saccharin, sodium glutamate, and vanilla essence [108]; acetaminophen by sodium bicarbonate, citric acid and cherry flavour [41]; and caffeine using starch, lactose, and mannitol [109]. The oils, surfactants, polyalcohols and lipids tend to increase the viscosity of released content in the mouth and coat the taste buds. Thus, they are potential taste masking agents. Formulations with a large excess of lecithin or lecithin like substances are claimed to control bitter taste in pharmaceuticals. Also, carbohydrates can be used as a coating material to mask the taste of orally administered drugs. Various forms of proteins have also been used extensively for taste masking. Moreover, ion exchange resins are utilised to stabilise the sensitive components, to sustain the drug release, to disintegrate tablets, and to mask taste of the formulation.

4.3. Formulation of FDOFs [38, 122]

The distinct advantages like larger surface area (which leads to rapid disintegration and dissolution in the oral cavity) and thus increased bioavailability makes polymer films better formulations over other oral formulations for the delivery of poorly soluble [123]. PF allow rapid and controlled wetting in the oral or buccal environment; are convenient, easy to swallow. They offer an improved acceptability and compliance among the geriatric and paediatric patients. PF offers manufacturing advantages also including continuous manufacturing capabilities that enable full product characterisation, when incorporated with in-line monitoring using process analytical technologies [123]. Even though, the interest in pharmaceutical films have increased based on publications and patents [124 - 133], more research is required in order to overcome potential limitations and in turn, increase the general patient acceptance.

FDOFs contains the API in a thin film form with an area of 5-20 cm^2 whose immediate dissolution (in water or saliva respectively) is reached through a special matrix from water-soluble polymers. The API up to a single dose of 15 mg can be incorporated and important factors such as formulation considerations (plasticisers, *etc.*) have been reported to affect the mechanical properties of the films, such as shifting the glass transition temperature to lower temperature [134].

4.3.1. Drugs/APIs

Various classes of drugs (like antiulcer, antiasthamatics, antitussives, anti microbial, expectorants, antihistaminics, NSAID's, *etc.*) can be formulated as FDOFs [17, 38, 135, 136].

4.3.2. Film Forming Polymers

More attention in medical and nutraceuticals is towards the use of water-soluble polymers to be utilised as film formers as they achieve rapid disintegration, good mouth feel and provide good mechanical strength to the films. The disintegration rate of the polymers can also be controlled by controlling the molecular weight of polymer film bases.

Common water soluble film forming polymers are lycoat NG73 (granular hydroxypropyl starch), HPMC, hydroxyethyl cellulose, Methyl cellulose A-3, A-6 and A-15, Pullulan, CMC Cekol 30, PVP K-90, pectin, gelatin, sodium alginate, hdroxypropylcellulose, polyvinyl alcohol, maltodextrins and Eudragit RD-10 [17, 38, 129, 137, 138]. Polymerised rosin has been reported as a novel film forming polymer [38, 129, 139].

Other than the above mentioned polymers, water soluble gums (like gum arabic, xanthan gum, tragacanth, acacia, carrageenan, guar gum, locust bean gum, pectin or alginates) and water soluble polysaccharides (such as polydextrose, dextrin, and dextran) can also be used [17, 140, 141].

4.3.3. Plasticisers

The addition of plasticiser provides mechanical strength, improves its flexibility and reduce the brittleness of the films so formed and changing their concentration affects their mechanical properties [17, 38, 123, 129]. The commonly used plasticisers are glycerol, propylene glycol, low molecular weight polyethylene glycols, phthalate derivatives (like dimethyl, diethyl and dibutyl phthalate), citrate derivatives (such as tributyl, triethyl, acetyl citrate, triacetin) and castor oil Plasticisers reduce the glass transition temperature of the polymer. Plasticiser is selected on the basis of its compatibility with the polymer and also the type of solvent employed in the casting of film. By its use, the better flow and strength of polymer can be achieved [142, 143]. The plasticisers are used in the concentration of 0–20% w/w of dry polymer weight [123, 144] and their inappropriate use may lead to film cracking, splitting and peeling of the strip [145 - 147], and may have an adverse effect on the absorption rate of the drug [148]. The plasticiser should decrease the glass transition temperature of polymer in the range of 40-60°C for non aqueous solvent system and below 75 °C for aqueous systems [147, 149].

4.3.4. Surfactants

Surfactants are added to the film as solubilising, wetting or dispersing agent so that the film dissolves within seconds and release its active agent immediately. The commonly used additives are sodium lauryl sulfate, benzalkonium chloride, bezthonium chloride, span, polyethylene ether, *etc*. [17, 38]. One of the most important surfactant is Poloxamer 407 (usually available in flakes), may be used as solubilising, wetting and dispersing agent [144].

4.3.5. Flavour

As the formulation is to be utilised for oral use and it will disintegrate there only, the flavour is an important component. The perception for the flavours changes from individual to individual depending upon the age and liking.

The flavour choice varies from individual to individual, with age and the type of drug to be incorporated in the formulation. As an example, geriatric population like mint or orange flavours while younger generation like flavours of fruit punch, raspberry *etc*. The flavour acceptance of the oral disintegrating or dissolving formulation by an individual by and large also depend on the initial flavour quality which is observed in few seconds (after the product has been consumed) and the after taste of the formulation (which lasts for at least about 10 min) [97, 123].The flavours such as foam reducing flavouring agents like menthol, cherry menthol, cinnamint, spearmint, peppermint, orange flavour, natural raspberry or their combinations can be added to have a good mouth feel effect [17, 140]. The oils and extracts derived from various parts of the plant may serve as a flavouring agent either alone or in the combination. The examples are peppermint oil, cinnamon oil, spearmint oil, oil of nutmeg (flavour oils); vanilla, cocoa, coffee, chocolate and citrus (fruity flavours); apple, raspberry, cherry, pineapple (fruit essence type). The usual concentration is 10% w/w flavours for oral formulations. Additionally, cooling agents like monomethyl succinate can be added to improve the flavour strength and to enhance the mouth-feel effect of the product. Also, WS3, WS23 and Utracoll II be used in conjunction with flavours for cooling effect in the formulation [150, 151].

4.3.6. Colour

D&C colours, EU colours, natural colours and custom pantone-matched colours may be utilised to impart colour to FDOFs.

4.3.7. Stabilising and Thickening Agents

The purpose of stabilising and thickening agent is to improve the viscosity and consistency of dispersion or solution of the strip preparation solution or suspension before casting. The natural gums like xanthan gum, locust bean gum, carrageenan and cellulosic derivatives can also be used (up to 5%w/w) as thickening agents and stabilising agent [123, 151].

4.3.8. Sweetening Agents

The sweeteners (both natural and artificial) play a very important role in the formulation, especially for paediatric formulation. They improve the palatability of FDOFs as they are intended to be disintegrated or dissolved in the oral cavity. The classical example of sweeteners is sucrose (derived from cane or beet in the form of liquid or dry state), dextrose, fructose, glucose, liquid glucose and maltose. The perception of sweetness is more rapid for fructose as compared to sucrose and dextrose and it is sweeter than sorbitol and mannitol and thus used widely as a sweetener. Other sweetners include polyhydric alcohols (sorbitol, mannitol, isomalt and maltitol) and they can provide good mouth-feel and cooling sensation also. Polyhydric alcohols are also less carcinogenic and do not have bitter after taste which is a vital aspect in formulating oral preparations. The sweetness property of most of the polyols is less than half of that of sucrose except xylitol and maltitol which have similar sweetness as that of sucrose (scale of 0.8–1.0). However, the use of natural sugars in such preparations needs to be restricted in people who are on diet or in the case of diabetic patients [123, 152, 153]. Therefore, artificial sweeteners have gained more popularity in food and pharmaceutical preparations. Saccharin, cyclamate and aspartame are the first generation of the artificial sweeteners followed by acesulfame potassium, sucralose, alitame and neotame which come under the second generation artificial sweeteners. Acesulfame-K and sucralose have more than 200 and 600 time sweetness. Neotame and alitame have more than 2000 and 8000 time sweetening power as compared to sucrose. Rebiana which is a herbal sweetener, derived from plant *Stevia rebaudiana* (South American plant) has more than 200–300 time sweetness [154]. The disadvantage of these artificial sweeteners is the after taste effect. This disadvantage of artificial sweeteners can be reduced by mixing or blending the natural and artificial sweetener. The flavour qualities of these artificial sweeteners are different from the natural sweeteners and may sometimes are not acceptable by patients who are accustomed to the natural sugars. The amalgamation of sweeteners may lead to synergism and improvement in the taste of the formulations [153]. Generally sweeteners are used in the concentration of 3-6% w/w either alone or in combination [151].

4.3.9. Saliva Stimulating Agents

The purpose of saliva stimulating agents is to enhance the disintegration and to get rapid drug release [123, 155] by increasing the rate of production of saliva. The acids used in the preparation of food can generally be utilised as salivary stimulants (2-6% w/w) like, citric acid, malic acid, lactic acid, ascorbic acid and tartaric acid (alone or in combination). Citric acid is the most preferred amongst them.. The sweeteners (like food grade sugars as well as synthetic sugars) can also act as salivary stimulants . Such sweeteners include glucose, fructose, xylose, maltose and lactose [123, 156]. To measure the stimulation, the amount of resting flow and stimulated flow at equal time under same conditions are measured and compared. The stimulant action of sweeteners is dependent on the sweetness value, like fructose has the sweetness value of 1.1 as compared to 0.7 of glucose and 1.0 of sucrose. The artificial sweetener is preferred over natural sugars because lower concentration is required and multiple uses don't result in dental caries in individuals [123, 156].

5. PACKAGING AND STORAGE

Being prone to humidity, the manufacturing as well as storage of FDDF requires special attention. Therefore special packages are generally used for their packaging and storage such as single pouch, blister card with multiple units, multiple unit dispenser and continuous roll dispenser. The choice of the package depends on the use as well as marketing objectives [15]. Usually such fast dissolving dosage forms are stored at cool temperature unless otherwise directed. Some dosage forms may be required to be stored in cold temperature, although in most cases stringent control of humidity is necessary, which may otherwise affect the integrity and hence the release rate of drug.

CONCLUSIONS

FDDFs have overcome many limitations associated with the conventional drug delivery systems. A successful FDDF product has a good taste and offers rapid drug release. Field of FDDFs is continuously growing and offers considerable benefits to the patient, formulator as well as the manufacturer. Paying a close attention to these advancements, pharmaceutical manufacturer may utilise it for product line extensions. Higher pace of FDDF patents armed with advanced technologies will certainly bring about a better healthcare system with an efficient therapeutic management and patient compliance. Moreover, development of novel pharmaceutical excipients may gift some more novel technologies in future.

REFERENCES

[1] Jeong SH, Fu Y, Park K. Frosta: a new technology for making fast-melting tablets. Expert Opin Drug Deliv 2005; 2(6): 1107-16. [http://dx.doi.org/10.1517/17425247.2.6.1107] [PMID: 16296813]

[2] Gisel EG. Oral-motor skills following sensorimotor intervention in the moderately eating-impaired child with cerebral palsy. Dysphagia 1994; 9(3): 180-92. [http://dx.doi.org/10.1007/BF00341263] [PMID: 8082327]

[3] Andersen O, Zweidorff OK, Hjelde T, Rødland EA. [Problems when swallowing tablets. A questionnaire study from general practice]. Tidsskr Nor Laegeforen 1995; 115(8): 947-9. [Problems when swallowing tablets. A questionnaire study from general practice]. [PMID: 7709385]

[4] Shukla D, Chakraborty S, Singh S, Mishra B. Mouth Dissolving Tablets I:An Overview of Formulation Technology. Sci Pharm 2009; 77: 309-26. [http://dx.doi.org/10.3797/scipharm.0811-09-01]

[5] Prajapati BG, Ratnakar N. A Review on Recent patents on Fast Dissolving Drug Delivery System. Int J Pharm Tech Res 2009; 1(3): 790-8.

[6] Lindgren S, Janzon L. Prevalence of swallowing complaints and clinical findings among 5079-yea--old men and women in an urban population. Dysphagia 1991; 6(4): 187-92. [http://dx.doi.org/10.1007/BF02493524] [PMID: 1778094]

[7] Porter SC. Novel drug delivery: Review of recent trends with oral solid dosage forms. Am Pharm Rev 2001; 4: 28-35.

[8] Jaccard TT, Leyder J. Une nouvelle forme galénique: le lyoc. Ann Pharm Fr 1985; 43(2): 123-31. [A new galenic form: lyoc]. [PMID: 4091454]

[9] Fix JA, Ed. Advances in quick-dissolving tablets technology employing Wowtab. IIR Conference on Drug Delivery Systems. Washington DC, USA. 1998.

[10] Virely P, Yarwood R. Zydis–a novel, fast dissolving dosage form. Manuf Chem 1990; 61: 36-7.

[11] Wilson CG, Washington N, Norman S, Greaves JL, Peach JM, Pugh K. A gamma scintigraphic study to compare oesophageal clearance of Expidet™ formulations, tablets and capsules in supine volunteers. Int J Pharm 1988; 46(3): 241-6. [http://dx.doi.org/10.1016/0378-5173(88)90084-1]

[12] Wilson CG, Washington N, Peach J, Murray GR, Kennerley J. The behavior of a fast dissolving dosage form (Expidet) followed by g-scintigraphy. Int J Pharm 1987; 40: 119-23. [http://dx.doi.org/10.1016/0378-5173(87)90056-1]

[13] Nagpal K, Singh SK, Mishra DN. Intellectual Property Rights and Patents Laws. Indian Scenario Pharma Buzz 2008; 3(10): 32-5.

[14] Nagpal K, Singh SK, Mishra DN. Intellectual Property Rights and Patents Laws. Indian Scenario Pharma Buzz 2008; 3(9): 14-28.

[15] Sharma R, Rajput M, Prakash P. Sharma s. Fast Dissolving Drug Delivery System - A Review. Int Res J Pharm 2011; 2(11): 21-9.

[16] Sandri G, Bonferoni MC, Ferrari F, Rossi S, Caramella C. Differentiating Factors between Oral Fast-

Dissolving Technologies. Am J Drug Deliv 2006; 4(4): 249-62.
[http://dx.doi.org/10.2165/00137696-200604040-00007]

[17] Goel H, Rai P, Rana V, Tiwary AK. Orally disintegrating systems: innovations in formulation and technology. Recent Pat Drug Deliv Formul 2008; 2(3): 258-74.
[http://dx.doi.org/10.2174/187221108786241660] [PMID: 19075912]

[18] Wehling F, Schuehle S. Base coated acid particles and effervescent formulation incorporating same. Patent US 5503846, 1996.

[19] Wehling F, Shuehle S, Madamala N. Effervescent dosage form with microparticles. Patent US 5178878, 1993.

[20] Ito A, Sugihara M. Development of oral dosage form for elderly patients: use of agar as base of rapidly disintegrating oral tablets. Chem Pharm Bull (Tokyo) 1996; 44(11): 2132-6.
[http://dx.doi.org/10.1248/cpb.44.2132] [PMID: 8945779]

[21] Cherukuri SR, Myers GL, Battist GE, *et al.* Process for forming quickly dispersing comestible unit and product therefrom. Patent US 5587172, 1996.

[22] Fuisz RC. Ulcer prevention method using a melt-spun hydrogel. Patent US 5622717, 1997.

[23] Fuisz R, Cherukuri SR. Cherukuri SR, Process and apparatus for making tablets and tablets made there from . Patent US 5654003, 1997.

[24] Myers GL, Battist GE, Fuisz RC. Delivery of controlled-release systems. Patent US 5567439, 1996.

[25] Myers GL, Battist GE, Fuisz RC. Apparatus for making rapidly dissolving dosage units. Patent US 5871781, 1999.

[26] Myers GL, Battist GE, Fuisz RC. Process and apparatus for making rapidly dissolving dosage units and product therefrom. Patent US 5622719, 1997.

[27] Seager H. Drug-delivery products and the Zydis fast-dissolving dosage form. J Pharm Pharmacol 1998; 50(4): 375-82.
[http://dx.doi.org/10.1111/j.2042-7158.1998.tb06876.x] [PMID: 9625481]

[28] Taste masking and ODTs: AdvaTab® Orally Disintegrating Tablets. , [Accessed on 10 Sep 2016]; Accessed from: http://www.adarepharma.com/pharmaceutical-technologies/taste-masking-and-odts/advatab.html

[29] Giri TK, Tripathi DK, Majumdar R. Formulation aspects in the development of orodispersible tablets: an overview. Int J Pharm Pharm Sci 2010; 2(3): 38-42.

[30] Shangraw R, Mitrevej A, Shah M. A new era of tablet disintegrants. Pharm Technol 1990; 4: 49-57.

[31] LyocTM Orally Disintegrating Tablet Technology: Product Brochure: Cima Labs Inc , 2008 [Accessed on 10 Sep 2016]; Accessed from http://www.cimalabs.com/assets/Lyocword.pdf

[32] Kuno Y, Kojima M, Ando S, Nakagami H. Evaluation of rapidly disintegrating tablets manufactured by phase transition of sugar alcohols. J Control Release 2005; 105(1-2): 16-22.
[http://dx.doi.org/10.1016/j.jconrel.2005.01.018] [PMID: 15955365]

[33] Alhusban F, Perrie Y, Mohammed AR. Formulation of multiparticulate systems as lyophilised orally disintegrating tablets. Eur J Pharm Biopharm 2011; 79(3): 627-34.
[http://dx.doi.org/10.1016/j.ejpb.2011.05.014] [PMID: 21693189]

[34] Sano S, Iwao Y, Kimura S, Itai S. Preparation and evaluation of swelling induced-orally disintegrating tablets by microwave irradiation. Int J Pharm 2011; 416(1): 252-9.
[PMID: 21763765]

[35] Aguilar-Díaz JE, García-Montoya E, Suñe-Negre JM, Pérez-Lozano P, Miñarro M, Ticó JR. Predicting orally disintegrating tablets formulations of ibuprophen tablets: an application of the new

SeDeM-ODT expert system. Eur J Pharm Biopharm 2012; 80(3): 638-48. [http://dx.doi.org/10.1016/j.ejpb.2011.12.012] [PMID: 22245156]

[36] Reddy LH, Ghosh B. Fast dissolving drug delivery systems: A review of the literature. Indian J Pharm Sci 2002; 64: 331-6.

[37] Siddiqui MD, Garg G, Sharma PK. A short review on "a novel approach in oral fast dissolving drug delivery system and their patents. Adv Biol Res (Faisalabad) 2011; 5(6): 291-303.

[38] Arya A, Chandra A, Sharma V, Pathak K. Fast dissolving oral films: an innovative drug delivery system and dosage form. Int J Chem Tech Res 2010; 2(1): 576-83.

[39] Bioprogress , [Accessed on 11 Sep 2016]; Accessed from http://www.moneyam.com/InvestorsRoom/posts.php?tid=4097from=1699

[40] McCarty JA. Fast dissolving buccal tablet. Patent US 5073374, 1991.

[41] Wehling F, Schuehle S, Madamala N. Effervescent dosage form with microparticles. Patent US 5178878, 1993.

[42] Wehling F, Schuehle S, Madamala N. Pediatric effervescent dosage form. Patent US 5223264, 1993.

[43] Allen LV, Wang B, Davies JD. Rapidly dissolving oral dosage form. Patent EP0743850 (A1), 1996.

[44] Alkire TG, Sanftleben RA, Schuehle SS. Taste masking microparticles for oral dosage forms. Patent US 5607697, 1997.

[45] Gergely G, Gergely T, Gergely I, *et al.* Granular product or tablet containing an effervescent system and an active pharmaceutical substance, as well as a method for its preparation. Patent US 5792473, 1998.

[46] Acosta-Cuello TR, Ouali A. Fast-melt tablet and method of making same. Patent US 5807578, 1998.

[47] Katzner LD, Jones B, Khattar J, *et al.* Blister package and packaged tablet. Patent US 6155423, 2000.

[48] Pather SI, Khankari RK, Eichman JD, *et al.* Sublingual buccal effervescent. Patent US 6200604, 2001.

[49] Khankari RK, Hontz J, Chastain SJ, *et al.* Rapidly dissolving robust dosage form. Patent US 6221392, 2001.

[50] Makooi-Morehead WT, Buehler JD, Landmann BR. Formulation of fast-dissolving efavirenz capsules or tablets using super-disintegrants. Patent US 6238695, 2001.

[51] Green R, Kearney P. Process for preparing Fast dispensing solid oral dosage form. Patent Application US 2001/0055611 A1, 2001.

[52] Karali TT, Kontny MJ, Le TT. Oral fast-melt dosage form of a cyclooxygenase-2 inhibitor. Patent WO2002015886 A3, 2002.

[53] Khankari RK, Hontz J, Chastain SJ. Organoleptically pleasant in-mouth rapidly disintegrable potassium chloride tablet. Patent US 6365182, 2002.

[54] Siebert JM, Khankari RK, Kositprapa U, *et al.* Orally disintegrable tablet forming a viscous slurry. Patent US 6368625, 2002.

[55] Johnson ES, Clarke A, Green RD. Oral fast-dissolving compositions for dopamine agonists. Patent Application US 2002/0156056 A1, 2001.

[56] Aylward JT, DeMey CF. Apparatus for handling and packaging friable tablets. Patent Application US 2002/0194815 A1, 2002.

[57] Furitsu H. Tablets immediately disintegrating in the oral cavity. Patent US 6743443 B1, 2004.

[58] Ogasawara K, Sogo K, Yamamura T. Rapidly disintegrating tablet and process for producing the same. Patent EP 1552851 A1, 2005.

[59] Suga T, Nakano T. Tablet quickly melting in oral cavity. Patent EP 1595533 A1, 2005.

[60] Jeong S, Kimura S, Fu Y, *et al.* Fast melting tablets having taste masking and sustained release properties. Patent WO2006101536 A1, 2006.

[61] Casey SM. Delivery and formulations of mast cell stabilizers. Patent Application US 2006/0280788 A1, 2006.

[62] Monteith D, Borderies P. Rapidly absorbing oral formulations of PDE5 inhibitor. Patent Application US 2007/0031349 A1, 2007.

[63] Tomoya Akutagawa MN. Intraorally rapidly disintegrating tablet. Patent Application US 2009/0117182 A1, 2007.

[64] Amborn J, Tiger V. Apparatus for handling and packaging friable tablet. Patent EP 1591360 B1, 2007.

[65] Hinrichs WL. Formulation for fast dissolution of lipophilic compounds. Patent EP 1572157 B1, 2009.

[66] Fukushima T, Shimizu T, Yoshida T. Tablet quickly disintegrating in the oral cavity and method for producing the same. Patent WO/2009/151072, 2009.

[67] Sugimoto M, Kitaoka K. Orally rapidly disintegrating tablet, and process for producing same. Patent WO/2010/061846, 2010.

[68] Fu Y, Pai CM, Park SY, *et al.* Highly plastic granules for making fast melting tablets. Patent US 7749533, 2010.

[69] Szamosi J, Kinter KS, Li VH, *et al.* Fast dissolving tablet. Patent US 7799342, 2010.

[70] Ahmed SU, Li L, Chowdhury TA. Non-effervescent, orally disintegrating solid pharmaceutical dosage forms. Patent US 7811604, 2010.

[71] Ahmed SU, Sethia S, Chowdhury TA. Orally disintegrating solid dosage forms comprising progestin and methods of making and use thereof. Patent US 7867515, 2011.

[72] Tanaka N, Nagai Y, Kawaguchi H, *et al.* Composition for rapid disintegrating tablet in oral cavity. Patent Application US 20110091546, 2011.

[73] Hallgren A, Swenson RMW. Immediate release tablet formulations. Patent US WO/2011/060290, 2011.

[74] Kashid N, Mukherji G. Mouth dissolving pharmaceutical composition and process for preparing the same. Patent US 8048449, 2011.

[75] Ohta M, Hayakawa E, Ito K, *et al.* Intrabuccally rapidly disintegrating tablet and a production method of the tablets. Patent US 8071128, 2011.

[76] Leung S-H, Leone RS, Kumar LD. Fast dissolving orally comsumable films. Patent US 6596298, 2003.

[77] Kulkarni N, Kumar LD, Sorg A. Fast dissolving orally consumable films containing an antitussive and a mucosa coating agent. Patent Application US 2003/0206942 A1, 2003.

[78] Kulkarni N, Kumar LD, Sorg A. Fast dissolving orally consumable films containing a sweetener. Patent Application US 2003/0211136 A1, 2003.

[79] Leung S-H, Leone RS, Kumar LD, *et al.* Fast dissolving orally consumable films Patent US 7407669, 2008.

[80] Bess WS, Kulkarni N, Ambiket SH. Fast dissolving orally consumable films containing a taste masking agent. Patent US 7648712, 2010.

[81] Wrenn SE, Marun MC. Dissolvable tobacco film strips and method of making the same. Patent US 7946296, 2011.

[82] Kuhlman K, Buehler MG. Electronic tongue. Patent US 6730201, 2004.

[83] Burgmans T. Method and apparatus for simulating taste sensations in a taste simulation system. Patent WO/2005/072821, 2005.

[84] Harada T. Taste recognition system and recognition method. Patent US 7090805, 2006.

[85] Sato T, Hirono J, Hamana H, *et al.* Chemical sensor system. Patent Application US 2007/0054266 A1, 2007.

[86] Xiaoping W, Shuyue Z, Shaoping D, *et al.* Electrochemical electronic tongue based on wide-bard pulse voltammetry. Patent CN 101071117, 2007.

[87] Son J-Y, Lee Y-H, Kim M-G, *et al.* Portable apparatus for storing taste and odor. Patent Application US 2009/0292469 A1, 2009.

[88] Kugimiya Y, Kobayashi Y, Cheng R, *et al.* Taste recognition apparatus and taste recognition system using the same. Patent US 7858036 B2, 2010.

[89] Fung YS, Sun H, Mo Z, *et al.* Electronic tongue sensor. Patent US 8004152, 2011.

[90] Sugihara M, Hidaka M, Saitou A. Discriminatory features of dosage form and package. Jpn J Hosp Pharm Tech 1986; 12: 322-8. [http://dx.doi.org/10.5649/jjphcs1975.12.322]

[91] Lies MC, Atherton AD, Copping NM. Freeze-dried dosage forms and methods for preparing same. US Patent 5188825, 1993.

[92] Ghosh TK, Pfister WR. Drug delivery to the oral cavity: molecules to market. Taylor & Francis 2005. [http://dx.doi.org/10.1201/9780849398513]

[93] Habib W, Khankari R, Hontz J. Fast-dissolve drug delivery systems. Crit Rev Ther Drug Carrier Syst 2000; 17(1): 61-72. [http://dx.doi.org/10.1615/CritRevTherDrugCarrierSyst.v17.i1.20] [PMID: 10755211]

[94] Hamilton EL, Luts EM. Advanced Orally disintegrating tablets bring significant benefits to patients and product life cycle. Drug Deliv Technol 2005; 5(1): 34-7.

[95] Chang RK, Guo X, Burnside BA, Couch RA. Fast dissolving tablets. Pharm Tech 2002; 24: 52-8.

[96] Divate S, Kavitha K, Sockan GN. Fast disintegrating tablets – an emerging trend. Int J Pharma Sci Rev Res 2011; 6(2): 18-22.

[97] Brown D. Orally disintegrating tablets: Taste over speed. Drug Deliv Tech 2001; 3(6): 58-61.

[98] Aurora J, Pathak V. Oral disintegrating technologies:Oral disintegrating dosage forms: An overview. Drug Deliv Technol 2005; 5(3): 50-4.

[99] Chandrasekhar R, Hassan Z, Alhusban F, Smith AM, Mohammed AR. The role of formulation excipients in the development of lyophilised fast-disintegrating tablets. Eur J Pharm Biopharm 2009; 72(1): 119-29. [http://dx.doi.org/10.1016/j.ejpb.2008.11.011] [PMID: 19073253]

[100] Patidar A, Mishra P, Main P, *et al.* A review on- recent advancement in the development of rapid disintegrating tablet. Int J Life Sci Pharma Res 2011; 1(1): 7-P16.

[101] Bhowmik D, Chiranjib B, Pankaj K, Chandira RM. Fast dissolving tablet: an overview. J Chem Pharm Res 2009; 1(1): 163-77.

[102] Guyot-Hermann AM, Ringard DJ. Disintegration mechanisms of tablets containing starches. Hypothesis about the particle-particle repulsive force. Drug Dev Ind Pharm 1981; 7(2): 155-77. [http://dx.doi.org/10.3109/03639048109057708]

[103] Yamamoto Y, Fujii M, Watanabe K, *et al.* Effect of powder characteristics on oral tablet disintegration. Int J Pharm 2009; 365(1-2): 116-20.
[http://dx.doi.org/10.1016/j.ijpharm.2008.08.031] [PMID: 18804156]

[104] Saroha K, Mathur P, Verma S, *et al.* Mouth dissolving tablets: An overview on future compaction in oral formulation technologies. Der Pharmacia Sinica 2010; 1(1): 179-87.

[105] Fuisz RC. Taste masked medicated pharmaceuticall. Patent US US5028632A, 1991.

[106] Brideau ME. Fast dissolving dosage forms containing taste-masking agents. Patent WO9533446, 1995.

[107] Pearlman R, Jenkins H, Serafini T. Combination therapy of arthritis with tranilast. Patent Application US 20100158905A1, 2009.

[108] Hidemi M, Yoshihiko K, Yukio S. Theophylline-containing liquid agent. Patent JPH05124963, 1993.

[109] Matsubara Y, Kawajiri A, Ishiguro F. Granule with suppressed bitterness. Patent JP 02056416, 1990.

[110] Malik K, Arora G, Singh I. Taste masked microspheres of ofloxacin: formulation and evaluation of orodispersible tablets. Sci Pharm 2011; 79(3): 653-72.
[http://dx.doi.org/10.3797/scipharm.1104-11] [PMID: 21886910]

[111] Malik K, Arora G, Singh I. Locust bean gum as superdisintegrantformulation and evaluation of nimesulide orodispersible tablets. Polim Med 2011; 41(1): 17-28. b
[PMID: 21739929]

[112] Subramanian S, Sankar V, Manakadan AA, Ismail S, Andhuvan G. Formulation and evaluation of Cetirisine dihydrochloride orodispersible tablet. Pak J Pharm Sci 2010; 23(2): 232-5.
[PMID: 20363705]

[113] Swamy PV, Divate SP, Shirsand SB, Rajendra P. Preparation and evaluation of orodispersible tablets of pheniramine maleate by effervescent method. Indian J Pharm Sci 2009; 71(2): 151-4.
[http://dx.doi.org/10.4103/0250-474X.54284] [PMID: 20336216]

[114] Abed KK, Hussein AA, Ghareeb MM, Abdulrasool AA. Formulation and optimization of orodispersible tablets of diazepam. AAPS PharmSciTech 2010; 11(1): 356-61.
[http://dx.doi.org/10.1208/s12249-010-9387-y] [PMID: 20232267]

[115] Ibrahim HK, El-Setouhy DA. Valsartan orodispersible tablets: formulation, *in vitro/in vivo* characterization. AAPS PharmSciTech 2010; 11(1): 189-96.
[http://dx.doi.org/10.1208/s12249-009-9354-7] [PMID: 20112137]

[116] Goel H, Vora N, Tiwary AK, Rana V. Formulation of orodispersible tablets of ondansetron HCl: investigations using glycine-chitosan mixture as superdisintegrant. Yakugaku Zasshi 2009; 129(5): 513-21.
[http://dx.doi.org/10.1248/yakushi.129.513] [PMID: 19420882]

[117] Sharma V, Philip AK, Pathak K. Modified polysaccharides as fast disintegrating excipients for orodispersible tablets of roxithromycin. AAPS PharmSciTech 2008; 9(1): 87-94.
[http://dx.doi.org/10.1208/s12249-007-9026-4] [PMID: 18446466]

[118] Singh J, Philip AK, Pathak K. Optimization studies on design and evaluation of orodispersible pediatric formulation of indomethacin. AAPS PharmSciTech 2008; 9(1): 60-6.
[http://dx.doi.org/10.1208/s12249-007-9018-4] [PMID: 18446462]

[119] Fini A, Bergamante V, Ceschel GC, Ronchi C, de Moraes CA. Fast dispersible/slow releasing ibuprofen tablets. Eur J Pharm Biopharm 2008; 69(1): 335-41.
[http://dx.doi.org/10.1016/j.ejpb.2007.11.011] [PMID: 18182280]

[120] Puttewar TY, Kshirsagar MD, Chandewar AV, *et al.* Formulation and evaluation of orodispersible

tablet of taste masked doxylamine succinate using ion exchange resin. J King Saud Univ Sci 2010; 22(4): 229-40.
[http://dx.doi.org/10.1016/j.jksus.2010.05.003]

[121] Singh SK, Mishra DN, Jassal R, *et al.* Fast disintegrating combination tablets of omeprazole and domperidone. Asian J Pharm Clin Res 2009; 2(4): 54-62.

[122] Sievens-Figueroa L, Bhakay A, Jerez-Rozo JI, *et al.* Preparation and characterization of hydroxypropyl methyl cellulose films containing stable BCS Class II drug nanoparticles for pharmaceutical applications. Int J Pharm 2012; 423(2): 496-508.
[http://dx.doi.org/10.1016/j.ijpharm.2011.12.001] [PMID: 22178619]

[123] Dixit RP, Puthli SP. Oral strip technology: overview and future potential. J Control Release 2009; 139(2): 94-107.
[http://dx.doi.org/10.1016/j.jconrel.2009.06.014] [PMID: 19559740]

[124] Li H, Gu X. Correlation between drug dissolution and polymer hydration: a study using texture analysis. Int J Pharm 2007; 342(1-2): 18-25.
[http://dx.doi.org/10.1016/j.ijpharm.2007.04.024] [PMID: 17548178]

[125] Mendoza-Romeroa L, Pinon-Segundo E, Nava-Arzaluz M, *et al.* Comparison of pharmaceutical films prepared from aqueous polymeric dispersions using the cast method and the spraying technique. Colloids Surf A Physicochem Eng Asp 2009; 337: 109-16.
[http://dx.doi.org/10.1016/j.colsurfa.2008.12.004]

[126] Matthews KH, Stevens HN, Auffret AD, Humphrey MJ, Eccleston GM. Formulation, stability and thermal analysis of lyophilised wound healing wafers containing an insoluble MMP-3 inhibitor and a non-ionic surfactant. Int J Pharm 2008; 356(1-2): 110-20.
[http://dx.doi.org/10.1016/j.ijpharm.2007.12.043] [PMID: 18280068]

[127] Boateng JS, Auffret AD, Matthews KH, Humphrey MJ, Stevens HN, Eccleston GM. Characterisation of freeze-dried wafers and solvent evaporated films as potential drug delivery systems to mucosal surfaces. Int J Pharm 2010; 389(1-2): 24-31.

[128] Garsuch V, Breitkreutz J. Comparative investigations on different polymers for the preparation of fast-dissolving oral films. J Pharm Pharmacol 2010; 62(4): 539-45.
[http://dx.doi.org/10.1211/jpp.62.04.0018] [PMID: 20604845]

[129] El-Setouhy DA, Abd El-Malak NS. Formulation of a novel tianeptine sodium orodispersible film. AAPS PharmSciTech 2010; 11(3): 1018-25.
[http://dx.doi.org/10.1208/s12249-010-9464-2] [PMID: 20532710]

[130] Perumal VA, Lutchman D, Mackraj I, Govender T. Formulation of monolayered films with drug and polymers of opposing solubilities. Int J Pharm 2008; 358(1-2): 184-91.
[http://dx.doi.org/10.1016/j.ijpharm.2008.03.005] [PMID: 18430529]

[131] Bess WS, Kulkarni N, Ambike SH, *et al.* Fast dissolving orally consumable films containing a taste masking agent. Patent US 7648712, 2010.

[132] Yang RK, Fuisz RC, Myers GL, *et al.* Method of making self-supporting therapeutic active-containing film. Patent US 7824588, 2010.

[133] Yang RK, Fuisz RC, Myers GL, *et al.* Process for forming an ingestible thin film with non-sel--aggregating uniform heterogeneity. Patent US US 7910031, 2011.

[134] Vollmer U, Galfetti P. Rapid film: Oral thin films as an innovative drug delivery system and dosage form. Drug Dev Report 2006; 64-7.

[135] Mashru RC, Sutariya VB, Sankalia MG, Parikh PP. Development and evaluation of fast-dissolving film of salbutamol sulphate. Drug Dev Ind Pharm 2005; 31(1): 25-34.
[http://dx.doi.org/10.1081/DDC-43947] [PMID: 15704855]

[136] Gohel MC, Sharma R, Soniwala MM. Development of taste masked film of Valdecoxib for oral use. Indian J Pharm Sci 2007; 69: 318-20.
[http://dx.doi.org/10.4103/0250-474X.33174]

[137] Cilurzo F, Cupone IE, Minghetti P, Selmin F, Montanari L. Fast dissolving films made of maltodextrins. Eur J Pharm Biopharm 2008; 70(3): 895-900.
[http://dx.doi.org/10.1016/j.ejpb.2008.06.032] [PMID: 18667164]

[138] Shimoda H, Taniguchi K, Nishimura M, *et al.* Preparation of a fast dissolving oral thin film containing dexamethasone: a possible application to antiemesis during cancer chemotherapy. Eur J Pharm Biopharm 2009; 73(3): 361-5.
[http://dx.doi.org/10.1016/j.ejpb.2009.08.010] [PMID: 19735731]

[139] Fulzele SV, Satturwar PM, Dorle AK. Polymerized rosin: novel film forming polymer for drug delivery. Int J Pharm 2002; 249(1-2): 175-84.
[http://dx.doi.org/10.1016/S0378-5173(02)00529-X] [PMID: 12433446]

[140] Fuisz RC, Fuisz JM, Myers GL. Polymer-based films and drug delivery systems made therefrom. Patent WO 2008100375 A3, 2008.

[141] Kulkarni AS, Deokule HA, Mane MS, *et al.* Exploration of different polymers for use in the formulation of oral fast dissolving strips. J Curr Pharm Res 2010; 2(1): 33-5.

[142] Sakellariou P, Rowe RC. Interactions in cellulose derivative films for oral drug delivery. Prog Polym Sci 1995; 20: 889-942.
[http://dx.doi.org/10.1016/0079-6700(95)00008-4]

[143] Banker GS. Film coating theory and practice. J Pharm Sci 1966; 55(1): 81-9.
[http://dx.doi.org/10.1002/jps.2600550118] [PMID: 5918657]

[144] Rowe RC, Sheskey PJ, Owen SC. A handbook of pharmaceutical excipients. Pharmaceutical Press 2006.

[145] Rowe RC, Forse SF. The effect of polymer molecular weight on the incidence of film cracking and splitting on film coated tablets. J Pharm Pharmacol 1980; 32(8): 583-4.
[http://dx.doi.org/10.1111/j.2042-7158.1980.tb13003.x] [PMID: 6106700]

[146] Rowe RC, Forse SF. The effect of film thickness on the incidence of the defect bridging of intagliations on film coated tablets. J Pharm Pharmacol 1980; 32(9): 647-8.
[http://dx.doi.org/10.1111/j.2042-7158.1980.tb13022.x] [PMID: 6107367]

[147] Rowe RC, Forse SF. The effect of plasticizer type and concentration on the incidence of bridging of intagliations on film-coated tablets. J Pharm Pharmacol 1981; 33(3): 174-5.
[http://dx.doi.org/10.1111/j.2042-7158.1981.tb13744.x] [PMID: 6116761]

[148] Singh P, Guillory JK, Sokoloski TD, Benet LZ, Bhatia VN. Effect of inert tablet ingredients on drug absorption. I. Effect of polyethylene glycol 4000 on the intestinal absorption of four barbiturates. J Pharm Sci 1966; 55(1): 63-8.
[PMID: 5918653]

[149] Browhn GL. Formation of films from polymer dispersions. J Polm Sci 1956; 22(102): 423-34.
[http://dx.doi.org/10.1002/pol.1956.1202210208]

[150] McGregor R, Homan H, Gravina S. Fast dissolving film delivery of nucleotides that inhibit the unpleasant taste of bitter tasting medications. Patent Applicaiton WO 2004019885 A2, 2004.

[151] Leung S-H, Leone RS, Kumar LD. Fast dissolving orally consumable films. Patent US 6596298, 2003.

[152] Mennella JA, Beauchamp GK. Optimizing oral medications for children. Clin Ther 2008; 30(11): 2120-32.
[http://dx.doi.org/10.1016/j.clinthera.2008.11.018] [PMID: 19108800]

[153] Hutteau F, Mathlouthi M, Portmann MO, *et al.* Physicochemical and psychophysical characteristics of binary mixtures of bulk and intense sweeteners. Food Chem 1998; 63(1): 9-16. [http://dx.doi.org/10.1016/S0308-8146(97)00243-4]

[154] Prakash I, Dubois GE, Clos JF, Wilkens KL, Fosdick LE. Development of rebiana, a natural, non-caloric sweetener. Food Chem Toxicol 2008; 46 (Suppl. 7): S75-82. [http://dx.doi.org/10.1016/j.fct.2008.05.004] [PMID: 18554769]

[155] Chapdelaine AH, Zyck DJ, Dzija MR. Edible film formulations containing maltodextrin. Patent US 6740332, 2004.

[156] Israel K, Leo M. Salivary stimulant. Patent US 4820506, 1989.

CHAPTER 6

Excipients for Fast Dissolving /Disintegrating Tablets

Vikas A. Saharan*

Department of Pharmaceutics, School of Pharmaceutical Sciences, Sardar Bhagwan Singh Post Graduate Institute of Biomedical Sciences and Research, Balawala, Dehradun 248161, Uttarakhand, India

Abstract: Excipients play important functional roles in dosage form manufacturing. Disintegration and dissolution of dosage form and sometimes the active ingredient is greatly influenced by the use of excipient(s) like diluents and superdisintegrants in the formulation. With the advent of FDDF technologies, several directly compressible excipient systems have been introduced by excipient industry to ease fast disintegrating/dissolving tablet (FDT) manufacturing by the process of direct compression. These excipient systems have supplied a royalty free, licensee free and a low cost solution for FDT manufacturing to drug product manufacturers. Advancements in disintegrants and disintegration enhancers have also helped in formulating quicker disintegrating dosage forms. Some new excipients have been used to overcome bitter taste of drugs, improve compressibility of saccharides and as diluents in formulating FDTs. Some excipients have been modified and provided in special for their exclusive use in formulating FDTs. This chapter provides an updated review on some of the excipient/excipient for their potential use formulating FDTs.

Keywords: Diluent, Mannitol, MCC II, Microcrystalline cellulose, Parteck® ODT, Pharmaburst®, Polymer, Prosolv® ODT, Saccharides, Superdisintegrant, Taste masking.

1. INTRODUCTION

FDTs share same excipients which have been used in preparing conventional tablets. However, lyophilisation processes may require formulation of dispersion and thus excipients required are similar to those excipients which are used conventionally for making dispersions. This chapter provides a comprehensive

* **Corresponding author Vikas A. Saharan:** Department of Pharmaceutical Sciences, Sardar Bhagwan Singh Post Graduate Institute of Biomedical Sciences and Research (www.sbspgi.edu.in), Balawala, Dehradun 248161, Uttarakhand, India; Tel: +91-135-2686246; Mobile: +91-8439820796; Fax: +91-135-2686246; E-mail: vikas.pharmaceutics@gmail.com

view on selected categories of excipients, which are of considerable importance in achieving fast disintegration/dissolving properties in tablets. These excipients can be grouped into superdisintegrants, water soluble excipients and coprocessed excipients.

One of the important quality attributes to qualify the status of FDT for a tablet is its faster disintegration, which shall be less than 60 s as per USP or at the most 180 s as per European Pharmacopoeia. Addition of high amounts of superdisintegrant may achieve this faster limit of disintegration but with this problem of poor hardness and high friability may crop up. Hence quality by design concept shall be applied for optimising the mechanical strength of the tablet and faster disintegration properties. Various superdisintegrants, like crospovidone, sodium starch glycolate (SSG), croscarmellose sodium (CCS), low substituted hydroxypropylcellulose (L-HPC), *etc.*, have been used to induce faster disintegration in tablets. These superdisintegrants have found widely used in FDTs manufactured by direct compression, wet/dry granulation and compression-moulding methods.

When a matrix of water soluble excipients is compressed or compressed/moulded at low pressure, the resulting FDT will dissolve quickly in mouth due to soluble nature of fillers in the composition. Sugar based excipients have been widely employed for making quickly soluble rather than quickly disintegrating type tablets. Sweetness of these fillers also helps in masking bitter/saline or other obnoxious taste of the drug. Most of the sugar and sugar alcohols are non-compressible and their compression properties are required to be improved. Excipients manufacturers have seen the demand of drug product manufactures and accordingly provides various compressible grades of sugar based excipients.

Direct compression of tablets is very popular among drug product manufacturers due to the use of least number of processing steps in it. Hence, most of the diluents are now available in directly compressible grades. For making specialised tablets, like FDTs, coprocessed excipients have been manufactured, which can possibly avoid the transfer of costly proprietary/patented FDT technology, costly formulation development and time consuming in optimising formulations. Some coprocessed excipients require a single step of mixing API with lubricant/glidant and coprocessed excipient before compression to FDTs, *e.g.* Pharmaburst®, Parteck® ODT, Prosolv® ODT *etc.*

2. SUPERDISINTEGRANTS

Addition of large amounts of superdisintegrant(s) to a direct compressible tablet can increase disintegration/dissolution of the tablet. In this approach, the type of disintegrant and its amount included in the formulation are of prime importance. The most popular superdisintegrants used for formulating FDTs are CCS, L-HPC, crospovidone and SSG. Some less explored superdisintegrants are Indion 414, modified polysaccharides or gums, novel combinations like glycine-chitosan, chitosan alginate complex and *Plantago ovata* mucilage. Some of the literature reports on use of various superdisintegrants in directly compressed FDTs are provided in Table **1**.

Table 1. Use of superdisintegrants and various diluents in FDTs prepared by direct compression.

Drug	Diluent	Disintegrant	Ref.
Acetaminophen and ascorbic acid	Avicel PH-M series and spherical sugar granules	L-HPC	[1]
Ascorbic acid and nifedipine	Mannitol	Crospovidone	[2]
Buspiron	Microcrystalline cellulose (MCC) (Avicel PH 102) and Pearlitol SD 200	Crospovidone, CCS and SSG	[3]
Carvidilol solid dispersion with PVP	MCC and mannitol	Crospovidone, SSG, CCS and polacrilin potassium	[4]
Celecoxib solid dispersion with sorbitol		SSG	[5]
Chlorpromazine HCl	MCC and mannitol	Crospovidone, CCS, SSG, L-HPC and pregelatinised starch	[6]
Cinnarizine	Avicel PH102 and mannitol	Crospovidone	[7]
Clonazepam	MCC and mannitol	Crospovidone, CCS and SSG	[8]
Clozapine	Avicel PH102 and mannitol	Kollidon CL and Explotab	[9]
Dicyclomine HCl, roxithromycin, montelukast sodium	Avicel PH102	Indion 414, CCS, SSG and crospovidone	[10]
Epinephrine	MCC (Avicel PH 301)	L-HPC	[11]
Ethenzamide	MCC	L-HPC	[12]
Famotidine	Spray dried lactose, mannitol and Avicel PH 101	SSG, Ac-Di-Sol and L-HPC	[13]
Famotidine	Dibasic calcium phosphate (DCP)	Ac-Di-Sol, crospovidone and SSG	[14]
Famotidine	MCC, xylitol and sucrose stearic acid esters	CCS	[15, 16]
Fexofenadine	Avicel PH102 and mannitol	Ac-Di-Sol, crospovidone and SSG	[17]
Flutamide	Ludipress, mannitol and Avicel PH102	SSG	[18]

(Table 1) contd.....

Drug	Diluent	Disintegrant	Ref.
Gliclazide	MCC and DCP	Crospovidone and CCS	[19]
Glipizide	MCC or DCP	Crospovidone and CCS	[20]
Glyburide/PEG 6000/Surfactant ternary solid dispersion	MCC and lactose monohydrate	Maize starch and pregelatinised starch	[21]
Granisetron HCl	MCC and mannitol	CCS, SSG and crospovidone	[22]
Hydrochlorthiazide	MCC	CCS and crospovidone	[23]
Ibuprofen solid dispersion with PEG 4000	Avicel PH 102	Primogel and Ac-Di-Sol	[24]
Lamotrigene	Mannitol and Avicel PH102	CCS, SSG and crospovidone XL-10	[25]
Losartan potassium	MCC and mannitol	Polyplasdone XL 10, CCS and Explotab	[26]
Meclizine	MCC (Avicel PH102 and Avicel PH301)	L-HPC	[27]
Meclizine	Mannitol and maltodextrin	CCS	[28]
Melatonin	Mannitol	PVP	[29]
Meloxicam	Pearlitol SD 200 and MCC	Polyplasdone XL 10, CCS and Explotab	[30]
Meloxicam PEG solid dispersion	MCC (RanQ102)	Ac-Di-Sol	[31]
Meloxicam-β-cyclodextrin complex	Co-spray dried MCC and mannitol (Avicel HFE-102)	SSG, CCS and crospovidone	[32]
Omeprazole and Domperidone	Mannitol	Kollidon CL, SSG and Ac-Di-Sol	[33]
Ondansetron HCl	Spray dried lactose	Glycine-Chitosan, CCS and crospovidone	[34]
Oxcarbapezine	Mannitol and DCP	Crospovidone and CCS	[35]
Oxycarbazepine	Avicel PH102	Polyplasdone XL10, Primojel and Ac-Di-Sol	[36]
Piroxicam	MCC and mannitol	Crospovidone and SSG	[37]
Rosiglitazone	MCC and lactose	SSG, Crosspovidone and CCS	[38]
Roxithromycin	MCC and spray dried lactose	Treated agar and treated guar gum	[39]
Salbutamol sulphate	Avicel PH102	Primojel (SSG), crospovidone (Polyplasdone R-XL) and CCS (Ac-Di-Sol),	[14]
Salbutamol sulphate	MCC and mannitol	SSG, CCS and Indion 414	[40]
Salbutamol sulphate	MCC and Mannitol	CCS, SSG and crospovidone	[41]
Salbutamol sulphate	Mannitol	SSG	[42]
Sildenafil citrate	MCC and starch	SSG and CCS	[43]
Tinidazole taste masked microspheres with Eudragit E100	MCC	SSG	[44]

(Table 1) contd.....

Drug	Diluent	Disintegrant	Ref.
Tizanidine HCl taste masked granules with Eudragit E100	MCC and mannitol	SSG, CCS and crospovidone	[45]
Valdecoxib and Metoclopramide	Mannitol and MCC	SSG, Ac-Di-Sol and Kollidon CL	[46]
Valsartan	MCC	Crospovidone, Ac-Di-Sol and SSG	[47]
Zidovudine and Lumivudine Fixed Dose Combination	Avicel PH102	Explotab	[48]

Direct compressible FDT formulation contains high level of superdisintegrants which may range from 10-20% by weight or even higher than this amount or lower in some cases [49]. At high levels superdisintegrant may affect mouthfeel, tablet hardness and friability of FDTs [13]. Hence, apart from disintegrant action, several other properties like compactability, mouthfeel, flow, particle size and distribution, particle shape and morphology and flowability are equally important in selecting a superdisintegrant for FDTs [49]. On the other hand, the properties of drug, amount of drug and presence of other additives are also paramount importance in determining quality attributes of FDTs.

Pharmaceutical disintegrants act mainly by following mechanism [50]:

i. *Capillary/wicking action*: Disintegrant absorbs water through pores in the tablet that enlarges the pores and reduces the binding forces between the tablets.
ii. *High swellability*: Disintegrant absorbs water resulting in increased swelling pressure that causes the tablet to disintegrate.
iii. Act by both capillary action and high swellability process.

As per force equivalent concept, disintegration efficiency is the ability of a disintegrant to convert absorbed water into swelling force referred to as disintegrating force [51]. A critical concentration of disintegrant is desired to optimise disintegration of tablet. At disintegrant concentration below this critical limit, disintegration time of tablet relates inversely to the disintegrant concentration and at concentration higher than critical concentration, the disintegration time either remains constant or may increase.

Followings are the factors affecting disintegration/dissolution of FDTs:

i. Type and amount of disintegrant
ii. Combination of disintegrants and their mechanism of action
iii. Water absorption capacity of the formulation

iv. Hardness and size of tablets
v. Nature of drug substance
vi. Nature of other tablet excipients
vii. Particle size distribution of diluents
viii. Porosity and pore size distribution

MCC and L-HPC have been widely used as diluent and disintegrant combination in preparing FDTs. MCC:L-HPC ratios of 8:2-9:1 gave best results to achieve fastest disintegrating times in tablets [1, 27, 52]. FDTs produced at a compression force of 300 kg rapidly disintegrated (within 30 s) *in vitro* and in the oral cavity [53]. Watanabe *et al.* (1995) formulated FDTs having disintegration time less than 30 s from crystalline cellulose and L-HPC. The combination of crystalline cellulose and L-HPC increased the porosity of tablets by promoting osmotic capillary action [27]. Ishikawa *et al.* (1990) prepared taste masked FDTs of oxybutynin and pirenzipine using MCC as diluent and L-HPC as disintegrant in 8:2 ratio [54]. FDTs of acetaminophen and ascorbic acid were prepared by direct compression using a special grade of MCC (Avicel PH-M series, particle size 7-32 μm) as diluent and L-HPC as disintegrant in the ratio of 9:1 [55]. Particle size is an important parameter in the clinical acceptance of FDTs. Sensory evaluation by volunteers showed superiority of such tablets, when compared with tablets with normal grade MCC (PH-102). Fluidity problem was solved by adding nonpareil spheres (crystalline sugar granules of sucrose and starch in ratio 7:3).

MCC particles are relatively smaller with large degree of circularity when compared to L-HPC (larger particles, fibrous). Number of contact points per unit cross sectional area of the fracture place of pure MCC tablet is larger in comparison to tablets prepared from L-HPC. Furthermore, stronger hydrogen bond interaction is present in MCC tablet when compared to hydrogen bond interaction in L-HPC tablet. The presence of three hydroxypropyl ether groups in amorphous region of L-HPC facilitate faster water uptake. A proper MCC/L-HPC system is able to give the desired tensile strength and porosity and ultimately quick disintegration [53]. FDTs prepared by direct compression of diluents and different levels of disintegrants showed that FDTs are produced at low compression forces. Improving the robustness of such tablets by increasing compression force reduces the porosity [56]. Ethenzamide FDT consisting of excipients MCC, lactose, erythritol and sodium carboxymethyl cellulose were made by direct compression [57]. Optimum combination of tablet porosity and formulation was obtained by superimposing the contour diagrams of tablet tensile strength and disintegration time. Erythritol granules (fluidised bed granulation with water) and L-HPC blend was compressed to prepare FDTs. Fine micronised grades (15 μm) gave tablets of greater hardness, when compared with the original larger size (40 μ) [58].

Co-grinding of crospovidone with D-mannitol in a vibration rod mill, followed by addition of crospovidone, D-mannitol and magnesium stearate and subsequent tableting was found very effective in improving hardness of resulting FDTs [2]. Crospovidone was used to assist grinding of D-mannitol. The size reduction of D-mannitol increased the specific surface area leading to an increase in hardness of tablets. The method was also found very effective with other saccharides and disintegrants. Dissolution rate of nifedipine improved remarkably when FDTs of nifedipine, prepared by this method, were tested in dissolution studies.

Disintegration and dissolution of directly compressed FDTs are based on the use of water soluble excipients or faster acting disintegrant(s). Faster dissolution and oral disintegration time of 11.4 s were achieved in famotidine FDTs prepared using mannitol and L-HPC when compared to formulations containing Avicel PH 101 and spray dried lactose and other disintegrants like Ac-Di-Sol and SSG [13].

Chitosan-glycine mixture was used as disintegrant-disintegrant accelerator combination in preparing FDTs of ondansetron HCl by a direct compression process [34]. FDTs containing 5.5% w/w of chitosan and 43.3% w/w of glycine disintegrated in 29±2 s in the oral cavity. Chitosan-alginate (1:1) interpolymer complex and chitin was used as a novel superdisintegrant in preparing FDTs of ondansetron HCl [59] and salbutamol sulphate [60]. The chitosan-alginate complex was prepared by coacervation phase separation method. A combination of chitin (10% w/w), glycine (40% w/w) and chitosan-alginate interpolymer complex (3% w/w) was found to exhibit excellent superdisintegrant action in FDTs of ondansetron HCl. FDTs of salbutamol sulphate containing 50% w/w of glycine, 10% w/w of chitosan-alginate complex and 15% w/w of chitin disintegrated quickly than FDTs containing other concentrations. Faster disintegration of FDTs was achieved due to swelling of chitosan-alginate complex by glycine transported aqueous medium to different parts of the tablets. A mathematical model was developed to study the effect of swelling index, water sorption, effective pore radius and hardness of tablet to correlate with disintegration time of FDTs [61].

MCC (60% w/w) and *Plantago ovata* mucilage (8% w/w) was used to achieve 11 s wetting time, 8 s *in vitro* disintegration and 86% water absorption ratio in FDTs of prochlorperazine maleate [62]. FDTs containing MCC and directly compressible mannitol (Pearlitol SD 200) as diluents were prepared by direct compression. The obtained results from the *Plantago ovata* mucilage were as good as those of crospovidone.

2.1. Wet Granulation

Wet granulation involves preparation of granules from raw materials with the aid of a binder solution/slurry prior to compression of tablets. Modification of materials' properties is easier in the wet granulation, when compared to dry granulation or direct compression. Control of compressibility and disintegration, essential in making FDTs, by altering the manufacturing conditions is feasible and rather easy in wet granulation. A binder solution or slurry helps with the formation of interparticle bonds and growth of granules for enhancing the hardness of the resulting tablets. Some of the literature reports on preparation of FDTs are shown as Table **2**.

Table 2. Use of diluents, disintegrants and binders in various FDTs prepared by wet granulation methods.

Drug	Diluent	Disintegrant	Binder	Ref
Acetaminophen and codeine phosphate	Mannitol	Ac-Di-Sol	Gelucire 44/14 and Kollidon VA64	[63]
Acetaminophen	Mannitol	CCS and sodium carboxymethylcellulose	PEG-6-stearate	[64]
Acetylsalicylic acid		Carmellose, carmellose sodium, carmellose calcium and L-HPC	Acid treated yeast cell wall	[50]
Buspiron	MCC (Avicel PH 102) and Pearlitol SD 200	Crospovidone, CCS and SSG		[3]
Carbamazepine	Monohydrate lactose	Crospovidone	PEG	[65]
Diazepam solid dispersion with PEG 4000/6000	MCC (Avicel PH 102) and lactose monohydrate	CCS	Starch paste	[66]
Glyburide/PEG 6000/Surfactant ternary solid dispersion	MCC and lactose monohydrate	Maize starch	Pregelatinised starch	[21]
Meclizine	Mannitol	CCS	Maltodextrin solution	[28]
Meloxicam	MCC, dextrose and β cyclodextrin	Crospovidone and CCS	Starch mucilage	[67]
Oxacarbazepine	Avicel PH102	Ac-Di-Sol	Starch	[68]

(Table 2) contd.....

Drug	Diluent	Disintegrant	Binder	Ref
	D-mannitol and corn starch		pregelatinised starch, D-sorbitol, macrogol 4000, hypromellose, hydroxylpropylcellulose and povidone	[69]
	Maltrin QD580 and Mannogem EZ Spray		Sucrose	[70]
	Corn starch	Amino acids (L-alanine, glycine, L-lysine HCl and L-tyrosine)	L—HPC	[71]

3. SUGAR BASED EXCIPIENTS

Sugar based excipients, *e.g.* mannitol, sorbitol, dextrose, fructose, maltose, isomaltose, maltitol, xylitol, lactiol, starch hydrolysate and polydextrose are widely used as bulking agents. Nearly all formulations of FDTs contain sugar based materials. FDTs prepared by lyophilisation, floss, moulding and direct compression methods utilise sugar based excipients as fillers/binders/sweeteners. High sweetness and aqueous solubility of these polyols offers a pleasing mouthfeel, good taste and taste masking effect. For incorporation into FDTs, sugar based excipients are required to possess good compressibility and/or compactibility.

Mannitol, among other polyols, has been extensively used and studied sugar based excipient for preparing FDTs (See Table **1** and Table **2**). Mannitol is used as diluent-binder alone or in combination with MCC or other sugar alcohol/saccharide. Mannitol is a non-cariogenic, sugar-free, slightly sweet, non-hygroscopic substance. It has an excellent aqueous solubility of 17 g/100 mL at 20°C. These properties coupled with its great physical and chemical stability make it an excipient of choice for making FDTs, chewable and effervescent tablets. In tablets, it provides superior organoleptic properties due to its sweetness, cooling sensation on dissolution (negative heat of solution), and superior mouthfeel, when it dissolves in the oral cavity. Its versatile properties enable it as an ideal diluent (10-90%) for preparing FDTs by almost any of the conventional method or by freeze-drying [72]. Mannitol, as a diluent, offers moisture barrier and protect the drug from degradation [72, 73]. It is available commercially with different excipient manufacturers as Pearlitol (Roquette), Mannogem, Emporve and C*pharm manidex [72]. Mannitol is constituent of nearly all coprocessed excipients like Ludiflash®, Pearlitol® Flash, Prosolv® ODT, F-Melt®, Parteck® ODT and Pharmaburst® 500, which have been especially developed for FDTs

[74]. Mannitol as a filler-binder excels among other fillers due to its excellent physicochemical characteristics and its suitability to current emerging technologies for FDTs [75, 76].

4. COPROCESSED EXCIPIENTS

A tablet formulation is composed of various excipients with diverse functions like diluents, disintegrant, binder, glidant, lubricant, *etc*. Two or more than two functions of excipients can be combined by suitably processing excipients by one or combination of two or more methods like granulation, fluidised bed drying, coating, melt extrusion, solvent evaporation, milling, crystallisation, *etc*. Simultaneous processing of two or more excipients to develop composite excipient is referred to as coprocessing and the resulting composite excipient is termed as coprocessed excipient or excipient formulation or excipient system. Sometimes, coprocessed excipients are also termed as multifunctional, high functionality and performance excipients. Coprocessed excipients are designed to physically modify their properties in such a manner that cannot be achieved by simple physical mixing and without altering their chemical structure/composition.

Table 3. Use of coprocessed excipients in preparing FDTs by direct compression.

Drug	Coprocecessed Excipient	Other Excipients	Ref.
Amlodipine	F-melt®	Magnesium stearate	[77]
Baclofen	Ludiflash®	Calcium stearate, aspartame, aerosol and sodium lauryl sulphate	[78]
Benzocaine	F-melt®, Pearlitol® Flash, Ludiflash® and Prosolv® ODT	Magnesium stearate	[79]
Cefopodoxime proxetil complex with Kyron T	Pharmaburst®	MCC, Kyron T (various grades), talc, saccharin, orange flavour and disintegrant (crospovidone or CCS or SSG)	[80]
Cetirizine dihydrochloride	Ludiflash®	Avicel PH101, Aerosil 200, magnesium stearate and sodium stearyl fumarate (SSF)	[81]
Gliclazide	Ludiflash®	MCC, sodium saccharine, magnesium stearate and talc	[82]
Hydrochlorthiazide	Parteck® ODT, Ludiflash®, Pearlitol® Flash, Prosolv® ODT and Pharmaburst® 500	SSF	[74]
Ibuprofen, diclofenac sodium and diltiazem HCl	F-melt® Type C and Type M	SSF	[83]

(Table 3) contd.....

Drug	Coprocecessed Excipient	Other Excipients	Ref.
Mirtazapine and Kleptose HPB complex	Ludiflash® and Pearlitol®	Kyron T314, Avicel PH101 and magnesium stearate	[84]
Rifampin	F-melt®	Avicel PH102, Ac-Di-Sol, cherry flavour and magnesium stearate	[85]
Sildenafil citrate	Pharmaburst® 500	Magnesium stearate, sucralose, mango flavour and colloidal silicon dioxide	[86]
Sildenafil citrate and Poloxamer 188 solid dispersion	Pharmaburst® 500	Peppermint, xylitol and magnesium stearate	[87]
Tramadol HCl	Pharmaburst®	Colloidal anhydrous silica, magnesium stearate, aspartame and tutti frutti flavour	[88]
	Ludiflash®	Cocoa powder	[89]
	Ludiflash® and Parteck®	Magnesium stearate and Kollidon (several grades), Avicel PH102 and Ac-Di-Sol	[90]
	Ludiflash®	Magnesium stearate and SSF	[91]
	RxCipient® FM1000 and Parteck®	SSG and magnesium stearate	[92]

Faster disintegration and adequate mechanical strength are two important quality attributes of FDTs. Keeping in view of this, diluents and superdisintegrants have been combined by subjecting them simultaneously to prepare coprocessed excipient, which will require the addition of minimum other excipients in a direct compression process. Uses of coprocessed excipients in developing FDTs are shown in Table **3**.

An ideal bulk coprocessed excipient for preparing FDTs must possess following attributes:

- Quick disintegration/dissolution in the mouth within a few seconds without leaving any residue or any gritty sensation
- Pleasant mouthfeel and ability to mask the bitter taste of drug
- Enables high drug loading
- Sugar free, non-cariogenic and compatible ingredients
- Good flowability, no segregation of active ingredient and directly compressible to yield a mechanically strong and robust tablet
- Provide flexibility in the formulation development
- Shall remain unaffected by changes in extreme environmental conditions of humidity or temperature
- Economically cheaper, low costing on sourcing, storage, manufacturing,

analysis and packaging.

Numerous directly compressible coprocessed excipient systems for FDTs available in the market include Pharmaburst®, F-Melt®, Ludiflash®, Parteck® ODT, Pearlitol® Flash, Prosolv® ODT, *etc*. Pharmafreeze® has been developed for manufacturing FDTs by lyophilisation. Most of these excipient systems utilise sugar alcohol(s) and a superdisintegrant. A few of these excipients systems also utilise glidant for improving flow properties. Number of components in their compositions may vary from 2-5. Regulatory work increases with the increase in excipients' number in the coprocessed excipient formulation [93]. Widely used sugar alcohol is mannitol due to its sweet taste, a pleasant mouth feel, non-hygroscoic, stable and its compatibility with most of the drugs. In a nutshell, based on excipient functionalities, these excipient systems may be described as binder-disintegrant, filler-disintegrant-binder or filler-disintegrant-binder-glidant combinations.

Sugar alcohol/saccharide in these excipient systems is not robust enough to suppress bitter taste of drugs. Hence, sweeteners and/or flavours are also added to these excipient systems, while preparing FDTs of bitter tasting drugs. Optionally bitter drugs may be encapsulated or processed with some other technique for taste masking before adding to these excipient systems for making FDTs. Lubricants/glidants are also required to be added with these excipient systems so as to obtain better flow properties in the formulation to prevent sticking to tablet tooling. The processing steps of direct compression of FDTs with superdisintegrants are shown in Fig. (**1**).

The choice of excipient system shall be based on its compatibility towards the components of the excipient system and the drug. However, in some cases it is also desirable to check residual solvents and impurities, which may adversely impact stability of the drug product. Impurities that may interact with one drug may not do so with other drugs. In one study, Prosolv® ODT was found incompatible with benzocaine [79]. In accelerated stability studies at 40°C and 75% RH, it was found that over time the Prosolv® ODT was responsible for degradation of benzocaine to N-formylbenzocaine. Prosolv® ODT excipient system contains silicified MCC and crospovidone that may be a potential source of organic acid and aldehyde impurities. The formyl and acetyl species was anticipated as the main cause for degradation of benzocaine, an amine drug. However, benzocaine degradation was only observed under conditions of high relative humidity and temperature, indicating that the degradation was related to the adsorbed water by the excipients. Another Prosolv® ODT component, fructose (critical relative humidity 64%) or crospovidone (which can swell on water uptake) was capable to absorb moisture under high humidity conditions that may result in migration of impurities at high humidity conditions.

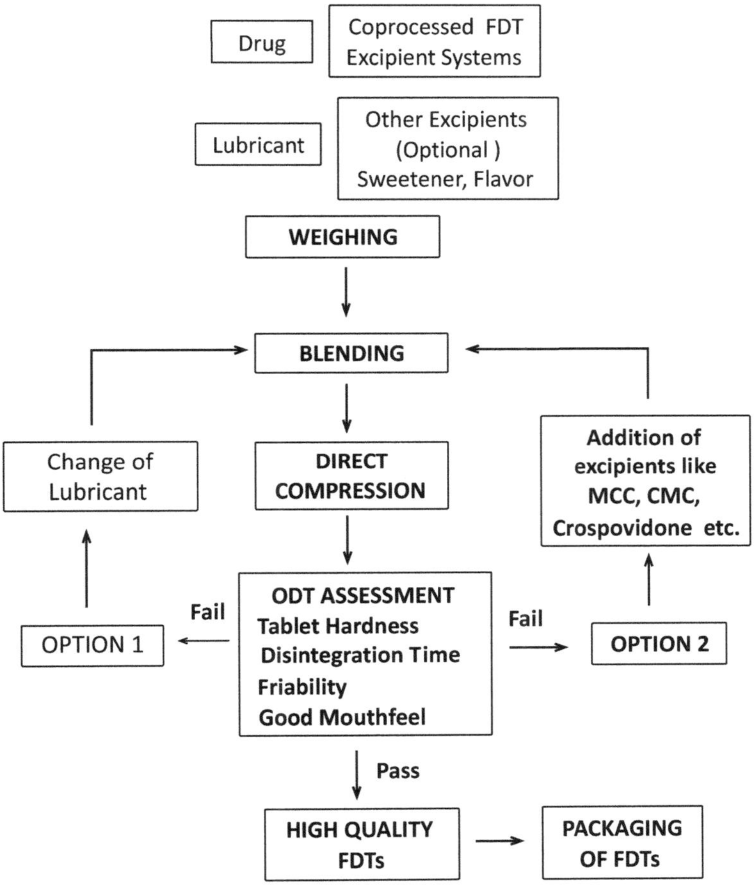

Fig. (1). Direct compression tableting and with coprocessed FDT excipient system and optimisation of tablet properties.

FDTs/ODTs shall be pharmaceutically elegant not only at the time of manufacturing but also during its entire shelf life. Physical appearance of ODTs with different excipient systems may vary due to their composition. When tablets of benzocaine were prepared with F-melt® were subjected to accelerated stability studies for 6 months, the diameter of F-Melt® tablets increased 2 and 1 mm for tablets that were compressed to a hardness of 100 N or at a compression force of 20 kN, respectively [79]. Crospovidone (a superdisintegrant and a component of F-melt®) can take up water under high humidity conditions leading to increase in size of tablets.

Hence, the choice of an excipient system is crucial when number of components in the excipient system increases. A formulator has to carefully scrutinise the compatibility of the drug with individual components of the excipient system giving special emphasis to impurities, residual solvents, and moisture uptake properties at normal and accelerated stability conditions.

4.1. Pharmaburst™

Pharmaburst™ (SPI Pharma, Wilington, DE, US; http://www.spipharma.com/) is a proprietary and patented coprocessed excipient system used to prepare FDTs having rapid oral disintegration and low adhesion onto punch faces during tableting. This excipient combines various useful properties of its constituent excipients, *viz.* mannitol, crospovidone, sorbitol and precipitated silicon dioxide [74]. This fast disintegrating excipient system is prepared by coprocessing of these excipients in a fluidised bed apparatus [94, 95]. Dry mixing of Pharmaburst® with drug, lubricant and flavour and subsequent direct compression on a conventional tablet machine can produce FDTs under normal humidity and temperature conditions. Tablets made with Pharmaburst® depending on the size and hardness will generally dissolve within 30-60 s. Tablets prepared with Pharmaburst® do not require special packaging and could be either packaged in blister packs or high density polyethelyne bottles.

Pharmaburst® is an "off the shelf" excipient system for manufacturing FDTs in-house quickly and cost effectively. However, other FDT technologies may require a third party manufacturer and are marketed under a license, making the process more expensive. When used in the formulation at levels 50% or higher, Pharmaburst® gives an excellent creamy mouth feel as the tablet dissolves flushing down the taste masked granules of the drug, without exhibiting any grittiness. Quick Melt (80 mg) Children's Non-Asprin Pain Reliever/Fever Reducer (Marlex Pharmaceuticals, located in New Castle, Delaware, USA) utilises SPI Pharma's Pharmaburst® quick dissolve technology. Pharmaburst® has been used in FDT formulations of tramadol HCl [88], cefopodoxime proxetil [80] sildenafil citrate [86] and sublingual tablets of sildendafil citrate [87].

4.2. Pharmafreeze™

SPI Pharma (http://www.spipharma.com/), in conjunction with Oregon Freeze Dry, Inc (www.ofd.com/), provides Pharmafreeze™, an ODT technology platform, for pharmaceutical applications using lyophilisation (freeze-dried) technology [96]. This technology enables the manufacture of ODTs that dissolve in less than 5 s [97]. The advantages of the patented process include a more robust matrix duet to controlled collapse during drying, yet quick dissolving tablets [98]. Drug loading of 1-250 mg/tablet at 1.0 mL fill volume is claimed with this technology. It also provides dosage flexibility when coupled with Pharmacaps® taste masking technology. FDTs of sublingual, gastrointestinal and rectal delivery can be fabricated. The drying process protects the form and functionality of thermolabile drugs.

This patented technology utilise a mixture comprising sufficient amounts of API, gum, carbohydrate base, and solvent to form a partially collapsed matrix network when the mixture is frozen and vacuum dried to remove the solvent above a collapse temperature of the matrix for a sufficient period of time to form the matrix [98]. Other components of the formulation are flavour, surfactant and sweetener. The gum may be guar, acacia, xanthan, tragacanth gum or carrageenan. The carbohydrate may be selected from dextrose, mannitol, sucrose, maltose, lactose, corn syrup solids or maltodextrin. The partial drying of the matrix is performed at temperature below its equilibrium freezing point. Vacuum drying is performed at temperature greater than the collapse temperature, instead of freeze drying it below the collapse temperature of the matrix, which is used conventionally in freeze drying. The patented process is capable of improving structural integrity in tablets and offers faster disintegration in saliva.

4.3. Prosolv®ODT/ODT G2

Prosolv® ODT and Prosolv® ODT G2 are coprocessed, proprietary (JRS Pharma http://www.jrs.de/, www.jrspharma.de) excipient systems consisting of mannitol, fructose, MCC, crospovidone and colloidal silicon dioxide [74, 79, 99, 100]. Average particle size of Prosolv® ODT is 100 µm and bulk density is 0.45 g/cm^3. It has been used in formulating Orally Disintegrating Mini Tablets (ODMTs) as child appropriate dosage form as it is a based on coprocessed mannitol [74]. Prosolv®:mannitol based excipient system has been found suitable for direct compression to FDTs having high mechanical strength, rapid disintegration and dissolution [101]. Prosolv® ODT G2 is a second generation excipient system for manufacturing ODTs characterised by creamy, smooth and cool mouth feel. Prosolv® ODT/ODT G2 provides a pleasing, convenient and discreet form of administration for drugs and nutritional ingredients without the need for water.

4.4. Parteck®ODT

Parteck® ODT (Merck; www.merckmillipore.in) is a proprietary excipient system for manufacturing FDTs by direct compression. Parteck®ODT is a blend of spray-granulated CCS and D-mannitol [102]. D-mannitol acts as filler-binder and CCS offers faster disintegration. It exhibits low hygroscopicity below 2% when it is stored at below 80% relative humidity at 25°C. Low hygroscopic nature makes it a suitable choice for moisture-sensitive drugs. Physical properties of Parteck® ODT are shown in Table **4**. Some of the recommendations for other excipients in a sample formulation are shown in Table **5**.

Table 4. Characteristic properties of Parteck® ODT [103].

Characteristic	
Appearance	White and colourless
Bulk density	0.55–0.65 g/mL
Tapped density	0.70–0.80 g/mL
Mean particle size distribution (measured by laser diffraction, D 0.50)	70–120 µm
Angle of repose	33–38°
pH value (of a 5% aqueous solution, partially dissolved)	5.0 –7.0
BET surface area (measured by nitrogen adsorption)	2.4–3.5 m^2/g
Recommended Lubricant	Magnesium stearate (1%)
Storage/Shelf life	25°C; 2 Years

Table 5. A sample formulation with Parteck® ODT [103].

Ingredient	Amount
Active ingredient	4–50%
Parteck®ODT	30–80%
Colloidal silicon dioxide	0.2–1.0%
Magnesium stearate	0.25–1.0%
Alternative lubricant (SSF)	0.5–2.0%
Sweetener & Flavour	Optional (If taste masking is not achieved by Parteck ODT)

Parteck ® ODT has been found insensitive towards changes in lubricant in placebo tablets and, therefore, it provides flexibility to drug product manufacture to resolve specific formulation problems [93].

4.5. PanExcea® ODT (MC 200G)

PanExcea® ODT (MC 200G) (http://jtbaker.com/; www.avantormaterials.com) is an excipient system for making ODTs or chewable tablets. It is composed of mannitol (75%) and calcium silicate (25%). This ODT matrix facilitate quick oral disintegration of a tablet and offers good taste, texture and mouthfeel to the formulation [104]. Drug products may be directly formulated with the drug. It can also accommodate dilution with other excipients and/or addition of other auxiliary excipients, as required. The physical properties of PanExcea® ODT (MC 200G) are provided in Table **6**.

Table 6. Some important characteristic properties of PanExcea® ODT (MC 200G) [104].

Characteristic	
Appearance	Odourless, white crystalline powder and dense spherical particles
Bulk density	0.64 g/cc
Tapped density	0.80 g/cc
Loss on drying	Less then 6%
Angle of repose	Less than 35 degrees
Flowability index	Greater than 85
Compressibility (Carr's Index)	19.4
Hausner ratio	Less than 1.35
Particle Size (D50)	103 μm
Loss on drying	0.04
Stability/Expiry	24 months

RubiODT® technology (Rubicon Research; http://www.rubicon.co.in/) is based on direct compression of taste masked API with a PanExcea® ODT [105]. The unique particle geometry and the composition of RubiODT® enable drug loading capacities up to 650 mg. This technology is suitable for drugs having different solubility profiles and bitter taste as it can be coupled with RubiCoat® taste masking technology and can also deliver drug in a controlled or sustained or delayed release manner. It employs use of conventional equipment for manufacturing and packaging.

4.6. Pearlitol® Flash

Pearlitol® Flash (Roquette; www.roquette.com, www.roquettepharma.com), an excipient system for ODTs, is a combination of mannitol and maize starch by coprocessing [79]. Pearlitol® Flash has been designed for direct compression processes and excellent flow properties and a good compactibility. Compression force of 15 kN is sufficient to obtain tablets with suitable hardness, friability and disintegration time [106]. Pearlitol® Flash is a self-disintegrating compound and thus there is no requirement of superdisintegrant. With this excipient system, 0.4% w/w lubricant is recommended in a direct compression process for a better tasting tablet, as a high level of lubricant can result in unpleasant taste. Tablets prepared with Pearlitol® Flash provide oral disintegration in less than 60 s and the *in vitro* Pharmacopoeial disintegration occurs in less than 3 minutes.

4.7. Ludiflash®

Ludiflash® (BASF, http://www.pharma-ingredients.basf.com) is a coprocessed formulation of D-mannitol (90%), polyvinyl acetate (5%) and crospovidone (5% Kollidon CL SF) obtained by granulation with Kollicoat® SR 30D [79, 107]. Mannitol, a sugar alcohol with sweet taste, is used as fast dissolving filler [108]. Crospovidone is a superdisintegrant responsible for faster disintegration even in very low amount of water as present in saliva and thereby provides pleasant, smooth and creamy mouthfeel in mouth. Polyvinyl acetate is a hydrophobic binder. All the components of Ludiflash® comply with the standards prescribed in pharmacopoeial monographs. Ludiflash® possess good flowability, high cohesion, almost no segregation of drug and least water absorption [108, 109].

With Ludiflash®, it is recommended to prepare FDTs by direct compression or dry granulation. FDTs should be compressed at 50–90 MPa since this pressure results in rapid disintegration and mechanically stable tablets [110]. Tablet characteristics remain unaffected by the speed of tableting speed. FDTs of loperamide and caffeine were prepared with Ludiflash® by direct compression at an optimum compression pressure of 60-110 MPa [111]. Resulting tablets were quickly disintegrating and mechanically stable. Ludiflash® can also be used for manufacturing FDTs by wet granulation. Some important properties of Ludiflash® are provided in Table **7**.

Table 7. Characteristic properties and recommendations for Ludiflash® [112].

Characteristic	
Colour	White to off white
Angle of repose	Nearly equal to 38°C
Solubility	Does not dissolve completely in water nor in organic solvent
Bulk density	0.40-0.52 g/mL
pH (5% in water, partially dissolved)	5.5-6.5
Particle size distribution	>0.400 mm (max. 20%); <0.200 mm (45-90%); 0.063 mm (15-45%)
Storage	Should not exceed 25°C
Recommended Lubricant	Magnesium stearate and SSF
Recommended drug load	Preferably up to 20%
Recommended disintegrant (extra granular)	5-10% Kollidon CL-SF

(Table 7) contd.....

Characteristic	
Recommended sweetener	Aspartame (0.3-0.7%); saccharin sodium (0.05-0.1%)
Recommended flavour	Vanilla (about 0.5%); L-menthol (0.1-0.3%)
Recommended effervescence	Citric acid and sodium bicarbonate (0.5% both)
Compression force	50-90 MPa (=3-6 kN compression force for a 10 mm tablet)

Ludiflash® is safe for paediatric use [113] and, therefore, used in formulating ODMTs for children [74]. ODMTs are easy to administer in children and offers great flexibility in altering doses [74]. ODMTs containing Ludiflash® are characterised with low friability, high compactability and quick simulated wetting-test time.

Orally dispersible granules from Ludiflash® or its combination with Kollidon CL-SF could be prepared by roller compaction [114]. The addition of Kollidon CL-SF reduced the dependency of applied compression force on particle size distribution and the amount of fines. Large amounts of Kollodon CL-SF, however, may cause unpleasant feeling in mouth due to absorption of huge amounts of saliva. Colour may be added to ODTs by either by coating Ludiflash® particles or by adding to the whole powder blend [114]. The later approach was found more efficient in achieving colour uniformity. However, a third approach of adding colour to Kollikoat SR 30D dispersion, during the production of Ludiflash®, has also been used.

Ludiflash® has shown superior organoleptic properties, faster disintegration and quick drug release from FDTs of baclofen prepared by a direct compression method [78]. However, in these tablets Aerosil® was used as lubricant.

Two different placebo FDTs (250 mg weight and diameter of 9.0 mm) containing Ludiflash® and other containing Ludiflash® with cocoa powder were prepared by direct compression [89]. When these tablets were tested in healthy volunteers to estimate clinical significant disintegration time, tablets containing Ludiflash® disintegrated in 10-20 s and tablets containing Ludiflash® and cocoa powder disintegrated in 23-34 s. However, this small difference in disintegration time was not statistically significant.

Particle size of water insoluble disintegrants is an important parameter when mouth feeling of FDTs is concerned [90]. Superfine crospovidone was found superior disintegrant for FDTs based on Ludiflash® and Parteck® ODT. Superfine crospovidone was pleasant tasting and pleasant feeling in the mouth, when FDTs disintegrated in mouth.

In FDTs, prepared with Ludiflash® by a direct compression, more hydrophilic SSF (0.5%) showed shorter disintegration times at all compression forces (2.5 to 25 kN), when compared to the more lipophilic magnesium stearate (0.5%), but surprisingly hardness was found almost identical in both cases [111].

4.8. F-melt®

F-melt® is a proprietary co-spray-dried excipient system of Fuji Chemical Industry Co., Ltd, Japan (www.fujichemical.co.jp/english/medical/medicine/f-melt/index.html, www.f-melt.com). F-melt® is developed from five different commponents consisting of carbohydrates (mannitol, xylitol, MCC), disintegrants (crospovidone) and inorganic excipients (magnesium aluminosilicate, DCP anhydrous) [79]. F-melt® is manufactured and made available in three different grades Type M, Type C and F1. Type M and Type C are designed for pharmaceutical industry, whereas F1 and Type C are developed for nutraceutical industry. Type C provides faster disintegration and Type M is used to achieve higher flowability and to improve quality of tablets. These two grades differ in their inorganic contents. Type C contains anhydrous DCP (Neusilin®), whereas grade M has porous magnesium aluminometasilicate (Fujicalin®) in its composition [83]. Comparative physical properties of these three grades are provided in Table **8**.

Table 8. Various grades and their properties of F-Melt®. (www.f-melt.com) [115].

Property / Parameter	Type M	Type C	F1
Appearance	White to pale yellow powder		
Loss on drying	1.80%	1.30%	5.90%
Loose bulk density	0.56 g/mL	0.54 g/mL	
Tapped density	0.65 g/mL	0.65 g/mL	
Mean particle size distribution	122.3 µm	120.8 µm	139 µm
Angle of repose	32.9°	34.2°	31°
ODT disintegration time	30 s		
Tablet hardness	50 N		
Drug loading	More than 50% possible		
Shelf life (Years)	3	3	1
Ingredients	D-Mannitol, xylitol, MCC, crospovidone and magnesium aluminometasilicate (Neusilin®)	D-Mannitol, xylitol, MCC, crospovidone and DCP anhydrous (Fujicalin®)	Waxy Rice Starch, MCC and DCP anhydrous (Fujicalin®)

(Table 8) contd.....

Property / Parameter	Type M	Type C	F1
Applications	Pharmaceutical and nutraceutical	Pharmaceutical	Dietary supplements

F-melt® can be blended with drug and lubricant followed by direct compression to prepare FDTs. A compression force from 10-15 kN is recommended to prepare placebo FDTs having disintegration time within 34-39 s and friability below 1% w/w. Tablets prepared with F-Melt® type C provides shorter disintegration time and better mechanical resistance than tablets consisting F-Melt® type M. However, the addition of drug, especially at high dose, may alter the quality of FDTs. Hence, an optimisation of the formulation with right lubricant and additional excipients may be required to further improve upon the quality of FDTs. Pleasant mouthfeel can be increased upon addition of corn starch, MCC and CMC [116]. Disintegration time of tablets can be increased by replacing magnesium stearate by SSF.

Drug solubility and its dose can have a great impact on hardness of the FDTs prepared with F-melt. It has been observed that increasing the dose of water soluble drug can adversely impact mechanical resistance of the tablet and prolong disintegration time [83]. An interaction between ibuprofen (200 mg amount per tablet) and F-melt type C (at 1:1 ratio) was observed resulting in unusual tablet with disintegration time of more than 120 min. The disintegration time of similar tablets with F-Melt® type M was about 15 min. The interaction between calcium ions coming from F-Melt® type C and carboxylic group of ibuprofen resulted in such longer disintegration time. However, no such interaction between F-Melt® type M and ibuprofen was observed due to absence of calcium ions in type M. In one study, 5 formulations out of 90 qualified the faster disintegration criterion of FDTs [83]. Obtained results emphasised that drug solubility, dose of drug and grade of F-melt® used in the formulation have great impact on quality of tablets prepared.

In a study with amolodipine FDTs, F-Melt® (as disintegrating agent) gave best results in terms of disintegration time (8 s) and magnesium stearate (lubricant) offered superior flow properties in the formulation [77]. Bitter taste was masked with mannitol/aspartame (sweetener) and use of peppermint flavour.

4.9. Disintequik™ ODT

Disintequik™ ODT (Sheffield Bio-Science's, http://www.sheffieldbioscience.com/) is a coprocessed fast dissolving tableting excipient for use in FDTs. It requires addition of drug, flavour and lubricant followed by compression to produce FDTs. It has been optimised to provide superior mouthfeel, while preserving ideal flow, disintegration and tablet hardness characteristics.

Disintequik™ MCC/MCC 25 is a co-processed lactose and MCC excipient system designed for tableting by direct compression and to achieve faster disintegration of tablets in the oral cavity [117, 118]. Coprocesssing has synergistically combined the properties of the lactose and MCC and thus eliminated blending issues, resulting in a uniform formulation. Disintequik™ MCC is more fluid, more compressible and produces tablets with higher mechanical strength, when compared to tablets prepared with lactose and MCC blend. Small quantities of API may be added directly and subsequently compressed without the requirements of preparing granulations. Coprocessing has thus brought together the superior binding abilities of lactose and quick disintegrating action of MCC together in a single product.

5. NATURAL POLYMERS

Natural polymers have been widely used for their disintegrating and filling properties in formulating FDTs. Natural polymers are non-toxic, biodegradable, eco-friendly, cost-efficacious and devoid of any side effects. The disintegrating properties of polymers obtained from *Lepidium sativum*, *Plantago ovata*, gum karaya, guar gum, mango peel pectin, fenugreek seed mucilage, *etc.* have been investigated for faster disintegration/dissolution properties in FDTs (Table **9**). These natural superdisintegrants are expected to provide faster disintegration/dissolution of FDTs leading to quicker onset, faster bioavailability and efficacious therapy coupled with improved patient compliance.

Table 9. Use of natural polymers as disintegrant/fillers in FDTs.

Natural Polymer	FDT Technology	Concentration (% w/w)	Drug	Disintegration Time (s)	Ref.
Aegle marmelos gum and modified *Aegle marmelos* gum	Direct compression	41.7	Aceclofenac	16, 18	[119]
Banana powder	Direct compression	2, 6, 8	Lornoxicam	18.23-22.34	[120]
Chitin and chitosan	Wet granulation	3	Cinnarizine	60	[121]
Chitin with Chitosan-Alginate: glycine	Direct compression	Chitosan-Alginate: glycine (30:70); chitin (5-20%)	Metoclopramide	16-28	[59]
Chitin–silicon dioxide coprecipitates	Direct compression	1, 5, 10, 20	Placebo Avicel and Lactose (70:30)	10-50	[122]

(Table 9) contd.....

Natural Polymer	FDT Technology	Concentration (% w/w)	Drug	Disintegration Time (s)	Ref.
Chitosan and silicon dioxide	Wet granulation	2.57	Metformin HCl	< 10	[123]
Chitosan–alginate based complex	Wet granulation	5-50	Phenytoin sodium	42-154	[124]
Fenugreek seed mucilage	Direct compression	4	Metformin hydrochloride	15.6	[125]
Karaya gum and natural agar	Dry granulation	2.5, 5, 7.5, 10	Ondansetron HCl	11-39	[126]
Lallemantia reylenne seed powder	Direct compression	2.5, 5, 7.5, 10	Nimesulide	11-22	[127]
Lepidium sativum mucilage		5–15	Nimesulide	17	[128]
Locust bean gum	Direct Compression	2.5-10	Nimesulide	13-20	[129]
Mangifera indica gum powder	Direct compression	2-10	Metformin HCl	40-64	[130]
Modified polysaccharides (Cogrinded treated agar / Cogrinded treated guar gum with mannitol)	Direct compression	5	Roxithromycin	35.1-44.3	[39]
Mucilages of *Hibiscus rosasinensis* Linn and treated agar	Direct compression	3, 6, 9, 12	Famotidine	12-46	[131]
Mucilage from seeds of *Lepidium sativum*	Direct compression	10	Nimesulide	37-47	[128]
Mucilage from *Trigonella foenum-graceum* seeds	Direct compression	2, 4, 6, 8, 10	Metformin HCl	17.3-63.6	[125]
Ocimum gratissimum mucilage powder and *Ocimum gratissimum* seed powder	Direct compression	5, 10, 15, 20	Metformin HCl	40-68	[132]
Plantago ovata husk	Direct compression	2.5, 3, 3.75	Amlodipine besylate	25, 23, 22	[25]
Plantago ovata husk	Direct compression	5	Ciprofloxacin HCl	42	[133]
Plantago ovata mucilage	Direct compression	2.5, 5, 7.5, 10	Aceclofenac	12-180	[134]
Plantago ovata mucilage	Direct compression	2-8	Prochlorperazine maleate	11-47	[135]

(Table 9) contd.....

Natural Polymer	FDT Technology	Concentration (% w/w)	Drug	Disintegration Time (s)	Ref.
Plantago ovata seed powder, mucilage and husk	Direct compression	3, 4, 5	Fexofenadine HCl	31-56	[14]
Plantago ovata seed mucilage	Direct Compression	3-7	Amlodipine besylate	11.69-21.52	[136]
Plantago ovata, gum karaya and guar gum	Direct compression	5	Granisetron HCl	17.1	[137]
Soy polysaccharide	Direct compression	2, 6, 8	Lornoxicam	10.33-17.23	[120]
Treated agar powder	Direct compression		Placebo tablets	5-6	[138]

Some of these natural polymers have been approved by regulatory agencies for their inclusion in food or drugs [139]. Chitosan, guar gum and locust bean gum are listed in Code of Federal Regulations (CFR21) and thus designated as GRAS (Generally Recognised as Safe). Gum karaya has been included in Food Chemicals index. Gellan gum (E418) is approved in Europe as a food additive and included in Food Chemicals Codex, JECFA and USP/NF, European Directive, *etc*.

6. SOME OTHER EXCIPIENTS

6.1. Avicel PH 101/PH102

In most of the directly compressible FDTs, MCC is used either alone or with mannitol or other saccharide (Table **1**). It acts as a good binder as well as it can add to faster disintegration.

6.2. MCC Sanaq® Burst

MCC Sanaq® Brust, also referred to as MCC II, is a polymorph of MCC I. MCC Sanaq® Burst is a multifunctional excipient with filler, binder and disintegrant properties for its use in direct compression, ODT and fast dissolving pellets [140]. It is pure MCC (100%) with better taste than the other types of cellulose, directly compressible and offer faster disintegration in pellets and tablets. With all these properties, it has a great potential to become a diluent of choice in FDTs and fast disintegrating pellets [141]. It can avoid the use of a separate disintegrant in fast disintegrating pellets or FDTs. MCC Sanaq® Burst has been used in developing fast disintegrating pellets by wet-extrusion/spheronisation [142]. Pellets made from MCC II have shown relatively faster disintegration and drug release when compared to MCC I pellets.

6.3. RxCipients® FM1000

RxCipients® FM1000, developed by Huber Health & Nutrition (www.hubermaterials.com or www.rxcipients.com), is used in preparing FDTs for faster oral disintegration. Tablets containing FM1000 can disintegrate in the mouth in 5-30 s. RxCipients® FM1000 is calcium silicate coated with a carbohydrate [143]. Huber has been issued a patent for RxCipients® FM1000 and its use [144].

RxCipients® FM1000 is used as disintegration promoter in FDTs where it can act alone or in the presence of other superdisintegrants to prepare tablets that disintegrate quickly in mouth. It has been recommended at 12.5% in ODTs of ibuprofen (200 mg) and dipenhydramine HCl (25 mg).

Rubicon has developed an ODT technology which uses RxCipients® FM1000 as a directly compressible excipient, calcium silicate coated with a carbohydrate [145]. Rubicon's ODT technology is successful in achieving optimal mechanical strength and quick oral disintegration in 60 s.

6.4. Eudragit® E

Eudragit® E100 is a cationic copolymer based on dimethylaminoethyl methacrylate, butyl methacrylate and methyl methacrylate (Fig. **2**) with a ratio of 2:1:1 and supplied as colourless to yellow tinged granules with a characteristic amine odour [146]. Eudragit® E PO is a solid substance obtained from Eudragit® E 100 and supplied as white powder (Dv50<50µm) with characteristic amine odour [146]. Eudragit® E 12,5 is a solution of Eudragit®E 100 containing 12.5% (w/w) Eudragit® E in a solvent mixture of isopropyl alcohol and acetone (60:40 ratio) [146]. Eudragit® E 12,5 is supplied as a low viscosity light yellow coloured liquid with a characteristic odour of solvents.

Eudragit® E is soluble below pH 5 in gastric fluids and permeable at pH above 5 in the intestinal fluids. Its glass transition temperature is 45°C (±5°C). Several successful attempts of taste masking with Eudragit E are enlisted in Table **10**.

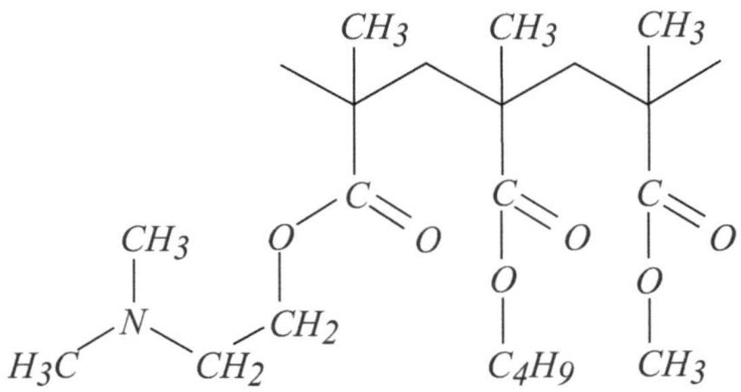

Fig. (2). Chemical structure of Eudragit E.

Table 10. Use of Eudragit EPO/E in taste masking of bitter drugs for preparing FDDFs.

Drug	Taste Masking Method	Excipient/Polymer	FDDF and Preparation Method	Ref.
Baclofen	Wet granulation/coating	Eudragit EPO, dextrates, HP-β-CD and PVP-K30	FDT, Wet granulation	[147]
Berberine HCl	Fluidised bed coating	Eudragit E100	FDT, Direct compression: superdisintegrant addition	[148]
Clindamycin HCl	Coating on MCC beads	Eudragit EPO	FDT, Direct compression: superdisintegrant addition	[149]
Donazepil HCl	Microsphere by spray drying	Eudragit EPO	FDT, Direct compression: Superdisintegrant addition	[150]
Ibuprofen	Solid dispersion by hot melt extrusion	Eudragit EPO	FDT, Direct compression: superdisintegrant addition	[151]
Lornoxicam	Solid dispersion by solvent evaporation	Eudragit EPO	FDT, Direct compression: superdisintegrant addition	[152]
Naratriptan HCl and naproxen	Coating	Eudragit E	FDT, Freeze drying	[153]
Ornidazole	Microspheres by solvent evaporation	Eudragit E100	FDT, Direct compression: superdisintegrant addition	[154]
Paracetamol	Fluidised bed coating	Eudragit EPO	FDT, Wet granulation method	[155]
Pioglitazone	Coating, sweetener, salt	Eudragit EPO, aspartame and sodium chloride	FDT	[156]
Prednisolone	Microspheres by solvent evaporation	Eudragit E100	FDT, Direct compression: superdisintegrant addition	[157]
Pyridostigmine bromide	Solid dispersion by solvent-evaporation deposition	Eudragit EPO	FDT	[158]
Sumatriptan succinate	Coating by spray drying	Eudragit EPO	FDT, Direct compression followed by sublimation	[159]

6.5. Kollicoat®Smartseal 30 D

Chemically Kollicoat® Smartseal 30 D (BASF) is a copolymer (Fig. **3**) of diethylaminoethyl methacrylate and methyl methacrylate [160]. When it is applied as coating on drug particles, pellets or granules, it provides protection from unpleasant taste and moisture. It offers quick release of the drug in the stomach without affecting the bioavailability/bioequivalence of drug.

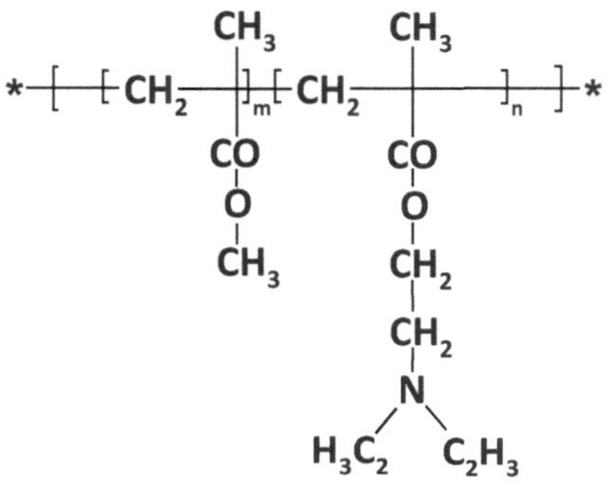

Fig. (3). Chemical structure of Kollicoat® Smartseal [143].

It is commercially available as an aqueous milky white to yellowish liquid dispersion for taste masking and moisture barrier applications. Dispersion (30% solid content) containing diethylaminoethyl methacrylate and methyl methacrylate is stabilised with approximately 0.8% sodium lauryl sulphate and 0.6% cetostearyl ether [160]. Glass transition temperature of this copolymer is 63°C. Recommended minimum film forming temperature is 57°C. Due to high lipophilicity of this copolymer, water can not act as plasticiser. Mean particle size, as determined by laser scattering is 150 nm, approximately.

The film coating offered by this polymer remains insoluble in saliva (pH 6.8-7.2). It is insoluble in neutral or basic media for more than two hours. Presence of tertiary amino group in its structure makes it soluble in acidic media at pH of 5.5 or below by protonation. A coating level of 2-6 mg/cm^2 is recommended for efficient taste masking purpose [160]. Its pH dependent solubility makes it efficient as a taste masking agent without affecting the onset of action and bioavailability of drugs.

Kollicoat® Smartseal can be applied on granules or pellets without any agglomeration up to relatively high concentration of 20% and coated pellets maintain their properties upon storage at stress conditions. Taste masking capability of Kollicoat® Smartseal is exemplified in coating of caffeine pellets and theophylline granules [161]. At 18% coating level, taste masking of theophylline was achieved. At lower levels (6%), slight bitter taste was perceived by taste panel. Paracetamol granules have been coated with Kollicoat® Smartseal 30 D at 3% level to achieve taste masking and used in preparing taste masked FDTs [162].

CONCLUSIONS

Fillers, binders and disintegrants play critical roles in formulating FDTs. Excipients have been developed to combine one or more functionality and thus new coprocessed excipients have come up for their exclusive use in FDTs. Coprocessed excipients are helpful in reducing processing steps in manufacturing of FDTs. Manufacturing of FDTs, initially developed from freeze drying methods, is now shifting towards cheaper and cost-effective direct compression methods and the whole credit goes to the availability of newer grades of excipients and coprocessed excipients. Disintegrants have been more advanced to achieve faster disintegration and therefore referred to as superdisintegrants, which are traditional disintegrants in formulations of FDTs. Taste masking agents are essential in formulating FDTs of bitter drugs. IERs, Eudragit® E/EPO and aqueous coatings are available to suppress bitter taste. Advent of new excipients has led to development of new formulations like fast disintegrating pellets, which provide excellent dosing flexibility in paediatrics.

REFERENCES

[1] Ishikawa T, Mukai B, Shiraishi S, *et al.* Preparation of rapidly disintegrating tablet using new types of microcrystalline cellulose (PH-M series) and low substituted-hydroxypropylcellulose or spherical sugar granules by direct compression method. Chem Pharm Bull (Tokyo) 2001; 49(2): 134-9. [http://dx.doi.org/10.1248/cpb.49.134] [PMID: 11217097]

[2] Shu T, Suzuki H, Hironaka K, Ito K. Studies of rapidly disintegrating tablets in the oral cavity using co-ground mixtures of mannitol with crospovidone. Chem Pharm Bull (Tokyo) 2002; 50(2): 193-8. [http://dx.doi.org/10.1248/cpb.50.193] [PMID: 11848208]

[3] Rajitha K, Shravan KY, Adhukondalu D, *et al.* Formulation and evaluation of orally disintegrating tablets of buspirone. Int J Pharm Sci Nanotechnol 2006; 1: 327-34.

[4] Singh H, Mishra SK, Varma R, *et al.* Formulation and evaluation of mouth dissolving tablets of carvedilol. Int J Pharma Bio Sci 2011; 2.

[5] Tiwari V, Kinikar DJ, Pillai K, *et al.* Preparation and evaluation of fast dissolving tablets of celecoxib. J Curr Pharm Res 2010; 4: 4-11.

[6] Gudas GK, Manasa B, Rajesham V, *et al.* Formulation and evaluation of fast dissolving tablets of Chlorpromazine HCl. J Pharm Sci Technol 2010; 2: 99-102.

[7] Patel BP, Patel JK, Rajput GC, Thakor RS. Formulation and evaluation of mouth dissolving tablets of cinnarizine. Indian J Pharm Sci 2010; 72(4): 522-5. [http://dx.doi.org/10.4103/0250-474X.73930] [PMID: 21218071]

[8] Shirsand SB, Suresh S, Swamy PV, Kumar DN, Rampure MV. Design and evaluation of fast dissolving tablets of clonazepam. Indian J Pharm Sci 2008; 70(6): 791-5.

[http://dx.doi.org/10.4103/0250-474X.49125] [PMID: 21369444]

[9] Masareddy RS, Kadia RV, Manvi FV. Development of mouth dissolving tablets of clozapine using two different techniques. Indian J Pharm Sci 2008; 70(4): 526-8. [http://dx.doi.org/10.4103/0250-474X.44611] [PMID: 20046788]

[10] Amin P, Prabhu N, Wadhwani A. Indion 414 as superdisintegrant in formulation of mouth dissolve tablets. Indian J Pharm Sci 2006; 68: 117. [http://dx.doi.org/10.4103/0250-474X.22983]

[11] Rawas-Qalaji MM, Simons FE, Simons KJ. Fast-disintegrating sublingual tablets: effect of epinephrine load on tablet characteristics. AAPS PharmSciTech 2006; 7(2): E41. [http://dx.doi.org/10.1208/pt070241] [PMID: 16796358]

[12] Bi Y, Sunada H, Yonezawa Y, Danjo K, Otsuka A, Iida K. Preparation and evaluation of a compressed tablet rapidly disintegrating in the oral cavity. Chem Pharm Bull (Tokyo) 1996; 44(11): 2121-7. [http://dx.doi.org/10.1248/cpb.44.2121] [PMID: 8945778]

[13] Abdelbary A, Elshafeey A, Zidan G. Comparative effects of different cellulosic-based directly compressed orodispersable tablets on oral bioavailability of famotidine. Carbohydr Polym 2009; 77: 799-806. [http://dx.doi.org/10.1016/j.carbpol.2009.02.030]

[14] Khinchi MP, Gupta MK, Bhandari A. Effect of various super disintegrants on drug release of orally disintegrating tablet. Int J Pharma Res and Dev 2010; 2.

[15] Koseki T, Onishi H, Takahashi Y, Uchida M, Machida Y. Development of novel fast-disintegrating tablets by direct compression using sucrose stearic acid ester as a disintegration-accelerating agent. Chem Pharm Bull (Tokyo) 2008; 56(10): 1384-8. [http://dx.doi.org/10.1248/cpb.56.1384] [PMID: 18827375]

[16] Koseki T, Onishi H, Takahashi Y, Uchida M, Machida Y. Preparation and evaluation of novel directly-compressed fast-disintegrating furosemide tablets with sucrose stearic acid ester. Biol Pharm Bull 2009; 32(6): 1126-30. [http://dx.doi.org/10.1248/bpb.32.1126] [PMID: 19483329]

[17] Solanki SS, Dahima R. Formulation and evaluation of fexofenadine mouth dissolving tablet. Dhaka Univ J Pharm Sci 2009; 8: 167-70.

[18] Elkhodairy KA, Hassan MA, Afifi SA. Formulation and optimisation of orodispersible tablets of flutamide. Saudi Pharm J 2014; 22(1): 53-61. [http://dx.doi.org/10.1016/j.jsps.2013.01.009] [PMID: 24493974]

[19] Shinde AJ, Paithane MB, More HN. Development and in-vitro evaluation of fast dissolving tablets of gliclazide. Int J Drug Dev Res 2010; 2: 724-9.

[20] Patel B, Patel D, Parmar R, *et al.* Development and invitro evaluation of fast dissolving tablets of glipizide. Int J Pharm Pharm Sci 2009; 1: 145-50.

[21] Cirri M, Maestrelli F, Corti G, Mura P, Valleri M. Fast-dissolving tablets of glyburide based on ternary solid dispersions with PEG 6000 and surfactants. Drug Deliv 2007; 14(4): 247-55. [http://dx.doi.org/10.1080/10717540601067802] [PMID: 17497357]

[22] Venkatalakshmi R, Sasikala C, Swathi R, *et al.* Formulation and evaluation of granisetron hydrochloride mouth dissolving tablet. Int J Pharm Sci 2009; 1: 336-41.

[23] Rangole US, Kawtikwar P, Sakarkar D. Formulation and *in vitro* evaluation of rapidly disintegrating tablets using hydrochlorothiazide as a model drug. Res J Pharm Tech 2008; 1: 349-52.

[24] Jain SK, Shukla M, Shrivastava V. Development and *in vitro* evaluation of ibuprofen mouth dissolving tablets using solid dispersion technique. Chem Pharm Bull (Tokyo) 2010; 58(8): 1037-42.

[http://dx.doi.org/10.1248/cpb.58.1037] [PMID: 20686256]

[25] Patil C, Das S. Effect of various superdisintegrants on the drug release profile and disintegration time of Lamotrigine orally disintegrating tablets. Afr J Pharm Pharmacol 2011; 5: 76-82. [http://dx.doi.org/10.5897/AJPP10.279]

[26] Kakade SM, Mannur VS, Ramani KB, *et al.* Formulation and evaluation of mouth dissolving tablets of losartan potassium by direct compression techniques. Int J Res Pharm Sci 2010; 1: 290-5.

[27] Watanabe Y, Koizumi K, Zama Y, Kiriyama M, Matsumoto Y, Matsumoto M. New compressed tablet rapidly disintegrating in saliva in the mouth using crystalline cellulose and a disintegrant. Biol Pharm Bull 1995; 18(9): 1308-10. [http://dx.doi.org/10.1248/bpb.18.1308] [PMID: 8845832]

[28] Elnaggar YS, El-Massik MA, Abdallah OY, Ebian AE. Maltodextrin: a novel excipient used in sugar-based orally disintegrating tablets and phase transition process. AAPS PharmSciTech 2010; 11(2): 645-51. [http://dx.doi.org/10.1208/s12249-010-9423-y] [PMID: 20405257]

[29] Muñoz H, Castan H, Clares B, Ruiz MA. Obtaining fast dissolving disintegrating tablets with different doses of melatonin. Int J Pharm 2014; 467(1-2): 84-9. [http://dx.doi.org/10.1016/j.ijpharm.2014.03.054] [PMID: 24699354]

[30] Swamy P, Areefulla S, Shirsand S, *et al.* Orodispersible tablets of meloxicam using disintegrant blends for improved efficacy. Indian J Pharm Sci 2007; 69: 836. [http://dx.doi.org/10.4103/0250-474X.39448]

[31] Shenoy VS, Pandey S. Meloxicam-PEG6000 solid dispersions in rapidly disintegrating tablets: preparation, *in vitro* and *in vivo* characterisation. Asian J Pharm Sci 2008; 3: 142-50.

[32] Obaidat AA, Obaidat RM. Development and evaluation of fast-dissolving tablets of meloxicam-β-cyclodextrin complex prepared by direct compression. Acta Pharm 2011; 61(1): 83-91. [http://dx.doi.org/10.2478/v10007-011-0005-7] [PMID: 21406346]

[33] Singh SK, Mishra DN, Jassal R, *et al.* Fast disintegrating combination tablets of omeprazole and domperidone. Asian J Pharm Clin Res 2009; 2: 74-82.

[34] Goel H, Vora N, Tiwary AK, Rana V. Formulation of orodispersible tablets of ondansetron HCl: investigations using glycine-chitosan mixture as superdisintegrant. Yakugaku Zasshi 2009; 129(5): 513-21. [http://dx.doi.org/10.1248/yakushi.129.513] [PMID: 19420882]

[35] Kalia A, Khurana S, Bedi N. Formulation and evaluation of mouth dissolving tablets of oxcarbazepine. Int J Pharm Pharm Sci 2009; 1: 12-23.

[36] Rizwanulla Madhubabu A. Preparation and evaluation of oxcarbazepine fast dissolving tablets. Int J Pharma Professional's Res 2011; 2: 201-5.

[37] Kiran NR, Palanichamy S, Rajesh M, *et al.* Formulation and evaluation of orodispersible piroxicam tablets. J Pharm Sci Res 2010; 10: 615-21.

[38] Arjun G, Prasad MS, Santhosha D, *et al.* Formulation and evaluation of rosiglitazone mouth dissolving tablet. Int J Pharma Bio Sci 2010; 1: 1-9.

[39] Sharma V, Philip AK, Pathak K. Modified polysaccharides as fast disintegrating excipients for orodispersible tablets of roxithromycin. AAPS PharmSciTech 2008; 9(1): 87-94. [http://dx.doi.org/10.1208/s12249-007-9026-4] [PMID: 18446466]

[40] Kumar A, Singh A, Saharan V. A comparative study of different proportions of superdisintegrants: formulation and evaluation of orally disintegrating tablets of salbutamol sulphate. Turk J Pharm Sci 2017; 14(1): 40-8.

[41] Thakur RR, Sardana V. Formulation optimisation and evaluation of orally disintegrating tablets of salbutamol sulphate by cost-efficient direct compression method. IJPI's J Pharmaceut Cosmetol 2011; 1: 77-89.

[42] Sharma D. Formulation development and evaluation of fast disintegrating tablets of salbutamol sulphate for respiratory disorders. ISRN pharmaceutics 2013. [http://dx.doi.org/10.1155/2013/674507]

[43] Kumar S, Sachdeva M, Bajpai M. Formulation and evaluation of mouth dissolving tablets sildenafil citrate. J Pharm Sci Technol 2010; 2: 202-6.

[44] Shishu KK, Rishi V. Development of taste-masked fast disintegrating tablets of tinidazole. Asian J Pharm Sci 2009; 4: 39-45.

[45] Zade P, Kawtikwar P, Sakarkar D. Formulation, evaluation and optimisation of fast dissolving tablet containing tizanidine hydrochloride. Int J Pharm Tech Res 2009; 1: 34-42.

[46] Mishra DN, Bindal M, Singh SK, Vijaya Kumar SG. Spray dried excipient base: a novel technique for the formulation of orally disintegrating tablets. Chem Pharm Bull (Tokyo) 2006; 54(1): 99-102. [http://dx.doi.org/10.1248/cpb.54.99] [PMID: 16394558]

[47] Jain C, Naruka P. Formulation and evaluation of fast dissolving tablets of valsartan. Int J Pharm Pharmaceut Sci 2009; 1: 219-26.

[48] Kayitare E, Vervaet C, Ntawukulilyayo JD, Seminega B, Bortel V, Remon JP. Development of fixed dose combination tablets containing zidovudine and lamivudine for paediatric applications. Int J Pharm 2009; 370(1-2): 41-6. [http://dx.doi.org/10.1016/j.ijpharm.2008.11.005] [PMID: 19059324]

[49] Camarco W, Ray D, Druffner A. Selecting superdisintegrants for orally disintegrating tablet formulations. Pharm Technol 2006; 30: s28.

[50] Ozeki T, Yasuzawa Y, Katsuyama H, *et al.* Design of rapidly disintegrating oral tablets using acid-treated yeast cell wall: a technical note. AAPS PharmSciTech 2003; 4(4): E70. [http://dx.doi.org/10.1208/pt040470] [PMID: 15198565]

[51] Caramella C, Ferrari F, Bonferoni MC, *et al.* Disintegrants in solid dosage forms. Drug Dev Ind Pharm 1990; 16: 2561-77. [http://dx.doi.org/10.3109/03639049009058547]

[52] Ishikawa T, Watanabe Y, Utoguchi N, Matsumoto M. Preparation and evaluation of tablets rapidly disintegrating in saliva containing bitter-taste-masked granules by the compression method. Chem Pharm Bull (Tokyo) 1999; 47(10): 1451-4. [http://dx.doi.org/10.1248/cpb.47.1451] [PMID: 10553641]

[53] Bi Y, Sunada H, Yonezawa Y, Danjo K, Otsuka A, Iida K. Preparation and evaluation of a compressed tablet rapidly disintegrating in the oral cavity. Chem Pharm Bull (Tokyo) 1996; 44(11): 2121-7. [http://dx.doi.org/10.1248/cpb.44.2121] [PMID: 8945778]

[54] Ishikawa T, Watanabe Y, Utoguchi N, Matsumoto M. Preparation and evaluation of tablets rapidly disintegrating in saliva containing bitter-taste-masked granules by the compression method. Chem Pharm Bull (Tokyo) 1999; 47(10): 1451-4. [http://dx.doi.org/10.1248/cpb.47.1451] [PMID: 10553641]

[55] Ishikawa T, Mukai B, Shiraishi S, *et al.* Preparation of rapidly disintegrating tablet using new types of microcrystalline cellulose (PH-M series) and low substituted-hydroxypropylcellulose or spherical sugar granules by direct compression method. Chem Pharm Bull (Tokyo) 2001; 49(2): 134-9. a [http://dx.doi.org/10.1248/cpb.49.134] [PMID: 11217097]

[56] Gupte S, Kumbale R, Khankar R. Evaluation of superdisintegrants in fast dissolve dosage form

prepared by direct compression. AAPS Annual Meeting and Exposition. Indianapolis, Indiana. 2000.

[57] Bi YX, Sunada H, Yonezawa Y, Danjo K. Evaluation of rapidly disintegrating tablets prepared by a direct compression method. Drug Dev Ind Pharm 1999; 25(5): 571-81. [http://dx.doi.org/10.1081/DDC-100102211] [PMID: 10219525]

[58] Obara S, Tanno F. Application of low-substituted hydroxypropylcellulose to tablets that rapidly disintegrate in oral cavity. AAPS Annual Meeting and Exposition. Indianapolis, Indiana. 2000.

[59] Goel H, Tiwary AK, Rana V. Fabrication and optimization of fast disintegrating tablets employing interpolymeric chitosan-alginate complex and chitin as novel superdisintegrants. Acta Pol Pharm 2011; 68(4): 571-83. [PMID: 21796940]

[60] Kharade S, Bhutkar M. Novel superdisintegrants interpolymeric chitosan-alginate complex and chitin in the formulation of orodispersible tablets. IJPRD 2013; 5: 87-94.

[61] Goel H, Arora A, Tiwary AK, Rana V. Development and evaluation of mathematical model to predict disintegration time of fast disintegrating tablets using powder characteristics. Pharm Dev Technol 2011; 16(1): 57-64. [http://dx.doi.org/10.3109/10837450903479996] [PMID: 20028210]

[62] Shirsand SB, Suresh S, Para MS, Swamy PV, Kumar DN. Plantago ovata mucilage in the design of fast disintegrating tablets. Indian J Pharm Sci 2009; 71(1): 41-5. [http://dx.doi.org/10.4103/0250-474X.51952] [PMID: 20177454]

[63] Popa G, Ochiuz L, Stoleriu I, *et al.* Binder and superdisintegrant influence on the properties of orally disintegrating high doses acetaminophen tablets. Farmacia 2010; 58: 303-7.

[64] Abdelbary G, Prinderre P, Eouani C, Joachim J, Reynier JP, Piccerelle P. The preparation of orally disintegrating tablets using a hydrophilic waxy binder. Int J Pharm 2004; 278(2): 423-33. [http://dx.doi.org/10.1016/j.ijpharm.2004.03.023] [PMID: 15196646]

[65] Perissutti B, Rubessa F, Moneghini M, Voinovich D. Formulation design of carbamazepine fast-release tablets prepared by melt granulation technique. Int J Pharm 2003; 256(1-2): 53-63. [http://dx.doi.org/10.1016/S0378-5173(03)00062-0] [PMID: 12695011]

[66] Giri TK, Sa B. Statistical evaluation of influence of polymers concentration on disintegration time and diazepam release from quick-disintegrating rapid release tablet. Yakugaku Zasshi 2009; 129(9): 1069-75.

[67] Suresh VK, Ranjit K, Nikunj P. Formulation and evaluation of fast disintegrating meloxicam tablets and its comparison with marketed product. Int J Pharm Pharmaceut Sci 2011; 3.

[68] Malke S, Shidhaye S, Kadam V. Formulation and evaluation of oxcarbazepine fast dissolve tablets. Indian J Pharm Sci 2007; 69: 211. [http://dx.doi.org/10.4103/0250-474X.33145]

[69] Mimura K, Kanada K, Uchida S, Yamada M, Namiki N. Formulation study for orally disintegrating tablet using partly pregelatinised starch binder. Chem Pharm Bull (Tokyo) 2011; 59(8): 959-64. [http://dx.doi.org/10.1248/cpb.59.959] [PMID: 21804239]

[70] Fu Y, Jeong SH, Park K. Fast-melting tablets based on highly plastic granules. J Control Release 2005; 109(1-3): 203-10. [http://dx.doi.org/10.1016/j.jconrel.2005.09.021] [PMID: 16260059]

[71] Fukami J, Ozawa A, Yoshihashi Y, Yonemochi E, Terada K. Development of fast disintegrating compressed tablets using amino acid as disintegration accelerator: evaluation of wetting and disintegration of tablet on the basis of surface free energy. Chem Pharm Bull (Tokyo) 2005; 53(12): 1536-9. [http://dx.doi.org/10.1248/cpb.53.1536] [PMID: 16327184]

[72] Rowe RC, Sheskey PJ, Cook WG. Handbook of Pharmaceutical Excipients. UK: Pharma Press 2012.

[73] Gupte A, Reynolds C, Mizell J. A case study of using common low moisture fillers in the roller compacted tablets. Accessed from http://www.metricsinc.com/wp-content/uploads/2012/07/Anshul_ Gupte-2012.pdf Accessed on 23 July 2014.

[74] Stoltenberg I, Breitkreutz J. Orally disintegrating mini-tablets (ODMTs)a novel solid oral dosage form for paediatric use. Eur J Pharm Biopharm 2011; 78(3): 462-9. [http://dx.doi.org/10.1016/j.ejpb.2011.02.005] [PMID: 21324357]

[75] Ohrem HL, Schornick E, Kalivoda A, Ognibene R. Why is mannitol becoming more and more popular as a pharmaceutical excipient in solid dosage forms? Pharm Dev Technol 2014; 19(3): 257-62. [http://dx.doi.org/10.3109/10837450.2013.775154] [PMID: 23528124]

[76] Bolhuis GK, Rexwinkel EG, Zuurman K. Polyols as filler-binders for disintegrating tablets prepared by direct compaction. Drug Dev Ind Pharm 2009; 35(6): 671-7. [http://dx.doi.org/10.1080/03639040802587799] [PMID: 19274511]

[77] Moghimi FJ, Asgharian R. S Mortazavi H. Formulation of amlodipine 5 mg oral disintegrating tablets and evaluation of its physicochemical properties. Res Pharm Sci 2012; 7: S352.

[78] Reza HM, Islam T, Shohel M, *et al.* Formulation design and evaluation of baclofen mouth dissolving tablets. Eur J App Sci 2012; 4: 110-6.

[79] Köllmer M, Popescu C, Manda P, Zhou L, Gemeinhart RA. Stability of benzocaine formulated in commercial oral disintegrating tablet platforms. AAPS PharmSciTech 2013; 14(4): 1333-40. [http://dx.doi.org/10.1208/s12249-013-0015-5] [PMID: 23990120]

[80] Raichur V, Khanum A, Pandit V, *et al.* Formulation and development of taste masked orally disintegrating tablets (ODTs) of cefpodoxime proxetil using ion exchange resins. Indo American J Pharmaceut Res 2014; 4: 151-65.

[81] Katewongsa P, Phaechamud T. Cetirizine dihydrochloride tablets comprising two different lubricants with highly loaded colloidal silicon dioxide. J Met Mat Min 2012; 22.

[82] Babu MK, Kumari SM, Sulthana MR, *et al.* Development and optimization of gliclazide sublingual tablets by using co-processed excipient to treat type II diabetes. World J Pharm Res 2014; 3: 3416-23.

[83] Krupa A, Jachowicz R, Pędzich Z, Wodnicka K. The influence of the API properties on the ODTs manufacturing from co-processed excipient systems. AAPS PharmSciTech 2012; 13(4): 1120-9. [http://dx.doi.org/10.1208/s12249-012-9831-2] [PMID: 22941425]

[84] Darwish MK. Application of quality by design principles to study the effect of coprocessed materials in the preparation of mirtazapine orodispersible tablets. Int J Drug Deliv 2013; 5: 309-22.

[85] Roth WJ, Kissinger CB, McCain RR, *et al.* Assessment of juvenile pigs to serve as human pediatric surrogates for preclinical formulation pharmacokinetic testing. AAPS J 2013; 15(3): 763-74. [http://dx.doi.org/10.1208/s12248-013-9482-6] [PMID: 23595360]

[86] Hiremath R, Mohanta GP. Orodispersible sildenafil citrate tablets: design and evaluation of formulation variables. World J Pharm Pharm Sci 2013; 2: 1298-308.

[87] Zayed R, Kamel AO, Shukr M, El-Shamy Ael-H. An *in vitro* and *in vivo* comparative study of directly compressed solid dispersions and freeze dried sildenafil citrate sublingual tablets for management of pulmonary arterial hypertension. Acta Pharm 2012; 62(3): 411-32. [http://dx.doi.org/10.2478/v10007-012-0027-9] [PMID: 23470352]

[88] Ponugoti RS, Gonugunta CR. Formulation and evaluation of mouth dissolving tablets of tramadol hydrochloride. Trop J Pharm Res 2014; 13: 669-75. [http://dx.doi.org/10.4314/tjpr.v13i5.3]

[89] Yoshita T, Uchida S, Namiki N. Clinical disintegration time of orally disintegrating tablets clinically available in Japan in healthy volunteers. Biol Pharm Bull 2013; 36(9): 1488-93. [http://dx.doi.org/10.1248/bpb.b13-00353] [PMID: 23995661]

[90] Amelian A, Winnicka K. Effect of the type of disintegrant on the characteristics of orally disintegrating tablets manufactured using new ready-to-use excipients (Ludiflash or Parteck) by direct compression method. Afr J Pharm Pharmacol 2012; 6: 2359-67. [http://dx.doi.org/10.5897/AJPP12.459]

[91] Kruse S, Gebert S, Meyer-Bohm K. Compression characterization and lubricant sensitivity of orally disintegrating tablets based on Ludiflash. APV World Meeting. Barcelona, Spain. 2008.

[92] Pabari RM, Ramtoola Z. Application of face centred central composite design to optimise compression force and tablet diameter for the formulation of mechanically strong and fast disintegrating orodispersible tablets. Int J Pharm 2012; 430(1-2): 18-25. [http://dx.doi.org/10.1016/j.ijpharm.2012.03.021] [PMID: 22465631]

[93] Ohrem HL, Ognibene R. Is another ODT excipient necessary?. Pharm Technol 2009; 21.(9)

[94] Tillotson J, Propst C. Highly compactable and durable direct compression excipients and excipient systems. US Patent 8617588, 2013.

[95] Norman GT, Nuguru KS, Amin AF. Co-processed carbohydrate system as a quick-dissolve matrix for solid dosage forms. US Patent 7118765, 2006.

[96] SPI Pharma and Oregon Freeze Dry form alliance. Accessed from: http://www.pharmaceuticalonline.com/doc/spi-pharma-and-oregon-freeze-dry-form-allianc-0001 Accessed on 22nd July 2014.

[97] SPI Pharma - Streamlining ODT technology. Accessed from: http://www.worldpharmaceuticals.net/contractors/drug-delivery-systems/spi-pharma/ Accessed on 22nd July 2014.

[98] Pebley WS, Jager NE, Thompson SJ. Rapidly disintegrating tablet. US Patent 5298261, 1994.

[99] ODT excipient matrix - license and royalty free: Prosolv ODT. Accessed from: http://www.jrs-pharma.de/Pharma/wEnglisch/produktinfo/productinfo_prosolv_odt.shtml Accessed on 22nd July 2014.

[100] Prosolv ODT G2. Accessed from: http://highfunctionalityexcipients.com/prosolv-odt.html Accessed on 22nd July 2014.

[101] Gowda V, Pabari RM, Kelly JG, *et al.* Influence of Prosolv and Prosolv:Mannitol 200 direct compression fillers on the physicomechanical properties of atorvastatin oral dispersible tablets. Pharm Dev Technol 2015; 394-400. [PMID: 24397821]

[102] Technical Information Parteck ODT. Accessed from http://www.merckmillipore.com/IN/en/products/small-molecule-pharmaceuticals/formulation/solid-dosage-form/parteck-excipients/parteck-odt/rsmb.qB.oWQAAAFQ_bF2h03D,nav# Accessed on 22 July 2014.

[103] Merck. Technical Information 100490 Parteck ODT: Merck; 2009.

[104] PanExcea™ multi-functional & co-processed performance excipients. Accessed from: http://www.avantormaterials.com/Pharmaceutical/Products/Pharmaceutical-Excipients/PanExcea-Multi-Functional-and-Co-Processed-Performance-Excipients.aspx Accessed on 22nd July 2014.

[105] RUBIODT® | Rubicon Research. Accessed from: www.rubicon.co.in/drug-delivery-technologies/rubi-odt/ Accessed on 22nd July 2014.

[106] Dusautois C. Melt-in-the-mouth ODTs. Manuf Chem Pharma Feb. 2010.

[107] Buhler V. Pharmaceutical technology of BASF excipients. 3rd ed., BASF The Chemical Company 2008.

[108] Ludiflash: the taste of success. 2011. Accessed from: http://www.pharma-ingredients.basf.com/Documents/ENP/Brochure/EN/03_110801e_Brochure%20Ludiflash.pdf Accessed on 22nd July 2014.

[109] Orally disintegrating products. 2014. Accessed from: http://www.pharma-ingredients.basf.com/Excipients/Technologies/OrallyDisintegratingProducts.aspx Accessed on 22nd July 2014.

[110] Wichtner M, Meyer-Böhm K, Maschke A. Application related properties of a new fast dispersible excipient. In: CRS 34th Annual Meeting & Exposition; Long Beach, California. 2007.

[111] Kruse S, Gebert S, Meyer-Böhm K. Development of orally disintegrating tablets based on a new excipient. San Deago, CA, US: AAPS 2007.

[112] Ludiflash. Technical information. Lampertheim: BASF SE; 2012.

[113] Heberstrelt P, Osswald F, Wildmaier R. Ludiflash as excipient for pediatric use, In: 2nd Conferrence of European Paediatric Formulation Initiative. Berlin, Germany: EU PFI 2010.

[114] Agnese T, Cech T, Herting MG. Using Ludiflash in roll compaction to produce orally dispersible acetaminophen granules 2nd Conference Innovation in Drug Delivery. Aix-en-Provence, France. 2010.

[115] F-Melt brochure. 2011. Accessed from: http://www.harke.com/fileadmin/images/pharma/Broschueren/Fuji_F-MELT_Brochure_JUN2011.pdf Accessed on 22nd July 2014.

[116] Discover the new ways to improve ODT performace with Fuji F-Melt system. 2009. Accessed from: http://www.fujichemical.co.jp/images/whatsnew/uploads/2010/10/Fuji_Email%20Blast_F-MELT_FEB16_FINAL_v2.pdf Accessed on 22nd July 2014.

[117] Disintequik™ MCC. 2014. Accessed from: http://www.sheffieldbioscience.com/disintequik_mcc/ Accessed on 22nd July 2014.

[118] Disintequik™ MCC 25. 2014. Accessed from: http://www.sheffieldbioscience.com/disintequik_MCC25/ Accessed on 22nd July 2014.

[119] Kulkarni U, Raghavendra NG, Hariprasanna RC, *et al.* Formulation and development of aceclofenac fast dissolving tablets: effect of functionality of subliming agents. J App Pharm 2011; 2: 179-90.

[120] Taksande J, Murade S, Trivedi R, *et al.* Formulation and characterization of lornoxicam fast dissolving tablet using natural superdisintegrants. Int J Res Pharm Biomed Sci 2013; 4: 459-64.

[121] Nagar M, Yadav A. Cinnarizine orodispersible tablets: a chitosan based fast mouth dissolving technology. Int J Pharm Tech Res 2009; 1: 1079-91.

[122] Rashid I, Al-Remawi M, Eftaiha A, Badwan A. Chitin-silicon dioxide coprecipitate as a novel superdisintegrant. J Pharm Sci 2008; 97(11): 4955-69. [http://dx.doi.org/10.1002/jps.21354] [PMID: 18314884]

[123] El-Barghouthi M, Eftaiha A, Rashid I, Al-Remawi M, Badwan A. A novel superdisintegrating agent made from physically modified chitosan with silicon dioxide. Drug Dev Ind Pharm 2008; 34(4): 373-83. [http://dx.doi.org/10.1080/03639040701657792] [PMID: 18401779]

[124] Malviya R, Srivastava P. Preparation, characterization and application of chitosan-alginate based polyelectrolyte complex as fast disintegrating drug delivery carrier. Polim Med 2011; 41(3): 45-54. [PMID: 22046827]

[125] Kumar R, Patil S, Patil M, *et al.* Isolation and evaluation of disintegrant properties of fenugreek seed mucilage. Int J Pharm Tech Res 2009; 1: 982-96.

[126] Bansal N, Sharma G. Formulation and Evaluation of orally disintegrating tablets of Ondansetron Hydrochloride using Natural Superdisintegrants. Int J Pharm Tech Res 2011; 3: 1616-21.

[127] Malik K, Arora G, Singh I, Arora S. Lallemantia reylenne seeds as superdisintegrant: Formulation and evaluation of nimesulide orodispersible tablets. Int J Pharm Investig 2011; 1(3): 192-8. [http://dx.doi.org/10.4103/2230-973X.85973] [PMID: 23071942]

[128] Mehta KK, Patel HH, Patel ND. Comparative evaluation of natural and synthetic superdisintegrant for promoting nimesulide dissolution for fast dissolving technology. Int J Pharm Pharmaceut Sci 2010; 2(3): 102-8.

[129] Malik K, Arora G, Singh I. Locust bean gum as superdisintegrantformulation and evaluation of nimesulide orodispersible tablets. Polim Med 2011; 41(1): 17-28. [PMID: 21739929]

[130] Nayak R, Patil S, Patil M, *et al.* Evaluation of disintegrating properties of *Mangifera indica* gum. RGUHS J Pharm Sci 2011; 1: 11-21.

[131] Halakatti P, Omer S, Gulgannavar R, *et al.* Formulation and evaluation of mouth disintegrating tablets of Famotidine by using Hibiscus rosa-sinensis mucilage and treated agar. International Journal of Research in Ayurveda and Pharmacy 2010; 1: 497-505.

[132] Kumar R, Shirwaikar A, Shirwaikar A, *et al.* Studies of disintegrant properties of seed mucilage of Ocimum gratissimum. Indian J Pharm Sci 2007; 69: 753. [http://dx.doi.org/10.4103/0250-474X.39428]

[133] Setia A, Goyal N, Kansal S. Formulation and evaluation of Ciprofloxacin hydrochloride dispersible tablets using natural substances as disintegrates. Pelagia Research Library Der Pharmacia Sinica 2011; 2: 36-9.

[134] Chakraborty S, Khandai M, Singh SP. Comparative study on effect of natural and synthetic superdisintegrants in the formulation of fast dissolving tablets. International Journal of Green Pharmacy 2008; 2: 22-5. [http://dx.doi.org/10.4103/0973-8258.39158]

[135] Shirsand SB, Suresh S, Para MS, Swamy PV. Design of fast disintegrating tablets of prochlorperazine maleate by effervescence method. Indian J Pharm Sci 2009; 71(4): 447-51. [http://dx.doi.org/10.4103/0250-474X.57298] [PMID: 20502555]

[136] Ghenge G, Pande S, Ahmad A, *et al.* Development and characterisation of fast disintegrating tablet of Amlodipine besylate using mucilage of plantago ovata as a natural superdisintegrant. Int J Pharm Tech Res 2011; 3: 938-45.

[137] Goudanavar P, Hiremath D, Spandana D, *et al.* Development and evaluation of fast disintegrating Tablets of Granisetron HCl with natural and synthetic polymers. Asian J Pharm Res 2011; 1: 72-7.

[138] Ito A, Sugihara M. Development of oral dosage form for elderly patients: use of agar as base of rapidly disintegrating oral tablets. Chem Pharm Bull (Tokyo) 1996; 44(11): 2132-6. [http://dx.doi.org/10.1248/cpb.44.2132] [PMID: 8945779]

[139] Alam MT, Parvez N, Sharma PK. FDA approved natural polymers for fast dissolving tablets. J Pharmaceutics 2014.

[140] MCC SANAQ® burst. Accessed from: http://www.pharmatrans-sanaq.com/products/multifunctional-excipients/mcc-sanaq-burst/ Accessed on 22nd July 2014.

[141] Leuenberger H, Leuenberger MN, Puchkov M. Right rirst time: computer-aided scale-up for manufacturing solid dosage forms with a shorter time to market. Swiss Pharma 2010; 32: 3-13.

[142] Krueger C, Thommes M, Kleinebudde P. MCC SANAQ burst- a new type of cellulose and its suitability to prepare fast disintegrating pellets. J Pharm Innov 2010; 5: 45-57. [http://dx.doi.org/10.1007/s12247-010-9080-4]

[143] RxCipients FM1000. Rapid Disintegrating Excipients. 2010. Accessed from:

http://www.hubermaterials.com/userfiles/files/product-finder/saleslit/RxCIPIENTS%20FM1000%20May%202010.pdf Accessed on 23 July 2014.

[144] Withiam MC, Donald P, Edward T. Calcium metasilicates and methods for making. US Patent 6610266, 2003.

[145] Pilgaonkar P, Rustomjee M, Gandhi A. Orally disintegrating tablets. US Patent 8545890, 2013.

[146] Eudragit® E 100, Eudragit® E PO and Eudragit® E 12,5. Specifications and test methods. Dramstadt, Germany: Evonik Industries AG; 2014.

[147] Janardhan D, Sreekanth J, Kumar PT, *et al.* Formulation and evaluation of baclofen orally disintegrating tablets. Int JPharm Sci Nanotechnol 2010; 2: 733-8.

[148] Hu X, Li Y, Zhang E, *et al.* Preparation and evaluation of orally disintegrating tablets containing taste-masked microcapsules of berberine hydrochloride. AAPS PharmSciTech 2013; 14(1): 29-37. [http://dx.doi.org/10.1208/s12249-012-9880-6] [PMID: 23180226]

[149] Cantor SL, Khan MA, Gupta A. Development and optimization of taste-masked orally disintegrating tablets (ODTs) of clindamycin hydrochloride. Drug Dev Ind Pharm 2014; 1-9.

[150] Yan Y-D, Woo JS, Kang JH, Yong CS, Choi HG. Preparation and evaluation of taste-masked donepezil hydrochloride orally disintegrating tablets. Biol Pharm Bull 2010; 33(8): 1364-70. [http://dx.doi.org/10.1248/bpb.33.1364] [PMID: 20686233]

[151] Gryczke A, Schminke S, Maniruzzaman M, Beck J, Douroumis D. Development and evaluation of orally disintegrating tablets (ODTs) containing Ibuprofen granules prepared by hot melt extrusion. Colloids Surf B Biointerfaces 2011; 86(2): 275-84. [http://dx.doi.org/10.1016/j.colsurfb.2011.04.007] [PMID: 21592751]

[152] Jadon RS, Nayak S, Amlan S. Taste masking of lornoxicam by polymer carrier system and formulation of oral disintegrating tablets. Int J Drug Deliv 2011; 1.

[153] Stange U, Führling C, Gieseler H. Formulation, preparation, and evaluation of novel orally disintegrating tablets containing taste-masked naproxen sodium granules and naratriptan hydrochloride. J Pharm Sci 2014; 103(4): 1233-45. [http://dx.doi.org/10.1002/jps.23896] [PMID: 24532095]

[154] Shishu K, Kamalpreet , Kapoor VR. Development of taste masked oral formulation of ornidazole. Indian J Pharm Sci 2010; 72(2): 211-5. [http://dx.doi.org/10.4103/0250-474X.65018] [PMID: 20838525]

[155] Sharma D, Chopra R, Bedi N. Development and evaluation of paracetamol taste masked orally disintegrating tablets using polymer coating technique. Int J Pharm Pharm Sci 2012; 4: 129-34.

[156] Nakano Y, Maeda A, Uchida S, Namiki N. Preparation and evaluation of unpleasant taste-masked pioglitazone orally disintegrating tablets. Int J Pharm 2013; 446(1-2): 160-5. [http://dx.doi.org/10.1016/j.ijpharm.2013.02.019] [PMID: 23419665]

[157] Anand V, Kandarapu R, Garg S. Preparation and evaluation of taste-masked orally disintegrating tablets of prednisolone. Asian J Pharm Sci 2007; 2: 227-38.

[158] Tan Q, Zhang L, Liu G, *et al.* Novel taste-masked orally disintegrating tablets for a highly soluble drug with an extremely bitter taste: design rationale and evaluation. Drug Dev Ind Pharm 2013; 39(9): 1364-71. [http://dx.doi.org/10.3109/03639045.2012.718784] [PMID: 22994163]

[159] Sheshala R, Khan N, Darwis Y. Formulation and optimization of orally disintegrating tablets of sumatriptan succinate. Chem Pharm Bull (Tokyo) 2011; 59(8): 920-8. [http://dx.doi.org/10.1248/cpb.59.920] [PMID: 21804234]

[160] Kollicoat Smartseal 30D. Technical information. Lampertheim: BASF SE; 2011.

[161] Kolter F, Guth F, Angel M. Effective taste-masking based of the new coating dispersion Kollicoat Smartseal 30D. 38th Annual Meeting and Exposition of the Controlled Release Society. Maryland, US. 2011.

[162] Sujitha V, Bhattacharyya S, Geetha T. Preparation and evaluation of orally disintegrating taste masking tablet of paracetamol with Kollicoat Smart Seal 30 D. Der Pharmacia Lettre 2014; 6: 82-9.

CHAPTER 7

Taste Masking in Fast Dissolving/Disintegrating Dosage Forms

Vikas A. Saharan[1,*], **Vandana Kharb**[2] and **Anupama Singh**[1]

[1] *Department of Pharmaceutics, School of Pharmaceutical Sciences, Sardar Bhagwan Singh Post Graduate Institute of Biomedical Sciences and Research, Balawala, Dehradun 248161, Uttarakhand, India*

[2] *Sachdeva College of Pharmacy, Gharuan 140413, District Mohali, Punjab, India*

Abstract: Fast dissolving/disintegrating dosage forms (FDDFs) comprise dosage forms meant for dissolution/disintegration in saliva and subsequent swallowing of the formulation. FDDFs include fast dissolving/disintegrating tablets (FDTs), fast dissolving/disintegrating films (FDFs), fast dissolving/disintegrating pellets (FDPs) or fast dissolving/disintegrating granules (FDGs), *etc.* Drug release from such dosage forms starts from the oral cavity itself and, therefore, a part of total drug may be absorbed much before the drug reaches in the stomach. Early release of the drug in saliva, in close proximity to taste buds, makes it desirable that the drug shall be presented in a taste masked form and palatability shall be improved to an extent that dosage form is highly acceptable among patients. Therefore, bitter or other unpleasant taste of the drug is a great challenge to formulate a taste masked FDDF formulation. An ideal taste masking technique should provide a good refreshing mouthfeel, pleasant taste and appealing flavour. On the other hand, an ideal taste masking technique shall not impart grittiness, reduction in bioavailability and a large increase in the size of the dosage form. Approaches for taste masking are generally categorised into physical, chemical and organoleptic (physiological). The technology of taste masking is highly proprietary and extensively patented. Physical/chemical methods of masking the undesirable taste work synergistically with organoleptic approaches for improving the overall palatability of pharmaceutical formulations. Hence, several proprietary taste masking technologies utilise synergistic/additive effect of two or more approaches for taste masking. This chapter provides a comprehensive overview on taste masking methods, proprietary and/or patented technologies, giving special emphasis on their application in FDDFs.

* **Corresponding author Vikas A. Saharan:** Department of Pharmaceutics, School of Pharmaceutical Sciences, Sardar Bhagwan Singh Post Graduate Institute of Biomedical Sciences and Research (www.sbspgi.edu.in), Balawala, Dehradun 248161, Uttarakhand, India; Tel: +91-135-2686246; Mobile: +91-8439820796; Fax: +91-135-2686286; E-mail: vikas.pharmaceutics@gmail.com

Vikas Anand Saharan (Ed.)

Keywords: Adsorption, Aqueous solubility, Bitter, Bitterness threshold, Coating, Complexation, Cyclodextrin, Extrusion, Granulation, Microencapsulation, Multiple emulsion, Prodrug, Resin, Rheology, Salt, Solid dispersion, Taste inhibitor, Taste modifier.

1. INTRODUCTION

Taste masking approaches restrict the movement of bitter or other undesirable taste of the drug from the dosage form to the taste buds. However, complete/drastic restriction on drug release from dosage form may sometime pose additional issues like prolonging onset of action and reduction in bioavailability. Hence, in practice, dosage form is designed and optimised to have an adequate control on drug release without compromising rate and extent of absorption. Approaches for masking taste can be broadly classified in three categories: physical, chemical and organoleptic (physiological) [1]. Physical methods of taste masking use barrier approach in reducing the contact of the drug with taste receptors present in taste buds. Chemical approaches utilise complexation with cyclodextrins, ion-exchange resins (IER) and other excipients and ion-pairing, wherein the drug is housed or bound in a manner that release of the drug in the oral cavity is prevented and when such a complex reaches in stomach/intestine, complex breaks apart to make the drug available for absorption. Some other chemical approaches used in taste masking are formation of salts and prodrugs of bitter tasting drugs, which in turn are either poor water soluble or reduce interaction of drug with taste receptors. Organoleptic taste masking require use of sweeteners, taste modifiers and taste inhibitors/modifiers, which act on taste buds by either competing with the drug for receptor site or by desensitising taste buds or by providing their strong sweet sensation/taste by interacting with taste buds. Strong sweet taste and use of flavours produces overshadowing effect, which increases the palatability of the formulation. Use of sweeteners and flavours is an age old concept in taste masking, which is still applied in most of the formulations in addition to other physical and chemical methods. Drugs differ relatively on extent of bitterness/unpleasant taste and other physicochemical properties complicating the situation and thus no single approach of taste masking can be applied universally to all the drugs and to all the dosage forms. Optimisation studies are always required to find some best compositions to achieve acceptable masking of the bitter taste.

2. PHYSICAL APPROACHES

Physical modifications in formulations can mask the taste of unpleasant drug by either preventing the drug to interact with the taste buds or delaying the reach of the drug to taste buds. These physical approaches of modifying formulations are also referred to as barrier methods. With these physical methods, the target of a formulation scientist is to reduce the drug release in oral cavity so that drug release shall remain lower than the bitterness threshold concentration. Bitterness threshold concentration can be identified for any bitter substance by organoleptic evaluation in human volunteers with a series of drug solutions varying in their concentrations. The highest drug concentration that does not elicit bitter taste is referred to as bitterness threshold concentration [2, 3]. A suitable control on drug release/dissolution of the drug from the formulation is used to maintain drug concentration lower than bitterness threshold concentration in the oral cavity. Physical approaches for reducing bitterness or other undesirable taste are coating, microencapsulation, granulations, solid dispersions, rheological modifications, microparticulates, multiple emulsions and adsorption.

2.1. Coating and Preparation of Microcapsules, Microspheres, Granules and Other Particulates

Applying polymer coating onto drug particles is an efficient mean of reducing the release of the drug below bitterness threshold in the oral cavity. Polymer coatings are applied on drug particles by spray coating in a pan or by fluidised bed coating. Alternatively, drugs may be incorporated into pellets, microspheres or microcapsules. These approaches allow the drug particles to be swallowed before attaining the threshold bitter concentration in the mouth. Coating and microencapsulation methods have disadvantages of a long term contact of drug with a liquid medium during manufacturing or storage at high humidity conditions, resulting in the release of a part of the drug in the liquid medium before the oral administration of the formulation. Furthermore, the applied polymer coat may weaken, soften, rupture or cracks may appear when coated drug particles or microcapsules are subjected to high pressures used in compressing tablets. Thus, it becomes an important pre-requisite to check whether the applied pressure is sufficient to withstand by microparticulates.

Coating/microencapsulation/granulation methods have been extensively used to overcome the problem of the unpleasant taste of the drug and render formulations palatable (Table **1**).

Table 1. Coating, microencapsulation and granulation methods for taste masking in FDDFs.

Drug	Taste Masking Method	Excipient/Polymer	FDDF and Preparation Method	Ref.
Acetaminophen	Fluidised bed coating	Kollicoat IR	FDT, dry coated tablets	[4]

(Table 1) contd.....

Drug	Taste Masking Method	Excipient/Polymer	FDDF and Preparation Method	Ref.
Prednisolone	Microspheres by solvent evaporation	Eudragit E100	FDT, direct compression: superdisintegrant addition	[5]
Clindamycin HCl	Coating on MCC beads	Eudragit EPO	FDT, direct compression: superdisintegrant addition	[6]
Cetirizine HCl	Fluidised bed coating	Eudragit RL30-D	FDT, direct compression: superdisintegrant addition	[7]
Berberine HCl	Fluidised bed coating	Eudragit E100	FDT, direct compression: superdisintegrant addition	[8]
Ambroxol HCl	Microspheres	Pectin	FDT, direct compression: Superdisintegrant addition	[9]
Baclofen	Wet granulation/coating	Eudragit EPO, dextrates, HP-β-CD and PVP K30	FDT, wet granulation	[10]
Nicorandil	Drug loaded particulates	Myristyl alcohol and stearyl alcohol	FDT, direct compression: superdisintegrant addition	[11]
Furosemide	Mixing, coating, mixing/coating granulation	Maltitol	FDT, compression of taste masked granules	[12]
Furosemide	Wet granulation	Yoghurt powder	FDT, wet granulation	[13]
Furosemide	Dry granulation	Yoghurt powder, maltitol and mannitol	FDT, dry granulation	[14]
Scopolamine HCl	Microspheres by ionotropic gelation and spray coating nanoparticles	Chitosan	FDT, wet granulation	[15]
Famotidine	Spray drying	Aquacoat ECD30, Eudragit NE30D and triacetin	FDT	[16]
Famotidine	Coating by spray drying	Aquacoat ECD30 and triacetin	FDT, wet granulation: mannitol + maltose granules compression	[17]
Pioglitazone	Coating, sweetener, salt	Eudragit EPO, aspartame and sodium chloride	FDT	[18]

(Table 1) contd.....

Drug	Taste Masking Method	Excipient/Polymer	FDDF and Preparation Method	Ref.
Paracetamol	Fluidised bed coating	Eudragit EPO	FDT, wet granulation method	[19]
Sumatriptan succinate	Coating by spray drying	Eudragit EPO	FDT, direct compression followed by sublimation	[20]
Lansoprazole	Enteric coating the layered granule in fluidised bed dryer (FBD)	Copolymer dispersions of methacrylic acid, copolymer dispersion of methyl methacrylate and ethyl acrylate, glyceryl monostearate emulsion, citric acid and triethyl citrate	FDT, granulation in FBD followed by mixing and compression	[21 - 24]
Ornidazole	Microspheres by solvent evaporation	Eudragit E100	FDT, direct compression: Superdisintegrant addition	[25]
Naratriptan HCl and naproxen	Coating	Eudragit E	FDT, freeze drying	[26]
Famotidine	Suspension spray coating, sweetener and flavour	Ethylcellulose	FDT, direct compression	[27]
Famotidine	Granulation by spray drying	Eudragit EPO, colloidal silicon dioxide, PEG 400	FDT, direct compression with Pharmaburst®	[28]
Model bitter drug (threshold value 30 mg/L), solubility 0.5 mg/mL at 20 °C	Fluidised bed coating	Ethylcellulose aqueous dispersion (Celioscoat EC-30A)	FDT, direct compression: superdisintegrant addition	[29]
Donazepil HCl	Microsphere by spray drying	Eudragit EPO	FDT, direct compression: superdisintegrant addition	[30]
Acetaminophen and imipramine	Salting-out taste-masking system (Multi layer coating)	Methylcellulose, povidone, Na_2CO_3, HPMC, Eudragit RS100, triethylcitrate and talc	FDT	[31]

Apart from masking bitter taste, microencapsulation/coating techniques offers odour masking, enhancing stability, incorporation of liquids into solids and developing controlled release formulation. Microencapsulation or coating of particles provides one of the best control on taste of the drug when formulated as liquid orals, granules, powders for reconstitution and FDDFs. Sometimes, microencapsulation and coating may result in lengthening of the dissolution time and thereby significantly affect the onset of action and bioavailability. However, a proper selection of coating material, thickness of coat, coating liquid composition may overcome the issues of rate and extent of absorption.

Taste masking has been achieved by spray coating a cationic copolymer (esters of methacrylic acid and dimethylaminoethyl methacrylate) onto bitter drug to formulate sprinkles, suspension, FDTs, chewable tablets or effervescent tablets [32]. Coating on a water soluble bitter tasting drug by coacervated polymeric material results into an adequate control required for taste masking [33].

In one interesting study, an attempt was made to simultaneous address taste masking and stabilisation concerns of lansoprazole in FDT formulation. Lansoprazole is an acid labile drug and incompatible with several excipients. Lansoprazole was coated with seven different layers to overcome the issues of bitter taste, stability concern and problem of breakage of enteric layer on compression [21 - 23]. These seven layers comprised of the core, drug layer, an intermediate layer, three enteric layers and an over coating layer. A core of lactose monohydrate-microcrystalline cellulose (MCC) was prepared and coated with six other layers, one by one, in a rotating fluidised-bed granulator. The enteric-coated microgranules, MCC, mannitol, low-substituted hydroxypropyl cellulose (L-HPC), crospovidone, magnesium stearate and other ingredients were mixed and compacted in a rotary tablet machine. FDTs of lansoprazole comprising enteric-coated microgranules disintegrated rapidly in the mouth and quickly released the drug in simulated intestinal fluid. Developed FDTs of lansoprazole (15 and 30 mg) were found bioequivalent to lansoprazole capsules [24].

2.1.1. Microcaps®

Microcaps® (Actavis; www.actavis.com, earlier Aptalis Pharmaceutical Technologies and much earlier Eurand) is a proprietary and patented taste masking technology of Actavis. This technology is equally effective and applicable to both poorly water soluble drugs and water insoluble drugs, with even at their highest doses. It uses a coacervation based microencapsulation process to encapsulate drug particles or granules and, thereby, offers consistent polymer coatings varying in porosities and thickness on coated microparticles of size150-300 µm [34]. This technology is also useful in preparing sustained/controlled release drug delivery systems. Coating on a water soluble drug by coacervated polymeric material (30-65% w/w) results in a taste masked microcapsule [33]. Coating materials may be selected from ethyl cellulose, cellulose acetate butyrate, cellulose acetate phthalate, polymethacrylates, carboxymethylethylcellulose, hydroxypropylmethyl cellulose phthalate, polylactic acid and their combinations. In a patent, effervescent microcapsules have been prepared to overcome bitter taste of the drug using a coacervating medium including cyclohexane as the solvent, ethylcellulose as the encapsulating polymer and a phase inducing polymer [35]. Naproxen and ibupforen have been taste masked in microcapsules prepared by coacervation using sodium sulphate aqueous solution as a coacervating agent, and gelatin and cellulose acetate phthalate as encapsulating materials [36]. Uniform coating around bitter drug particles acts as an inert barrier between the taste buds and the drug and a stabilisation barrier between the incompatible excipient and the drug. Sometimes, coating may hinder the absorption and thereby onset of action and bioavailability. To overcome this issue, porosity of the coating membrane may be increased by incorporating gastrosoluble inorganic or organic pore formers selected from calcium carbonate, calcium succinate, calcium phosphate, calcium saccharide, calcium tartrate, ferric hydroxide, ferric acetate, ferric phosphate, magnesium carbonate, magnesium phosphate, magnesium citrate, magnesium hydroxide and their mixtures [37]. As the coated particles reach into stomach after swallowing, pores are generated in the coating by the action of gastric fluid on microcapsules. These pores accelerate the delivery of immediate release drugs into the stomach and also ensure desired bioavailability/bioequivalence.

2.1.2. Cima's Patented Taste Masking Methods

Cima's FDT technologies, OraSolv® and DuraSolv®, use taste masked drug microparticles. The core of these microparticles consists of a drug and a saccharide which provides sweetness and a cooling sensation in the mouth. Coating on the core of microparticle reduces dissolution of drug in the mouth resulting in masking the undesired taste of the drug [38]. Cima's OraSolv® tablets use an effervescent couple to achieve supplemental taste masking for improving palatability.

2.1.3. Micromask™

Micromask™ (Particle Dynamics International, LLC's http://www.particledynamics.com/, previously KV Pharmaceuticals Inc.) involve spin congealing or casting of melt solutions or dispersions of the drug in a molten blend of wax (melting point 50-200°C), hydrophobic polymer and other excipients to produce drug loaded matrix microspheres, which are highly pliable and deformable [39]. This technology does not use any solvent and regarded as safe, fast and efficient. Taste/odour masking in chewable, sachet and quick-dissolve products can be achieved with Micromask™.

2.1.4. Taste Masking in Flashtab® Tablets

Flashtab® technology (Ethypharm, S.A., Paris, France; http://www.ethypharm.com) utilises coated multiparticles of the drug for effective taste masking, gastroresistance or controlled release [40]. In a patent issued to Ethypharm, core particles, consisting of the drug and acidic compound (*e.g.* citric acid), are coated with pH sensitive polymer soluble at pH of 5 or less (Eudragit E100) and permeable at pH above 5 [41]. The coated microparticles are prepared by Wurster spray coating in a fluidised bed.

2.1.5. Taste Masking in Zydis® Tablets

Zydis® formulations are prepared by freeze drying of a dispersion of drug and water-soluble matrix, thereby creating highly porous and friable tablets. In many instances when unpleasant tasting drug cannot be taste masked using flavours and sweeteners, alternate approaches of taste masking such as coating and complexation are used [42]. Complexation of IER and extremely bitter water soluble drugs renders the drug insoluble. For water insoluble drugs, bitterness can be masked by the use of microencapsulation techniques such as spray drying, spray-congealing or coacervation. A coating method has been developed that facilitates the use of large coated particles (>200 μm) without sedimentation or significant alteration of the properties of Zydis® tablet [43].

2.2. Rheological Modifications

Rheological modifications are used for improving the palatability of FDTs, FDF, suspensions, syrups and powders or granules for reconstitution. Several reported attempts on use of rheological modifications for bitterness reduction are provided in Table **2**. The viscosity of liquid formulations can be increased with the help of carbohydrates or gums or hydrocolloids, which act as a pseudo-barrier by lowering the diffusion of bitter drug and subsequent delay in dissolution/release of the drug from the dispersant leading to delay in the reach of the drug to the taste buds. The presence of sweeteners and flavours additionally improve the taste and overall acceptance of oral formulations.

In one instance, FDTs upon disintegration resulted in slurry with viscosity of 25,000 to 500,000 cp. High viscosity of the slurry retarded the spread of insoluble materials including the drug in a patients mouth from coated particles of the drug [44]. Less efficient mixing was observed in polymeric solutions when compared to granular solutions due to greater entanglements among polymeric chains resulting in reduction in release of bitter drug molecules to taste buds, finally leading to variations in mouth-feel attributes [45].

2.3. pH Control

Some drugs have pH dependent solubility making them either less soluble or higher soluble at pH value other than the salivary pH of 5.9. Formulating bitter drug at a pH of its minimum solubility in water is a beneficial approach for controlling the bitterness in pharmaceutical formulations. Controlling the pH leads to insufficient solubilisation of the drug resulting in equilibrium concentrations less than the bitterness threshold. This approach of adjusting pH is helpful in formulating palatable products with severely acidic (sour) or severely basic (bitter) drugs [46]. For drugs having good solubility at high pH, maintaining a low pH in the formulation renders it insoluble. Conversely, high pH is helpful in maintaining drug in suspension form, if the drug possesses good solubility at low pH. If the drug is insoluble at very high pH or very low pH, drug dissolution at salivary pH 5.9 would always be above taste threshold and it would not be feasible to use this approach for masking the bitter taste. When adjusting pH, following considerations shall be given to:

i. the pH at which drug is least soluble in the selected liquid medium;
ii. the bitterness threshold of the drug;
iii. the lowest buffer strength needed to prevent delayed release and therefore undesirable after taste;
iv. the pH stability profile of the drug;
v. the compatibility of the drug with buffer components and other excipients used in the formulation; and
vi. the physical, chemical and microbial stability of the drug in the liquid medium at selected pH.

Basic substances, such as sodium bicarbonate, sodium carbonate, calcium carbonate or sodium hydroxide, have been used in FDTs as solubilisation inhibitors, which acts by increasing the pH as granules of the drug (*e.g.* sildenafil) dissolve in aqueous medium/saliva [47]. This phenomenon reduces the amount of the drug in solution form, thereby reducing the chances of drug molecules to interact with taste buds.

Osmotic rupture of the coated drug particles or microcapsules upon suspending in the liquid medium is one major drawback when basic substances are incorporated within the coated drug particles. A product formulated in this manner will not remain taste masked for longer durations. It has also been observed that upon swallowing a pH adjusted formulation, some residue of the drug still remains in mouth that will dissolve rapidly when pH of the saliva equilibrates itself to the normal pH, giving bad aftertaste.

2.4. Solid Dispersions

Solid dispersions are dispersions in solid state prepared from one or more drug in a carrier or matrix by fusion (melting), solvent or combination of fusion and solvent method [48]. Solid dispersions of drugs have been prepared with insoluble matrices or bland matrices or excipients having sweet taste for masking the undesirable taste in pharmaceutical formulations. Generally, water-soluble carriers result in fast drug release rates. Depending on the active drug's degree of bitterness and percentage solubility, the choice of matrix or carrier shall be made to meet the required end points. Solid dispersions of primaquine phosphate and artemether were prepared with mono-ammonium glycyrrhisinate pentahydrate using solvent evaporation method [49, 50]. Solid dispersions with aminoalkyl methacrylate copolymer (Eudragit EPO) were prepared by solvent evaporation and solvent-precipitation for lornoxicam [51] and pyridostigmine bromide [52], respectively. FDTs comprising taste masked solid dispersions were prepared by direct compression with directly compressible diluents, superdisintegrants and other excipients.

Hot melt extrusion/extrusion-precipitation/extrusion techniques have been applied in preparing taste masked granules, which can be incorporated into FDTs. Most of these studies have used aminoalkyl methacrylate copolymer (Eudragit E100/Eudragit EPO) for taste masking of bitter drugs, *viz.* ibuprofen [53], hyoscine butylbromide [54], metoclopramide HCl [55], pirenzipine HCl [56], oxybutynin [56], chlorpheniramine maleate [57] and promethazine HCl [58].

2.5. Adsorption

Adsorption of bitter tasting medicaments on silicates suppresses bitter taste in tablets, liquid orals and chewable dosage forms. The drug becomes readily available, when the complex reaches in the acidic medium of the stomach. Drug adsorbates can be prepared by either slurry technique or by conventional granulation. Drug is first dissolved in an inert solvent followed by mixing with the adsorbent. Later, solvent is removed by drying and adsorbates in solid powder form are obtained.

Basic drugs like loperamide hydrochloride, phenylpropanolamine, dextromethorphan, diphenhydramine were adsorbed onto silicates, like calcium and/ or magnesium silicates, magnesium trisilicate and magnesium aluminium silicate, for achieving taste masking in liquid or solid formulations meant for oral ingestion [59 - 61]. Increasing magnesium oxide content in the complex and decreasing aluminium oxide content over conventional magnesium aluminium silicate provides merits of a more strong interaction between drug and adsorbent. Medicaments were more strongly held by magnesium oxide content, rather than the aluminium oxide content [62].

2.6. Multiple Emulsions

Reverse water-in-oil microemulsion of ranitidine hydrochloride have been prepared for improving the palatability of oral formulations [63]. The external phase of the lipid microemulsion prevents direct contact of the dissolved drug in the aqueous phase to the taste buds of the tongue, thereby masking the bitter taste.

In an another approach, microemulsions were adsorbed onto solid particles to formulate palatable solid dosage forms, wherein drug remained in a solid form yet maintained its inherent microemulsion or self emulsifying form [64]. Oral administration of the developed dosage form rapidly converts to microemulsion form giving the advantage of rapid dissolution. Palatable nonaqueous ibuprofen formulations were prepared by microemulsification [65]. Lecithin and ibuprofen dissolved in propylene glycol were dispersed in an oil phase. Excipients such as taste masking materials, sweeteners and flavouring agents were added to improve the palatability of the developed formulations. Gabapentin was incorporated into a gelatin gel, wherein an inner layer was surrounded by an outer oil layer to form microspheres [66]. Prepared microspheres were homogenised in an aqueous phase to obtain taste masked microspheres or spheres-in-oil in water emulsions.

3. CHEMICAL APPROACHES

Chemical modifications of the drug like making a prodrug or a salt or a complex with IER or cyclodextrin or other polymer or excipient reduces bitterness by decreasing either water solubility or makes the drug unavailable to taste buds. Effervescence, a chemical reaction, is also used in masking bitter taste and improving palatability of FDTs, especially in effervescent tablets and granules.

3.1. Effervescence

Evolution of gas (carbon dioxide) in the form of bubbles from a liquid is termed as effervescence. Gas is generated in liquid by a chemical reaction between effervescent couples, maintained in an anhydrous form, so that they may be activated in water or saliva. An effervescent couple contains a carbonate or bicarbonate, chosen among sodium and/or potassium hydrogen carbonates and bicarbonates, calcium carbonate, magnesium carbonate and amino acid carbonates, and a pH neutralising agent from the group consisting of L-tartaric acid, citric acid, lactic acid, maleic acid, fumaric acid, aspartic acid, ascorbic acid and amino acids. Addition of water to an effervescent formulation or water from saliva starts the effervescent reaction leading to the formation of carbon dioxide, which evolves rapidly in the form of bubbles. The effervescence from sparkling liquid helps to mask the taste of medicaments due to their topical anaesthetic effect. Oral topical anaesthetics like benzocaine, spilanthol and sweeteners may be additionally used along with effervescence for reducing the strong bitter taste of medicaments [67]. The effervescent formulation must be consumed soon as it is mixed with water. Inulin increases the effervescence time, which would allow a subject to ingest the effervescent drink over a longer period of time [68]. The use of effervescent formulations to administer medicaments provides the advantage of rapid dissolution and/or disintegration of the medicament in the oral cavity and thereafter quick dissolution of drug or drug release in the gastrointestinal tract. Effervescent effect in an ODT for administering vitamins to paediatrics results in materially enhanced acceptance of the tablets by children [69]. Rapid dissolution and/or dispersion of effervescent formulation presents drug in an easy to administer form to patients, who do not like tablets or find difficulty in swallowing tablets. Effervescence has been used for promoting pregastric absorption (buccal, sublingual or gingival absorption) of active ingredients from the oral cavity [70]. Such increase can rise from one or all of the following mechanisms:

i. Reduction in the viscosity of mucous leading to decrease in the thickness of the mucosal layer;
ii. Alteration in tight junction between cells;
iii. Facilitating change in the structure of the cell membrane; and
iv. Enhancing hydrophobicity inside the cell membrane.

OraVescent®, OraSolv® and DuraSolv® technologies of Cima labs, use effervescent technology for increasing the transport of active ingredients across mucosal membrane and formulating taste masked active ingredients in orally disintegrating tablets (ODTs). A slight change of 0.5 to 1 pH unit in the microenvironment at the oral mucosal contact area aids as permeation enhancer in ODTs [71]. Effervescence from ODT formulations have stimulatory effect on production of saliva leading to the availability of additional water to assist in effervescent action and subsequent disintegration of the dosage unit for easy oral administration in patients.

Difficulty of maintaining stability of hydrophobic compounds is another limitation with taste masked effervescent formulations. Another problem associated with the use of effervescent compositions has been the inability to incorporate acid-sensitive drugs because these compositions will hydrolyse or decompose when they come in contact with the acid of the effervescent system. Additionally, hydrophobic particles of the drug, contained within the effervescent composition, tend to leach out when mixed with water and deposit along the bottom or sides of the glass. Loratadine is an example of a hydrophobic active agent, which is difficult to formulate in an effervescent composition. Furthermore, effervescent compositions are not a preferred composition for formulating hygroscopic medicaments. Hygroscopic medicaments take up and absorb moisture. When hygroscopic compounds in effervescent formulations are exposed to moisture, they are quickly inactivated.

3.2. Inclusion Complexes with Cyclodextrins

Cyclodextrins consist of glucose units linked in a ring configuration. These may be defined as cyclic oligosaccharides of D-glucopyranose units joined by α-(1,4) linkages. Cyclodextrins are prepared by enzymatic reaction of glucosyl transferase on starch hydrolysates, which creates a cyclic truncated cone structure of glucopyranose units. The interior structure of cyclodextrins is lipophilic cavity and exterior surface is hydrophilic. The parent cyclodextrins are the naturally occurring α, β and γ form consisting of 6, 7 and 8 glucopyranose units and cavities of diameter 5.7°A, 7.8°A and 9.5°A, respectively. Cyclodextrins can entrap drug or other compounds in their lipophilic cavity without forming any covalent bond. Such a guest-host linkage between the entrapped molecule and cyclodextrin is referred to as inclusion complexation. Entrapped molecule may reside completely or partially in the cavity of cyclodextrin. Some specific applications of inclusion complexation are solubilisation of poorly water soluble drugs, stabilisation of sensitive drugs, reduction in volatility of drug, and masking obnoxious odours and undesirable taste of drugs. Several successful attempts for masking taste by forming inclusion complexes of bitter drugs are presented in the Table **2**.

Table 2. Some studies on complexation with cyclodextrins for masking bitter taste of drugs.

Drug	Taste Masking Method	Excipient/Polymer	FDDF and Preparation Method	Ref.
Clozapine	Cyclodextrin complexation	Hydroxypropyl-β-cyclodextrin (HP β CD)	FDT, direct compression	[74]

(Table 2) contd.....

Drug	Taste Masking Method	Excipient/Polymer	FDDF and Preparation Method	Ref.
Diazepam	Cyclodextrin complexation	HP β CD	FDT, direct compression: Superdisintegrant addition	[75]
Dimenhydrinate	Cyclodextrin complexation and sweetener	HP β CD, Sulfobutylether--cyclodextrin (SBE β CD), maltodextrin and saccharin sodium	FDF, solvent casting	[76]
Famotidine	Kneading and freeze drying	SBE β CD and polyvinyl pyrrolidone (Povidone) K30	FDT	[77]
Famotidine	Cyclodextrin complexation	Carboxymethyl β CD, SBE β CD	FDT, direct compression: superdisintegrant addition	[78]
Levocetirizine dihydrochloride	Cyclodextrin complexation	HP β CD	FDF, solvent casting	[79]
Lisinopril	Cyclodextrin complexation	β CD	FDT, direct compression	[80]
Meloxicam	IER and cyclodextrin complexation	HP β CD and resin	FDT, direct compression	[81]
Risperidone	Cyclodextrin complexation	Methyl-β-cyclodextrin	FDT, Direct compression: superdisintegrant addition	[82]
Triclosan	Cyclodextrin complexation and flavour	HP β CD and eugenol	FDF, Solvent casting	[83]

Cyclodextrin form complexes with the drug in aqueous environment that limit or reduce the contact of uncomplexed drug with the taste buds. Often these complexes have improved taste over the uncomplexed drug. Hydrophobic drug molecule displaces water molecules within the cavity leading to the formation of a thermodynamically stable system. The degree and stability of complexation depends on how well the guest molecule, or portions of it, fit within the cavity of the cyclodextrin. The exterior of the cyclodextrin molecule is hydrophilic, which can enhance the aqueous solubility of the complex and thereby the solubility of the guest molecule. A molar ratio of more than 1:5 dissolved cyclodextrin to the dissolved drug was found effective in masking the bitterness [72]. Contrary to this, molar ratio of 1:0.20 to 1:0.75 of ibuprofen salt and β-cyclodextrin was reported for masking the bitter taste [73].

Kneading, co-crystallisation, spray drying and simple dry mixing methods have been used in preparing drug-cyclodextrin complex based taste masked formulations [84]. More economical simple grinding and blending methods have also been proved effective in forming the complexes for their use in formulating taste masked chewable tablets, granules and FDTs [85].

In one unique attempt, physical mixture of amorphous cyclodextrin (particle size.<150μm) and coated taste-masked drug particles have been used in formulating chewable tablets in which the drug is present in a dissolution retarded form and cyclodextrin is present in a dissolution enhanced form [86]. A dissolution enhanced form of β-cyclodextrin was prepared by making a solid amorphous dispersion of β-cyclodextrin and hydroxypropyl methyl cellulose in a spray dryer. Drug microparticulates are coated by melt-congealing, granulation or extrusion-spheronisation. These studies have revealed that taste masking of drugs with cyclodextrins can be improved when a molar excess of dissolved cyclodextrin is maintained, in the buccal cavity, relative to the number of moles of the dissolved drug. Manipulating the dissolution rates of the drug and the cyclodextrin can maintain this molar excess of cyclodextrin.

3.3. Complexation with Ion-Exchange Resins

IERs have been extensively used to formulate taste masked FDTs, FDF, palatable suspensions and chewable tablets (Table **3**). Strong acid (sulphonated styrene divinylbenzene copolymer products) or weak cation exchange resins (CER) (carboxylated styrene divinylbenzene copolymer products) are used to mask bitter taste of drugs. Strong acid CER functions equally at all pH values, while weak acid CER are effective only at pH over 6. Weakly basic anion exchange resins (AER) are suitable below pH 7 [87]. Drug-IER complexes provide a sustained release effect in addition to the taste masking effect. The drug can be complexed with IER by a batch or a column method. IER binds the drug ionically and extra unbound drug and ions are washed off. Complexes of drug with IER are also called resinates. Purified resinate are used in preparation of various types of taste masked formulations. In suspensions, pH of the formulation must be maintained at such a level that complex should not degrade or dissociate. IER keeps the entire drug out of the solution in the complex form. Using IER complexation, it is possible to mask the taste in the vicinity of taste buds as the drug (in free form) cannot have a direct contact with taste buds [88]. Drug is ionically bound to IER and gives taste of IER, which can be easily masked by the use of flavours or sweeteners. Immediately after ingestion, ions in the body (especially in the stomach) cause rapid disintegration of IER-drug complex and dissolve/release the drug in the gastric contents for absorption [89]. IER may sometimes reduce the release of the drug from the complex resulting in drastic reduction in bioavailability. However, an appropriate IER selection for complexation may overcome this problem. It has been observed that less cross-linked IER do not hamper drug release adversely and, therefore, considered more suitable for masking the bitter taste. Pullulan edible films were taste masked by using sulfonated polymer IER comprising polystyrene cross-linked with divinylbenzene [90].

Table 3. IERs as agents for masking bitter taste of drugs.

Drug	Excipient/Polymer	FDDF and Preparation Method	Ref.
Ambroxol HCl	Indion 204, Indion234 and mint flavour	FDT, direct compression	[91]
Chlorpheniramine maleate	Indion 234	FDT, direct compression	[92]
Dextromethorphan HBr	Amberlite IRP69 and sodium polystyrene sulfonate	FDT, direct compression: Superdisintegrant addition	[93]
Donepezil HCl	Amberlite IRP64	FDT, direct compression: superdisintegrant addition	[94]
Doxylamine succinate	Indion 234, Indion 204 and Indion 414	FDT, direct compression: Superdisintegrant addition	[95]
Itopride	Indion 234 and Tulsion 335	FDT, wet granulation	[96]
Levocetirizine dihydrochloride	Tulsion-335, poly Kyron T-134 and Indion 204	FDT, wet compression	[97]
Meloxicam	IER and HP β CD	FDT, direct compression	[81]
Metoclopramide HCl	Indion 204 and Indion 214	FDT, direct compression: superdisintegrant/water soluble saccharide addition	[98]
Ondansetron HCl	Eudragit EPO	FDT, direct compression: superdisintegrant addition	[99]
Ondansetron HCl	Indion 234	FDT, sublimation	[100]
Ondansetron HCl	Indion 234	FDT, direct compression	[101]
Phencynonate HCl	Resin	FDT	[102]
Risperidone	Amberlite IRP64	FDT, direct compression with saccharides and superdisintegrants	[103]
Roxithromycin	Indion 214, Amberlite IRP64 and Carbopol 934P	FDT, direct compression	[104]
Tramadol HCl	Tulsion 335	FDT, direct compression: superdisintegrant addition	[105]

3.4. Ion-Pair Complexes

Ion-pair complexation is a non-covalent bonding of two oppositely charged molecules. The unpleasant taste of a positively charged drug, that is soluble in the mouth, can be masked by ion pairing it with a negatively charged component to form an insoluble precipitate. Mixed ternary ionic complex could be formed among unpleasant tasting active ingredient, which carries one cationic ionisable group, one negatively charged polymer comprising at least one anionic group and one positively charged polymer comprising at least one cationic group. In practice, solution of the drug in a solvent is mixed with a dispersing agent and ion-pairing agent to generate ion-pair complex. When taken orally, the API is released from the complex by the action of gastric or intestinal juices.

Caffeine forms 1:1 and 1:2 molecular complexes with gentisic acid and have improved taste due to slow release of the drug [106]. The fominoben/theophylline complex was prepared by refluxing a solution of fominoben hydrochloride and theophylline sodium salt in equimolar proportions in an alcoholic solvent, while at the same time dehydrating the reflux stream. In a slightly alkaline (pH 8) or slightly acidic (pH 6) medium the complex dissociated very rapidly into its component principles, fominoben and theophylline. This circumstance was very favourable when a syrupy neutral (pH 7) suspension of the complex was administered to a subject, the gastric acidity rapidly liberated fominoben and converted the later to hydrochloride which was absorbed and utilised as conventional fominoben hydrochloride [107].

An ion-pair complex of diphenhydramine and alpha-helical poly(glutamic acid) was found equally effective as sucralose in masking the bitter taste of diphenhydramine [108]. Further, diphenhydramine-poly(glutamic acid) complexes were found stable in weakly acidic or neutral (pH>5) media and used as novel oral formulations with improved taste and sustained release profile.

Extended release properties of dextromehorphan tannate are useful in an antitussive composition in a liquid oral formulation [109]. A paediatric suspension containing ion-pair complex of pamoic acid and chloroquine was assessed bitterless [110]. Phenylephrine, pyrilamine and dextromethorphan were dissolved in a solvent and mixed with a dispersing agent and tannic acid to generate tannate salts, which were further processed without purification or isolation to tablets and suspension [111]. Docusate interacts with 7-[2-[4-[4-(methoxyethoxy)phen-l]1-piperazinyl]ethyl]-2-(2-furanyl)-7H-pyrazolo[4,3-e]triazolo[1,5-c]p-rimidin-5-amine as an ion pair reagent at pH 2 and form an insoluble, hydrophobic complex [112].

3.5. Crystalline Complexes/Co-crystallisation

Crystalline complex formation provides an effective approach to mask bitter taste. Propiverine-salicylic acid crystalline complex is substantially less bitter than propiverine hydrochloride [113]. Prepared complexes are useful and valuable for the preparation of FDTs and improving patient compliance for substances with bitter tastes. Novel cocrystal consisting of acetaminophen and trimethylglycine exhibits improved tableting and potential to suppress the bitter taste of acetaminophen [114].

3.6. Complexation with Polymers and Other Molecules

A chlorhexidine complex, for inclusion in oral hygiene compositions such as dentrifices, was formulated by complexing chlorhexidine (a divalent, cationic antiseptic) with an anionic polymer such as algin or carboxymethylcellulose. The powdered form of the complex was pulverised finely enough to form a stable aqueous dispersion [115].

Palatable dosage forms can be formulated from complexes of bitter drug with polymers prepared by *in situ* complexation [116]. Complex of bitter tasting drug with polymer having one or more free carboxylic groups, such as alkylmethacrylate-methacrylic acid copolymers or nonacrylic or an acrylic polymer or polyvinyl acetate phthalate and polyvinylpyrrolidone (PVP), were prepared for developing sustained release dosage form. PVP renders the complex insoluble in organic solvents and in acidic solutions, where parent polymers can dissolve. Famotidine, caffeine, sildenafil, loratadine and buspirone form complexes with monoammonium glycyrrhizin and 18-α or 18-β-glycyrrhizinic acid [117]. These complexes were prepared by spray drying or freeze drying and formulated in various dosage forms like intraoral FDF, intraoral fast dissolving wafer, osmotic tablet and liquid orals. A molar ratio 1:1 to 1:3 of glycyrrhizinic acid to drug was found optimum for ionic complexation. In these complexes, the nitrogen containing moieties like heterocyclic or acyclic amine, imine, amide, imide or nitrile were preferred. Xanthine, phenazone complexes with acesulfame H were rendered bitterless and found acceptable for their oral use [118].

3.7. Chemical Structure Modifications and Formation of Salts and Prodrugs

Chemical structure modifications and formation of salts and prodrugs decreases the solubility of the drug to levels lower than the taste threshold value leading to insufficient drug concentrations required for the activation of taste receptors [119]. Several successful attempts for chemical structure modifications and formation of salts and prodrugs for bitterness suppression are provided in Table **4**. The parent molecule is cleaved from its derivative either in the GIT or after absorption. However, it has also been observed that bitterness suppression can be achieved with water solubilising groups like n-arylanthranilic glyceryl esters [120] or by synthesising lincomycin esters [121, 122]. Chemical alterations might introduce groups or bind with such groups which are otherwise essential for interaction with taste receptor [123, 124]. Unwanted taste of drugs may be improved by altering the chemical structure of drugs. Some empirical rules relating taste and chemical structure relationships were enunciated by Sinkula and Yalkowsky [125]. It was observed that replacing carboxylic group with tetrahedral sulfonic group antagonised bitter and sweet taste responses of caffeine, quinine and naringine [126].

Table 4. Chemical structure modifications/salts/prodrugs for bitterness suppression.

Parent Molecule (Drug)	Salt/Derivative/Prodrug/Structure Modification	Mechanism of Bitterness Reduction	Ref.
Chloramphenicol	Palmitate ester	Low aqueous solubility	[129]
Penicillin	Ethylenediamine; N, N' dibenzylethylenediamine	Substantially insoluble or sparingly soluble salts	[130 - 132]
Erythromycin	Ethylsuccinate	Low aqueous solubility	[133]
Bacitracin	Zinc salt	Reduction in aqueous solubility	[134]
Basic antihistaminic drugs (Pyrrolidyl ethyl phenyl benzyl amine)	Stearyl sulphate and distearyl sulphate	Low aqueous solubility	[135]
Cyclizine	Pamoate salt	Low aqueous solubility	[136]
Tetracycline	Cyclohexyl sulphamate salt	Low aqueous solubility	[137]
Acetaminophen	Carbonate and carboxylic acid ester	Low aqueous solubility	[138]
Lincomycin	Phosphate ester	Prevent bitter taste receptor interaction	[139]
Erythromycin A	Aliphatic sulphates (n-octdecyl sulphate, n-hexadecyl sulphate and n-tetradecyl sulphate)	Low aqueous solubility	[140]
Homochlorcyclizine	Alkyl sulphate salts	Low aqueous solubility	[141]

(Table 4) contd.....

Parent Molecule (Drug)	Salt/Derivative/Prodrug/Structure Modification	Mechanism of Bitterness Reduction	Ref.
Dextropropoxyphene	Napsylate salt	Low aqueous solubility	[142]
Tetracycline	3,4,5-trimethoxybenzoate salt	Low aqueous solubility	[143]
Lincomycin and clindamycin	Phosphate ester	Prevent bitter taste receptor interaction	[144]
Quinine HCl	Pamoate salt	Poorly soluble salt	[127]
Sildenafil	Lactate	Improved solubility alleviated bitterness	[128]
Clindamycin	Dialkylcarbonate esters	Low aqueous solubility	[145]
Acetaminophen	2-(p-acetaminophenoxy)-tetrahydropyran (Prodrug)	Low aqueous solubility	[146]
Clindamycin	Palmitate ester	Prevent bitter taste receptor interaction	[147]
3-Hydroxymorphinans (nalbuphine, naloxone, naltrexone, oxymorphone, butorphanol and levallorphan)	Ester (3-phenolic hydroxyl group) (*e.g.* nalbuphine-3-acetyl salicylate and nalbuphine---pivalate) (Prodrugs)	Prevent bitter taste receptor interaction	[124, 148]
Nitrofurantoin	Alkylamine salts	Low aqueous solubility	[149]
Norfloxacin	Acetyloxyalkyl carbamate	Low aqueous solubility	[88]
Clindamycin	Phosphate ester	Prevent bitter taste receptor interaction	[150]
Erythromycin A and Erythromycin B	Enol ether ethyl succinate and 2'-ethyl succinate (Prodrug)	Low aqueous solubility	[151 - 153]
Cysteamine	Palmitate, stearate, oleate, elaidioate and decanoate (Prodrug)	Low aqueous solubility	[154, 155]
Prednisolone	Acetate salt	Low aqueous solubility	[156]

Quninine pamoate is a poorly water soluble salt and thus cannot elicit threshold bitter concentration in saliva [127]. Sildenfil lactate is bitterless and solubility is improved upon this salt formation [128]. These salts can be directly compressed to FDTs with the aid of suitable excipients. Hence, salts which are either poorly soluble or where salt formation render them bitterless are of extreme use in formulating FDTs by avoiding the use of other taste masking approaches.

γ-glutamylisation of amino acids, such as leucine, isoleucine, valine, phenylalanine and tyrosine, had reduced bitterness and induced sourness leading to increase in oral preference [157]. Bacterial γ-glutamyltranspeptidase was employed to hydrolyse amino acids at their N-terminal region. In another approach, the peptides were rendered bitterless by removing these amino acids, when treated with aminopeptidases obtained from *Aeromonas caviae* T-64 [158]. Furthermore, bitterness of peptides, amino acids, caffeine, quinine, minerals, *etc.,* can be reduced with the addition of poly γ-glutamic acid [159].

Organoleptically acceptable formulations containing S(+) ibuprofen, devoid of R(-)ibuprofen, were extremely useful for preparing palatable oral liquid formulations [160]. Similarly S(+) etodoloac is more favourable in oral formulations than the racemic mixture of etodolac [161]. Monohydrate of rokitamycin, which is less bitter than rokitamycin, was prepared by crystallising rokitamycin in an acidic aqueous solution [162]. Noscapine in salt form is characterized by a bitter taste rendering it unpalatable in a liquid form. Noscapine was maintained in the alkaloid form, which was relatively tasteless, resulting in a more palatable preparation for use in treating coughs [163].

4. PHYSIOLOGICAL (ORGANOLEPTIC) APPROACHES

With the advancements in understanding of receptor substrate interactions at bitter taste receptors and taste physiology, the exact physiological actions of different taste masking substances have been investigated at molecular level. Taste masking agents inhibit bitter sensation either by desensitisation of taste buds or inhibition or competition at bitter taste receptor. Sweeteners also bind to taste receptors present in taste buds resulting in blending or overshadow effect.

4.1. Desensitisation of Taste Buds

Physiological cooling agents are specific compounds and classes of compounds that are used in various formulations for mitigating organoleptic characteristics. The combination of modified release/cooling agents have also been employed in controlling bitterness and improving palatability of oral formulations. Cooling action of these agents has also been controlled by coating to modify the properties of cooling agents.

Spicy and a slight anaesthetic effect of clove oil, with supportive flavour components, has been found very effective in masking the bitter taste in effervescent tablets [164]. Taste masking has also been achieved with menthol, N-ethyl-p-menthane-3-carboxamide and sucralose in dextromethorphan oral compositions [165]. Menthyl lactate, N-ethyl-p-menthane-3-carboxamide, 3-1-

menthoxypropane-1,2,diol and menthone glycerol ketal were used with mint flavour to reduce bitterness in mint flavour [166].

4.2. Addition of Sweeteners and/or Flavours

Sucrose is a most common sweetener used in pharmaceutical formulations. However, sucrose is contraindicated as a sweetener in drug products meant for diabetic patients. The ongoing search for sugar substitute has resulted in the use of alternative high intensity artificial sweeteners and natural sugar substitutes. Sorbitol and xylitol are natural sugar substitutes found in berries, vegetables, fruit and mushrooms. To reduce production costs, these natural sweeteners are produced synthetically. Stevia extract, liquorice extract or their components have been used in providing synergistic association with flavours and sweeteners [167 - 169]. Small amounts of cyclodextrin (0.5-20% w/w), in a formulation containing stevia-derived sweet substance, is used to mask the bitter aftertaste of stevia [170].

Sweeteners are classified into two categories, *viz.* natural and artificial. Natural sweeteners are sucrose, fructose, glycerol, glucose, erythritol, lactitol, maltitol, mannitol, miraculin, monellin, sorbitol, stevia, tegatose, thaumatin, xylitol, hydrogenated starch hydrolysates, *etc.* Artificial sweeteners are aspartame, alitame, ayclamate, neohesperidine, neotame, saccharin, sucralose, isomalt, *etc.*

Use of effective amounts of artificial sweeteners with flavouring agents is considered the preferred and most straightforward approach for masking bitter taste in oral formulations [171]. Saccharin and cyclamate, as their alkali metal salts, have been used in various oral solutions, suspensions and tablets of various bitter drugs to overcome taste problem [172]. Oral taste masked formulations of penicillins were prepared by adding saccharin and cyclamate [173]. Saccharin and cyclamate in excessive concentration tend to display a bitter note to the taste. A 10:1 cyclamate: saccharin blend is used in countries, where both of these sweeteners are legal for their strong synergistic effect and masking of the off-taste of each sweetener by the other. Dihydrochalcone, neohesperidine dihydrochalcone or naringin dihydrochalcone, or a salt thereof or mixtures of dihydrochalcones, the sugar, the cream of tartar and the vanilla flavour compositions are many times as sweet as sugar and do not have any menthol-like aftertaste or any delayed sweetness effect [174]. Caramel in strength 0.6% w/v has been used for ameliorating the bitter taste of vegetable crude drug in liquid oral preparation [175].

Sugar alcohols are non-sugar sweeteners having sweetness less than sucrose and bulk properties similar to sugars. High intensity sweetener(s) can be additionally added to modify the sweetness profile of sugar alcohols. Developing a sweetener composition for masking bitter taste or to replace sugar and to achieve optimum sweetness is a highly proprietary process in pharmaceutical industries. Inclusion of 10% sorbitol reduces viscosity of 2% pectin sols and ensures newtonian flow properties and diffusion controlled kinetics. Polyhydric alcohols have been used in formulating taste masked dry granules of clindamycin [176]. Artificial sweeteners with polyhydric alcohols act synergistically on bitterness reduction [177]. Most of the ternary mixtures of sweeteners are synergistic and significantly greater than the average of the three self-mixtures [178]. Use of sweeteners in various FDDF formulations is exemplified in Table **5**.

Table 5. Sweeteners used for taste masking in different FDDF formulations.

Drug	Taste Masking Method	Excipient/Polymer	FDDF and Preparation Method	Ref.
Cetirizine HCl	Sweeteners and flavour	Aspartame and sucralose	FDF, solvent casting	[179]
Diclofenac potassium	Sweetener	Mannitol and sucrose	FDT	[180]
Diclofenac sodium	Sweetener and flavour	Sucralose, mint and liquorice flavour	FDF, film casting	[181]
Donepezil HCl	Sweetener	Ammonium glycyrrhizinate	FDT, wet granulation	[182]
Indomethacin	Sweetener	Mannitol	FDT, sublimation	[183]
Levocetirizine dihydrochloride	Sweetener	Aspartame and sucralose	FDF, solvent casting	[79]
Metformin HCl	Sweetener and flavour	Saccharin and vanillin	FDT, direct compression: superdisintegrant addition	[184]
Metformin HCl	Sweetener and flavour	Saccharin and mango flavour	Effervescent tablet by wet granulation	[185]
Nicotine hydrogen tartrate	Flavour	Milk and mint flavour	FDF	[186]
Ondansetron	Sweetener	Aspartame	FDT, wet granulation	[187]
Ranitidine	Flavour	Strawberry flavour	FDT	[188]
Tramadol HCl	Sweetener	Sucrose and mannitol	FDT, direct compression: superdisintegrant addition	[189]
Verapamil	Sweetener	Maltodextrin	Fast dissolving strips, solvent casting	[190]
Zingiber officinale extract	Sweetener	Maltodextrin and sucralose	FDF, solvent casting	[191]

Most of the marketed and developed FDDF products use sugar based excipients as fillers or use one or the other sweetener. Sugar and sugar alcohols, like mannitol and similar compounds, are most widely used due to their quick dissolution in saliva, pleasing mouthfeel, taste masking ability and negative heat of dissolution providing a pleasant, cooling and sweet sensation. Sweetness combined with the cooling sensation provide a satisfactory level of masking undesirable taste, which is sometimes not otherwise available [38]. Such a combination can be selected from the group consisting of sorbitol, mannitol, a mixture of menthol and artificial sweetener, a mixture of methyl salicylate or menthol and a sugar. Cima's taste masking technology uses this principle in preparing oral formulations for improving patient preferences [38].

Wowtab® uses high mouldability and low mouldability saccharides in improving their compressibility and developing FDTs [16]. Zydis® uses sweeteners and flavours to mask bitter or other obnoxious taste [42]. Shearform® (candy floss process), liquifloss and Ceform® technologies are also based on use of sugar and sugar alcohols in producing floss or microparticulates which are later compressed with other excipients to obtain FDTs [192 - 195]. DuraSolv® also uses large amounts of sugar and sugar alcohols as non-direct compression fillers [196, 197]. Solblet®/Exlub® also utilise sugar and sugar alcohol to prepare FDTs. In drug market and products in development phase, there is seldom any FDDF which does not use any sweetener or flavour in its composition. Sweeteners and flavours improve palatability and thus regarded as an important criterion in patient acceptability.

4.3. Taste Inhibitors and Taste Modifiers

Bitter substances are characterised by a great diversity in chemical structures from each other, when compared to other taste stimuli. Phosphatidic acid (PA), beta-lactoglobulin (beta-LG), phosphatidylinositol (PI) and PA-LG are specific and selective bitterness inhibitors [198]. These substances inhibit bitterness without affecting other tastes in the formulation. Their activity of bitter taste inhibition is in the order of PA-LG>PA>PI [198 - 202]. Bitter taste of quinine was effectively masked by adding lecithin fraction or taste inhibitors into granules and coating these granules. Receptor sites on membranes of taste cells for sugars, salts and acids are hydrophilic and those for bitter taste are hydrophobic. Bitter taste is perceived by electrostatic and hydrophobic interaction between the bitter substance, a positively charged molecule *e.g.* pseudoephedrine, and taste receptor membranes [198]. Bitterness inhibitors selectively bind to hydrophobic sites of the receptor on taste cell membranes leading to the suppression of bitter taste. PA-LG has been used extensively to identify and confirm the molecular mechanisms for perception of bitter taste and bitterness suppression in pharmaceutical formulations and food compositions. In one study, it was observed that 36.1% of the bitterness suppression effect of PA was due to adsorption, while bitterness suppression due to interaction at taste receptor site was found 45.6% [203]. Taste masked chloroquine and quinine in the form of stable plurilamellar vesicles of lipids of egg phosphatidylcholine were prepared by sonication [204]. Riboflavin-binding protein (RBP) from chicken egg inhibits bitter as well as sweet taste [205, 206]. The broad bitterness inhibition activity, when compared with ovalbumin and beta lactoglobulin, was the consequence of the ability of RBP to interact with taste receptors.

Different grades of Benecoat (BMI-60, BMI-40 andBMI-40L) are manufactured by Kao Corporation (Japan) and supplied as bitterness inhibitors for their use in masking bitterness in pharmaceutical formulations. These bitterness masking substances are specific to the taste cell's bitterness receptors [215]. Noncompliance, due to the bitterness, can be improved using flavoured Benecoat BMI-60. The most striking characteristic of flavoured BMI-60 is the ease of preparation compared with the manufacture of other pharmaceuticals such as jelly, gummy and candy done to mask bitterness. Taste acceptability of ground polymyxin bisulfate and bactramin C tablets was improved with the addition of flavoured BMI-60. Both adult and child volunteers have found the bitter taste of these two drugs markedly inhibited, making them clinically useful [216]. Acetaminophen chewable tablets containing 5% w/w Benecoat BMI-40 have been formulated [209]. Several other bitterness inhibitors used in formulating palatable formulations are given in Table **6**. For more discussion on these novel bitterness inhibitors readers are referred to a book chapter [1].

Table 6. Taste inhibitors used for bitterness suppression [1].

Drug	Taste Inhibitor	Mechanism	Ref.
Quinine hydrochloride	Tannic acid, phosphatidic acid	Adsorption on gustatory receptors	[203]
Caffeine and amarogentin	Homoeriodictyol and its sodium salt, sterubin and eriodictyol	Taste modifier	[207]
Amino acid solutions	L-arginine and NaCl	Binding at the receptor site	[208]
Chloroquine and quinine	Phosphatidylcholine	Bitterness inhibitor	[204]
Acetaminophen	Benecoat BMI-40	Bitterness inhibitor	[209]
B lactam antibiotic, paracetamol and caffeine	Extracts of *Herba santa* and hydroxyflavanones	Bitterness inhibitor	[210]

(Table 6) contd.....

Drug	Taste Inhibitor	Mechanism	Ref.
Caffeine	Hydroxybenzoic acid vanillylamides and closest structural relatives of homoeriodictyol	Bitterness inhibitor	[207]
Bitterness of amino acids, peptides, quinine caffeine and minerals	Poly-γ-glutamic acid	Bitterness inhibitor	[159]
Potassium chloride	Guanosine-5-monophosphate (GMP) and inosine-5-monophosphate (IMP),	Bitter blocker	[211, 212]
L-phenylalanine, salicin, naringin, caffeine, peptide and Gly-Leu	Alapyridane	Taste modulatory activity	[213]
Zinc sulphate	Quinine-HCl, tetralone, and denatonium benzoate	Peripheral oral and central cognitive bitterness reduction mechanisms	[214]

5. CONCLUSIONS

FDDFs utilise diverse methods in masking the unpleasant taste of the drug. A major portion of tablet composition is sugar or sugar alcohols, especially in directly compressible and other proprietary and patented FDTs. Sugar and sugar alcohols in large quantities provide sweet taste with a cooling sensation, which improves the palatability of the formulation. Further, FDDFs utilise small quantities of sweetener, preferably artificial as these formulations cannot hold large quantities of functional excipients due to the limitations of size. Coating, complexation, solid dispersions or other taste masking approaches can significantly increase the bulk and, therefore, are not recommended for use in FDDFs. Effervescence is another popular approach for improving the palatability and simultaneously providing quick disintegration of FDTs. Complexation with IERs is a useful approach for soluble drugs to render them insoluble. Cyclodextrins provides the opportunity of addressing taste issues simultaneously with stability and also improve the dissolution rates of poorly soluble drugs. Hydrophobic and terribly bitter drugs can rely on coating/microencapsulation methods for alleviating bitterness. Novel taste inhibitors and modifiers have been identified but require more explorations in FDDFs. In a nutshell, it is observed that properties of the dosage form and drug govern the selection of a suitable taste masking approach. Properties of importance are extent of bitter taste, dose, solubility and ionic character of the drug and properties of the dosage form like type, size and shape deserve special considerations. Use of physical/chemical approach coupled with organoleptic masking makes the best combination for addressing most difficult bitterness and palatability issues.

REFERENCES

[1] Kharb V, Saharan VA, Singh A. Bitterness Suppression of Oral Pharmaceuticals. In: Lynch EJ, Ed. The Sense of Taste. Petrov, AP: Nova Science Publishers 2011; pp. 237-76.

[2] Kharb V, Saharan VA, Dev K, Jadhav H, Purohit S. Formulation, evaluation and $3(^2)$ full factorial design-based optimization of ondansetron hydrochloride incorporated taste masked microspheres. Pharm Dev Technol 2014; 19(7): 839-52. [http://dx.doi.org/10.3109/10837450.2013.836220] [PMID: 24079338]

[3] Dev K, Kharb V, Singh A. A proposed methodology for *in vitro* evaluation of bitterness in drug solutions and *in vitro* drug release samples. J Pharm Innov 2014; 9(3): 183-91.

[4] Kondo K, Niwa T, Ozeki Y, Ando M, Danjo K. Preparation and evaluation of orally rapidly disintegrating tablets containing taste-masked particles using one-step dry-coated tablets technology. Chem Pharm Bull (Tokyo) 2011; 59(10): 1214-20. [http://dx.doi.org/10.1248/cpb.59.1214] [PMID: 21963629]

[5] Anand V, Kandarapu R, Garg S. Preparation and evaluation of taste-masked orally disintegrating tablets of prednisolone. Asian J Pharm Sci 2007; 2: 227-38.

[6] Cantor SL, Khan MA, Gupta A. Development and optimization of taste-masked orally disintegrating tablets (ODTs) of clindamycin hydrochloride. Drug development and industrial pharmacy 2015; 41(7): 1156-64.

[7] Douroumis DD, Gryczke A, Schminke S. Development and evaluation of cetirizine HCl taste-masked oral disintegrating tablets. AAPS PharmSciTech 2011; 12(1): 141-51. [http://dx.doi.org/10.1208/s12249-010-9569-7] [PMID: 21181510]

[8] Hu X, Li Y, Zhang E, *et al.* Preparation and evaluation of orally disintegrating tablets containing taste-masked microcapsules of berberine hydrochloride. AAPS PharmSciTech 2013; 14(1): 29-37. [http://dx.doi.org/10.1208/s12249-012-9880-6] [PMID: 23180226]

[9] Jacob S, Shirwaikar A. Preparation and evaluation of microencapsulated fast melt tablets of ambroxol hydrochloride. Indian J Pharm Sci 2009; 71(3): 276-84. [http://dx.doi.org/10.4103/0250-474X.56028] [PMID: 20490294]

[10] Janardhan D, Sreekanth J, Kumar PT, *et al.* Formulation and evaluation of baclofen orally disintegrating tablets. Int J Pharm Sci Nanotechnol 2010; 2: 733-8.

[11] Jin Y, Ohkuma H, Wang CF, Natsume H, Sugibayashi K, Morimoto Y. [Pharmaceutical evaluation of fast-disintegrant tablet containing nicorandil-loaded particles]. Yao Xue Xue Bao 2001; 36(7): 535-8. [PMID: 12585088]

[12] Kawano Y, Ito A, Sasatsu M, Machida Y. [Preparation of orally disintegrating tablets for masking of unpleasant taste: comparison with corrective-adding methods]. Yakugaku Zasshi 2010; 130(1): 75-80. [http://dx.doi.org/10.1248/yakushi.130.75] [PMID: 20046069]

[13] Kawano Y, Ito A, Sasatsu M, Machida Y, Onishi H. [Preparation and evaluation of taste masked orally disintegrating tablets with granules made by the wet granulation method]. Yakugaku Zasshi 2010; 130(12): 1737-42. [http://dx.doi.org/10.1248/yakushi.130.1737] [PMID: 21139401]

[14] Kawano Y, Ito A, Sasatsu M, Machida Y. Preparation of orally disintegrating tablets with taste-masking function: masking effect in granules prepared with correctives using the dry granulation method and evaluation of tablets prepared using the taste-masked granules. Yakugaku Zasshi 2010; 130(1): 81-6. [http://dx.doi.org/10.1248/yakushi.130.81] [PMID: 20046070]

[15] Li FQ, Yan C, Bi J, *et al.* A novel spray-dried nanoparticles-in-microparticles system for formulating scopolamine hydrobromide into orally disintegrating tablets. Int J Nanomedicine 2011; 6: 897-904. [http://dx.doi.org/10.2147/IJN.S17900] [PMID: 21720502]

[16] Mizumoto T, Tamura T, Kawai H, Kajiyama A, Itai S. Formulation design of taste-masked particles, including famotidine, for an oral fast-disintegrating dosage form. Chem Pharm Bull (Tokyo) 2008; 56(4): 530-5. [http://dx.doi.org/10.1248/cpb.56.530] [PMID: 18379103]

[17] Mizumoto T, Tamura T, Kawai H, Kajiyama A, Itai S. Formulation design of an oral, fast-disintegrating dosage form containing taste-masked particles of famotidine. Chem Pharm Bull (Tokyo) 2008; 56(7): 946-50. [http://dx.doi.org/10.1248/cpb.56.946] [PMID: 18591807]

[18] Nakano Y, Maeda A, Uchida S, Namiki N. Preparation and evaluation of unpleasant taste-masked pioglitazone orally disintegrating tablets. Int J Pharm 2013; 446(1-2): 160-5. [http://dx.doi.org/10.1016/j.ijpharm.2013.02.019] [PMID: 23419665]

[19] Sharma D, Chopra R, Bedi N. Development and evaluation of paracetamol taste masked orally disintegrating tablets using polymer coating technique. Int J Pharm Pharm Sci 2012; 4: 129-34.

[20] Sheshala R, Khan N, Darwis Y. Formulation and optimization of orally disintegrating tablets of sumatriptan succinate. Chem Pharm Bull (Tokyo) 2011; 59(8): 920-8. [http://dx.doi.org/10.1248/cpb.59.920] [PMID: 21804234]

[21] Shimizu T, Sugaya M, Nakano Y, *et al.* Formulation study for lansoprazole fast-disintegrating tablet. III. Design of rapidly disintegrating tablets. Chem Pharm Bull (Tokyo) 2003; 51(10): 1121-7. [http://dx.doi.org/10.1248/cpb.51.1121] [PMID: 14519914]

[22] Shimizu T, Nakano Y, Morimoto S, Tabata T, Hamaguchi N, Igari Y. Formulation study for lansoprazole fast-disintegrating tablet. I. Effect of compression on dissolution behavior. Chem Pharm Bull (Tokyo) 2003; 51(8): 942-7. [http://dx.doi.org/10.1248/cpb.51.942] [PMID: 12913232]

[23] Shimizu T, Kameoka N, Iki H, Tabata T, Hamaguchi N, Igari Y. Formulation study for lansoprazole fast-disintegrating tablet. II. Effect of triethyl citrate on the quality of the products. Chem Pharm Bull (Tokyo) 2003; 51(9): 1029-35. [http://dx.doi.org/10.1248/cpb.51.1029] [PMID: 12951443]

[24] Baldi F, Malfertheiner P. Lansoprazole fast disintegrating tablet: a new formulation for an established proton pump inhibitor. Digestion 2003; 67(1-2): 1-5. [http://dx.doi.org/10.1159/000070393] [PMID: 12743433]

[25] Shishu K, Kamalpreet , Kapoor VR. Development of taste masked oral formulation of ornidazole. Indian J Pharm Sci 2010; 72(2): 211-5. [http://dx.doi.org/10.4103/0250-474X.65018] [PMID: 20838525]

[26] Stange U, Führling C, Gieseler H. Formulation, preparation, and evaluation of novel orally disintegrating tablets containing taste-masked naproxen sodium granules and naratriptan hydrochloride. J Pharm Sci 2014; 103(4): 1233-45. [http://dx.doi.org/10.1002/jps.23896] [PMID: 24532095]

[27] Sugiura T, Uchida S, Namiki N. Taste-masking effect of physical and organoleptic methods on peppermint-scented orally disintegrating tablet of famotidine based on suspension spray-coating method. Chem Pharm Bull (Tokyo) 2012; 60(3): 315-9. [http://dx.doi.org/10.1248/cpb.60.315] [PMID: 22382410]

[28] Xu J, Bovet LL, Zhao K. Taste masking microspheres for orally disintegrating tablets. Int J Pharm 2008; 359(1-2): 63-9.
[http://dx.doi.org/10.1016/j.ijpharm.2008.03.019] [PMID: 18455893]

[29] Yaginuma Y, Yoshida N. Preparing rapid disintegrating tablets containing taste-masking microgranules. 2007. Accessed from: http://www.pharmtech.com/pharmtech/Dosage+Forms/Preparing-rapid-disintegrating-tablets-containing-/ArticleStandard/Article/detail/456151 Accessed on 2014 16 July.

[30] Yan Y-D, Woo JS, Kang JH, Yong CS, Choi HG. Preparation and evaluation of taste-masked donepezil hydrochloride orally disintegrating tablets. Biol Pharm Bull 2010; 33(8): 1364-70.
[http://dx.doi.org/10.1248/bpb.33.1364] [PMID: 20686233]

[31] Yoshida T, Tasaki H, Maeda A, Katsuma M, Sako K, Uchida T. Optimization of salting-out taste-masking system for micro-beads containing drugs with high solubility. Chem Pharm Bull (Tokyo) 2008; 56(11): 1579-84.
[http://dx.doi.org/10.1248/cpb.56.1579] [PMID: 18981609]

[32] Cumming KI, Harris E. Taste-masked formulations. US Patent 6153220, 2000.

[33] Friend DR, Ng S, Sarabia RE. Taste-masked microcapsule compositions and methods of manufacture. US Patent 6139865, 2000.

[34] Harmon T. Beyond the first generation of orally disintegrating tablets. Tablets and Capsules Sep 2006; 1-6.

[35] Bettman MJ, Percel PJ, Powell TC. Effervescent microcapsules. US Patent 5709886, 1998.

[36] Ghanta SR, Guisinger RE. Procedure for encapsulating ibuprofen. US Patent 5814332, 1998.

[37] Lai J-w, Venkatesh G, Qian KK. Taste-masked pharmaceutical compositions with gastrosoluble pore-formers. Patent EP2417969, 2012.

[38] Alkire TG, Sanftleben RA, Schuehle SS. Taste masking microparticles for oral dosage forms. US Patent 5607697, 1997.

[39] Cuca RC, Harland RS, Riley TC Jr, *et al.* Tastemasked pharmaceutical materials. US Patent 5494681, 1996.

[40] Cousin G, Bruna E, Gendrot E. Rapidly disintegratable multiparticular tablet. US Patent 5464632, 1995.

[41] Chenevier P, Marechal D. Taste-masking coated particles, process for the preparation thereof and orodispersible tablets containing said coated particles. US Patent 8663682, 2014.

[42] Seager H. Drug-delivery products and the Zydis fast-dissolving dosage form. J Pharm Pharmacol 1998; 50(4): 375-82.
[http://dx.doi.org/10.1111/j.2042-7158.1998.tb06876.x] [PMID: 9625481]

[43] Grother L, Gree R, Hall M. Taste masking a fast-dissolving freeze dried tablet form. Pharm Manuf Rev 1998; 22-7.

[44] Siebert JM, Khankari RK, Kositprapa U, *et al.* Orally disintegrable tablet forming a viscous slurry. US Patent 6368625, 2002.

[45] Ferry A-L, Hort J, Mitchell JR, *et al.* Viscosity and flavour perception: Why is starch different from hydrocolloids? Food Hydrocoll 2006; 20: 855-62.
[http://dx.doi.org/10.1016/j.foodhyd.2005.08.008]

[46] Morella AM, Pitman IH, Heinicke GW. Taste masked liquid suspensions. US Patent 6197348, 2001.

[47] Tian W, Langridge J. Fast dissolving and taste masked oral dosage form comprising sildenafil. Patent WO/2004/017976, 2004.

[48] Chiou WL, Riegelman S. Absorption characteristics of solid dispersed and micronized griseofulvin in man. J Pharm Sci 1971; 60(9): 1376-80.
[http://dx.doi.org/10.1002/jps.2600600919] [PMID: 5567588]

[49] Shah PP, Mashru RC. Formulation and evaluation of primaquine phosphate taste-masked rapidly disintegrating tablet. J Pharm Pharmacol 2008; 60(10): 1279-85.
[http://dx.doi.org/10.1211/jpp.60.10.0003] [PMID: 18812020]

[50] Shah PP, Mashru RC. Development and evaluation of artemether taste masked rapid disintegrating tablets with improved dissolution using solid dispersion technique. AAPS PharmSciTech 2008; 9(2): 494-500.
[http://dx.doi.org/10.1208/s12249-008-9066-4] [PMID: 18431657]

[51] Jadon RS, Nayak S, Amlan S. Taste masking of Lornoxicam by polymer carrier system and formulation of oral disintegrating tablets. Int J Drug Deliv 2011; 1: 27-31.

[52] Tan Q, Zhang L, Liu G, *et al.* Novel taste-masked orally disintegrating tablets for a highly soluble drug with an extremely bitter taste: design rationale and evaluation. Drug Dev Ind Pharm 2013; 39(9): 1364-71.
[http://dx.doi.org/10.3109/03639045.2012.718784] [PMID: 22994163]

[53] Gryczke A, Schminke S, Maniruzzaman M, Beck J, Douroumis D. Development and evaluation of orally disintegrating tablets (ODTs) containing Ibuprofen granules prepared by hot melt extrusion. Colloids Surf B Biointerfaces 2011; 86(2): 275-84.
[http://dx.doi.org/10.1016/j.colsurfb.2011.04.007] [PMID: 21592751]

[54] Khattab IS, Zaghloul AA I, Afouna MI. Studies on the development of rapidly disintegrating hyoscine butylbromide tablets. Drug Discov Ther 2007; 1(1): 61-4.
[PMID: 22504365]

[55] Randale SA, Dabhi CS, Tekade AR, Belgamwar VS, Gattani SG, Surana SJ. Rapidly disintegrating tablets containing taste masked metoclopramide hydrochloride prepared by extrusion-precipitation method. Chem Pharm Bull (Tokyo) 2010; 58(4): 443-8.
[http://dx.doi.org/10.1248/cpb.58.443] [PMID: 20410620]

[56] Ishikawa T, Watanabe Y, Utoguchi N, Matsumoto M. Preparation and evaluation of tablets rapidly disintegrating in saliva containing bitter-taste-masked granules by the compression method. Chem Pharm Bull (Tokyo) 1999; 47(10): 1451-4.
[http://dx.doi.org/10.1248/cpb.47.1451] [PMID: 10553641]

[57] Shishu, Bhatti AB, Singh T, Preparation of tablets rapidly disintegrating in saliva containing bitter taste masked granules by compression method. Indian J Pharm Sci 2007; 69: 80-4.
[http://dx.doi.org/10.4103/0250-474X.32113]

[58] Haware RV, Chaudhari PD, Parakh SR, Bauer-Brandl A. Development of a melting tablet containing promethazine HCl against motion sickness. AAPS PharmSciTech 2008; 9(3): 1006-15.
[http://dx.doi.org/10.1208/s12249-008-9133-x] [PMID: 18770049]

[59] Denick J Jr, Peters D, Talwar AK. Medicament adsorbates of analgesics with complex magnesium aluminum silicate and their preparation. US Patent US4761274, 1988.

[60] Magid L, Weiss M. Antitussive compositions and preparation. US Patent US3085942, 1963.

[61] Mackles L, Chavkin L. Tasteless forms of basic drugs prepared by adsorption *in situ*. US Patent US5811131, 1998.

[62] Denick J Jr, Peters D, Talwar AK, *et al.* Medicament adsorbates with complex magnesium aluminum silicate and their preparation. US Patent US4711774, 1987.

[63] Vandamme T. Reverse water-in-oil microemulsions as taste masking of bitter drugs Intended for oral administration. STP Pharma Practice 2003; 13: 8-12.

[64] Pather IS, Gupte SV, Khankari RK. Microemulsions as solid dosage forms for oral administration. US Patent US6280770, 2001.

[65] Geyer RP. Non-aqueous microemulsions for drug delivery. US Patent 5110606, 1992.

[66] Chaturvedi PP, Niranjan Z. Microsphere-in-oil emulsion. Patent WO/1992/014443, 1992.

[67] Niazi S, Shemesh A. Chewing gum containing a medicament and taste maskers. US Patent US4639368, 1987.

[68] Pandya M. Effervescent vitaceutical compositions and related methods. US Patent US6589555, 2003.

[69] Wehling F, Schuehle S, Madamala N. Pediatric effervescent dosage form. US Patent US5223264, 1993.

[70] Pather SI, Khankari RK, Eichman JD. Sublingual buccal effervescent. US Patent US6200604, 2001.

[71] Moe D, Vikas A, Habib W. Patent WO/2005/065317, 2005.

[72] Chu J, Hsing C, Friesen D, Lyon D. Taste masking formulation comprising the drug in a dissolution-retarded form and/or cyclodextrin in a dissolution-enhanced form. Patent WO/2006/011051, 2006.

[73] Hunter C, Yau D. Pharmaceutical composition. US Patent US5019563, 1991.

[74] Zeng F, Wang L, Zhang W, Shi K, Zong L. Formulation and in vivo evaluation of orally disintegrating tablets of clozapine/hydroxypropyl-β-cyclodextrin inclusion complexes. AAPS PharmSciTech 2013; 14(2): 854-60.
[http://dx.doi.org/10.1208/s12249-013-9973-x] [PMID: 23649995]

[75] Giri TK, Sa B. Preparation and evaluation of rapidly disintegrating fast release tablet of diazepam-hydroxypropyl-Î²-cyclodextrin inclusion complex. Pharmacol Pharm 2010; 1: 18.
[http://dx.doi.org/10.4236/pp.2010.11003]

[76] Preis M, Pein M, Breitkreutz J. Development of a taste-masked orodispersible film containing dimenhydrinate. Pharmaceutics 2012; 4(4): 551-62.
[http://dx.doi.org/10.3390/pharmaceutics4040551] [PMID: 24300370]

[77] Mady FM, Abou-Taleb AE, Khaled KA, *et al.* Enhancement of the aqueous solubility and masking the bitter taste of famotidine using drug/SBE-beta-CyD/povidone K30 complexation approach. J Pharm Sci 2010; 99(10): 4285-94.
[http://dx.doi.org/10.1002/jps.22153] [PMID: 20737636]

[78] Mady FM, Abou-Taleb AE, Khaled KA, *et al.* Evaluation of carboxymethyl-beta-cyclodextrin with acid function: improvement of chemical stability, oral bioavailability and bitter taste of famotidine. Int J Pharm 2010; 397(1-2): 1-8.
[http://dx.doi.org/10.1016/j.ijpharm.2010.06.018] [PMID: 20600734]

[79] Mahesh A, Shastri N, Sadanandam M. Development of taste masked fast disintegrating films of levocetirizine dihydrochloride for oral use. Curr Drug Deliv 2010; 7(1): 21-7.
[http://dx.doi.org/10.2174/156720110790396454] [PMID: 19863484]

[80] Shivanand P, Goyani VD. Formulation and evaluation of taste masked fast disintegrating tablets of Lisinopril. Int J Pharm Tech Res 2010; 2: 1639-43.

[81] Samprasit W, Akkaramongkolporn P, Ngawhirunpat T, *et al.* Formulation and evaluation of meloxicam oral disintegrating tablet with dissolution enhanced by combination of cyclodextrin and ion exchange resins. Drug Dev Ind Pharm 2014; 41(6): 1006-6.
[PMID: 24865111]

[82] Rahman Z, Zidan AS, Khan MA. Risperidone solid dispersion for orally disintegrating tablet: its formulation design and non-destructive methods of evaluation. Int J Pharm 2010; 400(1-2): 49-58. [http://dx.doi.org/10.1016/j.ijpharm.2010.08.025] [PMID: 20801200]

[83] Dinge A, Nagarsenker M. Formulation and evaluation of fast dissolving films for delivery of triclosan to the oral cavity. AAPS PharmSciTech 2008; 9(2): 349-56. [http://dx.doi.org/10.1208/s12249-008-9047-7] [PMID: 18431674]

[84] Szejtli J, Szente L. Elimination of bitter, disgusting tastes of drugs and foods by cyclodextrins. Eur J Pharm Biopharm 2005; 61(3): 115-25. [http://dx.doi.org/10.1016/j.ejpb.2005.05.006] [PMID: 16185857]

[85] Stroppolo F, Ciccarello F, Milani R. Oral pharmaceutical compositions containing cyclodextrins as taste masking agent. Patent United States Patent Application 20040115258, 2004.

[86] Friesen DT, Lyon DK, Ketner RJ. Taste making formulation comprising the drug in a dissolution-retarded form and/or cyclodextrin in a dissolution-enhanced form. US Patent 20080075784, 2008.

[87] Roy GM. Taste masking in oral pharmaceuticals. Pharm Tech 1994; 18(4): 85-91.

[88] Alexander J, Fromtling RA, Bland JA, Pelak BA, Gilfillan EC. (Acyloxy)alkyl carbamate prodrugs of norfloxacin. J Med Chem 1991; 34(1): 78-81. [http://dx.doi.org/10.1021/jm00105a013] [PMID: 1992156]

[89] Anand V, Kandarapu R, Garg S. Ion-exchange resins: carrying drug delivery forward. Drug Discov Today 2001; 6(17): 905-14. [http://dx.doi.org/10.1016/S1359-6446(01)01922-5] [PMID: 11522519]

[90] Bess WS, Kulkarni N, Ambike SH. Fast dissolving orally consumable solid film containing a taste masking agent and pharmaceutically active agent at weight ratio of 1:3 to 3:1. US Patent US7067116, 2006.

[91] Venkatesh D. CG GR, Formulation of taste masked oro-dispersible tablets of ambroxol hydrochloride. Asian J Pharm 2008; 2: 261. [http://dx.doi.org/10.4103/0973-8398.45043]

[92] Yewale CP, Rathi MN, Kore GG, Jadhav GV, Wagh MP. Formulation and development of taste masked fast-disintegrating tablets (FDTs) of Chlorpheniramine maleate using ion-exchange resins. Pharm Dev Technol 2013; 18(2): 367-76. [http://dx.doi.org/10.3109/10837450.2011.627870] [PMID: 22023351]

[93] Malladi M, Jukanti R, Nair R, Wagh S, Padakanti HS, Mateti A. Design and evaluation of taste masked dextromethorphan hydrobromide oral disintegrating tablets. Acta Pharm 2010; 60(3): 267-80. [http://dx.doi.org/10.2478/v10007-010-0025-8] [PMID: 21134862]

[94] Kim JI, Cho SM, Cui JH, Cao QR, Oh E, Lee BJ. *In vitro* and *in vivo* correlation of disintegration and bitter taste masking using orally disintegrating tablet containing ion exchange resin-drug complex. Int J Pharm 2013; 455(1-2): 31-9. [http://dx.doi.org/10.1016/j.ijpharm.2013.07.072] [PMID: 23933050]

[95] Puttewar T, Kshirsagar M, Chandewar A, *et al.* Formulation and evaluation of orodispersible tablet of taste masked doxylamine succinate using ion exchange resin. J King Saud Univ Sci 2010; 22: 229-40. [http://dx.doi.org/10.1016/j.jksus.2010.05.003]

[96] Gupta S, Hasnain MS, Agarwal S. Formulation and evaluation of oral disintegrating tablets of itopride hydrochloride using ion exchange resins as drug carrier. Asian J Pharm Sci 2012; 7: 207-18.

[97] Devireddy SR, Gonugunta CS, Veerareddy PR. Formulation and evaluation of taste-masked levocetirizine dihydrochloride orally disintegrating tablets. PDA J Pharm Sci Technol 2009; 63(6): 521-6.

[98] Dahima R, Sharma R. Comparative study of ion-exchange resin Indion 204 and Indion 214 for the taste masking of metoclopramide hydrochloride and formulation of rapid-disintegrating tablets. Asian J Pharm 2010; 4: 110.
[http://dx.doi.org/10.4103/0973-8398.68461]

[99] Khan S, Kataria P, Nakhat P, Yeole P. Taste masking of ondansetron hydrochloride by polymer carrier system and formulation of rapid-disintegrating tablets. AAPS PharmSciTech 2007; 8(2): 46.
[http://dx.doi.org/10.1208/pt0802046] [PMID: 17622121]

[100] Pandya S, Shah S. Optimization of effect of superdisintegrants and subliming agent on orodispersible tablet of Ondansetron resinate. Indian J Pharm Sci Res 2010; 1: 123-31.

[101] Bhoyar P, Biyani D, Umekar M. Formulation and characterization of patient-friendly dosage form of ondansetron hydrochloride. J Young Pharm 2010; 2(3): 240-6.
[http://dx.doi.org/10.4103/0975-1483.66796] [PMID: 21042478]

[102] Ge Z, Yang M, Wang Y, *et al.* Preparation and evaluation of orally disintegrating tablets of taste masked phencynonate HCl using ion-exchange resin. Drug Dev Ind Pharm 2014.
[PMID: 24785576]

[103] Shukla D, Chakraborty S, Singh S, Mishra B. Fabrication and evaluation of taste masked resinate of risperidone and its orally disintegrating tablets. Chem Pharm Bull (Tokyo) 2009; 57(4): 337-45.
[http://dx.doi.org/10.1248/cpb.57.337] [PMID: 19336927]

[104] Mundada A, Meshram D, Banbale H, *et al.* Formulation and evaluation of dispersible taste masked tablet of roxithromycin. Asian J Pharm 2008; 2: 116.
[http://dx.doi.org/10.4103/0973-8398.42499]

[105] Madgulkar AR, Bhalekar MR, Padalkar RR. Formulation design and optimization of novel taste masked mouth-dissolving tablets of tramadol having adequate mechanical strength. AAPS PharmSciTech 2009; 10(2): 574-81.
[http://dx.doi.org/10.1208/s12249-009-9237-y] [PMID: 19440844]

[106] Higuchi T, Pitman IH. Caffeine complexes with low water solubility: synthesis and dissolution rates of 1:1 and 1:2 caffeine-gentisic acid complexes. J Pharm Sci 1973; 62(1): 55-8.
[http://dx.doi.org/10.1002/jps.2600620109] [PMID: 4682933]

[107] Scapini G, Raimondi A, Poidomani P. Method of making a fominoben/theophylline complex. US Patent US4246407, 1981.

[108] Agresti C, Tu Z, Ng C, Yang Y, Liang JF. Specific interactions between diphenhydramine and alpha-helical poly(glutamic acid)a new ion-pairing complex for taste masking and pH-controlled diphenhydramine release. Eur J Pharm Biopharm 2008; 70(1): 226-33.
[http://dx.doi.org/10.1016/j.ejpb.2008.04.004] [PMID: 18514496]

[109] Chopdekar VM, Schleck JR, Desai HS. Dextromethorphan tannate. US Patent US6670370, 2003.

[110] Chandibhamar V, Yadav MR, Murthy RS. Studies on the development of taste-masked suspension of chloroquine. Boll Chim Farm 2004; 143(10): 377-82.
[PMID: 15881817]

[111] Kiel JS, Thomas HG, Mani N. Phenylephrine tannate, pyrilamine tannate, and dextromethorphan tannate salts in pharmaceutical compositions. Patent WO/2005/023236, 2005.

[112] Heimbecher SK, Kou JH, Kazakevich I. Pharmaceutical compositions. Patent United States Patent Application 20060009504, 2006.

[113] Ogata T, Tanaka D, Ozeki T. Enhancing the solubility and masking the bitter taste of propiverine using crystalline complex formation. Drug Dev Ind Pharm 2013.
[PMID: 23789589]

[114] Maeno Y, Fukami T, Kawahata M, *et al.* Novel pharmaceutical cocrystal consisting of paracetamol and trimethylglycine, a new promising cocrystal former. Int J Pharm 2014; 473(1-2): 179-86. [http://dx.doi.org/10.1016/j.ijpharm.2014.07.008] [PMID: 25010838]

[115] Keith AD. Chlorhexidine complex. US Patent US4980150, 1990.

[116] Kumar V. Palatable, sustained release drug granules. US Patent US6372259, 2002.

[117] Chen L, Tao L, Liang A. Water soluble and palatable complexes. US Patent US7125564, 2006.

[118] Burgard A. Xanthine and phenazone-acesulfame-H complexes having improved taste, process for their preparation and their use. US Patent US6849623, 2005.

[119] Wermuth CG, Gaignault J-C, Marchandeau C. Designing prodrugs and bioprecursors I: Carrier prodrugs. In: Wermuth CG, Ed. The Practice of Medicinal Chemistry. London, UK: Academic Press 1996; pp. 671-96.

[120] Sherlock MH. Glyceryl N substituted phenyl anthranilates in the treatment of inflammation. US Patent US3767811, 1973.

[121] Sinkula AA, Morozowich W, Lewis C, MacKellar FA. Synthesis and bioactivity of lincomycin---monoesters. J Pharm Sci 1969; 58(11): 1389-92. [http://dx.doi.org/10.1002/jps.2600581121] [PMID: 5349756]

[122] Morozowich W, Lamb DJ, Karnes HA, *et al.* Synthesis and bioactivity of lincomycin-2-phosphate. J Pharm Sci 1969; 58(12): 1485-9. [http://dx.doi.org/10.1002/jps.2600581213] [PMID: 5353265]

[123] Hussain MA, Aungst BJ, Koval CA, Shefter E. Improved buccal delivery of opioid analgesics and antagonists with bitterless prodrugs. Pharm Res 1988; 5(9): 615-8. [http://dx.doi.org/10.1023/A:1015958417047] [PMID: 3247326]

[124] Aungst BJ, Hussain MA. Use of prodrugs of 3-hydroxymorphinans to prevent bitter taste upon buccal, nasal or sublingual administration. US Patent US4673679, 1987.

[125] Sinkula AA, Yalkowsky SH. Rationale for design of biologically reversible drug derivatives: prodrugs. J Pharm Sci 1975; 64(2): 181-210. [http://dx.doi.org/10.1002/jps.2600640203] [PMID: 1127579]

[126] Muller GW, Culberson JC, Roy G, *et al.* Carboxylic acid replacement structure-activity relationships in suosan type sweeteners. A sweet taste antagonist. 1. J Med Chem 1992; 35(10): 1747-51. [http://dx.doi.org/10.1021/jm00088a008] [PMID: 1588556]

[127] Kayitare E, Vervaet C, Mehuys E, *et al.* Taste-masked quinine pamoate tablets for treatment of children with uncomplicated *Plasmodium falciparum* malaria. Int J Pharm 2010; 392(1-2): 29-34. [http://dx.doi.org/10.1016/j.ijpharm.2010.03.023] [PMID: 20230885]

[128] Jung S-Y, Kim D-W, Seo YG, Woo JS, Yong CS, Choi HG. Development of sildenafil-loaded orally disintegrating tablet with new lactate salt. Drug Dev Ind Pharm 2012; 38(5): 635-41. [http://dx.doi.org/10.3109/03639045.2011.621432] [PMID: 22010981]

[129] Edgerton WH. Chloramphenicol esters and method for obtaining same. US Patent US2662906, 1953.

[130] Lester SJ, Bruce WF. Penicillin salts of substituted alkylene diamines. US Patent US2627491, 1953.

[131] Lester SJ, Bruce WF. Heterocyclic diamines and salts thereof. US Patent US2876236, 1959.

[132] Richard B, Hans M, Kurt R. Dibenzylethylenediamine-penicillin v. US Patent US2820789, 1958.

[133] Murphy HW. Erythromycin compounds. US Patent US3040025, 1962.

[134] Hodge EB, Lafferty GJ. Zinc bacitracin-containing troche. US Patent US2803584, 1957.

[135] Rieckmann P. Water-insoluble salts of basic antihistaminic compounds, and process of making same. US Patent 3,124,592, 1964.

[136] Emanuel K, Lieberman HA. Composition comprising salt of 1, 1'-methylene-bis-(2-hydr-xy-3-naphthoic acid) and 1-diphenylmethyl-4-methyl-piperazine. US Patent US3188273, 1965.

[137] Robert BJ, Andre CG. Tetracycline cyclohexyl sulphamate and process for preparation. US Patent US3299124, 1967.

[138] Dittert LW, Caldwell HC, Adams HJ, Irwin GM, Swintosky JV. Acetaminophen prodrugs. I. Synthesis, physicochemical properties, and analgesic activity. J Pharm Sci 1968; 57(5): 774-80. [http://dx.doi.org/10.1002/jps.2600570510] [PMID: 5657533]

[139] Morozowich W, Sinkula AA. 7-Halo-7-deoxy-lincomycin derivatives. US Patent 3580904, 1969.

[140] Jones PH, Wiegand RG, Forest L. Erythromycin aliphatic sulfate. US Patent 3,558,594,

[141] Geiszler AO. Alkyl sulfate salts of 1-(p-chlorobenzhydryl)-4-methylhomopiperazines. US Patent US3558600, 1971.

[142] Gruber CM Jr, Stephens VC, Terrill PM. Propoxyphene napsylate: chemistry and experimental design. Toxicol Appl Pharmacol 1971; 19(3): 423-6.
[http://dx.doi.org/10.1016/0041-008X(71)90001-9] [PMID: 4936996]

[143] Caputo O, Cattel L, Nobili G. [Tests on the activity and stability of tetracycline 3,4,5,-trimethoxybenzoate]. Farmaco, Prat 1971; 26(1): 54-66.
[PMID: 5547566]

[144] Argoudelis AD, Coats JH. Methods and compositions for treating bacterial and protozoan infections. US Patent US3641244, 1972.

[145] Sinkula AA, Morozowich W, Rowe EL. Chemical modification of clindamycin: synthesis and evaluation of selected esters. J Pharm Sci 1973; 62(7): 1106-11.
[http://dx.doi.org/10.1002/jps.2600620711] [PMID: 4714118]

[146] Repta AJ, Hack J. Acetaminophen prodrug: 2-(p-acetaminophenoxy)tetrahydropyran. J Pharm Sci 1973; 62(11): 1892-4.
[http://dx.doi.org/10.1002/jps.2600621140] [PMID: 4758097]

[147] Birkenmeyer RD. 1'-(β-Hydroxyethyl)-1'-demethyl clindamycin 2-acylates. US Patent US3892730, 1975.

[148] Hussain AA. Method of administering narcotic antagonists and analgesics and novel dosage forms containing same. US Patent US4464378, 1984.

[149] Hans-georg R, Peter R. Tasteless n-(5-nitrofurfurylidene)-1-aminohydantoin salts. US Patent US3234220, 1966.

[150] Tobkes M, Diaz S, Krishnan L. Clindamycin phosphate synthesis. US Patent US5182374, 1993.

[151] Bhadra PK, Morris GA, Barber J. Design, synthesis, and evaluation of stable and taste-free erythromycin proprodrugs. J Med Chem 2005; 48(11): 3878-84.
[http://dx.doi.org/10.1021/jm049155y] [PMID: 15916440]

[152] Hassanzadeh A, Barber J, Morris GA, Gorry PA. Mechanism for the degradation of erythromycin A and erythromycin A 2-ethyl succinate in acidic aqueous solution. J Phys Chem A 2007; 111(40): 10098-104.
[http://dx.doi.org/10.1021/jp073030y] [PMID: 17880049]

[153] Hassanzadeh A, Gorry PA, Morris GA, Barber J. Pediatric erythromycins: a comparison of the properties of erythromycins A and B 2-ethyl succinates. J Med Chem 2006; 49(21): 6334-42.
[http://dx.doi.org/10.1021/jm0602312] [PMID: 17034139]

[154] McCaughan B, Kay G, Knott RM, Cairns D. A potential new prodrug for the treatment of cystinosis: design, synthesis and in-vitro evaluation. Bioorg Med Chem Lett 2008; 18(5): 1716-9. [http://dx.doi.org/10.1016/j.bmcl.2008.01.039] [PMID: 18249536]

[155] Anderson RJ, Cairns D, Cardwell W, *et al.* Design, Synthesis and Initial *In Vitro* Evaluation of Novel Prodrugs for the Treatment of Cystinosis. Letters in Drug Design. Discovery 2006; 3: 336-45.

[156] Asotra S, Gao S, Yacobi A. Oral suspension of prednisolone acetate. US Patent US7799331, 2010.

[157] Suzuki H, Kato K, Kumagai H. Enzymatic synthesis of gamma-glutamylvaline to improve the bitter taste of valine. J Agric Food Chem 2004; 52(3): 577-80. [http://dx.doi.org/10.1021/jf0347564] [PMID: 14759151]

[158] Izawa N, Tokuyasu K, Hayashi K. Debittering of Protein Hydrolysates Using Aeromonas caviae Aminopeptidase. J Agric Food Chem 1997; 45: 543-5. [http://dx.doi.org/10.1021/jf960784t]

[159] Shih I-L, Van Y-T. The production of poly-(gamma-glutamic acid) from microorganisms and its various applications. Bioresour Technol 2001; 79(3): 207-25. [http://dx.doi.org/10.1016/S0960-8524(01)00074-8] [PMID: 11499575]

[160] Humber LG, Reuter GL. Oral formulations of S(+)-ibuprofen. US Patent US5780046, 1998.

[161] Humber LG, Reuter GL. Oral Formulations of S(+)-etodolac. US Patent US5958445, 1999.

[162] Kinoshita K. Rokitamycin monohydrate crystal and process for producing the same. Patent WO/1994/005683, 1994.

[163] Bianculli VD. Process of making cough syrup with masked noscapine. US Patent US4029797, 1977.

[164] Pandya HB, Callahan TP. Taste masking for unplatable formulations. US Patent US5837286, 1998.

[165] Lee K. Oral compositions having improved consumer aesthetics. US Patent US6391886, 2002.

[166] Record D, Tyrpin H, Broderick K. Mint flavored chewing gum having reduced bitterness and methods for making same. US Patent US5372824, 1994.

[167] Mona IM, Wafaa AA. Synergistic effects of some alternative sweeteners on the unpleasant attributes of stevia sweetener and its application in some fruit drinks. Alex. J Food Sci Technol 2005; 2: 1-10.

[168] Catani SJ, Liao S. Synergistic sweetening compositions. US Patent 20100285201, 2010.

[169] Surana SJ, Gokhale SB, Rajmane RA, *et al.* Non-saccharide natural intense sweeteners – An overview of current status. Indian J Nat Prod Resour 2006; 5: 270-8.

[170] Shimizu T, Tatara M, Shimizu T. Sweetener comprising a stevia-derived sweet substance. US Patent 20070003679, 2007.

[171] Ulrich SA, Zimm KR, Francois MK. Taste masked liquid pharmaceutical compositions. US Patent US6806256, 2004.

[172] Macdonald LH. Sweetening composition. Patent GB810537 (A), 1959.

[173] Hoff D, Bauer K. Formulation for oral administration of penicillins having improved taste properties. US Patent US3872227, 1975.

[174] Eisenstadt ME. Neohesperidine dihydrochalcone sweetening compositions. US Patent US4085232, 1978.

[175] Shima K, Nakai K, Shinomiya S. Liquid preparation for internal use. Patent 2004.

[176] Walzade K, Kulkarni R, Kulkarni S. Oral compositions of clindamycin. Patent WO/2010/010568, 2010.

[177] Olinger PM, Alene F. Sweetening composition. Patent EP0259996, 1988.

[178] Schiffman SS, Sattely-Miller EA, Graham BG, Booth BJ, Gibes KM. Synergism among ternary mixtures of fourteen sweeteners. Chem Senses 2000; 25(2): 131-40.
[http://dx.doi.org/10.1093/chemse/25.2.131] [PMID: 10781019]

[179] Mishra R, Amin A. Formulation development of taste-masked rapidly dissolving films of cetirizine hydrochloride. Pharm Technol 2009; 33(2): 48-56.

[180] Comoglu T, Dogan A, Comoglu S, Basci N. Formulation and evaluation of diclofenac potassium fast-disintegrating tablets and their clinical application in migraine patients. Drug Dev Ind Pharm 2011; 37(3): 260-7.
[http://dx.doi.org/10.3109/03639045.2010.505929] [PMID: 20704458]

[181] Cilurzo F, Cupone IE, Minghetti P, Buratti S, Gennari CG, Montanari L. Diclofenac fast-dissolving film: suppression of bitterness by a taste-sensing system. Drug Dev Ind Pharm 2011; 37(3): 252-9.
[http://dx.doi.org/10.3109/03639045.2010.505928] [PMID: 20704459]

[182] Liew KB, Tan YT, Peh KK. Taste-masked and affordable donepezil hydrochloride orally disintegrating tablet as promising solution for non-compliance in Alzheimers disease patients. Drug Dev Ind Pharm 2014.
[PMID: 24495273]

[183] Singh J, Philip AK, Pathak K. Optimization studies on design and evaluation of orodispersible pediatric formulation of indomethacin. AAPS PharmSciTech 2008; 9(1): 60-6.
[http://dx.doi.org/10.1208/s12249-007-9018-4] [PMID: 18446462]

[184] Gandhi PP, Vaidya KA, Shelake GT, Yadav JD, Kulkarni PR. Formulation and evaluation of metformin hydrochloride fast disintegrating tablets by using polacrilin potassium NF from different sources as superdisntegrants. Int J Pharm Pharmaceut Sci 2010; 2: 55-7.

[185] Mohapatra A, Parikh RK, Gohel MC. Formulation, development and evaluation of patient friendly dosage forms of metformin, Part-III: Soluble effervescent tablets. Asian J Pharm 2008; 2: 177.
[http://dx.doi.org/10.4103/0973-8398.43306]

[186] Cilurzo F, Cupone IE, Minghetti P, *et al.* Nicotine fast dissolving films made of maltodextrins: a feasibility study. AAPS PharmSciTech 2010; 11(4): 1511-7.
[http://dx.doi.org/10.1208/s12249-010-9525-6] [PMID: 20936440]

[187] Sheshala R, Khan N, Chitneni M, Darwis Y. Formulation and *in vivo* evaluation of ondansetron orally disintegrating tablets using different superdisintegrants. Arch Pharm Res 2011; 34(11): 1945-56.
[http://dx.doi.org/10.1007/s12272-011-1115-y] [PMID: 22139694]

[188] Tolia V, Han C, North JD, Amer F. Taste comparisons for lansoprazole strawberry-flavoured delayed-release orally disintegrating tablet and ranitidine peppermint-flavoured syrup in children. Clin Drug Investig 2005; 25(5): 285-92.
[http://dx.doi.org/10.2165/00044011-200525050-00001] [PMID: 17532666]

[189] Patel K, Shete S, Belgamwar V, *et al.* Formulation design and optimization of taste-masked mouth-dissolving tablets of Tramadol hydrochloride. Asian J Pharm 2010; 4: 239.
[http://dx.doi.org/10.4103/0973-8398.72125]

[190] Kunte S, Tandale P. Fast dissolving strips: A novel approach for the delivery of verapamil. J Pharm Bioallied Sci 2010; 2(4): 325-8.
[http://dx.doi.org/10.4103/0975-7406.72133] [PMID: 21180465]

[191] Daud AS, Sapkal NP, Bonde MN. Development of *Zingiber officinale* in oral dissolving films: Effect of polymers on *in vitro, in vivo* parameters and clinical efficacy. Asian J Pharm 2011; 5: 183.
[http://dx.doi.org/10.4103/0973-8398.91995]

[192] Myers GL, Yang RK, Herman MR. Liquiflash particles and method of making same. US Patent 5683720, 1997.

[193] Myers GL, Battist GE, Fuisz RC. Process and apparatus for making rapidly dissolving dosage units and product therefrom. US Patent 5866163, 1999.

[194] Cherukuri SR, Myers GL, Battist GE. Process for forming quickly dispersing comestible unit and product therefrom. US Patent 5895664, 1999.

[195] Misra TK, Currington JW, Kamath SV. Fast-dissolving comestible units formed under high-speed/high-pressure conditions. US Patent 5869098, 1999.

[196] Khankari RK, Hontz J, Chastain SJ. Rapidly dissolving robust dosage form. US Patent 6221392, 2001.

[197] Khankari RK, Hontz J, Chastain SJ. Rapidly dissolving robust dosage form. US Patent 6024981, 2000.

[198] Kurihara K, Katsuragi Y, Matsuoka I, Kashiwayanagi M, Kumazawa T, Shoji T. Receptor mechanisms of bitter substances. Physiol Behav 1994; 56(6): 1125-32. [http://dx.doi.org/10.1016/0031-9384(94)90356-5] [PMID: 7878081]

[199] Katsuragi Y, Sugiura Y, Lee C, Otsuji K, Kurihara K. Selective inhibition of bitter taste of various drugs by lipoprotein. Pharm Res 1995; 12(5): 658-62. [http://dx.doi.org/10.1023/A:1016295122461] [PMID: 7479549]

[200] Katsuragi Y, Mitsui Y, Umeda T, Otsuji K, Yamasawa S, Kurihara K. Basic studies for the practical use of bitterness inhibitors: selective inhibition of bitterness by phospholipids. Pharm Res 1997; 14(6): 720-4. [http://dx.doi.org/10.1023/A:1012138103223] [PMID: 9210187]

[201] Katsuragi Y, Sugiura Y, Otsuji K, Kurihara K. Characteristics of phosphatidic acid-containing lipoproteins which selectively inhibit bitter taste: high affinity to frog tongue surface and hydrophobic model membranes. Biochim Biophys Acta 1996; 1289(3): 322-8. [http://dx.doi.org/10.1016/0304-4165(95)00154-9] [PMID: 8620015]

[202] Katsuragi Y, Yasumasu T, Kurihara K. Lipoprotein that selectively inhibits taste nerve responses to bitter substances. Brain Res 1996; 713(1-2): 240-5. [http://dx.doi.org/10.1016/0006-8993(95)01541-8] [PMID: 8724996]

[203] Nakamura T, Tanigake A, Miyanaga Y, *et al.* The effect of various substances on the suppression of the bitterness of quinine-human gustatory sensation, binding, and taste sensor studies. Chem Pharm Bull (Tokyo) 2002; 50(12): 1589-93. [http://dx.doi.org/10.1248/cpb.50.1589] [PMID: 12499596]

[204] Popescu MC, Mertz ET. Taste moderating composition. US Patent US5009819, 1991.

[205] Maehashi K, Matano M, Nonaka M, Udaka S, Yamamoto Y. Riboflavin-binding protein is a novel bitter inhibitor. Chem Senses 2008; 33(1): 57-63. [http://dx.doi.org/10.1093/chemse/bjm062] [PMID: 17846099]

[206] Maehashi K, Matano M, Saito M, Udaka S. Extracellular production of riboflavin-binding protein, a potential bitter inhibitor, by Brevibacillus choshinensis. Protein Expr Purif 2010; 71(1): 85-90. [http://dx.doi.org/10.1016/j.pep.2009.12.016] [PMID: 20045733]

[207] Ley JP, Krammer G, Reinders G, Gatfield IL, Bertram HJ. Evaluation of bitter masking flavanones from Herba Santa (Eriodictyon californicum (H. and A.) Torr., Hydrophyllaceae). J Agric Food Chem 2005; 53(15): 6061-6. [http://dx.doi.org/10.1021/jf0505170] [PMID: 16028996]

[208] Ogawa T, Nakamura T, Tsuji E, *et al.* The combination effect of L-arginine and NaCl on bitterness suppression of amino acid solutions. Chem Pharm Bull (Tokyo) 2004; 52(2): 172-7. [http://dx.doi.org/10.1248/cpb.52.172] [PMID: 14758000]

[209] Suzuki H, Onishi H, Hisamatsu S, *et al.* Acetaminophen-containing chewable tablets with suppressed bitterness and improved oral feeling. Int J Pharm 2004; 278(1): 51-61.
[http://dx.doi.org/10.1016/j.ijpharm.2004.02.031] [PMID: 15158948]

[210] Ley JP, Krammer G, Kindel G. Use of hydroxyflavanones for masking bitter taste. US Patent 20020188019, 2002.

[211] Zolotov S, Braverman O, Genis M. Low sodium edible salt composition and process for its preparation. US Patent US5853792, 1998.

[212] Salemme FR, Bakal AI, Barndt R. Compositions and methods for producing flavored seasonings that contain reduced quantities of common salt. Patent WO/2007/002015, 2007.

[213] Soldo T, Hofmann T. Application of hydrophilic interaction liquid chromatography/comparative taste dilution analysis for identification of a bitter inhibitor by a combinatorial approach based on Maillard reaction chemistry. J Agric Food Chem 2005; 53(23): 9165-71.
[http://dx.doi.org/10.1021/jf051701o] [PMID: 16277418]

[214] Keast RS, Breslin PA. Bitterness suppression with zinc sulfate and na-cyclamate: a model of combined peripheral and central neural approaches to flavor modification. Pharm Res 2005; 22(11): 1970-7.
[http://dx.doi.org/10.1007/s11095-005-6136-0] [PMID: 16132352]

[215] Ishimaru T, Hatanaka S, Miwa T, Furukawa M. Clinical bitterness masking test for phantogeusia. Chem Senses 2001; 26(1): 91-3.
[http://dx.doi.org/10.1093/chemse/26.1.91] [PMID: 11124220]

[216] Saito M, Hoshi M, Igarashi A, Ogata H, Edo K. The marked inhibition of the bitter taste of Polymyxin B sulfate and trimethoprim x sulfamethoxazole by flavored BMI-60 in pediatric patients. Biol Pharm Bull 1999; 22(9): 997-8.
[http://dx.doi.org/10.1248/bpb.22.997] [PMID: 10513631]

CHAPTER 8

Quality Assurance and Evaluation of Fast Dissolving/Disintegrating Dosage Forms

Vikas A. Saharan*

Department of Pharmaceutics, School of Pharmaceutical Sciences, Sardar Bhagwan Singh Post Graduate Institute of Biomedical Sciences and Research, Balawala, Dehradun 248161, Uttarakhand, India

Abstract: Quality assurance and evaluation of fast dissolving/disintegrating dosage forms (FDDFs) require conduct of various pharmacopoeial and non-pharmacopoeial tests and their compliance to acceptance limits. Dosage forms specific and non-specific tests include assessment for hardness, weight variation, assay, content uniformity, friability, disintegration, dissolution, *etc*. Highly porous nature of fast disintegrating/ dissolving tablets (FDTs) makes them brittle and fragile. Friability limits for FDTs are generally higher than the friability limits of conventional tablets. Newer tests, methodologies and equipments have been devised for evaluation of *in vitro* dis-integration/dissolution and to simulate *in vivo* conditions of the oral cavity. Drug dissolution/release studies are also required to be conducted in a manner so as to simulate *in vivo* oral conditions to ensure reproducibility of batches. The developed drug release tests and explored methodologies are correlated to *in vivo* disintegration/ dissolution for their wider acceptance and future incorporation in pharmacopoeia. Taste masking and palatability of FDDFs are evaluated during drug development and stability studies. Some of these evaluation tests have been incorporated in regulatory guideline and/or pharmacopoeia, while some others are in development phases. This chapter provides a comprehensive overview on various quality control/assurance tests for evaluation of FDTs and capsules.

Keywords: Capsule, Content uniformity, Disintegration, Dissolution, Drug release, FDT, Friability, Gamma-scintigraphy, Hardness, OD-mate®, ODT, ODT-101®, Palatability, Tablet, Taste, Texture analyser, Tricorptester®, Water absorption, Water content, Weight uniformity, Wetting time.

* **Corresponding author Vikas A. Saharan:** Department of Pharmaceutics, School of Pharmaceutical Sciences, Sardar Bhagwan Singh Post Graduate Institute of Biomedical Sciences and Research, Balawala (www.sbspgi.edu.in), Dehradun 248161, Uttarakhand, India; Tel: +91-135-2686246; Mobile: +91-8439820796; Fax: +91-135-2686286; E-mail: vikas.pharmaceutics@gmail.com

Vikas Anand Saharan (Ed.)

INTRODUCTION

Fast Dissolving/Disintegrating Dosage Forms (FDDFs) are a group of dosage forms characterised by their quick *in vitro/in vivo* oral disintegration/dissolution and include tablets, mini-tablets, capsules, pellets, films, *etc*. Faster dissolution/ disintegration in the oral cavity has some obvious advantages like administration without water and ease and comfort in swallowing by special populations, *viz.* paediatrics, geriatrics, psychotics, bed-ridden patients, *etc.*

US FDA, CDER Nomenclature Standards Committee defines an orally disintegrating tablet (ODT) as "*A solid dosage form containing medicinal substances which disintegrates rapidly, usually within a matter of seconds, when placed upon the tongue*" [1]. US FDA guidance document on ODTs has defined the upper limits for disintegration time and weight of ODTs. ODTs must disintegrate in 60 s or less when evaluated by official tablet disintegration apparatus of USP or other equivalent methods [2]. However, alternative methods, which are more discriminating and proven correlations between *in vitro* and *in vivo* disintegration, may also be used. Several discriminating *in vitro* disintegration test methods for ODT with strong *in vivo* correlation and evaluation of ODT have come up. Ideally, weight of ODTs should not be greater than 500 mg. Tablets weighing more than 500 mg are difficult, however not impossible, to achieve faster disintegration and patient acceptance. ODTs have been formulated and reported with higher drug loading to benefit patients and still meet the ODT definition, safety and patient compliance requirements [3, 4]. The limit of 500 mg is frequently questioned by several authors and sponsors [3 - 5]. However, ODTs weighing more than 500 mg should be justified on the basis of their performance in disintegration and patient acceptance.

FDTs and Fast Disintegrating Capsules (FDCs) are evaluated for pharmacopoeial evaluation tests like uniformity of dosage units, friability, assay and disintegration/dissolution of the dosage form and dissolution/release of the drug from the dosage form. However, due to obvious differences in manufacturing technologies for FDTs from conventional tablet manufacturing, the acceptance limits for these tests are different from the acceptance limits for conventional tablets. Several modifications have been adapted in testing methodologies to assess faster disintegration/dissolution of FDDFs. Wetting test has been modified and simulated for evaluating wetting of FDTs in the oral cavity and correlated to *in vivo* disintegration. Due to rapid disintegration/dissolution of FDDFs in mouth, pharmacopoeial tests for disintegration and/or dissolution do not correlate well with *in vivo* disintegration/dissolution of the dosage form. Drug dissolution/

release studies have been modified and adapted so that they can correlate well to *in vivo* drug dissolution/release studies. Some successful dissolution test methods have found their acceptance in regulatory guidelines and pharmacopoeia. New equipments/machines have been developed and successfully commercialised for testing FDDFs. Rapid disintegration/dissolution in mouth, buccal/sublingual absorption and administration without water have led to the need for development of novel tests, different test methodologies and market launches of several novel disintegration test apparatuses for FDTs.

2. QUALITY CONTROL AND QUALITY ASSURANCE TESTS

2.1. Uniformity of Weight

Tablets contain a defined amount of the drug based on the daily dosing frequency. Uniformity of weight is an important quality control test to ensure that weight of tablets should not differ from permissible weight variations as defined in the official pharmacopoeia [6]. This test shall be carried out according to the official pharmacopoeial procedure [7]. Generally, uniformity of weight test is performed with 20 tablets, weighing each tablet individually, followed by estimation of their average weight and finally calculating percent variation of individual tablet from the average weight.

2.2. Potency and Content Uniformity

Potency and content uniformity of tablets are also assayed as per procedures recommended in the pharmacopoeia. It is evaluated by an assay procedure or a developed analytical procedure capable of extracting the drug from the dosage form. Evaluation of potency involves use of 20 tablets followed by crushing them together, extracting the drug from the powder mixture and subsequent analysing of the amount of drug present in mass equivalent to one dosage unit. Evaluation of content uniformity require test of individual tablet for drug content. Tablets having low dose of drug (25%/25 mg) are essentially subjected to uniformity of dosage units by evaluating their content uniformity [8]. ODMTs are essentially low dose dosage forms due to their small size and use of large amount of co-processed excipients. Low-dose and cohesive nature of drug pose may pose serious blend uniformity issues in powder blends leading to content uniformity issues. Therefore, FDTs of low dose drugs and ODMTs are compulsorily examined to comply with the requirements of content uniformity as per pharmacopoeia [9, 10].

2.3. Crushing Strength and Hardness

Hardness of tablets, also referred to as diametrical crushing strength, is measured as the force required for crushing the tablet radially/diametrically. Hardness of a tablet is indicative of its tensile strength [6] and depends on physical properties of granules, like particle size, particle size distribution, their hardness and deformation under load, amount of binders used in granulation and most significantly the compression force used in tableting. High value of hardness may reduces disintegration and dissolution times, which may adversely affect absorption and bioavailability. Hardness testers, currently in use, for FDTs are Monsanto type [11], Pfizer type, Schleuniger (Tablet Tester 6D, Schleuniger, Germany) [12], Erweka (TBH 21, Erweka GmbH) [13] or Varian (Varian Hardness Tester, VK-200) [3] and other hardness testers like KHT-20N (Fujiwara Scientific, Japan) and TS-50N (Okada Seiko, Japan) [14]. Measurements of hardness in these testers are repeated for several (mostly 10/20) times and the average and standard deviation are reported.

2.3.1. Tensile Strength

Tensile strength of FDT is estimated from crushing strength measurements using hardness testers like TS-50N (Okada Seiko) [14] or Tablet Tester 6D (Schleuniger) [12], where in the plunger moves at a constant speed (20 mm/min) and radial compression force is measured for breaking the tablet. The equation 1 is used to calculate tensile strength of tablets.

$$T_s = 2F/(\pi dt) \tag{1}$$

Where, T_s is tensile strength, F is the measured force, t is thickness of the tablet and d is diameter of the tablet. The results of tensile strength is generally calculated and reported as the mean and standard deviation from 10/20 measurements.

2.3.2. Crushing Strength for ODMTs

Conventional tablet hardness tester is usually not sensitive enough to measure differences between ODMTs due to their small size and use of low compaction force in compressing ODMTs. Therefore, the radial crushing strength of ODMTs is determined with a texture analyser like TA-XT2i (Stable Micro Systems, Godalming, UK) [10]. In this texture analyser, a punch moves at 0.1 mm/s speed to a selected distance to crush ODMT in a radial direction. In practice, texture analyser is used to measure and record continuously a force-distance diagram for selected (generally 20) number of ODMTs per batch.

2.4. Tablet Friability and Brittleness of Capsules

Friability is referred to as the loss of fine particles adhered from the surfaces of tablets during their handling and transportation. Sometimes, tablets are fragmented or chipped and thus in a wider sense tablet defects arising due to handling and transportation are also observed while estimating friability. Poor cohesion properties among tablet components or insufficient binder in the tablet formulation may result in high friability. Friability test apparatuses, also called as friabilators, consist of one or two hollow circular plastic drums with each having a curved flat flap inside to lift tablets and fall from a defined height when the drum rotates.

2.4.1. Friability Test for FDTs

As per official procedures in pharmacopoeias, accurately weighed 20 tablets are subjected to 100 rotations at 25 rpm for 4 min in a plastic drum of the friability test apparatus [3, 6, 15]. When drum rotates, tablets are lifted to the top and allowed to fall from a distance of 15 cm. Tablets are taken out of the drum, dedusted to remove adhered powder particles from the surface of tablets and accurately weighed. Friability is calculated as the loss in weight of tablets and reported as percentage. Tablets are also individually inspected for breaking and chipping.

2.4.2. Friability Test for ODMTs

Small size and low mass of ODMTs makes them very similar to pellets rather than to conventional tablets. Friability of ODMTs is, therefore, estimated by a modified method, which is very similar to the method used for measuring friability of spheroids/pellets/granules [10]. About 1 g of ODMTs are filled into a multi-dose container and subjected to shaking in a mechanical shaker at a frequency of 200 vibrations/min. ODMTs are removed from the container and de-dusting is performed with the help of an air jet sieve for 1 min. The samples are weighed before and after the treatment and friability is calculated. Friability of less than 1% is acceptable for ODMTs.

2.4.3. Brittleness Test for FDCs

The brittleness of FDCs or brittle capsules is determined by Shinogi test [16 - 18]. In this test, a weight of 50 g is dropped from a distance of 10 cm onto 20 capsules. The percentage of broken capsule is determined and referred to as percentage brittleness.

2.5. Tablet Porosity

Tablet porosity (ε) is calculated from true density (ρ), volume (V) and mass (M) of the tablet using the equation 2 [11, 12]:

$$\varepsilon\ (\%) = (1\text{-}M/V\rho)\times 100 \quad \textbf{(2)}$$

Pycnometer is used to determine true density. Thickness and diameter of tablets are measured using micrometer. Volume of tablet is calculated from tablet dimensions. Tablets shall be weighed on an analytical balance.

Alternatively, mercury penetration porosimeter is used for the measurement of the pore volume and its distribution in FDTs [11, 14].

2.6. Time and Rate of Tablet Wetting

Wetting tests for FDTs have been devised for assessment of quick ingress of water in all parts of the tablet. Quick water uptake ensure faster disintegration/dissolution of FDTs. Initial tests have used only water as wetting medium, which is modified to contain dye for easy visualisation of wetting as the dye colour reaches to all parts of the tablet with complete wetting. Wetting tests have also been modified to simulate wetting of tablets in oral cavity and correct measurement of the end point for completeness of wetting.

2.6.1. Wetting Time & Water Absorption Ratio

Wetting time of FDTs is determined in a petri dish containing distilled water with or without a water soluble dye. In one protocol, 10 ml of distilled water coloured with eosin dye was placed in a 10 cm diameter petri dish [7]. FDT was kept in a petri dish and observed for the time in which water reached to the top surface of the tablet. This method was later modified by adding a tissue paper in the petri dish and placing tablet above wet tissue paper [15]. Other modifications in this test are the use of a folded tissue paper (two fold; 10.75×12 mm) and the use of a 6.5 cm diameter culture dish holding 6 ml water [14, 19].

Water absorption ratio (R) for FDTs is calculated from equation 3.

$$R = 100(W_a - W_b)/W_b \quad \textbf{(3)}$$

Where, W_a is initial weight of the tablet and W_b is the weight of the tablet at the end of the water absorption test.

2.6.2. Water Absorption Rate

Rate of water absorption by FDTs is an important quality control parameter related to the ability of the tablet for quick disintegration in water or any other liquid medium. An apparatus has been designed by Nogami *et al.* and Kuno *et al.* for estimation of water absorption rate [13, 20]. In this apparatus, a glass cup is connected to a graduated pipette *via* connecting tube. The level of water in glass cup is maintained just slightly above the glass filter on which tablet is kept for absorption of water. Rate of water absorbed by the tablet is measured as mL/s.

2.6.3. Simulated Wetting Test Time (SWT time)

SWT time is a modified procedure of assessing wetting time of FDTs [10]. This test simulates the physiological environment of wet human tongue without giving any regard to the movement of the tongue.

Corning 12-well microplate (having 22 mm diameter wells) has been used for estimation of simulated wetting test of FDTs [3]. An automatic pipette is used to add Sensient Blue #1 dye (0.1% w/w) to each well containing Whatman filter paper disc of 21 mm diameter. The volume of dye solution depends on the tablet size. Tablet is placed in each well over and above the wet filter paper disc. SWT time is the time measured for uniform diffusion of dye solution into the tablet and end point of wetting is measured as the time by which the entire surface of the tablet becomes homogenously blue.

A modified SWT time test is recommended for ODMTs due to their small size [10]. In this modified method, a 96-well plate is used. Each well contains a 5 mm diameter disc of Whatman filter paper wetted with 20 μl of a 0.1% (w/w) Brilliant Blue 85 E 133 solution. A single ODMT is placed over the wet paper disc with the help of a forcep. SWT time is determined as the time required in which blue dye solution completely wets the tablet. Complete wetting of tablet is visually observed as a uniform blue colour on all surfaces of the tablet. At least 10 tablets shall be used for estimating SWT time and results may be reported as average and standard deviation.

2.7. Disintegration

Pharmacopoeias define disintegration test as an important performance test for oral solid unit dosage forms to assess whether dosage form disintegrates within the specified time limit or not. Disintegration test is usually conducted in a defined liquid medium at experimental conditions recommended in the pharmacopoeia. Complete disintegration of the dosage form is defined as "*the state in which any residue of the unit, except fragments of insoluble coating or capsule shell, remaining on the screen of the test apparatus or adhering to the lower surface of the disk, if used, is a soft mass having no palpably firm core*" [21]. Disintegration is a prerequisite for drug dissolution, but it does not measure drug release.

Disintegration test has been recommended by ICH for dosage forms meant for immediate release to replace lengthy and time consuming dissolution testing, if the following three conditions are fulfilled [22, 23]:

1. Highly soluble drugs having dose/solubility volume less than 250 ml in pH range 1.2-6.8.
2. Rapid dissolution, more than 80% within 15 min, of the drug in dissolution media maintained at pH 6.8, 4.0 and 1.2.
3. A correlation has been established between disintegration and dissolution test for the dosage form.

Disintegration also plays important role in performance of chewable tablets and HPMC capsule and, therefore, in near future suitable test conditions are expected [24]. Similarly ODT, ODMT, FDC and other FDDFs also await disintegration test guidance from Pharmacopoeia or drug regulatory agencies. Till then, FDDFs are treated similar to conventional tablets for disintegration testing. When pharmacopoeial disintegration tests are performed with ODTs, it is observed that changes in the media composition, leading to altered viscosity and surface tension could not significantly alter disintegration times [25]. However, milk has been found to significantly increase disintegration time of ODTs.

As of now, no separate disintegration test methodology/equipment for FDDFs has been specified in any of the pharmacopoeia. When FDTs are subjected to pharmacopoeial disintegration testing, correlation between *in vitro* disintegration and *in vivo* disintegration in mouth are extremely difficult to obtain due to the use of large amount of disintegration medium (900 mL water) and vigorous oscillations, making experimental conditions extremely different from the conditions of human mouth [26, 27]. *In vivo* estimation of disintegration in human volunteers suffers disadvantages like low reproducibility, volunteer (tester) constraints and regulatory hindrances of exposing humans to the risks associated with administration of test drugs [26].

In vivo and *in vitro* correlation (IVIVC) suffers the disadvantage of huge variation in the amount of disintegration/dissolution medium used and amount of saliva in the mouth. In attempt to correlate *in vivo* and *in vivo* disintegration several methods and novel apparatus have been designed [28 - 30].

2.7.1. Pharmacopoeial Methods

FDA guidance on ODT recommends disintegration testing of ODTs using USP disintegration test method for conventional tablets [2]. Alternative methods of disintegration testing, which have been proven equivalent to the USP method, may be used provided they are more discriminating. *In vivo* disintegration/dissolution of an ODTs is limited due to the presence of small volume of saliva within the oral cavity. Disintegration/dissolution tests in pharmacopoeial apparatuses have to use extremely large volumes of disintegration/dissolution media (900 mL or 1 L) and vigorous hydrodynamic conditions, which makes difficult to correlate results with the results of *in vivo* disintegration/dissolution [31]. Though ODTs have been developed and designed to disintegrate/dissolve the dosage form quickly in the oral cavity for quick drug release followed with faster onset, disintegration still remains a rate-limiting step for absorption of drug [32]. However, such assumptions are only applicable to the drugs of BCS class I and III only. For drugs belonging to BCS class II and IV, dissolution of the drug will be the rate determining step for absorption.

Pharmacopoeial test methods have been used in various research reports for estimation of *in vitro* disintegration time of FDTs [6, 7, 33 - 35]. FDTs are placed in the tubes of a basket-rack assembly, which moves up and down at 29-32 cycles/min in a beaker containing 900 ml of distilled water maintained at 37±2°C. In a modified procedure, vertical agitation speed of basket-rack assembly is altered to 50 cycles/min [7]. Upward and downward stroke times are equal and the distance of stoke is between 53-57 mm. However, Pharmacopoeias may differ slightly in specifications for the basket-rack-assemblies, beakers and discs. Disintegration time is measured accurately by a digital stopwatch/watch for visually observing complete disintegration. Six tablets are usually evaluated for disintegration time and the results are presented as average value and standard deviations.

USP22-NF17 has specified 2 minute time as the maximum time within which sublingual tablets must disintegrate when disintegration test is conducted in USP disintegration apparatus without plastic discs [36]. Pharmacopoeial disintegrating testing of sublingual tablets and disintegrating time limit cannot be applied to ODTs due to their faster disintegration making it difficult to measure differences in disintegration and the effect of changes in formulation development studies.

2.7.2. Disintegration Test in Petri Dish

Several research reports have employed disintegration tests in a petri dish (10 cm diameter) as quick bench-top method for evaluating disintegration of FDTs [15]. This methodology does not involve the use of a tissue or filter paper and water soluble dye. Tablet is kept centrally in a petri dish containing 10 mL of water and the disintegration time is measured as the time to achieve full disintegration.

In some other research reports, petri dish is filled with aqueous solution (10 mL/6 mL) of a water soluble dye, *e.g.* cobalt II 6-hydrate chloride [37], eosin, *etc.* [38]. Circular tissue paper or Whatman filter paper (WH 1442090) of diameter10 cm is kept in the petri dish to soak dye solution [37]. Dish is tilted until all the paper is soaked and to remove air bubbles from it. Tablet is carefully placed centrally in the dish and the time to achieve full disintegration is measured. When tablets does not disintegrate, tablets are observed for rise of dye by capillary action in the tablet and the final point of disintegration is measured as the time required for complete wetting, which is confirmed by the reach of dye in all parts of the tablet. Six tablets are generally tested and observations are reported as their average and standard deviation. These disintegration tests have striking similarities to the tests conducted for evaluating wetting time.

2.7.3. Disintegration Test by Dropping a Small Amount of Disintegration Medium with Syringe onto Tablet

A quick, simple desktop disintegration test for FDTs utilises a disposable syringe for pouring small amount (1 mL/3 mL) of water directly on top of a tablet kept horizontally on any even levelled surface [39, 40]. At the end of 30 s, tablet is physically inspected for complete disintegration by sensing disintegrated tablets with fingers.

This test may be used as a fast screening method by analysts/formulation scientists/review scientists to make a decision of the correct labelling of FDT onto a dosage form. Failure of FDT to disintegrate in this screening method may lead to additional tests in laboratory to confirm the claim of FDT by a manufacturer.

2.7.4. Disintegration Test in a Tube Containing Small Amount of Water

An another simple method has been developed and used to assess disintegration of FDTs meant for sublingual administration [41, 42]. This method uses a 10 mL glass test tube of diameter 1.5 cm containing small amount of water to stimulate sublingual area of human tongue and small volume of saliva. Tablet is dropped into 2 mL of distilled water contained in a glass tube. The time required for complete disintegration of the tablet is observed visually and recorded with the help of a stopwatch [42]. Visual inspection may be enhanced by gentle rotation of the test tube at a 45° angle without agitating or disturbing non-disintegrated parts of the tablet.

2.7.5. Disintegration Test in a Cylinder Fitted with a Sieve

The disintegration time for FDTs may be measured in an assembly comprising 10 mesh sieve fitted in a cylindrical vessel, which is shaken in a temperature controlled water bath [28 - 30]. In this assembly water is filled upto a level that only 2 ml of the disintegration medium is available under the sieve and only 1 ml would remain over the sieve. Simulated saliva is used as the disintegration medium. The assembly is placed on a shaker in a 37°C water bath consisting of disintegrating medium. Tablet is placed on sieve, immersed into water and the shaker provides 150 back and forth motions per minute, horizontally. The disintegration time is measured as the time by which no residue of tablet remains over the sieve.

2.7.6. Disintegration by Dropping a Small Amount of Test Medium onto a Tablet Kept on a Sieve

A disintegration test method and a disintegration tester have been described in a Japanese patent for measuring the disintegration time of FDTs with a small amount of water [43]. This disintegration tester comprises a mesh (first mesh) for placing a tablet, a provision for dropping the test liquid from above the tablet onto the tablet, a temperature controlled bath for keeping the test liquid at a constant temperature and a feed pump for supplying the test liquid from the bath to the disintegration test. While assessing disintegration time, FDT is placed on a mesh and a disintegration test medium is dropped from above the tablet onto the tablet to disintegrate it. End-point of disintegration is visually observed and chronometer is used for recording time.

2.7.7. Disintegration Test by Dropping Test Medium Using a Flow Pump and Simultaneous Compression by a Load

This disintegration test assembly consists of two meshes, a ring-shaped weight and an incubator [44]. Tablet is placed on a lower mesh and the upper side of tablet is covered with a second mesh. Tablet covered with mesh from both side is fastened with slide rails and load (10, 20, 40 g ring-shaped weight) is kept on the upper mesh. Artificial saliva at 37°C is dropped from a height of 8 cm above the tablet through a tube of diameter 3.5 mm at 6 mL/min rate by a flow pump.

Disintegration of tablet is considered complete when upper mesh contacts the lower mesh. High correlation values (r^2 values of 0.88 to 0.96) were observed between *in vivo* and *in vitro* disintegration of FDTs.

2.7.8. Disintegration Test in a Wire Basket Kept in a Glass Beaker

An in-house disintegration test assembly, consisting of a wire basket positioned in 1 L glass beaker with the help of a support, was used for evaluation of disintegration time of FDTs [45]. The assembly was designed in such a manner that when it is filled with 900 mL of simulated salivary fluid (disintegration medium having pH 6.2), only 6 mL of the disintegration medium will remain in the basket. A magnetic stirrer with a magnetic bead was used to stir disintegrating medium at 25/50 rpm. A constant temperature of 37±2°C was maintained with the help of an inbuilt thermostat of magnetic stirrer. Tablet was placed in the wire basket and disintegration time was observed as the time by which all particles from wire basket moves out.

2.7.9. Disintegration Test in a Sinker Fastened to the Dissolution Vessel

A dissolution apparatus, consisting of paddle as stirring element and a sinker for holding tablet, has been used in estimating disintegration time of FDTs [14, 19, 46 - 48]. A cylindrical sinker made of cupric sieve (openings of 1.98 mm) is fastened in a dissolution vessel. The sinker is completely submerged in the disintegration medium and attached to the side wall of the dissolution apparatus. Purified water, 900 ml maintained at 37°C, is continuously stirred by a paddle at 100 rpm. Disintegration time is measured as the time when nothing remains in the sinker and all disintegrated particles or granules completely passes through the screen.

The modified paddle method was used to optimise rizatriptan benzoate ODT using factorial design and good IVIVC of disintegration was achieved [46]. A logarithmic relation between paddle speed and disintegration time was obtained [46].

2.7.10. Disintegrating Bath Equipped with a CCD Camera

A novel disintegration test was developed for continuous video recording of disintegration of tablets [49]. A CCD camera attached to a computer was used for capturing images and software was used for observing and analysing collected images. Disintegration was tested in distilled water as medium under mild agitation giving an advantage of minor product differentiations to be identified *via* disintegration testing.

The disintegration bath consists of a plastic cell partitioned into an inner and outer tank. Inner tank contained the stirring bar, the stainless steel fabricated grid and the disintegration medium. Outer tank was a water bath containing 200 mL of distilled water maintained at 37°C and circulated *via* a water pump. The grid was built with three tablets placed at equal distances from each other and a support restricted the movement of the tablets during the disintegration test.

An auto focus CCD camera (VR-KT75, Sharp) connected to a computer with Windows 98 operating system was used for recording the images of tablets undergoing disintegration. The CCD camera was positioned just above the grid of tablets for getting clear visuals and pictures that can be captured simultaneously, recorded and stored.

2.7.11. Disintegration Test in a X-ray Computed Tomography Chamber

A X-ray computed tomography chamber has been designed for disintegrating testing of FDTs [50]. The plastic chamber consists of a tablet holder, inner bath and outer bath. The outer bath (width 85 mm, length 122 mm, height 75 mm) is used to contain 400 mL of distilled water maintained at 37±2°C. The inner water bath (diameter 50 mm and length 60 mm) holds 27 mL of distilled water maintained at 37± 2°C. The inner water bath kept suspended on gum strings is placed in the outer water bath. The tablet holder, consisting of upper and lower cylinders (12 mm diameter, 10 mm length and 3.4 g weight) with 1×1 mm or 2×2 mm mesh screens, is connected to a plastic line and is placed in the inner bath. The holder is dropped into the test solution in the inner bath to start the disintegration test by releasing the plastic line. To simulate movements of tongue in mouth, the inner bath is vibrated with air bubbles at an air flow rate of 2000 mL/min, from zero, one, two or four tubes (3.0 mm in inner diameter) installed 5 mm from the bottom and 70 mm from the centre of the outside bath. This tablet disintegration tester is loaded on the X-ray computed tomography chamber.

X-ray computed tomography based disintegration test is able to quantitatively measure dynamic disintegration of FDTs and correlates well to *in vivo* disintegration studies. The residual percent area of tablet cross-section is evaluated based on cross-sectional images of tablets as visualised by X-ray computed tomography using exclusive computer software, during the disintegration test.

2.7.12. Disintegration by Compression of Wet Tablet with a Rotary Shaft

A rotary shaft has been employed to test disintegration time of FDTs by compressing wet tablets [51]. Purified water at 37°C is used as disintegration medium. The disintegration medium is maintained at a level sufficient to slightly immerse the FDT, when kept above the wire gauze. The compression force is adjusted by weight. The rotary shaft crushes the tablet resulting in disintegration of the tablet. Weights are used to adjust the compression force. In one protocol, the rotation speed of 10 rpm and weight of 15 g were used to measure disintegration time of FDTs [51].

2.7.13. Disintegration Test Using Distopper®

Pharmacopoeial disintegration test apparatus was equipped with Distopper® (Toyama Sangyo Co., Ltd., Osaka) for automatic electronic detection of disintegration of tablets [49]. Use of naked eye to for disintegration end point determination is not always accurate owing to adhesion of wet granules or part of tablet to the disintegration test apparatus. Distopper® overcomes this specific problem. Distopper® has been made available by Xebex International as an accessory to its pharmacopoeial disintegration tester (Model NT-600) [52].

The coefficient of variation values for disintegration time estimations were less than 20% with Distopper®. A correlation of ($r=0.60$ at $p<0.05$ was obtained for *in vitro* disintegration test using the Distopper® and the *in vivo* test using human volunteers [53]. When disintegration times were limited to within 30 s, the values of correlation increased to $r=0.75$ ($p<0.001$). In another study, *in vitro* disintegration time correlated well with the *in vivo* disintegration times ($r^2=0.88$) and the slope was very close to 1 for majority of FDTs (30 of 43 commercial FDTs).The developed method was capable to predict disintegration profiles in the oral cavity [54]. This method can be optimised to simulate disintegration mechanism in oral cavity enabling its application in evaluating FDTs during manufacturing, development and clinical assessments.

2.7.14. Disintegration Method based on The Kyoto-Model

In this methodology, FDT samples are classified on the basis of their water permeability and volume of water to be used in disintegration test [27]. The disintegration testing device includes, a metallic rod, a first loading means for applying a load centrally on the tablet, a hollow acrylic cylinder, a second loading means for applying a load to the periphery of the tablet and a supply means for delivering a test solution to the tablet [55]. The hollow acrylic cylinder includes four action parts extending from the lower edge thereof to the circumferential direction with intervals and the tip part of the action part is formed in an acute angle tip. The tablet is placed on a flat bottom test tube (a placement part) of a holder (made from a test tube having internal diameter of 22 mm and a flat bottom) *via* a water absorbent sheet/ filter paper of 21 mm diameter and maintained at 37°C by thermostat bath.

Tablet is not directly splashed in the medium instead a small amount (0.5 ml) of purified water at 37°C is filled in the test tube. Time needed by water to reach into all parts of the tablet is measured by observing complete wetting of upper surface and referred to as water permeation time. This is followed by estimation of disintegration properties of FDT by placing inner and outer weights on the tablet. Inner weight (30 g) is placed centrally on the upper surface and outer weight (100 g) is kept at the periphery of the upper surface. Inner weight is attached to a metallic rod of 0.5 mm diameter. Four wedge-shaped boards support outer weight. Test tube is filled with purified water, 0.5 mL or 5 mL. If water permeation time for the test tablet is 60 s or less, 0.5 mL of purified water is required. Water permeation time of more than 60 s for a test tablet will require use of 5 mL of purified water. Complete disintegration of tablet is identified as the time required by the tips of weights in touching the filter paper. The results of six determinations are presented as average and standard deviation. Correlation was observed between disintegration time by Kyoto method and disintegration in oral cavity, for 25 commercial prescription FDTs. Kyoto method is also capable to evaluate formulation changes and time dependent changes in quality of FDTs and thus easily applicable to the development stages and quality control.

2.7.15. Texture Analyser Based Methods

Texture analysers have been used in several research reports for estimating *in vitro* disintegration time of FDTs [32, 56, 57]. The analytical procedure includes the measurement of changes in structure of tablets undergoing disintegration. A stainless steel flat-bottom cylindrical probe crushes the tablet immersed in a disintegration medium, *viz.* simulated saliva or water. At one end, the tablet is attached to the probe *via* glue or a double side tape. At the other end, the probe is attached to a calibrated load cell (5 kg or other). The instrument maintains a measurable force for a defined time (generally 60 s) to disintegrate a tablet. Software is used to measure continuously and plot penetration distance as a function of time, when tablet is crushed in the disintegration medium by the cylindrical probe. The plot helps in identifying the starting point and end point of disintegration.

In a modified methodology, the tablet is introduced with a constant force to a filter paper immersed in water [57]. A rapid increase in the rate of movement of probe indicates start of disintegration of tablet, which continues until the tablet disintegrates completely. Complete disintegration of tablet is identified when rate of movement of probe ceases.

In one study, a texture analyser based disintegration method was developed and optimised for predicting *in vivo* disintegration of tablets [58]. This optimised method qualified successfully when tested with independent tablets.

A texture analyser, CT3 (Brookfield), has been employed for disintegration studies of FDTs. An acrylic probe of 25 mm diameter is used to compress tablet in a disintegration device. The disintegration device consists of a small test sieve, of diameter 38 mm and having aperture size 1.25 mm, positioned on a polystyrene plate. A pipette is used to add disintegration medium into the gap between the sieve and the polystyrene plate. Polystyrene plate prevents the disintegration medium to flow off the sieve. A sufficient volume (about 5.4 mL) of the disintegration medium is added to achieve a uniform layer above the mesh.

In practice, tablet glued on cyclindrical probe is moved at a constant speed to the disintegration device holding disintegration medium at 24±0.5°C. Load on plunger is increased to 20 g, when tablet touches the mesh. At predetermined speed of probe, load-displacement curves are recorded with software TexturePro CT (Brookfield). Disintegration endpoint is the time by which probe touches the mesh and it is easily detectable from the shape of the load-displacement curve.

2.7.16. Texture Analyser Probe and a Specially Designed Cup

A texture analyser, for applying and recording forces on probes, has been employed for estimating *in vitro* disintegration time of FDTs in a specially designed cup [26]. FDT is placed in a specially designed cup followed by applying a force onto the tablet surface until this force reaches to a limiting value of 3 N. Water (2 ml; representing saliva) is poured into the cup and the force-displacement data is recorded for 200 s. Time for complete disintegration of the tablet is determined from the collapse time, *i.e.* the time needed to decrease the initial force from 3 N to 1.5 N. Collapse time has been correlated well with oral disintegration time. This test method has a limitation on its application as it is applicable only to FDTs formulated with mannitol.

2.7.17. Modified Texture Analyser Equipped with a Cylindrical Probe and Perforated Grid

Texture analysers (TAXT2i, RHEO, France & TA-XDPlus, Stable Micro Systems) equipped with a flat-bottom cylindrical probe made of stainless steel (P/25, diameter 12 mm and 25 mm height) and calibrated with a 5 kg load-cell have been used for determination of *in vitro* disintegrating test of FDTs [32].

A perforated grid (having aperture of 1.5 mm diameter, diameter 30 mm, height 10 mm) with a provision of pressure equilibrium *via* four side gaps is positioned on a cylindrical platform capable of moving down, when force is applied on cylindrical platform through tablet. The cylinder housing grid and movable platform is filled with disintegration medium up to the top boarder of the grid. The surface of the grid is kept completely dry. An elastic spring with the help of a screw is used to suspend cylindrical platform through a distance of 1-5 mm from the bottom of the cylindrical housing.

When disintegration test is performed, the test tablet is kept carefully at the centre of the perforated grid, immediately below the probe [59]. In this condition the tablet does not touches the surface of disintegration medium. When a trigger force is applied through probe, the tablet placed on the cylindrical platform moves downwards due to contraction of the spring. With this contraction tablet comes in contact with the disintegration medium and disintegration of the tablet starts. A force of 50 g is maintained for 60 s with suitable prior settings in the texture analyser. Disintegration of tablet allows passing of disintegrated granules through apertures in the grid stimulating oral disintegration and subsequent swallowing.

Penetration distance is measured with the texture analyser during the process of disintegration of tablet in the medium. Texture analysis software is used to obtain time–distance profiles for identifying the initiation and termination of tablet disintegration. Results from *in vitro* disintegration using texture analyser have been correlated well to oral disintegration of tablets.

The developed methodology of disintegration testing using texture analyser is very precise, convenient and successful for FDTs. The operating structure efficiently mimics the conditions of human mouth resulting in good simulation of the oral cavity. The use of perforated grid successfully minimised operating errors, which arise from the use of adhesive tape in other methodologies developed for disintegration testing.

Good IVIVC in disintegration times was obtained when disintegration studies were conducted with modified methodology and test was conducted in artificial saliva. The method was proposed and recommended in formulation development studies.

2.7.18. Tablet Disintegration Rig for Texture Analyser

A new rapid tablet disintegration rig has recently been unveiled as an innovative probe developed by Stable Micro Systems for its texture analyser model TA.XT*Plus* [60]. The rig closely simulates the conditions of the oral cavity, permitting reliable assessment of the mechanical properties and disintegration behaviour and time, allowing important insight into efficacy and performance of FDTs. Its unique and registered design allows disintegration medium to approach the tablet from all surrounding areas. A double side adhesive tape is used to attach the dry tablet to a probe. The probe is equipped with channels for allowing disintegration fluid to flow from all surrounding areas of the tablet without letting off the contact of probe with the tablet. Probe is moved down into the disintegration medium allowing the reach of tablet to a perforated platform. A constant force is applied through texture analyser onto the tablet resulting in ingress of water and subsequent disintegration. Five different probe heads are supplied with the rig for rapid sample preparation before testing and quick interchange.

2.7.19. Electronic Sensing of Disintegration of Tablets

A novel disintegration test apparatus has been designed for electronically sensing the completeness of disintegration of FDTs [34]. In this apparatus, a weight is connected to a rotating shaft at one end and metallic sponge to the other. Both weight and metallic sponge are made up of a conductive material. The tablet is crushed with a rotating shaft on a perforated stainless plate having holes of 1 mm diameter and separated into two equal left and right halves. Two halves of stainless plates are attached to electrodes for measuring changes in electrical resistance, when the plate comes in contact with the weight.

FDT is placed on the stainless plate with multiple holes fitted at the centre of a guide frame. The level of purified water is adjusted to the level that it touches the bottom surface of the stainless plate. When weight is kept on the FDT, the stainless punched plate bends resulting in slight immersion of FDT in the medium. The rotating weight crushes the tablet resulting in disintegration of the tablet. The compression force is adjustable by varying the weights (10 or 15 g) and the rotation speed is adjustable between 10-50 rpm. The end point of the disintegration is an electric signal received, when the weight comes in contact with the stainless perforated plate.

2.7.20. ODT-101®

ODT-101® disintegration tester (Fig. **1a**) is a patent protected instrument of Eisai (Japan) and Toyama Sangyo (Japan) [61]. This ODT tester is capable to measure the tablet disintegration at the minimum of 1/100 s with good accuracy, precision and reproducibility, which make it a good quality control tool. The results obtained have been found in good correlation with *in vivo* disintegration of ODTs. Hence, this equipment seems promising in reducing reliance of ODT disintegration tests by human sensory testing.

Water bath (Fig. **1b**) consists of a pipe heater (300 W) with micro-computer PID controller, platinum sensor (Pt100 Ω) for providing a controlled temperature in range of 5°-59.9°C with an accuracy of ±0.1°C. Stirring is performed by a magnetic stirrer. A single straight shaft of diameter 10 mm, having a provision of lock-pin and a hanging portion at 5 mm diameter mounted *via* one-touch mounting, provides revolutions 5-140 rpm *via* a belt connected to a 10 W DC motor. A drive unit lifts/lowers the shaft with a provision of automatic stop at the specified positions. ODT-101® is supplied with accessories like five plummets, two fixing frame, fixing ring, sample stage, two detection sheets, flat bottom beaker, rotating shaft, level, two stirrers, four detection cables, drain pipe, a temperature sensor and a dot matrix printer.

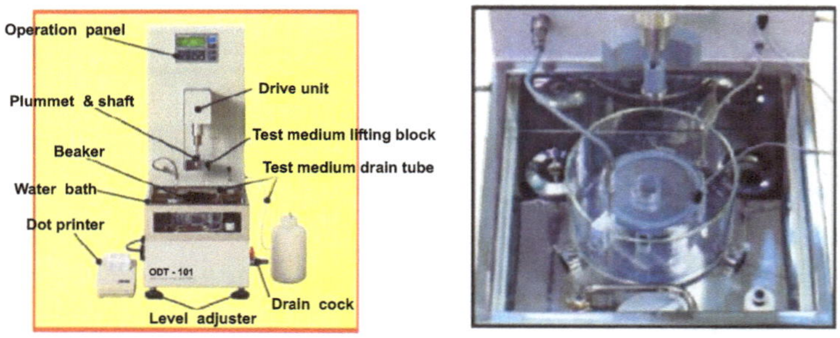

Fig. (1). ODT-101® (**a**) and top view (**b**) inside bath of ODT-101® [61].

In ODT-101® tester, purified water or simulated saliva maintained at 37 °C is used as the disintegration medium. When disintegration test is run, tablet is carefully kept on the wire gauze such that the lower surface of the tablet comes in contact with a small amount of the disintegration medium. Rotary shaft applies compression force resulting in disintegration of the tablet in the medium. Weights are used to adjust the compression force. A rotation speed of 25 rpm and weight of 15 g is considered satisfactory for testing ODTs. Disintegration time is measured electronically with an accuracy of 0.01 s and displayed in minutes or seconds on the operation panel.

ODT disintegration time assessed with ODT-101® has been found in good agreement with disintegration time measured in oral cavity of humans [62].

Further, the ODT-101® tester is helpful in formulation development studies for assessing the effect of various factors like porosity, weight, hardness and shape on disintegration time of ODTs. ODT-101® test has also been used to develop and compare other prototype in-house developed disintegration tester [63].

2.7.21. Tricorptester®

Tricorptester® (Fig. **2**) is an *in vitro* disintegration test apparatus developed by Okada Seiko, Japan. Tricorptester® consists two meshers, holders and a provision of dripping water onto FDT [64]. FDT is placed on a lower mesh. Upper mesh, in contact with tablet, is attached to holders and receives disintegration medium as drippings from above. Disintegration medium, mostly artificial saliva, maintained at 37°C is dripped at the rate of 6.0 mL/min from 80 mm height and a load of 40 g is considered sufficient for testing ODTs [65].

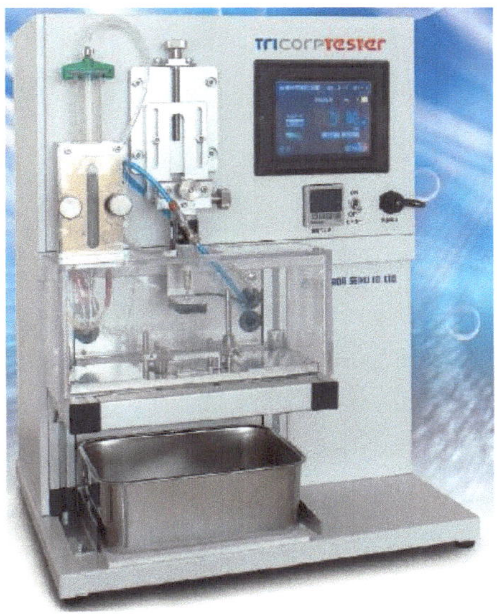

Fig. (2). Tricorptester® [66].

Tricorptester® is assembled as a compact structure and has a provision of touch sensitive control panel [66]. Disintegration test can start, end and other operations can be controlled quickly from the touch panel. Results of disintegration test can be confirmed on the touch panel and data can be transferred to a personal computer.

In one research report, disintegration times of FDTs from 26 different manufacturers have been measured between 4.40-30.4 s using Tricorptester® [64]. Tricorptester® gave a good simulation of disintegration in oral cavity and an IVIVC (r=0.79; p<0.001) was found acceptable. In another study, Tricorptester®

has been used in estimating *in vitro* disintegration time of FDTs of propiverine HCl [67].

2.7.22. OD-mate®

OD-mate® (Fig. **3**) is a disintegration tester developed as an outcome of research cooperation between Higuchi Inc. and Kyoto Pharmaceutical Industry Co., Ltd [69]. It is used for automation of *in vitro* disintegration testing of FDDFs like FDTs, ODMTs, *etc.* OD-mate® may be coupled with electronic tongue or taste sensor for an overall palatability assessment of FDDFs [68].

(a) **(b)**

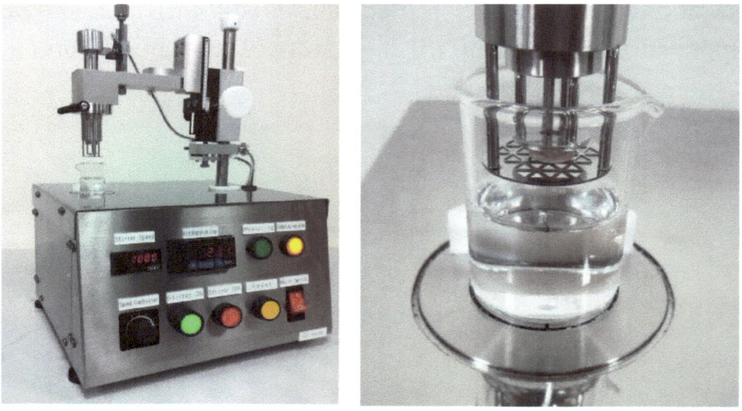

Fig. (3). OD-mate® developed by Higuchi Inc. Courtesy: Furuno Hiroyuki, Higuchi Inc.

Disintegration time of 10 different amlodipine ODTs were measured using the OD-mate® [70]. The OD-mate® was found useful for predicting the disintegration of amlodipine ODTs in the mouth. Good IVIVC between disintegration time in human oral cavity and disintegration time evaluated from OD-mate® has been achieved for amlodipine ODTs. In one assessment study, ODMTs of size 2 mm have also been evaluated for disintegration testing using OD-mate® [71]. Automation of disintegration test by commercial disintegration testers like OD-mate® gives precise results leading to better performances in quality control testing of FDDFs.

2.7.23. Electroforce® 3100 Test Instrument

ElectroForce Systems (TA Instruments, New Castle, DE) has designed a tabletop system, ElectroForce® 3100, for providing superior control resolution in applications requiring low force [72]. ElectroForce® 3100 instrument applies controlled forces on FDTs and measures displacement with time (Fig. **4**). The testing methodology aims to simulate disintegration/dissolution of FDTs in oral cavity.

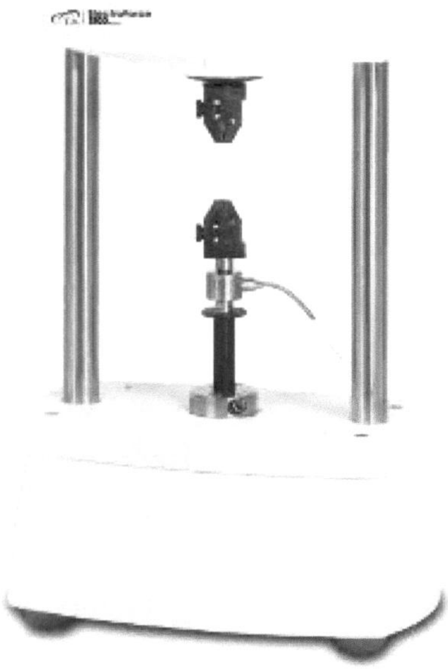

Fig. (4). Electroforce test instrument. Courtesy: Judy Stokes, TA Instruments, New Castle, DE.

FDT is kept on the lower plate of the ElectroForce® 3100 and the lower plate is lifted to attain a preload of less than 10 mN. To simulate *in vivo* disintegration, about 5 mL water at 37°C is placed around the FDT. Load is increased in a controlled manner to 10 mN at the rate of 0.1 N/s using WinTest® software. As tablet disintegrates, the equipment maintains a load of about 10 mN on tablet or its parts. The test is manually stopped soon after disintegration/dissolution of the tablet.

2.7.24. Disintegration Tester Assembly for Disintegration Time, Behaviour and Mechanism

A prototype disintegration tester has been developed estimating not only the disintegration time of FDTs but also the disintegration behaviour and mechanism, [63]. In this tester, FDTs absorb disintegration test medium through a screen followed by application of reciprocating shear stress, which mimics the motion of the tongue. The disintegration process is recorded dynamically using a CCD camera, which provides more insights about disintegration behaviour and mechanism. An accurate disintegration endpoint is estimated by image analysis *via* a CCD camera.

When estimating disintegration, a tablet is placed at the centre of a screen (screen opening, 1.70 mm) and an acrylic board (acrylic board loading, 20 g) is kept onto the tablet. The acrylic board is connected to a motor for reciprocal motion (rotation speed of 25 rpm, 10 mm width per reciprocal motion). Purified water, maintained at 37±2°C, is added to a tank under the screen using a syringe until purified water level touches the tablet. After the contact between the test medium and the tablet, the level of the test medium in the tank is maintained. The tablet absorbs the test medium and subjected to reciprocal shear stress leading to disintegration of the tablet. CCD camera, set vertically against the tablet, records visuals of the process of disintegration. The disintegration time is the time by which all granules of the tablet pass through the screen and nothing remains on screen, as measured from the recorded video.

A swelling-water absorption tester has also been designed by modifying the prototype disintegration tester. In this apparatus, a 15 mm×15 mm filter paper is positioned at the centre of a screen and the test medium (purified water at 20°C) is added to a tank under the screen using a syringe until the filter paper is completely wet. Excess water is removed from the filter paper and a tablet is placed at the centre. The water volume absorbed into the tablet is recorded at fixed time intervals using a graduated pipette set at the height of the screen, at room temperature.

2.8. Dissolution Testing

FDTs disintegrate quickly in the oral cavity resulting in a dispersion of the drug and excipients. Dissolution/release of the drug from tablet may start soon after disintegration of the tablet in the mouth or in the gastrointestinal tract, depending on the properties of the drug. Therefore, methodologies for testing *in vitro* dissolution have been largely derived from dissolution testing of tablets or suspensions. Regulatory authorities require bioequivalence testing of FDTs with immediate release tablet for granting market authorisations. Dissolution profiles of FDTs are expected to match with the reference listed drug product [73]. For FDTs, rotation of paddle at 100 rpm results too fast dissolution and thus slower speeds of rotation are recommended to obtain bioequivalent dissolution profiles. Paddle dissolution apparatus at 50 rpm is mostly preferred to conduct dissolution testing of FDTs [6, 73, 74]. However, higher speeds in the range of 50-75 rpm may be considered for large size tablets [73, 74]. Dissolution test conditions recommended for reference listed drug may initially be tried followed by other dissolution mediums like buffers at pH 7.8, 6.8 and 4.5 and 0.1 N HCl buffer [6, 73].

For FDTs having quick dissolution properties, FIPS recommends dissolution testing at a single time point [74]. Additionally, it is also recommended that a good discriminating disintegration method is sufficient for eliminating the need to conduct dissolution studies in routine quality control testing.

Taste masking plays an important role in dissolution method development, testing and setting specifications. Taste masking is achieved by various barrier approaches including granulations, adsorption, microencapsulation, solid dispersions, coating, microparticulates, multiple emulsions and rheological modifications. Dissolution method shall be developed for evaluation of the effect of polymer on the release of drug so that drug release at early time points (up to 5 minutes) may remains less than the threshold for bitterness sensation [73, 74]. Assessment of taste masking is feasible during drug development studies by simply performing release studies at early time points. For adequate taste masking, the release of drug shall be delayed as long as drug passes through mouth and subsequently a complete release of the drug in gastrointestinal tract. A dissolution criterion, like ≤10% dissolved in 5 minutes, depending on the intensity of bitterness of the drug, allows *in vitro* drug release studies to avoid human sensory evaluation for assessing taste masking properties of the formulations. Dissolution testing at early time point is also helpful in drug development studies, scale up and stability testing.

3. EVALUATION DURING DRUG DEVELOPMENT

3.1. Water Content/Moisture Analysis/Ice Crystals

3.1.1. Estimation of Water Content

Tablets are crushed and about 5 mg powder in an aluminium pan is placed in a thermogravimetric analyser for examining loss in weight with the rise of temperature up to 200°C at a rate of 5°C/min in nitrogen atmosphere [12].

3.1.2. Moisture Analysis

Karl Fischer titration is used to determine the residual moisture in FDTs [7]. Tablet is crushed to powder and transferred into a titration vessel filled with Karl-Fischer grade methanol, stirred for 3 minute and subsequently titrated with reagent (Hydranal Composite 5).

3.1.3. Morphology of Ice Crystals

The presence of ice crystals, their size and shape characteristics in lyophilised tablets provide important insights in optimising the lyophilisation process. Quantitative and qualitative estimation of morphology of ice crystals is performed by subjecting test tablets to X-ray microtomography [75].

3.2. Solid State Analysis

X-ray diffraction and differential scanning calorimetry (DSC) are used to identify nature of the solid state (amorphous or crystalline) of the drug incorporated in FDTs [7]. Scans of pure drug, physical mixture and FDT formulations are compared for characteristic peaks and their intensities. Reduction of characteristic endothermic peak of the drug in DSC signifies reduction in crystallinity in FDT. X-ray diffraction studies are used to estimate crystallinity relatively by comparing heights of representative peaks in diffraction patterns obtained from pure drug and drug in FDTs.

3.3. Surface Morphology

A scalpel is used to cut out a thin slice from the tablet. This thin slice, also referred to as cross-section sample, is examined by scanning electron microscope for observing surface morphology [7]. Micrographs of FDTs are helpful in visualising highly porous surfaces and inner structure of FDTs. High porosity in FDTs is essential for obtaining rapid access of water to all parts of the tablet allowing faster wetting, quick disintegration and subsequent faster dissolution.

3.4. *In vivo* Disintegration and Palatability

Healthy human volunteers are used in evaluating *in vivo* disintegration time. Generally five or six healthy volunteers are selected and FDTs are administered without water [7, 11, 12]. However, less than five or even a single human volunteer have been reported for assessment of *in vivo* disintegration time [13]. Ten or more healthy human volunteers have also been recruited for such studies [59, 27, 32]. Selection of number of volunteers depends on nature of the study, its purpose and statistical comparisons among test groups required. *In vivo* studies require approval from the Ethics Committee followed by obtaining written informed consent from each volunteer so that the study shall comply with Helsinki declaration. The oral disintegration time is recorded as time in which FDT completely dissolves/disintegrate in mouth and no lumps remain. In some protocols volunteers are asked to keep their tongue motionless [12], while in some other protocols they may be asked to move their tongue [7, 13]. Apart from *in vivo* disintegration time, roughness levels and bitterness may be evaluated simultaneously using healthy human volunteers [59].

3.4.1. Magnetic Marker Monitoring

Magnetic marker monitoring is used to examine *in vivo* disintegration phenomenon and fate in a magnetically marked dosage forms [76]. Black iron oxide (1.3 mg), as a magnetic label, is incorporated in dosage form. Healthy human volunteers swallow a capsule each time, on several different occasions, for studying behaviour of capsule undergoing *in vivo* disintegration. Measurement of magnetic moments successfully predicts *in vivo* disintegration, which may be compared to *in vitro* disintegration.

3.4.2. Gamma Scintigraphy

Gamma scintigraphy allows easy detection and monitoring of the passage of the formulation throughout the gastrointestinal tract [77, 78]. The design of suitable dosage forms for drugs having poor bioavailability is facilitated by simultaneous pharmacokinetic and scintigraphic profiles. Factors affecting oral/peroral delivery can be studied using a dual isotope technique. It also allows estimation of drug release characteristics of different orally administered dosage forms [78]. Dispersion/spreading of a dosage form in the oral cavity is an important characteristic for some dosage forms like sublingual tablets, lozenges, chewing gum and FDTs. Oral administration of 99mTc E-HIDA (N-(N'-(2,6-dimethyl-phenyl))carbamoylmethyl iminoacetic acid) labelled dosage forms has been used in evaluating spread of a test dosage form in mouth, oesphagous and gastric contents [79].

In one study, micronised ion exchange resin (Amberlite CG 400; quantity 10 mg) was used to adsorb 99mTc-pertechnetate (radioactivity dose 2-4 MBq) and later incorporated in Expidet® (12 mm ODT) formulation [80]. Two distinct patterns of behaviour were observed with Expidet® formulations, when these were swallowed whole or allowed to disintegrate in mouth followed by swallowing of the resulting dispersion. Oral dispersion of Expidet® formulation required several swallows to clear the mouth. On one occasion, formulation remained in lower part of oesophagus, which was later cleared by peristaltic waves without the need of administering water. A mean transit time of 2.7-14.1 s was observed with Expidet® formulations.

In another study, the Expidet® compositions containing 100 mg of ^{99m}Tc-labelled diethylenetriaminepentaacetic acid (99mTc-DTPA) dissolved completely within

15 s. However, the swallowing activity was observed in the oesophagus by 30 s to completely clear about 8% of the resin remaining in the glottal area [81]. This study established that FDTs have the potential to overcome the problem of difficulty in swallowing, especially in bed-ridden patients and in situations when easy access to water/fluid is not available.

A significant longer gastric residence time and a more uniform coating onto gastric mucosa was achieved with Expidet® formulation labelled with ^{99m}Tc resin when compared to liquid formulation or a conventional tablet [82].

3.5. Taste Evaluation

Taste, palatability and *in vivo* disintegration time are simultaneously estimated by performing human sensory tests in healthy human volunteers [6, 7, 27, 34, 35]. Usually 5 or 6 healthy human volunteers, in a taste panel, are employed for a good estimate [7, 34]. However, volunteers up to 14 or more have also been reported in such studies for better estimates and to achieve meaningful statistical comparisons [27, 32]. The volunteers are screened for hypersensitivity to the drug. Each human volunteer provide informed consent as per Declaration of Helsinki. Before proceeding with the test, distilled water is used to clean and rinse mouth by all volunteers. Volunteers are asked to place tablet on top of the tongue and close the mouth and immediately the time is recorded. In some protocols, movements of the tablet with tongue are allowed. However, in no case biting of tablet is permitted. Disintegration end point is the time required for complete disintegration of the tablet in mouth provided no noticeable residue of tablet, granule or fragment remains in the mouth. After sensing complete disintegration/dissolution of FDTs in mouth, volunteers are asked to report taste on a sensory scale, *e.g.* a five point or ten point sensory scale. After completion of the test, the contents of the mouth are spit out and volunteers rinse their mouth with distilled water. During whole taste assessment procedure, the volunteers are prohibited to swallow the saliva or the tablet. When assessing palatability, the volunteers are asked to assess the difficulty or easiness in swallowing the solution/dispersion of FDT formed in saliva.

Several taste sensing equipments, known as taste sensors/electronic tongues, have been commercially available to reduce reliance on the use of human volunteers in sensory analysis. The readers are directed to other reviews and articles for details on their working and methodologies for assessment of taste and palatability [83 - 87]. Astree 2 electronic tongue of AlphaMOS and SA 402 taste sensing system of Insent Inc are commercially available for taste assessment studies of FDTs [88]. A good correlation has been obtained between the bitterness intensity obtained in human volunteers *versus* the taste sensor evaluation [88].

3.6. Stability Studies

FDTs shall be stored for specified duration and temperature as recommended in ICH or country specific guidelines for accelerated/intermediate/long term stability testing. After opening the packages, physicochemical properties of FDTs are evaluated [89]. Their weight, diameter, thickness and colour differences are observed at initial stages and subsequent evaluation stages. Drug assay is performed to evaluate degradation of the drug. DSC and XRD tests are performed to evaluate changes in crystalline/amorphous state of the drug [7]. Changes in hardness, disintegration time, friability, dissolution rates are determined. *In vivo* disintegration time, taste, palatability and preference are evaluated by human sensory testing. ANOVA, test or other appropriate statistics shall be applied to compare results among different groups for statistical significant difference.

CONCLUSIONS

Market success and clinical acceptance of FDDFs are two driving forces for motivating launch of new apparatus/equipments for evaluation of FDDFs and development of innovative test methodologies. New methodologies have emerged from simple disintegration/swelling tests performed in a small beaker/petri plate to advance apparatuses consisting of temperature controlled bath and sieves having automated means of assessing test parameters. More advanced protocols have provision for visualising the disintegration phenomenon by a CCD camera or computer tomography. Texture analyser probes and disintegration rig have been especially designed for evaluating disintegration of FDTs. Commercial apparatus like ODT-101®, Tricorpteser® and OD-mate® have been successfully marketed. Commercial disintegration apparatus coupled with taste sensor are now providing *in vitro* means for assessing palatability. The current use of *in vitro* approaches for disintegration and palatability assessments have drastically reduced the reliance of human volunteers in sensory analysis of FDDFs.

REFERENCES

[1] FDA. CDER data standards manual (C-DRG-00201 Version 008). Accessed from: www.fda.gov/Drugs/DevelopmentApprovalProcess/FormsSubmissionRequirements/ElectronicSubmissions/DataStandardsManualmonographs/ucm071666.htm Accessed on 20th February 2015.

[2] FDA. Guidance for industry: orally disintegrating tablets. 2008. Accessed from: www.fda.gov/OHRMS/DOCKETS/98fr/FDA-2007-D-0365-gdl.pdf.

[3] Park J, Holman K, Bish G, *et al.* An Alternative to the USP Disintegration Test for Orally Disintegrating Tablets. Pharm Technol 2008; 32(8): 54-88.

[4] Park J, Wu S. Should Orally Disintegrating Tablets (ODTs) Have A Weight Limit? In: AAPS Annual Meeting and Exposition; San Diego, CA. 2007.

[5] McLaughlin R, Banbury S, Crowley K. Orally Disintegrating Tablets: The Effect of Recent FDA Guidance on ODT Technologies and Applications. Pharm Technol Sep. 2009; p. 33.

[6] Puttewar TY, Kshirsagar MD, Chandewar AV, *et al.* Formulation and evaluation of orodispersible tablet of taste masked doxylamine succinate using ion exchange resin. J King Saud Univ Sci 2010; 22: 229-40.
[http://dx.doi.org/10.1016/j.jksus.2010.05.003]

[7] Shoukri RA, Ahmed IS, Shamma RN. *In vitro* and *in vivo* evaluation of nimesulide lyophilized orally disintegrating tablets. Eur J Pharm Biopharm 2009; 73(1): 162-71.
[http://dx.doi.org/10.1016/j.ejpb.2009.04.005] [PMID: 19406232]

[8] Kukkar V, Anand V, Kataria M, *et al.* Mixing and formulation of low dose drugs: underlying problems and solutions. Thai J Pharm Sci 2008; 32: 43-8.

[9] Rahman Z, Zidan AS, Khan MA. Risperidone solid dispersion for orally disintegrating tablet: its formulation design and non-destructive methods of evaluation. Int J Pharm 2010; 400(1-2): 49-58.
[http://dx.doi.org/10.1016/j.ijpharm.2010.08.025] [PMID: 20801200]

[10] Stoltenberg I, Breitkreutz J. Orally disintegrating mini-tablets (ODMTs)a novel solid oral dosage form for paediatric use. Eur J Pharm Biopharm 2011; 78(3): 462-9.
[http://dx.doi.org/10.1016/j.ejpb.2011.02.005] [PMID: 21324357]

[11] Fukami J, Yonemochi E, Yoshihashi Y, Terada K. Evaluation of rapidly disintegrating tablets containing glycine and carboxymethylcellulose. Int J Pharm 2006; 310(1-2): 101-9.
[http://dx.doi.org/10.1016/j.ijpharm.2005.11.041] [PMID: 16434157]

[12] Sugimoto M, Maejima T, Narisawa S, Matsubara K, Yoshino H. Factors affecting the characteristics of rapidly disintegrating tablets in the mouth prepared by the crystalline transition of amorphous sucrose. Int J Pharm 2005; 296(1-2): 64-72.
[http://dx.doi.org/10.1016/j.ijpharm.2005.02.031] [PMID: 15885456]

[13] Kuno Y, Kojima M, Nakagami H, Yonemochi E, Terada K. Effect of the type of lubricant on the characteristics of orally disintegrating tablets manufactured using the phase transition of sugar alcohol. Eur J Pharm Biopharm 2008; 69(3): 986-92.
[http://dx.doi.org/10.1016/j.ejpb.2008.02.016] [PMID: 18396020]

[14] Sunada H, Bi Y. Preparation, evaluation and optimization of rapidly disintegrating tablets. Powder Technol 2002; 122: 188-98.
[http://dx.doi.org/10.1016/S0032-5910(01)00415-6]

[15] Gohel M, Patel M, Amin A, Agrawal R, Dave R, Bariya N. Formulation design and optimization of mouth dissolve tablets of nimesulide using vacuum drying technique. AAPS PharmSciTech 2004; 5(3): e36.
[http://dx.doi.org/10.1208/pt050336] [PMID: 15760070]

[16] Shionogi. Qualicaps Product Brochure Gelatin/PEG capsules. SQ 005-1998E, 1998.

[17] Ciper M, Bodmeier R. Preparation and characterization of novel fast disintegrating capsules (Fastcaps) for administration in the oral cavity. Int J Pharm 2005; 303(1-2): 62-71.
[http://dx.doi.org/10.1016/j.ijpharm.2005.07.004] [PMID: 16111845]

[18] Ciper M, Bodmeier R. Modified conventional hard gelatin capsules as fast disintegrating dosage form in the oral cavity. Eur J Pharm Biopharm 2006; 62(2): 178-84.
[http://dx.doi.org/10.1016/j.ejpb.2005.08.014] [PMID: 16260126]

[19] Bi Y, Sunada H, Yonezawa Y, Danjo K, Otsuka A, Iida K. Preparation and evaluation of a compressed tablet rapidly disintegrating in the oral cavity. Chem Pharm Bull (Tokyo) 1996; 44(11): 2121-7. [http://dx.doi.org/10.1248/cpb.44.2121] [PMID: 8945778]

[20] Nogami H, Nagai T, Fukuoka E, Sonobe T. Disintegration of the aspirin tablets containing potato starch and microcrystalline cellulose in various concentrations. Chem Pharm Bull (Tokyo) 1969; 17(7): 1450-5.
[http://dx.doi.org/10.1248/cpb.17.1450] [PMID: 5822503]

[21] Indian Pharmacopoeia 2007. Ghaziabad: Indian Pharmacopoeia Commission 2007.

[22] International Conference on Harmonisation; guidance on Q6A specifications: test procedures and acceptance criteria for new drug substances and new drug products: chemical substances. Notice. Fed Regist 2000; 65(251): 83041-63.
[PMID: 12356095]

[23] Gupta A, Hunt RL, Shah RB, Sayeed VA, Khan MA. Disintegration of highly soluble immediate release tablets: a surrogate for dissolution. AAPS PharmSciTech 2009; 10(2): 495-9. [http://dx.doi.org/10.1208/s12249-009-9227-0] [PMID: 19387843]

[24] Donauer N, Löbenberg R. A mini review of scientific and pharmacopeial requirements for the disintegration test. Int J Pharm 2007; 345(1-2): 2-8. [http://dx.doi.org/10.1016/j.ijpharm.2007.08.045] [PMID: 17935916]

[25] Anwar S, Fell JT, Dickinson PA. An investigation of the disintegration of tablets in biorelevant media. Int J Pharm 2005; 290(1-2): 121-7. [http://dx.doi.org/10.1016/j.ijpharm.2004.11.023] [PMID: 15664137]

[26] Popescu C, Zhou L, Joshi A. Selection of non-synthetic disintegrants for pharmaceutical and nutraceutical orally disintegrating tablets. Tablets and Capsules July 2010.

[27] Kakutani R, Muro H, Makino T. Development of a new disintegration method for orally disintegrating tablets. Chem Pharm Bull (Tokyo) 2010; 58(7): 885-90. [http://dx.doi.org/10.1248/cpb.58.885] [PMID: 20606331]

[28] Late SG, Yu Y-Y, Banga AK. Effects of disintegration-promoting agent, lubricants and moisture treatment on optimised fast disintegrating tablets. Int J Pharm 2009; 365(1-2): 4-11. [http://dx.doi.org/10.1016/j.ijpharm.2008.08.010] [PMID: 18778759]

[29] Fu Y, Jeong S, Callihan J. Preparation of fast-dissolving tablets based on mannose. Cary, NC, ETATS-UNIS. Oxford University Press 2006. [http://dx.doi.org/10.1021/bk-2006-0924.ch023]

[30] Fu Y, Jeong S, Kim J. Mannose-based fast dissolving tablets. US Patent 20060134195, 2006.

[31] Azarmi S, Roa W, Löbenberg R. Current perspectives in dissolution testing of conventional and novel dosage forms. Int J Pharm 2007; 328(1): 12-21. [http://dx.doi.org/10.1016/j.ijpharm.2006.10.001] [PMID: 17084051]

[32] Abdelbary G, Eouani C, Prinderre P, Joachim J, Reynier J, Piccerelle P. Determination of the *in vitro* disintegration profile of rapidly disintegrating tablets and correlation with oral disintegration. Int J Pharm 2005; 292(1-2): 29-41.
[http://dx.doi.org/10.1016/j.ijpharm.2004.08.019] [PMID: 15725551]

[33] Alhusban F, Perrie Y, Mohammed AR. Formulation of multiparticulate systems as lyophilised orally disintegrating tablets. Eur J Pharm Biopharm 2011; 79(3): 627-34. [http://dx.doi.org/10.1016/j.ejpb.2011.05.014] [PMID: 21693189]

[34] Harada T, Narazaki R, Nagira S, Ohwaki T, Aoki S, Iwamoto K. Evaluation of the disintegration properties of commercial famotidine 20 mg orally disintegrating tablets using a simple new test and human sensory test. Chem Pharm Bull (Tokyo) 2006; 54(8): 1072-5. [http://dx.doi.org/10.1248/cpb.54.1072] [PMID: 16880646]

[35] Watanabe Y, Koizumi K, Zama Y, Kiriyama M, Matsumoto Y, Matsumoto M. New compressed tablet rapidly disintegrating in saliva in the mouth using crystalline cellulose and a disintegrant. Biol Pharm Bull 1995; 18(9): 1308-10. [http://dx.doi.org/10.1248/bpb.18.1308] [PMID: 8845832]

[36] US Pharmacopeia and National Formulary. Rockville: United States Pharmacopeial Convention 1990.

[37] Ferran JS. Orally disintegrating tablets and process for obtaining them. US Patent 20060165781, 2006.

[38] Pandya VM, Patel DJ, Patel JK, *et al.* Formulation, characterization, and optimization of fast-dissolve tablets containing celecoxib solid dispersion. Dissolut Technol 2009; 16: 22-7. [http://dx.doi.org/10.14227/DT160409P22]

[39] Fang F, Adams R, Hahm H. Desktop Disintegration Test for Orally Disintegrating Tablets (ODT's): A Rapid and Simple Method for Observing the Disintegration Behavior for the Regulatory Review Scientists in the Evaluation of Drug Applications. Poster K-14. In: FDA Science Forum; Washington DC. 2006.

[40] Umaki Y, Nozaki S, Sugishita S, *et al.* [Is an oral disintegrating tablets a formulation that is easy to ingest for patients experiencing difficulty with eating and swallowing?]. Rinsho Shinkeigaku 2009; 49(2-3): 90-5. [http://dx.doi.org/10.5692/clinicalneurol.49.90] [PMID: 19348172]

[41] Rawas-Qalaji MM, Simons FE, Simons KJ. Sublingual epinephrine tablets *versus* intramuscular injection of epinephrine: dose equivalence for potential treatment of anaphylaxis. J Allergy Clin Immunol 2006; 117(2): 398-403. [http://dx.doi.org/10.1016/j.jaci.2005.12.1310] [PMID: 16461140]

[42] Rawas-qalaji M, Simons K, Xiaochen G. Fast-disintegrating epinephrine tablets for buccal or sublingual administration. US Patent 20070202163, 2007.

[43] Yohei H, Naohisa K, Toshiya K, *et al.* Tablet disintegration method and disintegration tester. Japan Patent 2006-205008, 2006.

[44] Hoashi Y, Tozuka Y, Takeuchi H. Development of a novel and simple method to evaluate disintegration of rapidly disintegrating tablets. Chem Pharm Bull (Tokyo) 2013; 61(9): 962-6. [http://dx.doi.org/10.1248/cpb.c13-00441] [PMID: 23995360]

[45] Khan S, Kataria P, Nakhat P, Yeole P. Taste masking of ondansetron hydrochloride by polymer carrier system and formulation of rapid-disintegrating tablets. AAPS PharmSciTech 2007; 8(2): 46. [http://dx.doi.org/10.1208/pt0802046] [PMID: 17622121]

[46] Que L, Wu W, Cheng X, Hu T. Evaluation of disintegrating time of rapidly disintegrating tablets by a paddle method. Pharm Dev Technol 2006; 11(3): 295-301. [http://dx.doi.org/10.1080/10837450600767649] [PMID: 16895840]

[47] Bi YX, Sunada H, Yonezawa Y, Danjo K. Evaluation of rapidly disintegrating tablets prepared by a direct compression method. Drug Dev Ind Pharm 1999; 25(5): 571-81. [http://dx.doi.org/10.1081/DDC-100102211] [PMID: 10219525]

[48] Bi Y, Yonezawa Y, Sunada H. Rapidly disintegrating tablets prepared by the wet compression method: mechanism and optimization. J Pharm Sci 1999; 88(10): 1004-10. [http://dx.doi.org/10.1021/js990061z] [PMID: 10514347]

[49] Morita Y, Tsushima Y, Yasui M, Termoz R, Ajioka J, Takayama K. Evaluation of the disintegration

time of rapidly disintegrating tablets *via* a novel method utilizing a CCD camera. Chem Pharm Bull (Tokyo) 2002; 50(9): 1181-6.
[http://dx.doi.org/10.1248/cpb.50.1181] [PMID: 12237533]

[50] Otsuka M, Yamanaka A, Uchino T, Otsuka K, Sadamoto K, Ohshima H. Quantitative evaluation of the disintegration of orally rapid disintegrating tablets by X-ray computed tomography. Chem Pharm Bull (Tokyo) 2012; 60(12): 1502-7.
[PMID: 23006519]

[51] Narazaki R, Harada T, Takami N, Kato Y, Ohwaki T. A new method for disintegration studies of rapid disintegrating tablet. Chem Pharm Bull (Tokyo) 2004; 52(6): 704-7.
[http://dx.doi.org/10.1248/cpb.52.704] [PMID: 15187391]

[52] Disintegation Tester Model NT 600. 2009. Accessed from: http://www.xebex.jp/Prod/cn8/nt.html Accessed on 20th February 2015.

[53] Ogata K, Takamura NS, *et al.* Evaluation on Disintegration Tests of Rapidly-Disintegrating Tablets. J Pharm Health Care Sci (Jp) 2001; 27: 553-8.
[http://dx.doi.org/10.5649/jjphcs.27.553]

[54] Keishi Y, Masashi N, Rie S, *et al.* Evaluation of oral disintegration time of rapidly disintegrating tablets (RDTs) by *in vivo* and *in vitro* disintegration testing. J Pharm Health Care Sci (Jp) 2006; 32: 1124-32.
[http://dx.doi.org/10.5649/jjphcs.32.1124]

[55] Akira S, Hiroyuki M, Tadashi M. Apparatus and method for testing disintegation of tablet. Japan Patent 2010-164415, 2010.

[56] el-Arini SK, Clas SD. Evaluation of disintegration testing of different fast dissolving tablets using the texture analyzer. Pharm Dev Technol 2002; 7(3): 361-71.
[http://dx.doi.org/10.1081/PDT-120005732] [PMID: 12229267]

[57] Fu Y, Jeong SH, Park K. Fast-melting tablets based on highly plastic granules. J Control Release 2005; 109(1-3): 203-10.
[http://dx.doi.org/10.1016/j.jconrel.2005.09.021] [PMID: 16260059]

[58] Szakonyi G, Zelkó R. Prediction of oral disintegration time of fast disintegrating tablets using texture analyzer and computational optimization. Int J Pharm 2013; 448(2): 346-53.
[http://dx.doi.org/10.1016/j.ijpharm.2013.03.047] [PMID: 23558313]

[59] Gryczke A, Schminke S, Maniruzzaman M, Beck J, Douroumis D. Development and evaluation of orally disintegrating tablets (ODTs) containing Ibuprofen granules prepared by hot melt extrusion. Colloids Surf B Biointerfaces 2011; 86(2): 275-84.
[http://dx.doi.org/10.1016/j.colsurfb.2011.04.007] [PMID: 21592751]

[60] Rapid Disintegration Tablet Rig replicates the *in vivo* conditions of the human mouth for FMT and OBT testing. 2012. Accessed from: http://texturetechnologies.com/blog/rapid-disintegration-tablet-rig-replicates-the-in-vivo-conditions-of-the-human-mouth-for-the-reliable-assessment-of-the-mechanical-properties-of-fast-melting-tablets-fmts-and-orally-disintegrating-t/ Accessed on 20th February 2015.

[61] ODT-101 Catalogue. 2009. Accessed from: http://www.xebex.jp/_userdata/ODT-101.pdf Accessed on 20th February 2015.

[62] Harada T, Narazaki R, Ohwaki T, *et al.* Effect of physical properties of orally disintegrating tablets on disintegration time as determined by a new apparatus. J Drug Deliv Sci Technol 2010; 20: 377-83.
[http://dx.doi.org/10.1016/S1773-2247(10)50062-5]

[63] Kondo K, Niwa T, Danjo K. Evaluation of disintegration properties of orally rapidly disintegrating tablets using a novel disintegration tester. Chem Pharm Bull (Tokyo) 2012; 60(10): 1240-8.
[http://dx.doi.org/10.1248/cpb.c12-00307] [PMID: 23036967]

[64] Yoshita T, Uchida S, Namiki N. Clinical disintegration time of orally disintegrating tablets clinically available in Japan in healthy volunteers. Biol Pharm Bull 2013; 36(9): 1488-93. [http://dx.doi.org/10.1248/bpb.b13-00353] [PMID: 23995661]

[65] Hoashi Y, Katayama N, Daidouji S. Method for producing orodispersible tablets. Patent EP2719377, 2014.

[66] Tricorptester (Information Brochure). 2006. Accessed from: http://www.okadaseiko.co.jp/ Accessed on 20th February 2015.

[67] Matsui R, Uchida S, Namiki N. Combination effect of physical and gustatory taste masking for propiverine hydrochloride orally disintegrating tablets on palatability. Biol Pharm Bull 2015; 38(1): 17-22. [http://dx.doi.org/10.1248/bpb.b14-00467] [PMID: 25744453]

[68] Uchida T, Hazekawa M, Ikezaki H. Prediction of bitterness for ten kinds of orally disintegrating tablets by taste sensor. In: AAPS Annual Meeting and Exposition, McCormick Place; Chicago. 2012.

[69] Orally disintegrating tablet tester OD-mate. 2015. Accessed from: http://www.higuchi-inc.co.jp/pharma/analysis/physical/odmate/ Accessed on 20th February 2015.

[70] Uchida T, Yoshida M, Hazekawa M, *et al.* Evaluation of palatability of 10 commercial amlodipine orally disintegrating tablets by gustatory sensation testing, OD-mate as a new disintegration apparatus and the artificial taste sensor. J Pharm Pharmacol 2013; 65(9): 1312-20. [http://dx.doi.org/10.1111/jphp.12101] [PMID: 23927469]

[71] Sieber D, Krampe R, Pein M. Critical evaluation of different disintegration testers for orodisperible minitablets regarding their correlation with *in vivo* data. In: AAPS Annual Meeting and Exposition; San Diego Convention Center, San Diego. 2014.

[72] Evaluation of orally disintegrating tablets (ODTs) using precision compressive loading. 2014. Accessed from: http://worldwide.bose.com/electroforce/assets/pdf/appBriefs/appbrief_ODT_062911_low.pdf Accessed on 20th February 2015.

[73] Klancke J. Dissolution testing of orally disintegrating tablets. Dissolut Technol 2003; 10(2): 6-9. [http://dx.doi.org/10.14227/DT100203P6]

[74] Siewert M, Dressman J, Brown CK, Shah VP. FIP/AAPS guidelines to dissolution/*in vitro* release testing of novel/special dosage forms. AAPS PharmSciTech 2003; 4(1): E7. [http://dx.doi.org/10.1208/pt040107] [PMID: 12916916]

[75] Hancock B, Mullerney M. X-ray microtomography of solid dosage forms. Pharm Technol 2005; 29(44): 92-100.

[76] Weitschies W, Karaus M, Cordini D, Trahms L, Breitkreutz J, Semmler W. Magnetic marker monitoring of disintegrating capsules. Eur J Pharm Sci 2001; 13(4): 411-6. [http://dx.doi.org/10.1016/S0928-0987(01)00140-3] [PMID: 11408156]

[77] Wilson CG, Washington N. Assessment of disintegration and dissolution of dosage forms *in vivo* using gamma scintigraphy. Drug Dev Ind Pharm 1988; 14: 211-81. [http://dx.doi.org/10.3109/03639048809151971]

[78] Wilding IR, Coupe AJ, Davis SS. The role of gamma-scintigraphy in oral drug delivery. Adv Drug Deliv Rev 2001; 46(1-3): 103-24. [http://dx.doi.org/10.1016/S0169-409X(00)00135-6] [PMID: 11259836]

[79] Christrup LL, Davis SS, Frier M, *et al.* Deposition of a model substance, 99m Tc E-HIDA, in the oral cavity after administration of lozenges, chewing gum and sublingual tablets. Int J Pharm 1990; 66: 169-74. [http://dx.doi.org/10.1016/0378-5173(90)90396-L]

[80] Wilson CG, Washington N, Norman S, *et al.* A gamma scintigraphic study to compare oesophageal clearance of "Expidet" formulations, tablets and capsules in supine volunteers. Int J Pharm 1988; 46: 241-6.
[http://dx.doi.org/10.1016/0378-5173(88)90084-1]

[81] Wilson CG, Washington N, Peach J, *et al.* The behaviour of a fast-dissolving dosage form (Expidet) followed by [gamma]-scintigraphy. Int J Pharm 1987; 40: 119-23.
[http://dx.doi.org/10.1016/0378-5173(87)90056-1]

[82] Washington N, Wilson CG, Greaves JL, *et al.* A gamma scintigraphic study of gastric coating by Expidet, tablet and liquid formulations. Int J Pharm 1989; 57: 17-22.
[http://dx.doi.org/10.1016/0378-5173(89)90258-5]

[83] Anand V, Kataria M, Kukkar V, Saharan V, Choudhury PK. The latest trends in the taste assessment of pharmaceuticals. Drug Discov Today 2007; 12(5-6): 257-65.
[http://dx.doi.org/10.1016/j.drudis.2007.01.010] [PMID: 17331891]

[84] Woertz K, Tissen C, Kleinebudde P, Breitkreutz J. Rational development of taste masked oral liquids guided by an electronic tongue. Int J Pharm 2010; 400(1-2): 114-23.
[http://dx.doi.org/10.1016/j.ijpharm.2010.08.042] [PMID: 20816732]

[85] Woertz K, Tissen C, Kleinebudde P, Breitkreutz J. Performance qualification of an electronic tongue based on ICH guideline Q2. J Pharm Biomed Anal 2010; 51(3): 497-506.
[http://dx.doi.org/10.1016/j.jpba.2009.09.029] [PMID: 19853397]

[86] Woertz K, Tissen C, Kleinebudde P, Breitkreutz J. Development of a taste-masked generic ibuprofen suspension: top-down approach guided by electronic tongue measurements. J Pharm Sci 2011; 100(10): 4460-70.
[http://dx.doi.org/10.1002/jps.22629] [PMID: 21607955]

[87] Woertz K, Tissen C, Kleinebudde P, Breitkreutz J. A comparative study on two electronic tongues for pharmaceutical formulation development. J Pharm Biomed Anal 2011; 55(2): 272-81.
[http://dx.doi.org/10.1016/j.jpba.2011.02.002] [PMID: 21353433]

[88] Okamotoa M, Sunada H, Nakano M, *et al.* Bitterness evaluation of orally disintegrating famotidine tablets using a taste sensor. Asian J Pharm Sci 2010; 4: 1-7.

[89] Hori K, Yoshida N, Okumura T, Okamura Y, Kawakami J. Method for the evaluation of the stability and usability after opening packages of orally disintegrating tablets: case of amlodipine besilate products. Yakugaku Zasshi 2010; 130(8): 1029-40.
[http://dx.doi.org/10.1248/yakushi.130.1029] [PMID: 20686207]

CHAPTER 9

Clinical Studies on Fast Dissolving/Disintegrating Dosage Forms

Prashant Mathur[1,*], **Arpita Jindal**[1], **Sokindra Kumar**[2] and **Vikas A. Saharan**[3]

[1] *Department of Clinical Pharmacy, Division of Pharmaceutical Sciences, Shri Guru Ram Rai Institute of Technology and Science, Dehradun, Uttarakhand, India*

[2] *RV Northland Institute of Pharmacy, Greater Noida, Uttar Pradesh, India*

[3] *Department of Pharmaceutics, School of Pharmaceutical Sciences, Sardar Bhagwan Singh Post Graduate Institute of Biomedical Sciences and Research, Balawala, Dehradun, Uttarakhand, India*

Abstract: Swallowing medication has always been a major problem among 50% of the population, especially in cases of elderly and children due to a fear of choking, resulting to an inappropriate medication adherence and in turn to non-compliance of dosage regimen. Swallowing problems are also seen in adult people who are bed-ridden or those who are busy in working or travelling, which makes them to forget or miss their doses as it requires water to swallow. This issue can be overcome by using FDDFs (Fast Dissolving/Disintegrating Dosage Forms), which have gained an immense popularity worldwide and a specific position in the field of novel drug delivery systems due to their easier administration and excellent palatability. FDDF has characteristics of both solid as well as liquid dosage form, as during storage and before administration it is solid in nature, a stability factor and as soon as it is placed in the mouth or beneath the tongue it rapidly gets transformed into its liquid form in the presence of saliva within a few seconds of its administration. The buccal mucosa is well supplied with both vascular and lymphatic systems and most importantly avoidance of intestinal or hepatic metabolism. The site and extent of absorption through buccal cavity are the important factors to be considered in developing FDDFs. The other factors like meta-bolising enzyme transporters involved, bioavailability and physicochemical properties of the drug are also important properties to be considered in developing FDDFs. FDDFs, as delivery systems, are widely used in treatment of allergies or emergency conditions which require a rapid therapeutic effect of the drug, *e.g.* sublingual tablet of nitroglycerin in case of angina attack. The disintegration time is also the important factor for classifying a drug product as FDDF, as generally, it is below 60 s in case of FDDF. Several FDDF drug products belonging to Fast

* **Corresponding author Prashant Mathur:** Department of Clinical Pharmacy, Division of Pharmaceutical Sciences, Shri Guru Ram Rai Institute of Technology and Science, Dehradun, Uttarakhand, India; Tel: +91-135-2726435; Mobile: +91-7895221122; Fax: +91-135-2721762; E-mail: prashantmats@yahoo.com

Vikas Anand Saharan (Ed.)

Dissolving/Disintegrating tablets (FDTs), Fast Dissolving/Disintegrating Oral Films (FDOFs) have been introduced in the market as a result of an increased patient demands and their market presence is expected to expand in the forthcoming years.

Keywords: Absorption, Bioavailability, Bioequivalence, Compliance, Clinical, Dysphagia, Film, Geriatric, ODT, Paediatric, Psychotic, Quality of life, Tablet.

1. INTRODUCTION

A drug delivery system is designed in a specific manner so that drug can reach to its target site or region in an appropriate concentration required to elicit desired therapeutic effect. Designing and developing a new drug or a drug delivery system has always been a tremendous challenge in the pharmaceutical industry [1]. Recently, the interest in designing the newer buccal route for drug delivery especially for metabolically unstable drugs has evolved drastically as the absorption of active ingredients from the oral cavity provides a direct passage for the drug into the systemic circulation [2]. Swallowing a tablet/capsule has been a major difficulty for paediatrics and geriatrics, leading to poor patient compliance. Dysphagia, *i.e.* difficulty in swallowing, is prevalent among all age groups [3]. According to a report, approximately 35% of the general population is suffering from dysphagia. Even 30-40% of elderly hospitalised subjects were found affected with some sort of dysphagia [4]. Size, surface, texture, odour and taste of tablets/capsules are the most frequent complaints for difficulty in swallowing. Paediatric and geriatric populations are more in need of conveniently swallowed dosage forms [5]. Some other studies have also revealed that majority of the population suffers from the problem of swallowing tablets or capsules [6]. These studies have shown an urgent requirement of novel dosage forms to overcome the problem of dysphagia. Easily dispersible dosage forms seem capable to overcome the problem of swallowing in paediatric and geriatric populations.

For the convenience of paediatric, geriatric and psychotic patients several FDDFs have been developed, *e.g.* FDDF would be a more suitable dosage form than antihistamine syrup for an 8-10 year old allergic child. Similarly, a woman of middle age with breast cancer undergoing radiation therapy would be more comfortable of placing the tablet beneath tongue or above the tongue for disintegration of tablet in the oral cavity [5]. Hence, FDDFs like FDTs, FDOFs may be most suitable choice for these patients [6]. FDDFs increase the patient compliance due to their quick disintegration/dissolution in the saliva within seconds and thereby eliminating the need of water for swallowing. These tablets, which can be placed in the mouth for their rapid dispersion/dissolution, are termed as "Orodispersible" as per the European Pharmacopoeia [7] and "Orally Disintegrating Tablets (ODTs)" according to USP/NF [8].

Recently, FDDFs have gained immense popularity all around the world and the family of FDDF is continuously expanding with dosage forms like FDOFs, Fast Disintegrating Pellets (FDPs), Orally Disintegrating Mini-Tablets (ODMTs) and Fast Disintegrating Granules (FDGs). To enhance the quality of life (QOL) of patients, these new types of FDDFs are being developed and marketed by many pharmaceutical companies [9]. Ease of administration, no need of swallowing with water, accurate dosing, better palatability, rapid onset of action, avoidance of first pass metabolism and increased bioavailability are some of the potential advantages of FDDFs over other oral solid unit dosage forms [2, 10]. Furthermore, the advantages of oral route over other routes of administration are also gaining the acceptance of FDDFs among all types of patient populations. Thus, in the recent years a multiple number of fast dissolving over-the-counter (OTC) and prescription drugs have entered into the market worldwide. Nitroglycerin was the first drug that showed substantial amount of absorption through oral mucosa, after which several other drug delivery forms through oral cavity had been developed. The development of the buccal drug delivery systems can be differentiated into two periods of its invention. The first period focuses on the development of sublingual tablets and oral solutions. Recently, refined by using new technologies such as sprays, patches and quick-dissolving solid matrices, the second period of invention was spawned over the last decade with the innovations of using highly permeable oral mucosa for targeted drug delivery [2].

Despite their tremendous popularity, FDDFs are often being confused with other solid dosage forms present in the market, which can also be consumed without water such as lozenges, chewable tablets, *etc*. Lozenges are meant to dissolve slowly in the mouth, whereas chewable tablets require manual chewing before swallowing. FDTs are far more different from such type of tablets as they get rapidly dissolved/dispersed in the mouth in the presence of saliva few seconds. The research, development and marketing of these new unconventional dosage forms or delivery systems are been regulated by U.S Congress, which is been enforced by the U.S Food & Drug Administration (FDA). Through the Federal Register, FDA proposes rules and regulations for assisting the management of approval process for new drug and drug products, which are later compiled in the U.S. Code of Federal Regulations (CFR) [11]. The relevant CFR sections that address different aspects of clinical pharmacology and biopharmaceutics informational needs for supporting a new product's approval are Part 201 of Title

21 (21 CFR 201) and Part 320 of Title 21 (21 CFR 320) entitled *Labelling* and *Bioavailability and Bioequivalence Requirements*, respectively [12]. The ICH guidelines and FDA regulations and guidance complement each other.

2. ENHANCED PREGASTRIC ABSORPTION AND RAPID ONSET OF ACTION

FDDFs instantly disintegrate in the saliva, when kept on or beneath the tongue, releases the active ingredients that gets dispersed or dissolved in to the saliva, which is then swallowed and the active ingredient is absorbed by normal absorption mechanisms from different parts of gastrointestinal tract. The disintegrated mass along with saliva moves down the oesophagus and gets absorbed while passing down to the stomach and then to small intestine. Partial absorption of drug from the oral cavity, as the disintegrated/dissolved particles with saliva moves downwards to the stomach, may produce quick onset of action.

Some FDDFs have been designed to achieve faster onset and improvements in bioavailability due to pregastric absorption of active ingredient from mucous membranes lined in the mouth, pharynx and oesophagus [13]. Faster disintegration/dissolution of FDDFs and subsequent immediate release of active ingredient may lead to faster rate of absorption and subsequently causing a rapid onset of action. Pregastric absorption increases bioavailability of active ingredient because active ingredient reaches directly into the circulatory system and bypasses first pass metabolism. This bioavailability benefit may sometimes be beneficial in reducing the overall dose of the active ingredient and minimising toxic effects [14 - 16].

FDTs of piroxicam are considered better due to its rapid onset of action, longer duration of action, less adverse effects and high tolerance in controlling post-surgical pain in spine [17], for the therapeutic management of subjects with acute low back pain [18] and in emergency renal colic treatment [19], where other drugs have some lag time to control the pain. Similarly, for the therapeutic management of moderate to severe migraine pain, the FDT formulation of sumatriptan was found more effective, well tolerated and onset of pain relief action started as early as 30 minutes with 50 mg dose and as early as 20 minutes with 100 mg dose [20]. A study on healthy, nonatopic white subjects revealed that ebastine 20 mg FDT showed a significantly higher inhibition of the response to histamine injection as compared to placebo and desloratidine 5 mg capsule after 1 and 5 days. An overall preference for the FDT formulation over capsule was acknowledged by most of the subjects [21]. In some clinical studies, significant increase in onset of action has been observed and reported with FDDFs (Table **1**).

Table 1. Clinical studies on FDDFs demonstrating faster onset of action and/or enhanced pregastric absorption.

Drug	Dosage Form	Compared with	Type of Study	Outcome of the Study	Ref.
Vardenafil	ODT	Film coated tablet	A *post hoc* integrated analysis on data from two 12 week, double blind, single dose (10 mg), multicenter, randomised, parallel-group, placebo-controlled phase III trials	ODT showed a rapid onset of action than film coated tablet	[22]
Zolmitriptan	Bioenhanced sublingual tablets	BEST-5® and Zomig®-ZMT ODT	Pharmacokinetic study in human volunteers	Significant increase in the rate and extent of sublingual absorption, less variations of T_{max} after sublingual, rapid onset of action	[23]
Zolmitriptan	ODT	Placebo	Randomised, double blind, parallel group trial; zolmitriptan 5 mg ODT (n=329) or matching placebo (n=341) to treat two migraine headaches of moderate or severe intensity	A migraine control as early as 30 minutes after dosing and good maintenance of effect for 24 hours with zolmitriptan 5 mg ODT	[24]

3. IMPROVEMENTS IN BIOAVAILABILITY

The bioavailability of an ingested drug from FDDFs may be higher than the bioavailability from its conventional dosage form. This happens due to the occurrence of pregastric absorption of drug from mouth, pharynx or oesophagus, as the saliva passes down to the stomach. The dispersible tablets are dissolved or dispersed in water prior to their oral administration, whereas FDDFs disintegrate or dissolve in saliva present in the oral cavity [25]. Moreover, as compared to the conventional oral formulations there may be a decrease in the first pass metabolism leading to an increase in bioavailability and/or quicker onset of action [26].

FDDFs, like FDTs and FDOFs, are capable to deliver drugs *via* sublingual/buccal route due to their ability for faster disintegration/dissolution and subsequently allowing quick dissolution/release of the drug in the saliva to make the drug available for absorption from oral/sublingual mucosa. Not every drug can be formulated as sublingual or buccal tablet. For efficient sublingual or buccal absorption, drug is expected to have a molecular weight of less than 500 D (as free base), log P value of 1-5, optimum water solubility and pKa value or pH be maintained for minimum ionisation [27]. Some clinical studies on improvement of bioavailability of drugs through FDDFs are presented in Table **2**.

Sublingual administration is mostly preferred for the treatment of hypertensive crisis, migraine, breakthrough cancer pain, erectile dysfunctions, angina pectoris, allergic rhinitis, allergic rhinoconjunctivitis and other allergies [27, 32]. Apomorphine, a non-narcotic morphine derivative and dopamine agonist, is used sublingually for the treatment of Parkinson's disease. When administered orally, apomorphine exhibit high first-pass hepatic metabolism [33], which can be avoided through its sublingual administration, significant interaction with food or other drugs is also reduced [34]. Oral strip formulation of apomorphine for sublingual administration has been designed for easy to administer and to rapidly, safely and reliably convert a patient from "off" to "on" status in all types of off episodes, including those experienced in the morning [35].

Table 2. Pharmacokinetic assessment for improvements in bioavailability of drugs administered through FDDFs.

Drug	Dosage Form	Compared with	Type of Study	Volunteers	Outcome of the Study	Ref.
Buprenorphine/ naloxone	Sublingual OX219 (Zubsolv®) (5.7/1.4 mg)	Suboxone® tablets (8/2 mg) and films	Open label, two period, randomised, crossover comparative bioavailability study	60 male and female healthy volunteers	Pharmacokinetics were equivalent in OX219 (at 30% lower dose) and Suboxone® tablets. OX219 was preferred over Suboxone® tablet and film formulations by 77.4% and 88.9% of subjects, respectively.	[14]
Diethylstilbestrol	FDOF	Capsule	Single dose bioequivalence study	12 healthy male volunteers	FDOF had a significantly high bioavailability.	[28]
Griseofulvin	Lyophilised dry emulsion tablet	Immediate release conventional tablet	Single dose (125 mg), randomised, open label, six period, crossover study, fasted and fed states	Nine healthy volunteers	Significant faster rate of absorption and AUC 43% larger from lyophilised dry emulsion tablets	[29]

(Table 2) contd.....

Drug	Dosage Form	Compared with	Type of Study	Volunteers	Outcome of the Study	Ref.
Nimesulide	ODT	Conventional tablet	Randomised crossover design	Healthy human subjects	Significantly higher ($p=0.012$) peak plasma concentration and shortened time to C_{max} by 1h ($p=0.029$). AUC was 62% larger with ODT	[30]
Sumatriptan succinate	ODT	Conventional oral tablet Imitrex®	Pharmacokinetic study	Healthy human subjects	Relative bioavailability was 132.34% relative to Imitrex®	[31]

Suprabioavailability of an FDT formulation of vardenafil was ascribed to partial pregastric absorption of vardenafil [36]. In a single dose crossover pharmacokinetic study, an increase of 21-44% in bioavailability of vardenafil was observed with a FDT formulation, when compared to a film coated tablet. However, geometric mean C_{max} remained same with both the formulations. When geometric mean $AUC_{0-\infty}$ and C_{max} of vardenafil were compared between men with erectile dysfunction aged ≥65 years and men of age <65 years, an increase of 41% and 24% in bioavailability was observed, respectively,

Zelapar® (Zydis® formulation of selegiline) ODT allows rapid pregastric absorption of selegiline from buccal mucosa and thereby prevents first pass metabolism and inhibition of gut monoamine oxidases (MAO). Zydis® formulation showed a 13 fold increase in selegiline bioavailability when compared to conventional tablet of selegiline (Eldepryl®) with the 10 mg dose, but the bioavailability of a metabolite was similar from both the formulations. The degree of monoamine oxidase type B (MAO-B) inhibition and the plasma concentration of selegiline were found similar from both the formulations, but the concentration of principal metabolites was markedly reduced with about one-eight dose of selegiline (1.25 mg) in Zydis® formulation [16]. Thus, decrease in concentration of a potential harmful metabolite and equal monoamine oxidase type B-inhibitory effect at a lower dose (Zydis® selegiline 1.25 mg) was found more useful in the treatment of Parkinson's disease due to safer and more predictable treatment [15]. Safe reduced daily off time was observed in a study, in Parkinson's disease patients when Zydis® selegiline at doses of 1.25 mg was used as adjunctive therapy with levodopa [37]. Similarly, sublingual tablets of zolmitriptan offered reduction in hepatic first pass effect and improvements in bioavailability [38].

An OX219 sublingual formulation (Zubsolv®), containing 5.7 mg of buprenorphine and 1.4 mg of naloxone, was found bioequivalent to Suboxone tablets containing 8 mg of buprenorphine and 2 mg of naloxone [14]. Equivalent systemic exposure from OX219 formulation was due to efficient sublingual absorption leading to reduction in gastrointestinal side effect (constipation) and availability of less buprenorphine for parenteral abuse.

In one interesting study, increase of 65% and 77% in bioavailability of griseofulvin, in the presence and absence of water, respectively, was observed when lyophilised dry emulsion tablets (125 mg) were compared to immediate release tablets [29]. A higher C_{max} (2 times) and higher t_{max} values (>3h) from lyophilised dry emulsion tablet indicated a faster rate of drug absorption from gastrointestinal tract. Surprisingly, the effect of meal was not significant in lyophilised tablets when administered with or without water.

Ulfon Lyoc® formulation (520 mg daily) containing aluminium were tested in patients with gastrointestinal symptoms and normal kidney functions for 30 days [39]. There was no increase in rate of absorption or significant increase in urinary excretion levels with Lyoc® formulations and the treatment was found safe, without any toxic effect.

4. RAPID *IN VIVO* DISPERSION AND MUCOSAL COATINGS

Zydis® FDDF is a unique freeze dried medicinal tablet in which drug is physically entrapped or dissolved within the matrix of a fast dissolving carrier formulation [40]. After placing into the mouth, there is an instantaneous disintegration of freeze dried structure releasing the drug, which get dissolved or dispersed into the saliva and subsequently absorbed through gastrointestinal tract [6]. Bioavailability of drug from Zydis® formulations may be significantly greater than those observed from standard or conventional dosage forms. Upon swallowing, Zydis® formulations coat the buccal mucosa and thereafter gastric mucosa uniformly [41 - 43]. Gastric residence time for a resin delivered through Expidet® formulation was found significantly greater than the resin administered through a tablet or suspension [41]. Furthermore, resin delivered through Expidet® formulation coat gastric mucosa more uniformly than a tablet or suspension. Mean gastric emptying times for tablet, liquid and Expidet® formulations were 2.3, 2.5 and 5.5 h, respectively. Gamma scintigraphic studies with Expidet® formulations established that Expidet® formulations cleared from the mouth easily without any oesophageal adhesion [43].

Another scinitgraphic study revealed that oesophageal transit of the resin incorporated in ODT was significantly prolonged [44]. Resin was evenly distributed throughout the stomach and about 20-25% remained for upto 5.5 h. Fast disintegration/dissolving property of ODT coupled with mucoadhesive nature of resin aided in rapid distribution and delayed clearance of the resin from stomach. Therefore, oral ODTs containing finely divided particles of ion exchange resins were recommended for topical treatment of the gastric mucosa in *Helicobacter pylori* infection.

5. PREFERENCE, ACCEPTANCE AND IMPROVEMENTS IN PATIENT COMPLIANCE

Many FDDF formulations have shown improved preference and good acceptance among patients. Good acceptance of FDDF formulations have considerably improved compliance to dosage regimens leading to improvements in clinical response. The improvements in patient compliance with FDDFs are due to their ease in oral administration without water, acceptable taste masking and pleasant flavour. Some clinical studies for improvements in preference/acceptance and/or patient compliance are presented in Table **3**.

A face-to-face interview based study on a new formulation of ebastine FDT was conducted in physicians (82) and patients (60), using placebo, to understand the strengths and perceived key attributes of the FDT formulation. Comfort of use (water is not needed and can be taken anywhere) and convenience were observed as two key attributes for the patient preference. The new FDT formulation was preferred by most of the physicians (54 out of 82) and patients (47 out of 60), because it was more convenient, easier to comply and perceived to offer a rapid onset of action [45]. In acute treatment settings, FDTs of olanzapine offered improvements in medication adherence and greater patient acceptance when compared to conventional tablet of olanzapine [47]. Further, treatment with FDTs was more cost effective than conventional tablets. In one study, all the patients of schizophrenia or schizoaffective disorder rated risperidone FDTs as very acceptable and the formulation was well tolerated [48]. In a preference and acceptance study with 186 patients, zolmitriptan ODT was reported more convenient and less disruptive by more than 80% patients, 60% preferred ODT over conventional sumatriptan tablets and 90% agree with the fact that ODT formulation can be taken whenever and wherever a migraine occurs [49].

A survey was conducted in the subjects diagnosed with allergic rhinitis or dermatitis or urticaria to assess the degree of acceptance of and preference for an FDT formulation [46]. Most of the patients were highly satisfied with the characteristics of the FDT formulation and preferred them for the treatment of allergies. Of the 7,686 patients, who participated in the survey, 9% considered the initial flavour and 83% considered the aftertaste to be very or quite satisfactory, 95% were very satisfied with the disintegration time, 79% were very satisfied with the form, 82% with the size, 72% with the packaging and 78% with the instructions for use. A significant high number of patients (93%) considered that being able to take the drug at any time or place was very important or fairly important and 94% patients considered the ease of use to be much better or better. If given the choice, 93% would choose an FDT formulation. About 88% patients would like to change their current antihistaminic drug for a new allergy drug in an FDT formulation.

Table 3. Clinical studies demonstrating benefits of preference, acceptance and compliance in delivering drugs through FDDFs.

Drug	Dosage Forms Tested	Type of Study	Volunteers	Outcome of the Study	Ref.
Buprenorphine/ naloxone	Sublingual OX219 (Zubsolv®) (5.7/1.4 mg), Suboxone tablets (8/2 mg) and films	Open label, two period, randomised, crossover comparative bioavailability study	60 male and female healthy volunteers	Pharmacokinetics was equivalent in OX219 (at 30% lower dose) and Suboxone® tablets. OX219 was preferred over Suboxone® tablet and film formulations by 77.4% and 88.9% of subjects, respectively.	[14]
Ebastine	FDT	Face to face interview with patients and physicians	60 Patients and 82 physicians	47 patients and 54 physicians preferred new FDT formulation	[45]
Ebastine	FDT formulation	Survey in patients	7686 patients suffering from allergic rhinitis or dermatitis and urticaria	If given an option, 93% would choose FDT formulation. About 80% would like to change their existing antihistaminic drug with a new FDT formulation	[46]
Olanzapine	ODT and conventional tablet	Cost effective study in acute treatment settings	100 schizophrenic patients	3 ODT formulations were found more cost effective.	[47]
Risperidone	ODT	Single centre, open label trial	10 schizophrenic patients	All patients rated risperidone ODTs as very acceptable	[48]

(Table 3) contd.....

Drug	Dosage Forms Tested	Type of Study	Volunteers	Outcome of the Study	Ref.
Zolmitriptan/ Sumatriptan	Zolmitriptan ODT (2.5 mg) and conventional oral sumatriptan tablets (50 mg)	Preference and acceptance study in patients	186 patients	> 60% among 186 patients preferred for ODT; > 80% of patients reported ODT as more convenient and less disruptive; approximately 90% of patients agreed ODT as a dosage form which can be taken wherever and whenever a migraine occurs	[49]

A study was conducted in 85 subjects to determine the compliance of antipsychotic medication, olanzapine as ODT formulation (Zyprexa® Zydis®) in acutely ill patients, who were non-compliant to conventional formulation.. Subjects, who were suffering with schizophrenia or schizoaffective disorder and met the criteria of medication non-compliance were given 10-20 mg/day dose of ODT formulation of olanzapine for upto 6 weeks [50]. Different rating scales to measure medication-taking and compliance attitudes, changes in psychopathology and nursing-care burden were used to assess improvements in compliance with medication along with the assessment of safety variables. In the positive and negative syndrome scale, a significant ($p<0.001$) improvement from the baseline was observed from first week to week 6. There was also a significant ($p<0.05$) improvement in different scales measuring other parameters like compliance with the medication, nursing care burden and attitude. The ODT was well tolerated and facilitated the acceptance regarding antipsychotic drug therapy.

6. BIOEQUIVALENCE

FDDFs of an approved drug are mostly developed as bioequivalent formulations to their conventional dosage forms. However, in some cases, pregastric absorption of the drug may lead to clinically significant improvements in bioavailability, which require confirmation by performing comparative bioavailability studies. Bioequivalence testing for generic FDDFs is essential for obtaining market authorisations from drug regulatory agencies. Several clinical studies have been reported wherein bioequivalence has been demonstrated either between FDDF product and conventional tablet or between FDDF product and the generic (first) FDDF product. For bioequivalent formulations, the 90% confidence interval for the ratio of geometric means of C_{max}, $AUC_{0-\infty}$, and AUC_{0-t} must remain within equivalence limits, *i.e.* 80%-125%. Bioavailability of the drug may be affected when FDDFs are knowingly or unknowingly administered with water or food. Hence, the effect of water and food must be assessed in bioequivalence trials.

If a drug incorporated in FDDF product is absorbed from gastrointestinal tract after swallowing and no part of the drug is absorbed from oral cavity, BCS biowaiver may be expected as per EMA guideline [51]. Else bioequivalence must be proved by conducting bioequivalence studies in humans [51].

6.1. Bioequivalence

Generally, FDDFs and conventional formulations of same dosage strength have similar pharmacokinetics and, therefore, demonstrate bioequivalence. For any change in pharmacokinetic parameters with the FDDF formulation, when compared to a conventional tablet, the safety and efficacy related issues associated for the concern indications should be justified [52]. Some clinical studies demonstrating bioequivalence between FDDFs and conventional dosage forms are presented in Table **4**.

Table 4. Pharmacokinetic assessment for bioequivalence for drugs administered through FDDFs and conventional dosage forms.

Drug	Dosage Forms Tested	Type of Study	Volunteers	Outcome of the Study	Ref.
Escitalopram	Single doses of escitalopram ODT (2×10 mg and 1×20 mg) and conventional tablets (2×10 mg)	Randomised, open label and 3 way crossover trial	Pharmacokinetic and statistical analysis of data from 29 men who completed all 3 treatments.	Bioequivalence was established	[53]
Finasteride	ODT and conventional tablet	Single dose, randomised, open label, 2 way crossover trial	24 men	Bioequivalence was established. A significant difference for T_{max} between ODT and conventional tablet	[54]
Flurbiprofen	ODT and conventional tablet	Randomised, single dose (50 mg), open label, 2 period, crossover study	Non-smoking Chinese male volunteers	ODT was found bioequivalent to conventional tablet	[55]
Levetiracetam	"Fast-melt" oral formulations by three-dimensional printing (3DP) technology and Immediate release tablets (Keppra®)	Three way crossover design to find relative bioavailability	33 in healthy male and female subjects	Equivalent rate and extent of absorption	[56]
Meclizine HCl	FDOF and Zentrip®	Bioequivalence study		FDOF showed bioequivalence to Zentrip®	[57]

(Table 4) contd.....

Drug	Dosage Forms Tested	Type of Study	Volunteers	Outcome of the Study	Ref.
Meloxicam	ODT and conventional tablet	Two randomised and crossover, studies with a 7 day or 14 day washout period	28 volunteers	Bioequivalence was established in fasting conditions	[58]
Metoclopramide	ODT and conventional tablet	Randomised, single dose (10 mg), crossover study	41 healthy volunteers	Bioequivalence established and treatment was well tolerated	[59]
Olanzapine	ODT and conventional tablet	Randomised, 3-way crossover study	10 healthy volunteers	No statistically significant differences in pharmacokinetic parameters was observed	[60]
Ondansetron	Oral film (Zuplenz®, Monosol Rx, Warren, NJ) and ODT (Zofran®, GlaxoSmithKline, Research Triangle Park)	3 individual open label and randomised studies under fasted, fed conditions and fasted with and without water	Study 1: 48 volunteers; Study 2: 48 volunteers; Study 3: 18 volunteers	Bioequivalence was established	[61]
Ondansetron HCl	RapidFilm® (orodispersible films) and Zydis® Lingual (ODT)	Randomised, single dose (8 mg), open, crossover two period (1 week washout period)	24 healthy human volunteers (Caucasian, 12 males and 12 females)	RapidFilm® was found bioequivalent to Zydis® Lingual	[62]
Risperidone	ODT and Conventional tablet	Randomised, open label, single dose (0.5 mg), 2 way crossover trial	Healthy volunteers	Bioequivalence with respect to the drug and its metabolite 9-hydroxy-risperidone	[63]
Sildenafil	ODT and film coated tablets	Randomised, open label, 2 period crossover study, at two doses 50 mg and 100 mg	53 subjects of ages of 20-50 years and within 20% of their ideal weight	Similar pharmacokinetic in both dosage form and at both doses	[64]
Tramadol	ODT (Zamadol® Melt) and conventional capsule	Bioequivalence study	20 healthy volunteers	Bioequivalence was established for tested formulations. Pharmacokinetics of tramadol and active metabolite O-desmethyl tramadol was found equal.	[65]

(Table 4) contd.....

Drug	Dosage Forms Tested	Type of Study	Volunteers	Outcome of the Study	Ref.
Zonisamide	ODT and conventional capsule	Open label, randomised sequence, single dose (300 mg ODT *vs* 100 mg capsule), 2 period, 2 treatment crossover studies	Healthy male volunteers of age 18 to 55 years; Study one: 36 male and study two: 40 male subjects	Zonisamide ODT met regulatory criteria for bioequivalence to the reference formulation	[66]

Bioequivalence of Ondansetron RapidFilm® (orodispersible films) and Zofran® Zydis® Lingual (ODT) was demonstrated through a randomised, single dose (8 mg), open, crossover two period (separated by 1 week washout period) clinical trial performed in 24 healthy human volunteers (Caucasian, 12 males and 12 females) by Labtec GmbH [62]. Prior to this, in a pivotal two way crossover study in 6 healthy human volunteers, bioequivalence between ondansetron RapidFilm® and Zofran® Zydis® Lingual (8 mg) was established [67].

A study was conducted to evaluate bioequivalence of an FDT formulation of ondansetron and a marketed conventional tablet of ondansetron available in the Brazilian market. FDT formulation showed log transformed values of C_{max} and AUC values between 80-125%, when assessed with confidence interval approach. Thus, bioequivalence was demonstrated between both the formulations of ondansetron [52]. Similarly, FDT and immediate release capsule formulation of zonisamide demonstrated bioequivalence, when tested in healthy male volunteers [68].

6.2. Water Effect

FDDFs offer a convenient alternative method of administration of tablets as they do not require water for ingestion. Ingestion without water is helpful in improving compliance in frequent travellers and in situations when patient has no access to water. Oral administration without water also improves acceptability of FDDFs and quality of life improves among patients suffering from nocturnal polyuria. However, FDTs may be, knowingly or unknowingly, administered with water. One important question which arise out of this situation is, whether administration with or without water would have any impact on bioavailability of the drug? Bioequivalence, with or without water administration of FDDF, is deemed essential when FDDF product is meant for absorption through the gastrointestinal tract and no absorption of drug takes place from oral cavity. Higher bioavailability from FDDF products, when administered without water, indicates pregastric/

sublingual absorption. Generally, 2 period bioequivalence study of FDDF product is considered sufficient when administration with or without water does not affect bioavailability or drug is not absorbed from any pregastric region. A 3 period study is recommended to assess the effect of water or fluid intake on bioavailability of FDDF product [51]. When bioequivalence of FDDF product is assessed by administering without water, EMA guideline recommends wetting of mouth with 20 ml of water before administering FDDF on the tongue. Furthermore, fluid intake is not allowed earlier than 1 h from administration of FDDF product. Some studies emphasising the effect of water on pharmacokinetics of drugs administered through FDDF are shown in Table **5**.

Sildenafil ODT and marketed sildenafil film coated oral tablets, administered orally with and without water, were assessed for bioequivalence through two randomised, open label, crossover, single dose (50 mg) studies in healthy men (n=36) of age ≥45 years [69]. Sildenafil ODTs administered with or without water, were found bioequivalent to marketed sildenafil film-coated oral tablets.

Table 5. Pharmacokinetic assessment for the effect of water/fluid intake while administering FDDFs.

Drug	Dosage Forms Tested	Type of Study	Volunteers	Outcome of the Study	Ref.
Sildenafil citrate	ODT and film coated tablets	Randomised, open label, crossover, single dose (50 mg), food effect study and bioequivalence study with and without water	Bioequivalence study in 36 subjects, effect of a standard high fat meal in 12 subjects	Equivalent systemic exposure of both tablets. High fat meals reduced the C_{max} by about 59% and a delay of t_{max} was about 0.6-4 h. Sildenafil ODT should be taken on an empty stomach.	[69]
Desmopressin	ODT	Interventional pilot study	6 female and 6 male patients of age 30-89 years (mean age 69 year; standard deviation 18)	Individualised dose titration recommended rather than fixed dose regimens	[70]

(Table 5) contd.....

Drug	Dosage Forms Tested	Type of Study	Volunteers	Outcome of the Study	Ref.
Fentanyl	Sublingual ODT	Study 1: No pretreatment; Study 2: Moistening of the oral cavity before dosing; Study 3: Administration of pilocarpine hydrochloride (saliva stimulant) before dosing	9 cancer patients with salivary gland hypofunction	The T_{max} was longer, the C_{max} was lower, the AUC_{0-30} lower, and the AUC_{last} lower in the phase involving no pretreatment	[71]
Ondansetron	Oral film (Zuplenz®, Monosol Rx) and ODT (Zofran®, GlaxoSmithKline	3 individual open label, randomised studies under fasted and fed conditions; and fasted with and without water	Study 1: 48 volunteers; Study 2: 48 volunteers; Study 3: 18 volunteers	Bioequivalence was established	[61]
Solifenacin	ODT (Vesicare®) and conventional tablets	Randomised crossover trial	30 healthy volunteers	ODT required less amount of water for ingestion and oral (clinical) disintegration time of ODT was 21.4 s	[72]

The availability of sufficient saliva in the oral cavity is considered essential for *in vivo* disintegration of FDDFs. Salivary gland hypofunction in diseases like oral cancer can often result in altered pharmacokinetics from ODTs or sublingual ODTs as it may significantly affect absorption of the drug from oral mucosa and subsequently affect clinical performance by either influencing onset of action or the bioavailability. In 3 pharmacokinetics studies with sublingual ODTs of fentanyl performed in 9 cancer patients, the effect of pretreatment of oral cavity with water (moistening) and the administration of a salivary stimulant (pilocarpine HCl) was compared with administration without any pretreatment [71]. A longer T_{max}, lower C_{max}, AUC_{0-30} and the AUC_{last} were observed in the pharmacokinetics when ODT was administered with no pretreatment. Use of salivary stimulant negatively influenced the pharmacokinetics, while pharmacokinetic profile was similar when oral cavity was moistened and a pretreatment of pilocarpine HCl before dosing.

6.3. Food Effect

Generally, food may have a similar effect on drug absorption, whether drug is administered as a conventional tablet or as FDDF. But when FDDF disintegrates in the mouth, drug get dissolved and swallowed with the saliva, there is still a significant amount of the drug is remaining, to be absorbed, in GI tract. This becomes important, particularly for the drugs which have a significant effect of food on absorption, efficacy, or safety, and is an issue of concern to be addressed. In these conditions following key points are need to be considered [2]:

- If the bioavailability of the conventional tablets is not affected by the food, the similar effect may be anticipated with the FDDF formulations. Thus, there is no need of conducting an investigation to study food effect in FDDF as long as absorption and metabolism remain unchanged from the conventional tablets.
- If the bioavailability of the conventional tablets is affected by the food, the study (as per FDA guidance on food effect studies) for the effect of food on the FDDF formulations may be conducted. In these studies, the FDDF formulations need to be administered without the water, as per, the nature and label instructions of the dosage form.

Food effect studies (Table **6**) have been reported with FDTs of sildenafil citrate [69], vardenafil [36], clozapine [73], alprazolam [74] and amphetamine [75].

Table 6. Effect of food on bioavailability of drugs administered through FDDFs.

Drug	Dosage Form	Type of Study	Volunteers	Outcome of the Study	Ref.
Alprazolam	ODT	Single dose (1 mg), randomised, open label, two period crossover study at fasted and fed state	16 healthy volunteers (7 men and 9 women) of age 20-50 years	Food had no effect on extent of absorption of alprazolam from ODT 1.0 mg. However, the rate of drug absorption decreased with food.	[74]
Amphetamine	Adzenys® XR-ODT™	Single dose (18.8 mg), open label, 3 period, 3 treatment, randomised, crossover, food effect study	42 adults were enrolled	Slight decrease in the d- and l-amphetamine C_{max} and approximately a 2-hour delay in T_{max} with food.	[75]
Clozapine	ODT	Randomised, open label, two way crossover study, fasted and fed state	24 healthy males of age 18-45 years; In period I, ODT 12.5 mg after an overnight fasting and in period II clozapine ODT 12.5 mg within 30 minutes of consuming a high-fat/calorie breakfast	Food decreased the rate of drug absorption from ODT and no effect on the extent of drug absorption. The C_{max} value for clozapine was 20% lower in the fed *versus* the fasted state.	[73]

(Table 6) contd.....

Drug	Dosage Form	Type of Study	Volunteers	Outcome of the Study	Ref.
Griseofulvin	Lyophilised emulsion tablet	Single dose (125 mg), crossover study in fasted and fed state, with and without water	9 healthy volunteers	Prominent effect of the high fat meal in immediate release tablets than in lyophilised emulsion tablets, when administered with or without water	[29]
Sildenafil citrate	ODT	Randomised, open label, crossover, single dose (50 mg), food effect study and a bioequivalence study with and without water	Bioequivalence study was conducted in 36 subjects. Effect of a standard high fat meal on the pharmacokinetics of sildenafil in 12 subjects	High fat meals reduced the C_{max} by about 59% and a delay of t_{max} was about 0.6-4 h. Sildenafil ODT should be taken on an empty stomach.	[69]
Vardenafil	ODT and film coated tablets	Randomised 4 fold crossover study; a phase I study to assess single and multiple dosing compared to single dosing of vardenafil film coated tablet; a pharmacokinetic study in phase III trial in men of broad age range.	In young and elderly men having erectile dysfunctions	Bioequivalence was demonstrated at multiple dosing. Administration of vardenafil ODT with food had no meaningful effect on the pharmacokinetics of vardenafil. Vardenafil ODT was well tolerated.	[36]

In a food effect study, it was concluded that sildenafil ODT should be taken on an empty stomach because high fat meals reduced the C_{max} by about 59% and a delay of t_{max} was about 0.6-4 h [69]. AUC values remained similar for treatments with food or without food. Pharmacokinetics of vardenafil was similar when vardenafil ODT was administered with or without food [36].

When compared with drug administration in the fasted state, co-administration of food was shown to decrease the rate of clozapine absorption from clozapine ODT (12.5 mg) as assessed by C_{max} but had no effect on the extent of clozapine absorption as assessed by AUC_{0-t} and $AUC_{0-\infty}$ [73]. The C_{max} value for clozapine was approximately 20% lower in the fed *versus* the fasted state. Thus, clozapine ODT was recommended to be administered at least 1 hour before meals or after a light meal. The reported adverse events in 24 healthy male subjects were consistent with those expected from healthy subjects taking oral clozapine.

Co-administration of food was shown to have no effect on extent of absorption of immediate release alprazolam ODT (1.0 mg) when compared with administration in the fasted condition [74]. However, the rate of drug absorption decreased with food. The C_{max} decreased by about 25% and a delay of about 1.5 h was observed in T_{max} in food effect studies, which had a minimal clinical implication.

In a recent study with amphetamine ODT formulation (Adzenys® XR-ODT™), a slight decrease in the C_{max} of d-and l-amphetamine and approximately a 2 h delay in T_{max} with food was observed [75].

7. SAFETY, EFFICACY AND TOLERABILITY STUDIES

Safety and efficacy of FDDFs are compromising when pregastric absorption or bypassing of hepatic first pass effect results in enormous increase in either C_{max} or bioavailability (AUC). Increase in rate and extent of absorption shall be adequately substantiated with a decrease in dose of the drug in FDDF formulation. There have been several literature reports recommending reduction in dose of drug in FDDF formulation for safety reasons [14 - 16]. FDDFs are essentially tested for safety, efficacy and tolerability in clinical trials when these formulations are either first market entry or administered for the first time by oral route. Some of these safety, efficacy and tolerability studies are shown in Table **7**.

Table 7. Clinical studies for evaluation of safety, efficacy and tolerability of FDDF drug products.

Drug	Dosage Form	Type of Study	Volunteers	Outcome of the Study	Ref.
Capecitabine	Rapidly disintegrating tablet	Phase I study to estimate the maximum tolerated dose; 3+3 phase I design	24 children of age 3-21 years with newly diagnosed intrinsic brainstem or high grade gliomas	Well tolerated at dose 650 mg/m^2	[76]
Desmopressin	ODT and intranasal desmopressin	Multicentre open label, dose titration study	20 patients, age 6-75 years	Sufficient antidiuretic control from ODT when compared to intranasal therapy. Well tolerated in long term treatment	[77]
Desmopressin	ODT	Multicentre, randomised, double blind, placebo controlled, parallel group study	261 patients of age 19-87 years	At a dose of 25 µg, desmopressin ODT was effective and well tolerated in females	[78]

(Table 7) contd.....

Drug	Dosage Form	Type of Study	Volunteers	Outcome of the Study	Ref.
Desmopressin	ODT	Phase II multicentre, randomised, placebo controlled, double blind, parallel group, comparative clinical trial	Subjects age 55-75 years with a mean of ≥2 voids per night	A lower dose of desmopressin was required in females (gender specific therapeutic window) and a reduced risk of hyponatraemia without compromising efficacy on reduction of nocturnal voids	[79]
Desmopressin	ODT and conventional tablet	Pooled analysis of three short term efficacy studies	351 patients completing treatment of 40-56 weeks	Efficacy was in favour of females (gender difference) with desmopressin ODT 25 µg	[80]
Desmopressin	ODT	Randomised, double-blind, parallel study at 50 µg and 75 µg doses	Full analysis set comprised 385 men	Desmopressin ODT was effective and well tolerated for the treatment of nocturia in men	[81]
Fentanyl	Sublingual ODT	A multicentre, prospective, open label study	182 enrolled and 177 completed the study	In cancer and non-cancer patients, rapid and consistent relief from breakthrough pain; treatment well tolerated and well accepted	[82]
Fentanyl	Sublingual ODT	Randomised, crossover, double blind, placebo controlled and non blind active drug controlled, comparative clinical trial	51 patients	Sublingual fentanyl at doses determined by a conversion ratio of 1/50 was effective and safe	[83]
Fentanyl	Sublingual ODT	A multicentre, randomised, placebo-controlled, double-blind phase III trial.	42 subjects	Doses determined by titration were effective and safe the treatment of breakthrough pain in cancer patients treated with strong opioid analgesics	[84]

(Table 7) contd.....

Drug	Dosage Form	Type of Study	Volunteers	Outcome of the Study	Ref.
Fentanyl	Sublingual fentanyl ODT	Non-randomised, open label, multicentre, Phase III study conducted in opioid tolerant patients	139 recruited patients	Sublingual fentanyl ODT was effective and well tolerated for the long term treatment of breakthrough pain in opioid tolerant cancer patients	[85]
Fentanyl	Sublingual fentanyl ODT	Randomised, placebo controlled, multicentre, phase III trial	A total of 131 opioid tolerant male and female patients of age ≥17 years with breakthrough pain entered the titration phase, of whom 61 were included in the primary efficacy analysis.	Sublingual fentanyl ODT was efficacious and well tolerated for the treatment of breakthrough pain in opioid tolerant patients with cancer	[86]
Fentanyl	Sublingual ODT	Multicentre, prospective, open label study	Total 182 patients were enrolled and 177 (97.2%) completed the study: 37 had breakthrough cancer pain and 145 had breakthrough non-cancer pain.	Sublingual fentanyl ODT provided rapid and consistent relief from breakthrough pain, both in cancer and non-cancer patients. Treatment was well tolerated and well accepted.	[82]
Fentanyl	ODT	Prospective, multicentre phase IV study	217 enrolled patients, 181 (83.4%) completed the observation period	ODT was effective and welltolerated in opioid tolerant cancer patients. Patients reported rapid onset of action in the majority of breakthrough pain episodes.	[87]
Grass allergen (75,000 SQ-T)	Orodispersible grass allergen tablet 75,000 SQ-T (Grazax®, ALK-Abelló A/S, Hørsholm, Denmark) and placebo	Randomised, double blind and placebo controlled	60 children aged 5-12 yearr suffering from grass pollen-induced rhinoconjunctivitis (with or without asthma)	Grazax® was well tolerated in children and considered suitable in paediatrics	[88]

(Table 7) contd.....

Drug	Dosage Form	Type of Study	Volunteers	Outcome of the Study	Ref.
Methylphenidate	Extended Release ODT (XR-ODT) and placebo	Randomised, multicentre, double blind, placebo controlled, parallel, laboratory classroom study	Children (n = 85) of age 6-12 years	XR-ODT was effective and well tolerated	[89]
Olanzapine	ODT and coated tablets	1 year, prospective, observational study	903 patients: 612 patients of schizophrenia, 291 patients of bipolar disorder	No significant difference was observed on discontinuation rates of the tested formulations	[90]
Piribedil	ODT and placebo	Single dose, double blind, double placebo, 3x3 crossover study	38 patients of age 60 ± 8 years, Parkinson's disease duration: 12 ± 6 years	Doses up to 60 mg of sublingual piribedil was found superior to placebo	[90]
Risperidone	ODT and intramuscular haloperidol	Randomised open, prospective study	124 patients with psychotic agitation in an emergency room or inpatient ward	ODT was equally effective and tolerable as intramuscular administration	[91]
Rizatriptan	ODT	Safety and tolerability of rizatriptan ODT was assessed	Open label study in paediatric migraineurs of age 6-17 years	Treatment was found safe and well tolerated in long term acute treatment of migraine	[92]

An investigation was conducted to assess the persistent efficacy of grass tablet immunotherapy (Grazax® Alk-Abello′ A/S, Hørsholm), in Denmark. A randomised, double blind and placebo controlled phase III trial [93] was designed. to evaluate the safety and efficacy of grass allergen immunotherapy, as daily treatment for 3 years. The patients with grass pollen induced moderate to severe allergic rhino conjunctivitis were treated with grass allergen tablets or placebo, for the total of 22 months period. A total of 351 patients with moderate (n =143 [41%]) or severe (n=208 [59%]) grass pollen allergy were included in the study. In the active drug group, there was an average decrease of 36% in the rhino conjunctivitis symptom score (P<0.0001) and average decrease of 46% in the rhino conjunctivitis medication score (P<0.0001), quite significant, as compared with the placebo group. Mean rhino conjunctivitis quality of life was 33% better (P<0.0001). A significant changes in allergen-specific immunoglobulin's coupled with clinical improvements was observed. No serious adverse events were reported with the test formulations and the treatment was well tolerated. Only 1% of patients, treated with active formulations, were affected with adverse events related withdrawal. Highly significant efficacy and progressive immunologic changes were observed with the test formulations over 2 years of continuous treatment.

In a randomised open prospective study on 124 patients with psychotic agitation in an emergency room or inpatient ward, ODT formulation of risperidone was found equally effective and tolerable as intramuscular administration of haloperidol [91].

Sufficient antidiuretic control from ODT formulation, when compared to intranasal therapy, of desmopressin was achieved [77]. The treatment was well tolerable in long-term in a multicentre open-label dose-titration study on 20 patients of 6-75 years age.

In a multicentre, prospective, open label study, fentanyl sublingual gave rapid and consistent relief from breakthrough pain in both cancer and non-cancer patients [82]. In another study, sublingual fentanyl was also found effective and well tolerated for the long-term treatment of breakthrough pain in opioid-tolerant cancer patients [85]. Recently, dose titration is recommended for breakthrough pain treatment in cancer patients treated with strong opioid analgesics [84].

In a randomised, multicenter, double-blind, placebo-controlled, parallel, and laboratory classroom study, an extended release formulation (XR-ODT) of methylphenidate was found effective and well tolerated in children of age 6-12 years [89].

A once daily FDDF of piroxicam was compared with the enteric coated tablets of diclofenac in patients with acute musculoskeletal disorders (sprains or tendinitis) [94]. It was a double blind, double dummy, parallel group, multicentre study carried out in 5 European countries by 24 investigators Patients (n=224) were randomised to take either diclofenac (50 mg) enteric-coated (EC) tablets (n=116 patients, three times a day, with meals for 2 days and then twice a day thereafter) or once-daily FDDF of piroxicam (40 mg) (n=108 patients with 40 mg for the first 2 days and 20 mg for the remaining period). A total of 4 participants in FDDF of piroxicam group and 7 in diclofenac enteric coated tablets group were lost to follow up. For all the parameters for efficacy measured, from baseline, a significant improvement ($P < 0.001$) in both the groups was observed at each follow-up visit. Parameters measured for efficacy were change in overall symptoms since the last visit, ability to resume a specific activity, pain on movement, tenderness on palpation and restriction of active motion. In cases of sprain injury, in both the treatment groups, majority of the patients and investigators acknowledged overall impression of the efficacy, as either good or excellent. But, in case of tendinitis majority of the patients and investigators, acknowledged the overall impression of the efficacy, as significantly better (P=0.02 and P=0.009, respectively) in the piroxicam FDDF group, than that of diclofenac treatment group. A low incidence of adverse events was observed in piroxicam FDDF (12%) group when compare to diclofenac (18%) treatment group. Adverse events related withdrawal of drug was 7% in the piroxicam FDDF treatment group and 5% in the diclofenac treatment group. FDDF of piroxicam was found to be comparable with the conventional enteric coated tablets of diclofenac in terms of tolerability and efficacy in the patients with acute musculoskeletal disorders.

CONCLUSIONS

FDDFs have successfully carved a niche for them amongst other oral dosage forms because of their numerous advantages over other oral delivery systems as these are more patient compliant, convenient to administer and carry, have better safety profile, lesser side effects, cost-effective and may offer greater bioavailability. It is evident from the recent clinical studies that FDDFs have faster onset of action in special patients groups like surgical patients or the subjects with migraine *etc.*, who are unable to swallow the conventional medication, because of improvement in the pregastric absorption of the active drug from buccal or sublingual route, or oesophageal and oropharyngeal membranes. There is also reduction in the amount of active drug, which may undergo the first pass metabolism, resulting into increased bioavailability and decreased incidences of side-effects. The faster disintegration of FDDF has made swallowing convenient and enhances absorption of drug from buccal cavity resulting in improved bioavailability. Improved patient compliance have been observed with many FDDFs formulations. These formulations are well tolerated and found as very acceptable to the users. Most of the patients were found highly satisfied with the characteristics of the FDDF formulations and would choose it for the treatment of their allergies and other acute ailments. There is no need of water for swallowing these formulations and shows a similar effect of food intake in drug absorption as with the conventional tablets. Bioequivalence of FDDF to conventional tablets is highly desired characteristic for obtaining their regulatory approval.

REFERENCES

[1] Devarajan P, Gandh A. *In vitro* and *in vivo* models for oral transmucosal drug delivery. In: Jain N, Ed. Advances in controlled and novel drug delivery. New Delhi: CBS Publishers and Distributors 2008; pp. 70-8.

[2] Ghosh TK, Chatterjee DJ, Pfister WR. Quick-Dissolving Oral Dosage Forms: Scientific and Regulatory Considerations from a Clinical Pharmacology and Biopharmaceutics Perspective. Drugs and the Pharmaceutical Sciences. Marcel Dekker 2005; 145: pp. 337-55.

[3] Fu Y, Yang S, Jeong SH, Kimura S, Park K. Orally fast disintegrating tablets: developments, technologies, taste-masking and clinical studies. Crit Rev Ther Drug Carrier Syst 2004; 21(6): 433-76. [http://dx.doi.org/10.1615/CritRevTherDrugCarrierSyst.v21.i6.10] [PMID: 15658933]

[4] Lindgren S, Janzon L. Dysphagia: Prevalence of swallowing complaints and clinical finding. Med Clin North Am 1993; 77: 3-5.

[5] Sastry SV, Nyshadham JR, Fix JA. Recent technological advances in oral drug delivery - a review. Pharm Sci Technol Today 2000; 3(4): 138-45.
[http://dx.doi.org/10.1016/S1461-5347(00)00247-9] [PMID: 10754543]

[6] Seager H. Drug-delivery products and the Zydis fast-dissolving dosage form. J Pharm Pharmacol 1998; 50(4): 375-82.
[http://dx.doi.org/10.1111/j.2042-7158.1998.tb06876.x] [PMID: 9625481]

[7] European Pharmacopoeia – edition 7.4. Strasbourg, France: European Directorate for the Quality of Medicines (EDQM); 2012.

[8] USP 35 NF 30. Rockville, Md., USA: The United States Pharmacopeial Convention Inc 2012.

[9] Okuda Y, Irisawa Y, Okimoto K, Osawa T, Yamashita S. A new formulation for orally disintegrating tablets using a suspension spray-coating method. Int J Pharm 2009; 382(1-2): 80-7.
[http://dx.doi.org/10.1016/j.ijpharm.2009.08.010] [PMID: 19686825]

[10] Prajapati BG, Ratnakar N. A review on recent patents on fast dissolving drug delivery system. Int J Pharm Tech Res 2009; 1: 790-8.

[11] Electronic Code of Federal Regulations. 2016. Accessed from http://www.ecfr.gov/cgi-bin/ECFR?page=browse Accessed on 11 Sep 2016.

[12] Title 21: Food and Drugs Chapter I:Food And Drug Administration, Department of Health and Human Services; Subchapter C- Drugs: General Part 201:Labeling. 2016. Accessed from https://www.accessdata.fda.gov/scripts/cdrh/cfdocs/cfcfr/CFRSearch.cfm?CFRPart=201 Accessed on 11 Sep 2016.

[13] Embleton JK. Method for treating ophthalmic disease through fast dispersing dosage forms. US Patent 6297240, 2001.

[14] Fischer A, Jönsson M, Hjelmström P. Pharmaceutical and pharmacokinetic characterisation of a novel sublingual buprenorphine/naloxone tablet formulation in healthy volunteers. Drug Dev Ind Pharm 2015; 41(1): 79-84.
[http://dx.doi.org/10.3109/03639045.2013.846365] [PMID: 24099551]

[15] Clarke A, Brewer F, Johnson ES, *et al.* A new formulation of selegiline: improved bioavailability and selectivity for MAO-B inhibition. J Neural Transm (Vienna) 2003; 110(11): 1241-55.
[http://dx.doi.org/10.1007/s00702-003-0036-4] [PMID: 14628189]

[16] Clarke A, Johnson ES, Mallard N, *et al.* A new low-dose formulation of selegiline: clinical efficacy, patient preference and selectivity for MAO-B inhibition. J Neural Transm (Vienna) 2003; 110(11): 1257-71.
[http://dx.doi.org/10.1007/s00702-003-0042-6] [PMID: 14628190]

[17] Pookarnjanamorakot C, Laohacharoensombat W, Jaovisidha S. The clinical efficacy of piroxicam fast-dissolving dosage form for postoperative pain control after simple lumbar spine surgery: a double-blinded randomized study. Spine 2002; 27(5): 447-51. [http://dx.doi.org/10.1097/00007632-200203010-00002] [PMID: 11880827]

[18] Nappi G, Micieli G, Tassorelli C, Viotti E, Altavilla T. Effectiveness of a piroxicam fast dissolving formulation sublingually administered in the symptomatic treatment of migraine without aura. Headache 1993; 33(6): 296-300. [http://dx.doi.org/10.1111/j.1526-4610.1993.hed3306296.x] [PMID: 8349471]

[19] Supervía A, Pedro-Botet J, Nogués X, *et al.* Piroxicam fast-dissolving dosage form *vs* diclofenac sodium in the treatment of acute renal colic: a double-blind controlled trial. Br J Urol 1998; 81(1): 27-30. [http://dx.doi.org/10.1046/j.1464-410x.1998.00505.x] [PMID: 9467472]

[20] Sheftell FD, Dahlöf CG, Brandes JL, Agosti R, Jones MW, Barrett PS. Two replicate randomized, double-blind, placebo-controlled trials of the time to onset of pain relief in the acute treatment of migraine with a fast-disintegrating/rapid-release formulation of sumatriptan tablets. Clin Ther 2005; 27(4): 407-17. [http://dx.doi.org/10.1016/j.clinthera.2005.04.003] [PMID: 15922814]

[21] Antonijoan R, García-Gea C, Puntes M, *et al.* Comparison of inhibition of cutaneous histamine reaction of ebastine fast-dissolving tablet (20 mg) *versus* desloratadine capsule (5 mg): a randomized, double-blind, double-dummy, placebo-controlled, three-period crossover study in healthy, nonatopic adults. Clin Ther 2007; 29(5): 814-22. [http://dx.doi.org/10.1016/j.clinthera.2007.05.001] [PMID: 17697901]

[22] Debruyne FM, Gittelman M, Sperling H, Börner M, Beneke M. Time to onset of action of vardenafil: a retrospective analysis of the pivotal trials for the orodispersible and film-coated tablet formulations. J Sex Med 2011; 8(10): 2912-23. [http://dx.doi.org/10.1111/j.1743-6109.2011.02462.x] [PMID: 21883954]

[23] El-Setouhy DA, Basalious EB, Abdelmalak NS. Bioenhanced sublingual tablet of drug with limited permeability using novel surfactant binder and microencapsulated polysorbate: *In vitro/in vivo* evaluation. Eur J Pharm Biopharm 2015; 94: 386-92. [http://dx.doi.org/10.1016/j.ejpb.2015.06.006] [PMID: 26086847]

[24] Spierings EL, Rapoport AM, Dodick DW, Charlesworth B. Acute treatment of migraine with zolmitriptan 5 mg orally disintegrating tablet. CNS Drugs 2004; 18(15): 1133-41. [http://dx.doi.org/10.2165/00023210-200418150-00007] [PMID: 15581383]

[25] Bhowmik D, Chiranjib B, Krishnakanth P, *et al.* Fast dissolving tablet: an overview. J Chem Pharm Res 2009; 1: 163-77.

[26] El-Kattan A, Varma M. Oral absorption, intestinal metabolism and human oral bioavailability. In: Paxton J, Ed. Topics on drug metabolism. Rijeka, Croatia: InTech 2012; pp. 1-34. [http://dx.doi.org/10.5772/31087]

[27] Sayeed VA, Ashraf M. Considerations in developing sublingual tablets: an overview. Pharm Technol 2014; 38.(11)

[28] Zhang H, Chen H, Li X-J, *et al.* Pharmacokinetics and safety profiles of novel diethylstilbestrol orally dissolving film in comparison with diethylstilbestrol capsules in healthy Chinese male subjects. Int J Clin Pharmacol Ther 2014; 52(5): 407-15. [http://dx.doi.org/10.5414/CP201989] [PMID: 24618069]

[29] Ahmed IS, Aboul-Einien MH, Mohamed OH, Farid SF. Relative bioavailability of griseofulvin lyophilised dry emulsion tablet *vs.* immediate release tablet: a single-dose, randomized, open-label, six-period, crossover study in healthy adult volunteers in the fasted and fed states. Eur J Pharm Sci 2008; 35(3): 219-25.
[http://dx.doi.org/10.1016/j.ejps.2008.07.002] [PMID: 18675344]

[30] Shoukri RA, Ahmed IS, Shamma RN. *In vitro* and *in vivo* evaluation of nimesulide lyophilized orally disintegrating tablets. Eur J Pharm Biopharm 2009; 73(1): 162-71.
[http://dx.doi.org/10.1016/j.ejpb.2009.04.005] [PMID: 19406232]

[31] Tayel SA, El Nabarawi MA, Amin MM. Comparative study between different ready-made orally disintegrating platforms for the formulation of sumatriptan succinate sublingual tablets. AAPS PharmSciTech 2016; 1-4.
[http://dx.doi.org/10.1208/s12249-016-0517-z]

[32] Pleskovic N, Bartholow A, Gentile DA, Skoner DP. The future of sublingual immunotherapy in the United States. Curr Allergy Asthma Rep 2015; 15(8): 44.
[http://dx.doi.org/10.1007/s11882-015-0545-x] [PMID: 26149585]

[33] LeWitt PA. Subcutaneously administered apomorphine: pharmacokinetics and metabolism. Neurology 2004; 62(6) (Suppl. 4): S8-S11.
[http://dx.doi.org/10.1212/WNL.62.6_suppl_4.S8] [PMID: 15037665]

[34] Mulhall JP. Sublingual apomorphine for the treatment of erectile dysfunction. Expert Opin Investig Drugs 2002; 11(2): 295-302.
[http://dx.doi.org/10.1517/13543784.11.2.295] [PMID: 11829718]

[35] Hauser RA, Olanow CW, Dzyngel B, *et al.* Sublingual apomorphine (APL-130277) for the acute conversion of OFF to ON in Parkinsons disease. Mov Disord 2016; 31(9): 1366-72.
[http://dx.doi.org/10.1002/mds.26697] [PMID: 27430123]

[36] Heinig R, Weimann B, Dietrich H, Böttcher MF. Pharmacokinetics of a new orodispersible tablet formulation of vardenafil: results of three clinical trials. Clin Drug Investig 2011; 31(1): 27-41.
[http://dx.doi.org/10.2165/11584950-000000000-00000] [PMID: 20925442]

[37] Löhle M, Storch A. Orally disintegrating selegiline for the treatment of Parkinsons disease. Expert Opin Pharmacother 2008; 9(16): 2881-91.
[http://dx.doi.org/10.1517/14656566.9.16.2881] [PMID: 18937619]

[38] Prajapati ST, Patel MV, Patel CN. Preparation and evaluation of sublingual tablets of zolmitriptan. Int J Pharm Investig 2014; 4(1): 27-31.
[http://dx.doi.org/10.4103/2230-973X.127737] [PMID: 24678459]

[39] Guillard O, Huguet F, Fauconneau B, Piriou A, Pineau A. Absence of gastrointestinal absorption or urinary excretion of aluminium from an allantoinate complex contained in two antacid formulations in patients with normal renal function. Eur J Clin Chem Clin Biochem 1996; 34(8): 609-12.
[PMID: 8877335]

[40] Vijetha KA, Padmaja B, Kumar GS, *et al.* Formulation and Characterization of Fast Dissolving Tablets of Isradipine by Using Different Technologies. Int J Pharm Res Biomed Anal 2012; 1: 1-10.

[41] Washington N, Wilson C, Greaves J, *et al.* A gamma scintigraphic study of gastric coating by Expidet, tablet and liquid formulations. Int J Pharm 1989; 57: 17-22.
[http://dx.doi.org/10.1016/0378-5173(89)90258-5]

[42] Wilson C, Washington N, Peach J, *et al.* The behaviour of a fast-dissolving dosage form (Expidet) followed by gamma-scintigraphy. Int J Pharm 1987; 40: 119-23.
[http://dx.doi.org/10.1016/0378-5173(87)90056-1]

[43] Wilson C, Washington N, Norman S, *et al.* A gamma scintigraphic study to compare oesophageal clearance of Expidet formulations, tablets and capsules in supine volunteers. Int J Pharm 1988; 46: 241-6.
[http://dx.doi.org/10.1016/0378-5173(88)90084-1]

[44] Burton S, Washington N, Steele RJ, Musson R, Feely L. Intragastric distribution of ion-exchange resins: a drug delivery system for the topical treatment of the gastric mucosa. J Pharm Pharmacol 1995; 47(11): 901-6.
[http://dx.doi.org/10.1111/j.2042-7158.1995.tb03268.x] [PMID: 8708983]

[45] Roger A, Fortea J, Artes M, *et al.* Attributes for preference of new fast dissolving tablet (FDT) formulation of ebastine in patients with allergy. Value Health 2005; 8: A23.
[http://dx.doi.org/10.1016/S1098-3015(10)67208-7]

[46] Roger Reig A, Plazas Fernández MJ, Galván Cervera J, Heras Navarro J, Artés Ferragud M, Gabarrón Hortal E. Acceptance survey of a fast dissolving tablet pharmaceutical formulation in allergic patients. Satisfaction and expectancies. Allergol Immunopathol (Madr) 2006; 34(3): 107-12.
[http://dx.doi.org/10.1157/13088176] [PMID: 16750120]

[47] Ozsogut B, Saylan M. Cost effectiveness model comparing fast dissolving olanzapine and conventional olanzapine tablets in the treatment of schizophrenia. Value Health 2006; 9: A314.
[http://dx.doi.org/10.1016/S1098-3015(10)63548-6]

[48] Chue P, Welch R, Binder C. Acceptability and disintegration rates of orally disintegrating risperidone tablets in patients with schizophrenia or schizoaffective disorder. Can J Psychiatry 2004; 49(10): 701-3.
[PMID: 15560318]

[49] Dowson AJ, Charlesworth BR. Patients with migraine prefer zolmitriptan orally disintegrating tablet to sumatriptan conventional oral tablet. Int J Clin Pract 2003; 57(7): 573-6.
[PMID: 14529055]

[50] Kinon BJ, Hill AL, Liu H, Kollack-Walker S. Olanzapine orally disintegrating tablets in the treatment of acutely ill non-compliant patients with schizophrenia. Int J Neuropsychopharmacol 2003; 6(2): 97-102.
[http://dx.doi.org/10.1017/S1461145703003389] [PMID: 12890301]

[51] Guideline on the investigation of bioequivalence European Medicines Agency. London: EMA 2010.

[52] Armando YP, Schramm SG, Silva MdeF, *et al.* Bioequivalence assay between orally disintegrating and conventional tablet formulations in healthy volunteers. Int J Pharm 2009; 366(1-2): 149-53.
[http://dx.doi.org/10.1016/j.ijpharm.2008.09.021] [PMID: 18848869]

[53] Nilausen DO, Zuiker RG, van Gerven J. The perception and pharmacokinetics of a 20-mg dose of escitalopram orodispersible tablets in a relative bioavailability study in healthy men. Clin Ther 2011; 33(10): 1492-502.
[PMID: 21999886]

[54] Chen L, Jiang X, Huang L, *et al.* Bioequivalence of a single 10-mg dose of finasteride 5-mg oral disintegrating tablets and standard tablets in healthy adult male Han Chinese volunteers: a randomized sequence, open-label, two-way crossover study. Clin Ther 2009; 31(10): 2242-8.
[http://dx.doi.org/10.1016/j.clinthera.2009.09.015] [PMID: 19922895]

[55] Liu Y-M, Liu G-Y, Liu Y, *et al.* Pharmacokinetic and bioequivalence comparison between orally disintegrating and conventional tablet formulations of flurbiprofen: a single-dose, randomized-sequence, open-label, two-period crossover study in healthy Chinese male volunteers. Clin Ther 2009; 31(8): 1787-95.
[http://dx.doi.org/10.1016/j.clinthera.2009.08.008] [PMID: 19808137]

[56] Boudriau S, Hanzel C, Massicotte J, Sayegh L, Wang J, Lefebvre M. Randomized comparative bioavailability of a novel three-dimensional printed fast-melt formulation of levetiracetam following the administration of a single 1000-mg dose to healthy human volunteers under fasting and fed conditions. Drugs R D 2016; 16(2): 229-38.
[http://dx.doi.org/10.1007/s40268-016-0132-1] [PMID: 27028750]

[57] Zhao Y, Quan P, Fang L. Preparation of an oral thin film containing meclizine hydrochloride: *In vitro* and *in vivo* evaluation. Int J Pharm 2015; 496(2): 314-22.
[http://dx.doi.org/10.1016/j.ijpharm.2015.10.008] [PMID: 26456247]

[58] Radicioni M, Connolly S, Stroppolo F, Granata G, Loprete L, Leuratti C. Bioequivalence study of a novel orodispersible tablet of meloxicam in a porous matrix after single-dose administration in healthy volunteers. Int J Clin Pharmacol Ther 2013; 51(3): 234-43.
[http://dx.doi.org/10.5414/CP201781] [PMID: 23380429]

[59] Fass R, Pieniaszek HJ, Thompson JR. Pharmacokinetic comparison of orally-disintegrating metoclopramide with conventional metoclopramide tablet formulation in healthy volunteers. Aliment Pharmacol Ther 2009; 30(3): 301-6.
[http://dx.doi.org/10.1111/j.1365-2036.2009.04045.x] [PMID: 19459829]

[60] Markowitz JS, DeVane CL, Malcolm RJ, *et al.* Pharmacokinetics of olanzapine after single-dose oral administration of standard tablet *versus* normal and sublingual administration of an orally disintegrating tablet in normal volunteers. J Clin Pharmacol 2006; 46(2): 164-71.
[http://dx.doi.org/10.1177/0091270005283839] [PMID: 16432268]

[61] Dadey E. Bioequivalence of ondansetron oral soluble film 8 mg (ZUPLENZ) and ondansetron orally disintegrating tablets 8 mg (ZOFRAN) in healthy adults. Am J Ther 2015; 22(2): 90-7.
[http://dx.doi.org/10.1097/MJT.0000000000000174] [PMID: 25581856]

[62] Reiner V, Giarratana N, Monti NC, Breitenbach A, Klaffenbach P. Rapidfilm: an innovative pharmaceutical form designed to improve patient compliance. Int J Pharm 2010; 393(1-2): 55-60.
[http://dx.doi.org/10.1016/j.ijpharm.2010.03.055] [PMID: 20363308]

[63] van Schaick EA, Lechat P, Remmerie BM, Ko G, Lasseter KC, Mannaert E. Pharmacokinetic comparison of fast-disintegrating and conventional tablet formulations of risperidone in healthy volunteers. Clin Ther 2003; 25(6): 1687-99.
[http://dx.doi.org/10.1016/S0149-2918(03)80163-7] [PMID: 12860492]

[64] Roh H, Son H, Lee D, *et al.* Pharmacokinetic comparison of an orally disintegrating film formulation with a film-coated tablet formulation of sildenafil in healthy Korean subjects: a randomized, open-label, single-dose, 2-period crossover study. Clin Ther 2013; 35(3): 205-14.
[http://dx.doi.org/10.1016/j.clinthera.2013.02.006] [PMID: 23497759]

[65] Tagarro I, Vauzelle-Kervroedan F, Díez MC. Pharmacokinetic assessment of a fast-release orodispersible tramadol tablet compared to a conventional tramadol capsule. Arzneimittelforschung 2004; 54(5): 293-7.
[PMID: 15212192]

[66] Maanen Rv, Bentley D. Bioequivalence of zonisamide orally dispersible tablet and immediate-release capsule formulations: results from two open-label, randomized-sequence, single-dose, two-period, two-treatment crossover studies in healthy male volunteers. Clin Ther 2009; 31(6): 1244-55.
[http://dx.doi.org/10.1016/j.clinthera.2009.06.012] [PMID: 19695391]

[67] Reiner V, Giarratana N, Breitenbach A. Ondansetron RapidFilm: an innovative pharmaceutical form to improve patient compliance. 49° Simposio A.F.I.. Italy: Palacongressi di Rimini, Rimini RN 2009.

[68] Maanen Rv, Bentley D. Bioequivalence of zonisamide orally dispersible tablet and immediate-release capsule formulations: results from two open-label, randomized-sequence, single-dose, two-period, two-treatment crossover studies in healthy male volunteers. Clin Ther 2009; 31(6): 1244-55. [http://dx.doi.org/10.1016/j.clinthera.2009.06.012] [PMID: 19695391]

[69] Damle B, Duczynski G, Jeffers BW, Crownover P, Coupe A, LaBadie RR. Pharmacokinetics of a novel orodispersible tablet of sildenafil in healthy subjects. Clin Ther 2014; 36(2): 236-44. [http://dx.doi.org/10.1016/j.clinthera.2013.12.010] [PMID: 24447534]

[70] Goessaert A-S, Everaert K, Hoebeke P, Vande Walle J. Pharmacokinetics and pharmacodynamics of the oral disintegrating tablet of desmopressin in adults with nocturnal polyuria: a pilot study. Adv Ther 2015; 32(9): 799-808. [http://dx.doi.org/10.1007/s12325-015-0247-8] [PMID: 26412224]

[71] Davies A, Mundin G, Vriens J, Webber K, Buchanan A, Waghorn M. The influence of low salivary flow rates on the absorption of a sublingual fentanyl citrate formulation for breakthrough cancer pain. J Pain Symptom Manage 2016; 51(3): 538-45. [http://dx.doi.org/10.1016/j.jpainsymman.2015.11.018] [PMID: 26706627]

[72] Uchida T, Krauwinkel WJ, Mulder H, Smulders RA. Food does not affect the pharmacokinetics of solifenacin, a new muscarinic receptor antagonist: results of a randomized crossover trial. Br J Clin Pharmacol 2004; 58(1): 4-7. [http://dx.doi.org/10.1111/j.1365-2125.2004.02097.x] [PMID: 15206986]

[73] Disanto AR, Golden G. Effect of food on the pharmacokinetics of clozapine orally disintegrating tablet 12.5 mg: a randomized, open-label, crossover study in healthy male subjects. Clin Drug Investig 2009; 29(8): 539-49. [http://dx.doi.org/10.2165/00044011-200929080-00004] [PMID: 19591515]

[74] Erdman K, Stypinski D, Combs M, Witt P, Stiles M, Pollock S. Absence of food effect on the extent of alprazolam absorption from an orally disintegrating tablet. Pharmacotherapy 2007; 27(8): 1120-4. [http://dx.doi.org/10.1592/phco.27.8.1120] [PMID: 17655512]

[75] Stark JG, Engelking D, McMahen R, Sikes C. A randomized crossover study to assess the pharmacokinetics of a novel amphetamine extended-release orally disintegrating tablet in healthy adults. Postgrad Med 2016; 128(7): 648-55. [http://dx.doi.org/10.1080/00325481.2016.1216716] [PMID: 27488574]

[76] Kilburn LB, Kocak M, Schaedeli Stark F, *et al.* Phase I trial of capecitabine rapidly disintegrating tablets and concomitant radiation therapy in children with newly diagnosed brainstem gliomas and high-grade gliomas. Neuro-oncol 2013; 15(6): 759-66. [http://dx.doi.org/10.1093/neuonc/nos315] [PMID: 23592571]

[77] Arima H, Oiso Y, Juul KV, Nørgaard JP. Efficacy and safety of desmopressin orally disintegrating tablet in patients with central diabetes insipidus: results of a multicenter open-label dose-titration study. Endocr J 2013; 60(9): 1085-94. [http://dx.doi.org/10.1507/endocrj.EJ13-0165] [PMID: 23811987]

[78] Sand PK, Dmochowski RR, Reddy J, van der Meulen EA. Efficacy and safety of low dose desmopressin orally disintegrating tablet in women with nocturia: results of a multicenter, randomized, double-blind, placebo controlled, parallel group study. J Urol 2013; 190(3): 958-64. [http://dx.doi.org/10.1016/j.juro.2013.02.037] [PMID: 23454404]

[79] Yamaguchi O, Nishizawa O, Juul KV, Nørgaard JP. Gender difference in efficacy and dose response in Japanese patients with nocturia treated with four different doses of desmopressin orally disintegrating tablet in a randomized, placebo-controlled trial. BJU Int 2013; 111(3): 474-84. [http://dx.doi.org/10.1111/j.1464-410X.2012.11547.x] [PMID: 23046147]

[80] Juul KV, Klein BM, Nørgaard JP. Long-term durability of the response to desmopressin in female and male nocturia patients. Neurourol Urodyn 2013; 32(4): 363-70. [http://dx.doi.org/10.1002/nau.22306] [PMID: 22972524]

[81] Weiss JP, Zinner NR, Klein BM, Nørgaard JP. Desmopressin orally disintegrating tablet effectively reduces nocturia: results of a randomized, double-blind, placebo-controlled trial. Neurourol Urodyn 2012; 31(4): 441-7. [http://dx.doi.org/10.1002/nau.22243] [PMID: 22447415]

[82] Guitart J, Vargas I, De Sanctis V, *et al.* Efficacy and safety of sublingual fentanyl orally disintegrating tablets in patients with breakthrough pain: multicentre prospective study. Clin Drug Investig 2013; 33(9): 675-83. [http://dx.doi.org/10.1007/s40261-013-0111-z] [PMID: 23881567]

[83] Shimoyama N, Gomyo I, Teramoto O, *et al.* Efficacy and safety of sublingual fentanyl orally disintegrating tablet at doses determined from oral morphine rescue doses in the treatment of breakthrough cancer pain. Jpn J Clin Oncol 2015; 45(2): 189-96. [http://dx.doi.org/10.1093/jjco/hyu182] [PMID: 25378647]

[84] Shimoyama N, Gomyo I, Katakami N, *et al.* Efficacy and safety of sublingual fentanyl orally disintegrating tablet at doses determined by titration for the treatment of breakthrough pain in Japanese cancer patients: a multicenter, randomized, placebo-controlled, double-blind phase III trial. Int J Clin Oncol 2015; 20(1): 198-206. [http://dx.doi.org/10.1007/s10147-014-0697-z] [PMID: 24839047]

[85] Nalamachu S, Hassman D, Wallace MS, Dumble S, Derrick R, Howell J. Long-term effectiveness and tolerability of sublingual fentanyl orally disintegrating tablet for the treatment of breakthrough cancer pain. Curr Med Res Opin 2011; 27(3): 519-30. [http://dx.doi.org/10.1185/03007995.2010.545380] [PMID: 21208151]

[86] Rauck RL, Tark M, Reyes E, *et al.* Efficacy and long-term tolerability of sublingual fentanyl orally disintegrating tablet in the treatment of breakthrough cancer pain. Curr Med Res Opin 2009; 25(12): 2877-85. [http://dx.doi.org/10.1185/03007990903368310] [PMID: 19814586]

[87] Überall MA, Müller-Schwefe GH. Sublingual fentanyl orally disintegrating tablet in daily practice: efficacy, safety and tolerability in patients with breakthrough cancer pain. Curr Med Res Opin 2011; 27(7): 1385-94. [http://dx.doi.org/10.1185/03007995.2011.583231] [PMID: 21561313]

[88] Ibañez MD, Kaiser F, Knecht R, *et al.* Safety of specific sublingual immunotherapy with SQ standardized grass allergen tablets in children. Pediatr Allergy Immunol 2007; 18(6): 516-22. [http://dx.doi.org/10.1111/j.1399-3038.2007.00556.x] [PMID: 17680910]

[89] Childress AC, Kollins SH, Cutler AJ, Marraffino A, Sikes CR. Efficacy, safety, and tolerability of an extended-release orally disintegrating methylphenidate tablet in children 612 years of age with attention-deficit/hyperactivity disorder in the laboratory classroom setting. J Child Adolesc Psychopharmacol 2016. [http://dx.doi.org/10.1089/cap.2015.0261] [PMID: 27183299]

[90] Kraemer S, Chartier F, Augendre-Ferrante B, *et al.* Effectiveness of two formulations of oral olanzapine in patients with schizophrenia or bipolar disorder in a natural setting: results from a 1-year European observational study. Hum Psychopharmacol 2012; 27(3): 284-94. [http://dx.doi.org/10.1002/hup.2224] [PMID: 22473831]

[91] Lim HK, Kim JJ, Pae CU, Lee CU, Lee C, Paik IH. Comparison of risperidone orodispersible tablet and intramuscular haloperidol in the treatment of acute psychotic agitation: a randomized open, prospective study. Neuropsychobiology 2010; 62(2): 81-6. [http://dx.doi.org/10.1159/000315437] [PMID: 20523078]

[92] Ho TW, Pearlman E, Lewis D, *et al.* Efficacy and tolerability of rizatriptan in pediatric migraineurs: results from a randomized, double-blind, placebo-controlled trial using a novel adaptive enrichment design. Cephalalgia 2012; 32(10): 750-65. [http://dx.doi.org/10.1177/0333102412451358] [PMID: 22711898]

[93] Dahl R, Kapp A, Colombo G. Sublingual grass allergen tablet immunotherapy provides sustained clinical benefit with progressive immunologic changes over 2 years. J Allergy Clin Immunol 2008; 121: 512-8.

[94] Auvinet B, Crielaard J, Manteuffel G, *et al.* A double-blind comparison of piroxicam fast-dissolving dosage form and diclofenac enteric-coated tablets in the treatment of patients with acute musculoskeletal disorders. Current Ther Res 1995; 56: 1142-53. [http://dx.doi.org/10.1016/0011-393X(95)85124-0]

CHAPTER 10

Fast Dissolving Oral Films

Mahaveer Singh and **Hemant R. Jadhav***

Department of Pharmacy, Birla Institute of Technology and Sciences, Vidya Vihar, Pilani 333031, Jhunjhunu, Rajasthan, India

Abstract: Ease of administration and patient compliance makes the oral route as the most popular route of administration, but difficulty in swallowing or dysphagia may limit the use of oral route in special populations like paediatrics, geriatrics, psychotics, cancer patients, *etc*. Unavailability of water and episodic attack of allergy also contributes to difficulties in swallowing tablets and capsules. Here the novel fast dissolving oral film (FDOF) technology gives new hope to overcome these problems. Oral films made from active ingredient and hydrophilic polymers are capable of rapidly dissolution/disintegration in the buccal cavity. A part of the drug is absorbed from buccal route providing the advantages of quicker onset, bypassing first pass effect and reducing gastric degradation or metabolism. These qualities have made oral film a very popular and convenient dosage form for paediatric, geriatric as well as adult populations. This chapter describes formulation aspects, preparation technologies and some important patents of FDOFs.

Keywords: Dysphagia, Fast dissolving oral film, Mucoadhesive, Nitroglycerin, Pullulan, Starch.

1. INTRODUCTION

Historically, the most important route of administration has been the oral route. Since the start of drug dispensing, oral cavity has been used as a site for drug delivery for most of the drugs. Way back in 1847, it was discovered that nitroglycerin gets absorbed from the oral cavity. It was just a start because oral cavity has been exploited a lot for either local or systemic use. The FDOF is a new drug delivery system to provide easy administration of medicines to patients having problem in swallowing or patients suffering from nausea/emesis. Films can be used for their local application, rapid release of drugs in systemic circulation and in various mucoadhesive systems to give release in controlled

* **Corresponding author Hemant R. Jadhav:** Department of Pharmacy, Birla Institute of Technology and Sciences, Vidya Vihar, Pilani 333031, Jhunjhunu, Rajasthan, India; Tel: +91-1596-515506; Mobile: +91-94146-48696; Fax: +91-1596-244183; E-mails: hemantrj@gmail.com, hemantrj@pilani.bits-pilani.ac.in

Vikas Anand Saharan (Ed.)

fashion [1, 2]. FDOFs are more convenient to use when compared to other dosage forms such as tablets and capsules. FDOFs avoid swallowing of unnecessary water and acceptable taste and palatability can be obtained with easier dosing accuracy and better handling. Therefore, FDOFs have attracted lots of attention and many pharmaceutical companies have come up with FDOFs as their new drug products [3, 4].

The FDOFs offer various advantages over oral drug delivery systems, a few of the advantages are as follows:

- FDOFs can be used to deliver drugs sublingually and by buccal route. This improves the onset of action and dosing frequency thereby enhancing safety and efficacy of the drug.
- Oral films dissolve quickly than other oral dosages forms and are also more stable when compared to liquid or gel type preparations.
- Improved dosing accuracy can be obtained with oral films because each strip contains a fixed amount of the drug.
- Due to ease of administration, oral films offer advantage of improved patient compliance. It gives special benefit to paediatric, geriatric and patients suffering from neurodegenerative diseases, where proper and complete dosing is difficult.
- FDOFs dissolve rapidly in saliva eliminating the need of water to swallow the medication and thereby solves the problem of administering oral medications to patients suffering from swallowing disorders, especially patients suffering from nausea, particularly receiving cancer chemotherapy and to those who are suffering from drug induced nausea and vomiting.
- FDOF drug delivery technology allows pharmaceutical companies to extend revenue lifecycles of drugs vulnerable to generic competition.
- FDOF offers a convenient method of drug administration where drug is an abuse deterrent film matrix that cannot be crushed or injected by patients, thereby it prevents drug abuse.
- FDOFs are of immense use in cough, cold, sore throat and erectile dysfunctions, when an immediate onset of action is desired.

Challenges/disadvantages of FDOF are given below:

- Due to size limitations, FDOFs cannot be prepared for drugs having high dose.
- FDOFs, being hygroscopic, need proper storage conditions (*e.g.* dry place).
- For product stability and safety, specialised packaging may be required.

2. FORMULATIONS OF FAST DISSOLVING ORAL FILMS

2.1. Film Forming Polymers

Polymers are the most important constituents as they form the base for FDOFs. The polymer to be used in oral films should be free from toxic, irritant and leachable impurities such as nitrosamines. There should be sufficient peel, shear and tensile strength in the polymer [4]. It should be readily available at a cheaper cost. Films obtained should be tough enough to withstand damages during handling and transportation. Robustness of a film depends on polymer type and composition [5, 6]. Up to 45% w/w polymer can be accommodated in FDOFs. Most commonly used polymers are pullulan, gelatin, hypromellose, maltodextrin, *etc*. Non animal originated polymers are very important as they are suitable for vegetarians and people with religious dietary restrictions. Some of these polymers are discussed in following sections.

2.1.1. Natural Film Forming Materials

2.1.1.1. Pullulan

Pullulan is a natural polysaccharide consisting of maltotriose units. Three glucose units of maltotriose are connected by α-1,4 glycosidic bonds and maltotriose units are connected to each other by a α-1,6 glycoside bond (Fig. **1**). Bender *et al.* (1959) named it "pullulan." The chemical structure of pullulan was resolved in 1960 [7]. Bender and Wallenfels (1961) discovered the enzyme pullulanase, which hydrolyses pullulan and converts pullulan to maltotriose. The α-1,4 and α-1,6 linkage pattern imparts structural flexibility and solubility to pullulan, resulting in distinct film and fibre forming characteristics. Pullulan is produced from starch by the action of fungus *Aureobasidium pullulans*. Other microbial sources for producing pullulan from starches include *Tremella mesenterica, Cytaria harioti, Cytaria darwinii* [8], *Cryphonectria parasitica* [9], *Teloschistes flavicans* [10] and *Rhodototula bacarum* [11]. Pullulan provides clear homogeneous films without structural modification to it. Low oxygen permeability and low water content are characteristics which make it most suitable for production of thin films [12]. It is easily soluble in both hot and cold water and makes clear and viscous solutions. It has high adhesion and film forming abilities as compared to other polymers. Pullulan is a nonionic polysaccharide, which is blood compatible, biodegradable, non-toxic, non immunogenic, nonmutagenic and non carcinogenic. Pullulan films are thermostable and possess anti-static and elastic properties and can be developed into compression mouldings.

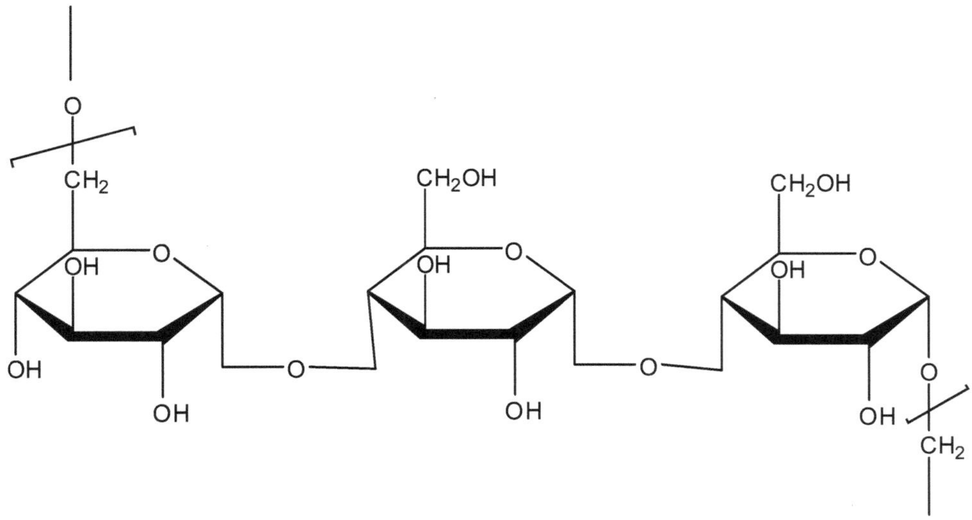

Fig. (1). Structure of maltotriose units of pullulan.

Films made from pullulan are highly water soluble, colourless, tasteless, odourless, transparent, flexible and heat sealable. Pullulan film offers 300 times stronger oxygen barrier than HPMC film and 9 times stronger than gelatin film of the same thickness [13].

2.1.1.2. Modified Starch

Modified starches are also popular for production of FDOFs. It is cheaper and used in combination with pullulan and reduces overall cost of the product. About 50-80% w/w of total polymer can be replaced by starch in production of oral films without affecting the desired properties. Out of total polymer 60-65% w/w of oral film is composed of a water soluble polymer. Starch is a water soluble polymer used in forming clear films, which readily adheres to the moistened skin. It dissolves quickly and releases active ingredient with added flavour [14, 15].

Starch is a major carbohydrate which is stored in plant tubers and seed endosperm. It is found as starch granules, each typically contain large numbers of amylopectin and amylose molecules (Fig. **2**). Amylose is considered to be responsible for the film-forming property of starch [16]. The major source of starch is corn (maize) and other sources are wheat, potato, tapioca and rice. Modification of starch results in improved functionality. Starch is used to produce biodegradable oral films, which can partially or entirely replace synthetic polymers. The starch films are transparent or translucent, odourless, tasteless and colourless [17]. Major disadvantage of starch film is its poor mechanical strength. Films made up of high amylose corn starch and potato starches were found to be more stable during aging. Films prepared from cassava starch resulted in good flexibility and low water permeability, indicating their potential application as edible film former. Starch films from oxidised potato starch with glycerol as a plasticiser have also been reported to provide good flexibility and better mechanical properties [18].

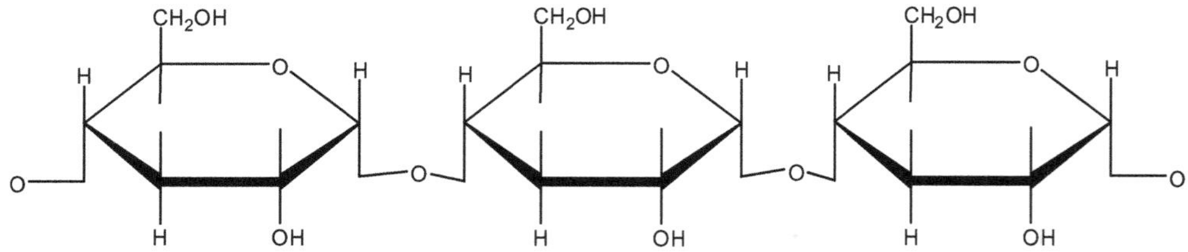

Fig. (2). Structure of starch.

2.1.1.3. Gelatin

Gelatin is a translucent, colourless, brittle (when dry) and odourless solid substance derived from collagen of skin and bones. Films made from gelatin are stable and easy to use for their preparation mixture in solvents like ethanol and water. On long term storage films made up of gelatin become yellowish. In the recent years, the gelatin films formed principally with fish gelatin have attracted great attention of researchers, because they eliminate some of the religious obstacles. Gelatin films dissolves rapidly, produces smooth mouth feel and are excellent carriers for flavours [19].

Gelatin, a mixture of peptides and proteins, is prepared by partial acid hydrolysis (type A gelatin) or by partial alkaline hydrolysis (type B gelatin) of protein fraction of animal collagen (Fig. **3**). The protein fractions consists amino acids joined by amide linkages to form linear polymers. Gelatin can also be prepared by the thermal denaturation of collagen, isolated from animal skin, bones and fish skin [20]. Film forming ability of gelatin depends on molecular weight, the higher the average molecular weight, better is the quality of the film. The molecular weight of gelatin depends mainly on the degree of collagen cross-linking and the extraction procedure used [21].

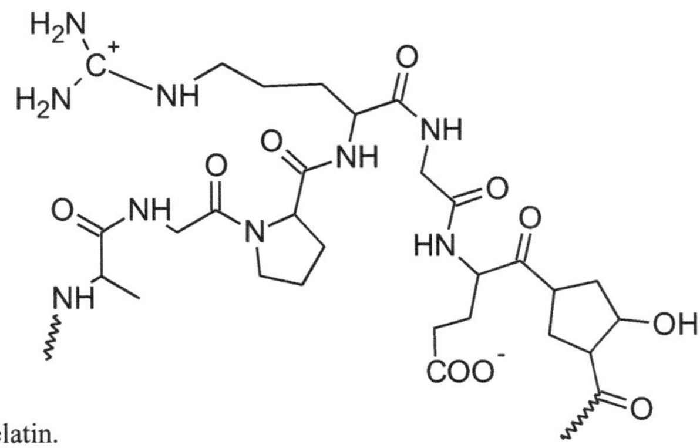

Fig. (3). Structure of gelatin.

2.1.1.4. Maltodextrin

Maltodextrin is prepared by partial hydrolysis of starch and is usually found as a creamy-white hygroscopic powder. It consists of 3 to 19 D-glucose units linked with α-1,4 glycosidic bond (Fig. **4**) [22]. Maltodextrins are classified by Dextrose Equivalent (DE) and have DE values 3-20. Higher DE value results in shorter glucose chains, higher sweetness and higher solubility [23]. Maltodextrin is used as film forming agent in mostly all kind of oral films. Films made up of maltodextrin are homogenous and have high drug loading capacity.

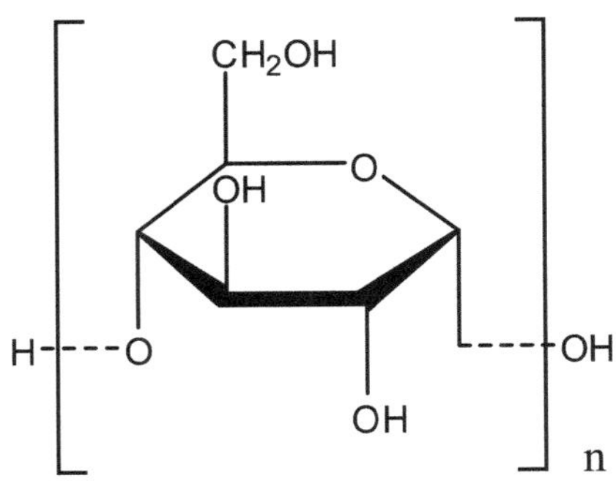

Fig. (4). Structure of maltodextrin.

2.1.1.5. Polymerised rosin

Rosin, a solid resin formerly called colophony or Greek pitch (*Pixgraeca*), is obtained from pines. It is produced by heating fresh liquid resin to evaporate the volatile terpene components [24]. Rosin and its esters are reported to have excellent film forming properties and can be used for enteric coating and delayed release of various drugs. Commercial polymerised rosin is made from gum rosin by polymerisation *via* suitable catalyst [25]. It has various excellent properties such as higher softening point, non-crystalline nature, good oxidation resistance and higher viscosity in organic solvents [26].

2.1.1.6. Lycoat®

Lycoat® NG 73 is an excellent film forming polymer. It is obtained from pea starch and prepared by suitable chemical and physical treatments [27]. Lycoat is a novel granular hydroxypropyl starch polymer, which is designed especially for FDOF. It is easily dispersible in water without forming any lump. It results in a homogenous solution as viscosity develops progressively by cooking. It can be used as the sole or in combination with other film forming polymer to formulate FDOFs [28].

2.1.1.7. Sodium Alginate

Sodium alginate consists of sodium salt of alginic acid, which is a mixture of polyuronic acids composed of residues of D-mannuronic acid and L-glucuronic acid (Fig. **5**). Alginate is a biomaterial produced by brown seaweeds (*Phaeophyceae*, mainly *Laminaria*) and serves as a good source of dietary fibre. It is found mostly in the cell walls of brown algae as calcium, magnesium and sodium salts of alginic acid [28]. Alginate has a very good potential to form oral film and coating component as it expresses various excellent colloidal properties like thickening, stabilising, suspending, film forming, gel producing and emulsion stabilising properties. The disadvantage of edible films prepared from alginate is poor water resistance because of their hydrophilic nature. The water permeability and mechanical strength are considered as moderate compared to other synthetic polymers films. Edible films, made from alginate, are appropriate to load additives and antibacterial compounds [29].

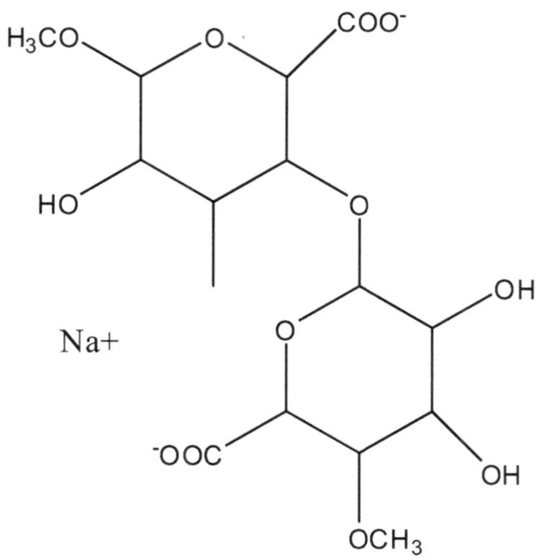

Fig. (5). Structure of sodium alginate.

2.1.1.8. Pectin

Pectin (Fig. **6**) is a structural polysaccharide, mainly extracted from citrus fruits and used in food as gelling agent. It is a high molecular weight complex anionic polysaccharide consisting β-1,4 linked d-galacturonic acid residues, where the uronic acid carboxylic groups are either fully (HMP, high methoxy pectin) or partially (LMP, low methoxy pectin) methyl esterified. It is a good film former with better drug carrying capacity and particularly suitable for low pH applications. Solubility and dissolution of the films in oral cavity depend on the molecular weight of the polymer [30, 31].

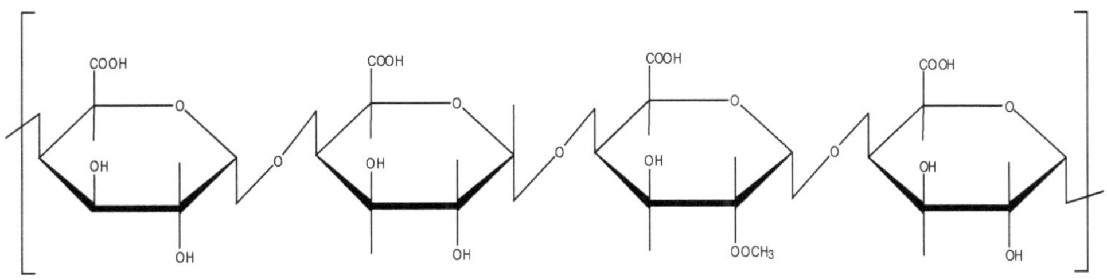

Fig. (6). Structure of pectin.

Table 1. Natural polymers used in oral films.

Polymer	Drug	Description	Ref.
Maltodextrin	Piroxicam	Maltodextrin with low dextrose equivalent was used by casting and extrusion method, it resulted in better tensile strength and swelling properties	[22]

(Table 1) contd.....

Polymer	Drug	Description	Ref.
Maltodextrin	Nicotine	Better tensile strength and faster disintegration resulted by using maltodextrin	[23]
Pullulan	Cetrizine HCl	Oral films with good mechanical properties, thickness and disintegration time	[32]
Pullulan	Pilocarpine HCl	Easy swelling quick disintegration	[33]
Sodium alginate	Levocetrizine HCl and salbutamol sulphate	Good films with faster dissolution and better mechanical strength	[34]
Gelatin	Montelukast sodium	Compositions containing gelatin as film former, PEG as plasticiser and MCC as disintegrating agent resulted in fast disintegrating oral films	[35]

Some of the above discussed polymers with their active pharmaceutical ingredient and advantages are give in Table **1**.

2.1.2. Synthetic Film forming Polymers

2.1.2.1. Hydroxypropyl Cellulose

Hydroxypropyl cellulose (HPC) is a non-ionic water soluble thermoplastic cellulose ether polymer (Fig. **7**). It may contain silica as anti-caking agent (not more than 0.6% w/w) and commercially available in wide range viscosity grades. It has relatively high glass transition temperature, so produced films are stiff and exhibit brittle fracture [36, 37]. Films formed with HPC have low elastic modulus and acceptable percent elongation. The films made up of HPC have good carrying capacity and reasonable clarity. HPC has better film forming property comparable to other polymers. It is chosen as the primary matrix-forming polymer because it is the only water soluble cellulose derivative of thermoplastic nature [37 - 39].

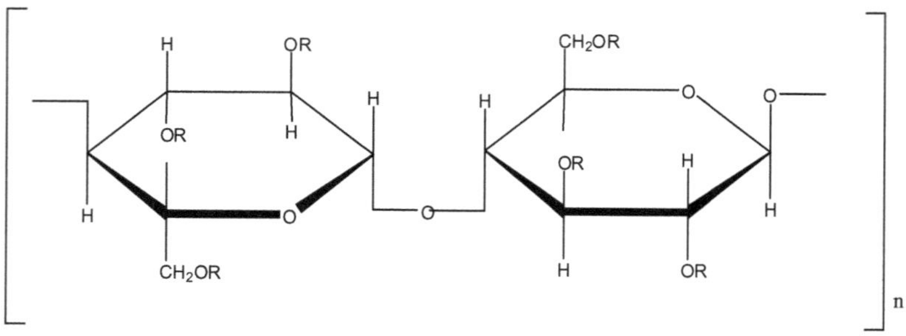

R= $CH_2CHOHCH_3$

Fig. (7). Structure of hydroxypropyl cellulose.

2.1.2.2. Hydroxy Propyl Methyl Cellulose

Hydroxy Propyl Methyl Cellulose (HPMC) or hypromellose is a partly O-methylated and O-(2-hydroxypropylated) cellulose (Fig. **8**). It has very good film forming properties Lower grades of HPMC like Methocel E3, E5 and E15 are specially used for film formation, as they have low viscosity. HPMC polymer has a high glass transition temperature. When it comes in contact with water, HPMC hydrates rapidly and forms gelatinous film which gives controlled release of the drug. HPMC forms highly transparent and flexible films from aqueous solutions [40]. Several studies have been performed on the influence of additives on physiochemical properties of HPMC films. It has been postulated that compounds of lipoidal nature, such as waxes, triglycerides (*e.g.* tristearin) and fatty acids (*e.g.* stearic and palmitic acid) are frequently incorporated into HPMC films leading to decrease in hydrophilicity and moisture transfer due to their high hydrophobicity [41].

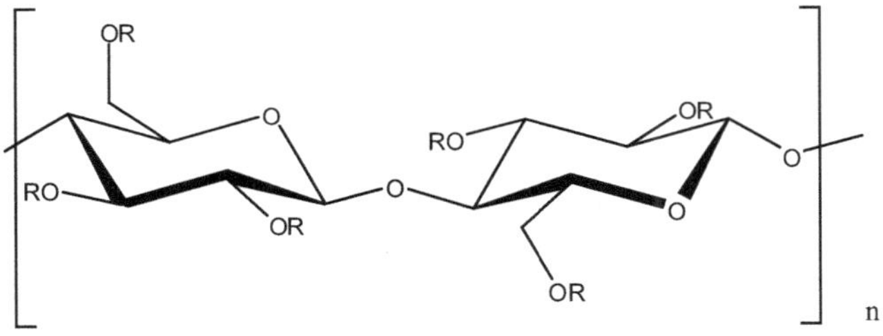

R= H, CH3, -CH_2-$CHOHCH_3$

Fig. (8). Structure of HPMC.

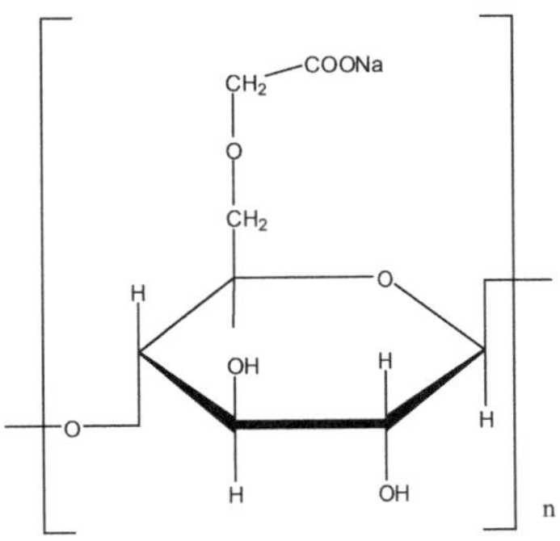

Fig. (9). Structure of sodium CMC.

2.1.2.3. Sodium Carboxy Methyl Cellulose

Sodium Carboxy Methyl Cellulose (sodium CMC) is prepared from cellulose by treatment with alkali and chloro acetic acid or its sodium salt. Sodium CMC is an anionic cellulose ether polymer and most commonly used in controlled release hydrophilic matrix systems (Fig. **9**). It is an inert and non-toxic polymer, which can accommodate high drug loadings [40, 41]. Formulations consisting of sodium CMC and other hydrophilic polymers such as HPMC and xanthan gum have good potential of delivering of drugs to high moistened surfaces such as the oral cavity. The enzymatically modified CMC is considered to have good film forming properties. Modified CMC can be used in combination with other film forming polymers for preparation of oral films [42]. Modified CMC rapidly precipitates, if mixture of water and ethanol are used.

2.1.2.4. Polyvinyl Alcohol

Polyvinyl alcohol (PVA) is prepared by the polymerisation of vinyl acetate to form polyvinyl acetate and followed by hydrolysis of polyvinyl acetate to polyvinyl alcohol (Fig. **10**). PVA has good film forming, emulsifying and adhesive properties. It is colourless, nontoxic and offers good tensile strength and flexibility to films. Commercial PVA grades are available with high degree of hydrolysis [43, 44].

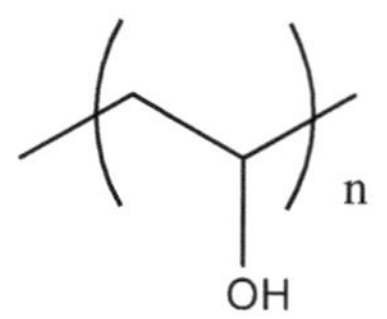

Fig. (10). Structure of PVA.

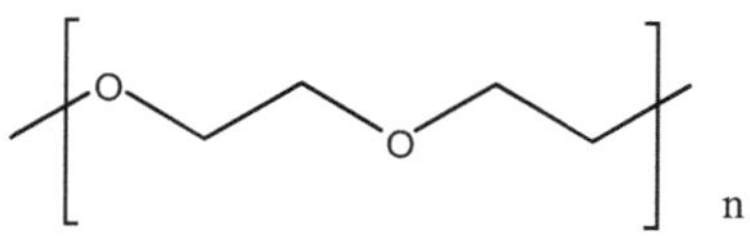

Fig. (11). Structure of PEO.

2.1.2.5. Polyethylene Oxide

Polyethylene Oxide (PEO) or Polyox is a synthetic polymer available over a wide range of molecular weights (Fig. **11**). Materials with molecular weights less than 100,000 are called as PEGs, whereas higher molecular weight polymers are classified as PEO. PEO are white, free-flowing hydrophilic crystalline powders with an average particle size around 150 µm. It is an inert and biocompatible polymer. Some important properties of PEO for their use in films are relatively high melting point, good structural integrity, low glass transition temperature, low toxicity and biocompatibility. It is a non-ionic and water soluble polymer having highly hydrophilic, good lubricating, binding and film forming properties [45].

2.1.2.6. Kollicoat®

Kollicoat®, a PVA-PEG graft copolymer, is specially developed as a coating polymer for immediate release tablets and oral films. PVA moiety is responsible for good film forming properties, whereas PEG part acts as an internal plasticiser providing excellent flexibility. Kollicoat® gives smart protection from unpleasant taste, fast release of medicament and is economical also. Kollicoat® delivers maximum quality in terms of function, stability, appearance and release. The molecule is hydrophilic, so readily soluble in water and plasticiser covalently binds in the molecule. In contrast to pure PVA films, the flexibility is maintained during storage due to prohibition of rearrangement of the molecules to a high level of order (crystallisation). Relative humidity does not affect the mechanical properties of the Kollicoat® films. Films formed of Kollicoat® are transparent in appearance [46].

2.1.2.7. Polyvinyl Pyrrolidine

Polyvinyl pyrrolidone (PVP), also commonly called Polyvidone or Povidone, is a water soluble polymer prepared from the monomer *N*-vinyl pyrrolidone (Fig. **12**). In solution, it has excellent wetting and film forming properties. It is biodegradable, non-toxic, chemically inert, thermostable, pH-stable, non-ionic and colourless. PVP films are brittle in nature; therefore, co-povidone is mixed with PVP for preparation of flexible oral films [47].

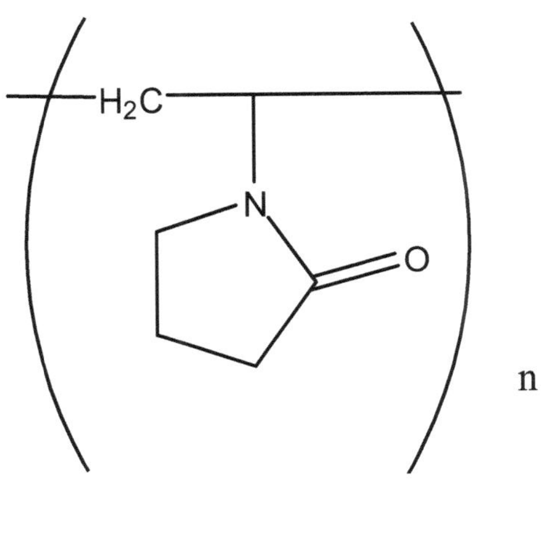

Fig. (12). Structure of PVP.

Synthetic polymers, as discussed above, have been successfully used in preparing FDOFs (Table **2**).

Table 2. Synthetic polymers used in oral films.

Polymer	Drug	Description	Ref.
HPC	Levocetrizine HCl	HPC in combination with HPMC resulted in better taste masking	[48]
HPMC	Verapamil	Combination of maltodextrin and HPMC gave desired thickness with better tensile strength	[49]
HPMC	Prochlorperazine	Acceptable stability and dissolution profile was achieved with the use of hypromellose (7.4% w/w) in combination with low substituted HPC (1.3% w/w) in preparing films.	[50]
PEO	Ondansetron HCl	Low viscosity grade HPMC gave good films	[51]
PVA	Rofecoxib	Use of PVA up to 4% w/w in a solvent casting method resulted in good mechanical properties and better disintegration of films.	[52]

2.2. Plasticisers

Plasticisers are vital ingredient of oral films, which improves flexibility and reduces brittleness by reducing glass transition temperature. Some plasticisers used in oral films are glycerol, propylene glycol, PEG, diethyl and dibutyl phthalate, tributyl, triethyl, acetyl citrate, castor oil, *etc*. The selection of a plasticiser for oral film depends on the solvent and the polymer to be used [53, 54]. Cellulosic hydrophilic polymers are plasticised with hydroxyl group containing PEG, propylene glycol, glycerol and polyol. Less cellulosic hydrophilic polymers are plasticised with esters of citric acid and phthalic acid. Studies have shown that malic acid is a superior plasticiser as compared to citric acid, oleic acid and tartaric acid. It does not crystallise out when the films are dried. In oral films, plasticisers are used at 0-20% w/w of the total polymer weight [55 - 59]. Flexibility of a plasticiser depends on the volatile nature of the plasticiser and the type of interaction between the plasticiser and the polymer. Plasticiser should be compatible with the polymer and other excipients [60, 61].

PEG 300 has been found to be a superior plasticiser when compared to PEGs having higher molecular weights [62]. Lower molecular weight PEGs form superior films with low water vapour permeation rate. Sorbitol has been found superior when compared to mannitol for gelatin films, since mannitol quickly crystallises out from the gelatin films [62]. Glycerin and propylene glycol are used as plasticisers for maltodextrin based oral films with in a concentration range of 16-20% w/w. Glycerin is considered better than propylene glycol, when the films are manufactured by solvent casting and hot melt extrusion methods [62].

Some drug molecules also act as plasticiser and affect transition temperature of the polymer by plasticisation. Sometimes, there are chemical interaction observed between the drug and the polymer. Dissolution rate of ibuprofen decreases because of hydrogen bonding when its concentration in the formulation increases above a certain limit [62, 63].

There are two mechanisms for plasticisation, internal plasticisation involving chemical interaction and external plasticising effect. External plasticising effect mechanism is preferred as it does not result in chemical interactive alterations in the product. Chemical structure and concentration of plasticisers play important roles in maintaining the glass transition temperature of the polymers and plasticisation effect [64, 65].

2.3. Active Pharmaceutical Ingredient

Size of film is always a limitation in oral film technology so molecules with high dose are difficult to incorporate in FDOF. Generally 5-30% w/w of API can be incorporated in the FDOF. Nutraceuticals up to 10% w/w of dry film weight can be incorporated in the oral film. If API is water soluble, it remains dissolved and if not, it remains uniformly distributed in the film. If polymer is water soluble and API is water insoluble than distribution of API is very critical while manufacturing FDOF. Size reduction technologies like milling, micronisation and nanonisation can be used to reduce the size of API and thereby improve texture, uniformity and dissolution of the oral film. If an API is bitter in taste, taste masking methods can be used to improve palatability [66, 67]. A few approaches for taste masking are mixing of API with pleasant taste excipient, complexation, matrixing, polymeric coating, microparticle formation, *etc*. Bitter taste of paracetamol was masked using lipid excipients such as lecithin [68]. The promising results have been found in the oral delivery of famotidine using spray drying techniques [69]. Chemical modification has been successively employed by Glaxo Smithkline for taste masking of ondansetron. A base was used for its *in situ* conversion in salt form. Salting out technology has been used for taste masking by salting out the layer, which contains salt and water soluble polymer [70, 71].

2.4. Sweetening Agents

Sweeteners are very important as FDOFs are required to disintegrate/dissolve in the oral cavity and a part of API may be absorbed from the oral cavity. In paediatric formulations, sweeteners are of prime importance as they improve palatability of oral films [72]. The sweeteners used in oral films can be natural and artificial. The important natural sweeteners used in FDOFs are sucrose, dextrose, fructose, glucose, maltose, *etc.* Apart from these, polyhydric alcohols such as sorbitol, mannitol and maltitol are also used as sweeteners. Sweeteners can be used alone or in combination to provide good taste and cooling sensation. Polyhydric alcohols vary in their sweetening capacity [73]. When natural sugars are used, the issue of increased sugar levels should be carefully considered for diabetic patients. Because of sugar level restrictions, artificial sweeteners have gained more attention now-a-days. Important artificial sweeteners are saccharin, aspartame, cyclamate, sucralose, alitame, neotame, *etc.* They differ in their sweetening capacity as compared to glucose. Some of the sweeteners are carcinogenic and gives bitter after taste [74].

2.5. Saliva Stimulating Agents

Saliva stimulating agents are added to oral films for increasing the rate of production of saliva. Increased saliva would aid in the faster disintegration and rapid dissolution of oral films. Citric acid, malic acid, lactic acid, ascorbic acid and tartaric acid are often used as salivary stimulants. Citric acid is the most preferred saliva stimulating agent used in oral films. These agents can be used alone or in combination between 2-6% w/w of weight of the oral film [75].

2.6. Flavouring Agents

It has been stated that age plays an important role in the taste fondness. The selection of flavour depends on the type of drug to be incorporated and the liking of particular age group. Mint flavour is usually added in products used for gastrointestinal tract (GIT) related ailments like indigestion and is most favoured by geriatrics. The quality of flavour soon after disintegration of the film plays a significant role in patient acceptance. Flavouring agents can be obtained from synthetic sources such as flavour oils, oleo resins *etc.* Extract derived from various parts of the plants like leaves, fruits and flowers can also be used as flavouring agents. Various flavour oil used in film formulation are peppermint oil, cinnamon oil, nutmeg oil, spearmint oil, *etc.* Some fruity flavours are vanilla, chocolate, cocoa, coffee, *etc.* Fruit essence types are raspberry, cherry, pineapple and apple. Generally up to 10% w/w flavours are added in the oral film formulations [76].

2.7. Colouring Agents

FD&C approved colours are used up to 1% w/w concentration in oral films. Natural colouring agents, pigments including titanium oxide, silicon dioxide, zinc dioxide and custom pantone-matched colours can be used in FDOF. These agents are incorporated when some of the formulation ingredients or drugs are present in insoluble or suspension form [77].

2.8. Stabilising and Thickening Agents

The stabilising and thickening agents are employed to improve the viscosity, consistency and stability of the solution/suspension used to prepare oral film. Natural gums like xanthan gum, locust bean gum, carragenan and cellulosic derivatives are preferentially used in concentrations up to 5% w/w [78]. Other ingredients such as surfactants and emulsifying agents can also be used in small amounts to improve overall quality of the oral film [79].

3. DRUG DELIVERY TECHNOLOGIES

There are different proprietary and patented technologies available for preparation of FDOFs. They offer faster dissolution and better delivery of medicament. Some of these important technologies are discussed below.

3.1. SoluLeaves™

SoluLeaves™ is an edible FDOF based on non-animal derived material. SoluLeaves™ technology, a BioProgress technology patented by Meldex International, has been designed to produce a large range of oral drug delivery films incorporated with colours and flavours. SoluLeaves™ films dissolve rapidly on contact with saliva, quickly releasing the active ingredients and flavours. These unique qualities make these films an excellent drug delivery system for a large range of products, which requires fast release in the oral cavity. For pharmaceutical uses, SoluLeaves™ FDOF system is particularly appropriate for paediatric or elderly patients, who have difficulty in swallowing tablets or capsules. The SoluLeaves™ FDOF delivery system can be used for low dosage applications including cough/cold, gastrointestinal, pain, and nutraceutical preparations. SoluLeaves™ films can also be designed to adhere to mucous membranes where it releases the active ingredient within 15 minutes.

Some salient features of SoluLeaves™ technology are as follows:

- A vegetable origin polymer based film that carries low levels of active ingredients and flavouring agents
- Fast dissolution in the oral cavity with enhanced taste masking
- Enhanced patient convenience with accurate dosing
- Flexible film with fast release and quick action

- Genetically Modified Organism (GMO) and gelatin free (suitable for vegetarians and people with religious dietary restrictions)
- Sugar free variant is suitable for diabetics
- Application for a wide range of vitamins, flavourings and for many pharmaceutical actives
- Suitable for paediatric and geriatric patients
- Suitable for oral delivery of herbal and pharmaceutical products.

SoluLeaves™ FDOF, as vitamin preparations such as vitamin C film strip, vitamin B complex thin film and as OTC products such as local anaesthetics for sore throat, cold and cough cure, are available commercially [79 - 81].

3.2. WaferTab™

WaferTab™ is a unique, innovative, effective and highly stable edible FDOF drug delivery system that carries APIs into an ingestible film strip. WaferTab™ was initially developed by Bioprogress, a subsidiary of Meldex International (UK) [82]. The WaferTab™ system provides quick dissolution and rapid release of API when the strip comes into contact with saliva in the oral cavity. API is integrated into a pre-manufactured film to enhance product stability. The film may be coloured as per the need and can be printed during manufacture for branding and coding. The WaferTab™ system lends itself to many opportunities for innovative new product design, enabling multiple films with different APIs to be combined together. WaferTab™ can be prepared in a variety of shapes and sizes and is an ideal method for delivery of APIs, which require rapid release or for use by patients having difficulty in swallowing traditional dosage forms.

Features of WaferTab™ are as under:

- Stable rapid dissolving oral film
- Enhanced taste masking with better convenience and portability
- GMO and gelatin free (suitable for vegetarians and people with religious dietary restrictions)
- Sugar free variant suitable for diabetic patients
- Aqueous based and solvent free
- Can be used for comparatively less stable pharmaceutical forms, particularly salt forms of the drug.

3.3. XGel™

XGel™ film is Meldex International's drug delivery technology. It is used in all its film systems including SoluLeaves™, FoamBurst® and WaferTab®. It uses existing drugs in formulating FDOF for more rapid onset of action and ease in swallowing. XGel™ film offers several other benefits for healthcare and pharmaceutical products. It uses non animal derived polymer, which are GMO free and generally regarded as safe (GRAS) such as cellulose, HPMC, CMC, *etc* [83]. XGel™ film can mask bad taste, can be coloured, layered and stable for enteric applications. The XGel™ film systems can be prepared to encapsulate any oral dosage form and is soluble in both cold and hot water.

3.4. FoamBurst™

FoamBurst™ is a special variant of the SoluLeaves™, which also uses XGel™ technology wherein an inert gas is allowed to pass into the film during production [84]. This results in a film with a honeycombed structure, which dissolves rapidly in the oral cavity. FoamBurst™ has attracted a great deal of interest from manufacturers of food and confectionary as a means of carrying and releasing flavours in the oral cavity.

3.5. RapidFilm®

RapidFilm® is a patented technology developed and commercialised by tesa Labtec GmBH and APR Applied Pharma Research [85]. This is a novel, non mucoadhesive and FDOF technology. The strip disintegrates and releases the drug into the oral cavity and leads to quick systemic absorption of drugs. RapidFilm® dissolves in a very small amount of liquid and, therefore, considered ideal for "medicines to go". It gives spontaneous disintegration and pleasant taste when it is placed in mouth and comes in contact with saliva. Extra liquid is not required to consume RapidFilm® and it gives release of drug in seconds. Ondansetron RapidFilm® 8 mg was found bioequivalent to Zydis® Lingual ODT 8 mg in a randomised, open, crossover, two-period study with a 1 week washout period [86]. Soon thereafter, in 2010 Ondansetron RapidFilm® received regulatory approval in 16 European countries [87] followed by expansion in other countries like China [87] and India [88].

3.6. VarsaFilm®

IntelGenx's rapid release oral film technology, VersaFilm®, is made up of a strip of thin polymeric film consisting of United States Pharmacopeia (USP) components, which are safe and approved by the FDA for use in food, pharmaceutical and cosmetic products [89]. This film technology is used in various breath enhancement strips and was initially developed for the instant delivery of mouth fresheners and flavours to food substrates. The film has various advantages over existing fast dissolving conventional dosage form. It is the application system of choice for indications requiring the immediate onset of actions like migraine, motion sickness, nausea, erectile dysfunction or seasonal allergies. Volatile drugs such as nicotine or nitroglycerin can also be delivered through these films.

3.7. PharmFilm®

MonoSol Rx's PharmFilm® gives an appearance of a postage stamp. These films are more stable, robust and fast dissolving. More API can be incorporated in it, as compared to RapidFilm®, enabling a wide range of products to be delivered from oral and buccal cavity [90]. MonoSol Rx's drug-delivery technology, called PharmFilm, is very much similar to Johnson & Johnson's popular breath freshener Listerine PocketPaks®. It is rapid dissolving, taste masked oral film, which offers fast onset and precise dosing to the patients whose medical condition makes conventional drug therapies (pills, injectable and gels) a challenge. One of the examples of this technology is ondansetron (Zuplenz®), which is prescribed to the cancer patients undergoing chemotherapy. It is a small, thin piece of film that's packaged in its own plastic packet. A patient can slip the film in his mouth and it will dissolve quickly in the oral cavity. Few products from various companies are given in Table **3**.

Table 3. Products from different companies along with their therapeutic applications.

S. No.	Company	Product	Ingredient	Application
1	Pfizer	Listerine PocketPaks®	Mint and Cinnamon flavours	Bad breath
2	Novartis	Triaminic thin strips	Diphenhydramine HCl	Cough and runny nose
3	Labtec	Rapid Film	Ondansetron	Chemotherapy induced emesis
4	Hughes Medical Corporation	Caffeine strips	Caffeine	Stimulant
5	Paladin Labs	Nicotine strips	Nicotine	To reduce smoking habit
6	Biofilm	Male vitality strip	Maca root extract	Aphrodisiac

4. MANUFACTURING METHODS

Various manufacturing methods, with almost similar processing steps, are used for production of oral films, depending on the solvent and properties of API. Typical process utilises following steps:

- Splitting of mass into strip
- Spreading of films on a platform
- Cross cutting of films
- Stacking or placing of strips
- Pouching individual strip or loading into container

Most commonly used manufacturing methods including printing of film are discussed below:

- Solvent casting
- Hot melt extrusion
- Semisolid casting
- Solid dispersion extrusion
- Rolling
- Printing

4.1. Solvent Casting

Solvent casting is almost a century-old film manufacturing technology. For pharmaceutical applications, the API is dispersed or dissolved in a volatile solvent to prepare a solution of polymers, plasticisers and other ingredients. This mixture, known as the film dope, is spread out onto a continuous roll of release media like plastic-impregnated paper. The coated media is finally passed through a drying apparatus to drive off the solvents. The dried film is then cut into small strips, packed and sealed in air tight pouches [91]. Solvent casting is operated at a lower temperature to eliminate solvent from a film containing heat sensitive API. Special safety equipment and procedures should be followed for flammable solvents. It is an ideal technology for manufacturing of oral films containing heat sensitive API's because the temperatures required to remove solvents are relatively low when compared to hot melt extrusion and any other process. The dried solvent cast films, containing traces of residual solvents, has to be checked for compendial compliance limits. Specific types of rollers are used for pouring the solution onto an inert base. Glass, plastic or teflon plates are mostly used as inert bases for film in solvent casting technology. Process transfer from laboratory production scale may encounter problems like irregular thickness and improper drying that needs to be essentially addressed. The commonly available sizes of films are 3×2 cm and 2×2 cm. Depending upon the characteristics of the film, single-unit containers and multiple-unit dispensers can be selected [92 - 94].

Some Precautions

- The physicochemical properties of API play very important role in selection of a solvent.
- Compatibility of API with excipient and polymer is very important.
- Moisture content should be controlled properly as it affects film properties.
- Temperature should be controlled properly as it plays a role in viscosity.

4.2. Hot Melt Extrusion

Hot melt extrusion is the most accepted technique for production of oral films. Currently this technique is applied for manufacturing of variety of dosage forms such as pellets, suppositories, transdermal delivery systems and oral films. Hot melt extrusion method is a process of applying heat and pressure to drug-polymer mixture to melt and force to flow through an orifice. Hot melt extrusion has fewer operation steps with better content uniformity and technology runs without using a solvent [95].

The equipment consists of an extruder with auxiliary equipments and monitoring tools. The extruder consist a feeding hopper, single or twin screw barrels and die. The auxiliary equipment consist heating cooling devices for barrel, convey belt to downstream the product, screw speed controller and temperature pressure gauze [96]. The extruder consist of rotating screws in barrel, which is manufactured in sections, bolted and clamped together. The end plate die determines the size of the product. The heat for melting of material is generated by heaters mounted on barrel walls and friction of material between rotating screw as well. Process involves following steps:

- Feeding of extruder
- Conveying of mass
- Size reduction
- Flow through die
- Downstream processing

Some of the important advantages of hot melt extrusion are as follows:

- No need to use solvent or water
- Less number of processing steps
- Compressibility properties of the API are not affected
- Better dispersion mechanism for poorly water soluble APIs
- Results in more uniform dispersion of the fine particles because of intense mixing and agitation

- Less energy required in comparison to high-shear methods
- Minimum product waste with scale up possibilities
- Good control over operating parameters

A comparison of solvent casting and hot melt extrusion methods is provided in Table **4**.

Table 4. Comparisons of solvent casting and hot melt extrusion methods [95, 96].

Solvent Casting	Hot Melt Extrusion
Thermostable and thermolabile API can be used	Only thermostable can be used
Solvent required	Not required
Hydrous process	Anhydrous process
Rollerand coaters required	Extruder required
Scale up is difficult	Easy scale up
High chances of air entrapment	Low chances of air entrapment

4.3. Semisolid Casting

Semisolid casting involves preparation of a base from a water soluble film forming polymer by adding to it the solution of acid insoluble polymer like cellulose acetate phthalate or butyrate. Plasticiser in an appropriate amount is also incorporated to obtain a gel. This mass is casted into films or ribbons using controlled temperature sources. The average thickness of the film is about 0.015-0.05 inches. The ratio of the acid insoluble polymer to film forming polymer should be 1:4 [97].

4.4. Solid Dispersion Extrusion

In this technique, a solid dispersion of one or more API with an inert carrier is prepared in the presence of a hydrophilic polymer such as PEG. The API is dissolved in an appropriate amount of a liquid solvent and a solution is incorporated in melt of PEG without removing the solvent. This polymer mixture is extruded to provide thin films of variable sizes. In this method, immiscible compounds are extruded with API and solid dispersions are prepared and subsequently films are shaped in dies [98].

4.5. Rolling Method

It is a simple method in which solution or suspension is rolled onto a carrier to get thin films of desired shape and size after drying. The solvent remains water mainly or a hydro alcoholic mixture. The drying of film is done while it is rolled and then cut into desired pieces. In this method, there is a premix of all ingredients except API. Polymer, solvent and other excipients are added to a feed tank, the desired amount of drug is added to the mixer and blend is mixed properly. After proper mixing, the blend is fed to a pan by metered devices and subsequently films are formed on the substrate with the help of rollers [99].

4.6. Printing of Films

Printing technologies for film based drug delivery systems include flexographic, inkjet printing and 3D printing. Inkjet technology precisely and accurately deposits small liquid base on digital predesign pattern [100]. After designing a printing pattern desired ratio of API and excipients can be deposited on a carrier substrate. Three dimensional (3D) printing includes preparation of 3D objects. Sequential layers of material can be deposited and the objects created can be of virtually any shape. These objects are produced with the help of computer-aided design 3D model. Additive manufacturing (AM) technologies include stereolithography, sintering, melting, fused deposition modeling or fused filament fabrication, *etc*. Inkjet technologies can be considered as 3D techniques when it uses 3D objects formed from multiple layering.

5. EVALUATION

Most challenges are faced when a final film formulation is scaled up from bench to production scale. Optimisation at every step, such as mixing, casting, rolling and drying, is very important. Wet strip thickness and drying always affect final film. For drying, different industries are using different driers, *e.g.* bow type and hot flue type dryer. Cutting of strip should also be perfect or else it may result in inaccurate doses. For packing of strips or films aluminium foils are most useful.

Finally, product is examined critically for all parameters like thickness, dryness, tensile strength, percent elongation, tear resistance, Young's modulus, folding endurance, disintegration time, assay and organoleptic characteristics.

5.1. Film Thickness

Thickness is directly related to the content present in an oral film and uniform thickness in the specified reference range gives an indication of quality and accuracy of doses [101]. In FDOFs, thickness should lie in range 5-500 μm. Thickness can vary with the use of film in the oral cavity, *e.g.* buccal and sublingual films have 500 μm and 200 μm thickness, respectively. Thickness of film can be measured by micrometer screw gauze at two to three locations of the film.

5.2. Dryness/Tack test

Dryness is a measure of certain physical and chemical changes including solvent evaporation, oxidation, polymerisation, which are mostly time dependent. Various stages of drying in oral films may be subjective and may be affected by various factors such as temperature, humidity, light and air These variables must be minimised to produce proper films. Dryness at different levels can be checked in the drying process. Various parameters in stage of drying are set-to-touch time, dust- free time, dry-to-touch time, dry-hard time, dry-through-time, dry-to-recoat time and print-free time [102].

5.3. Tensile Strength

Soft materials with low tensile strength are not abrasion resistant. Polymers have sufficient tensile strength to abrasion resistance. Tensile strength can be measured by auto stripping tester as it is the maximum force applied at which film breaks and can be calculated by Equation **1** [103].

$$\text{Tensile Strength} = (\text{Load at failure/Strip thickness}) \times \text{Strip width} \quad \textbf{(1)}$$

5.4. Film Elongation (%)

One important basic parameter in the study of the mechanics of deformable bodies is the resistive property of materials. When gauge marks or extensometers are used for defining a specific test section, only this length is used in the calculation, otherwise the distance between the grips can be used as the initial gauge length. The result is expressed in percent and reported to two significant figures usually. Percent elongation depends on plasticiser content in the film and can be calculated by Equation **2** [103].

$$\text{Elongation (\%)} = (\text{Increase in length/Initial length}) \times 100 \quad \textbf{(2)}$$

5.5. Tear Resistance

Tear resistance of a polymer film is a function or property of its final resistance to rupture. The resistance of a film to tear not only depends on thickness but also on geometry of the film. Maximum stress, near the onset of tearing, in Newton's or pound-force is measured by applying force [104].

5.6. Young's Modulus

Young's modulus measures the resistance of elastic materials to deformation under a specified load. A stiff or hard material will have high Young's modulus and changes the size very slightly at load, *e.g.* diamond. But a flexible material like polymer changes their shape to a larger extent and has a low Young's modulus. Stiffness can be said as opposite to elasticity. A stiff material requires high load to deform it. Stiffness depends on Young's modulus of the material, the loading of material, and shape and size of the film. Specific stiffness can be measured by dividing Young's modulus by the density (Equation **3**) [105].

$$\text{Young's Modulus} = (\text{Slope} \times 100/\text{Strip thickness}) \times \text{Cross head speed} \qquad \textbf{(3)}$$

5.7. Folding Endurance

The number of folds a film can withstand is referred to as folding endurance. Folding endurance can be measured by repeated folding of the strip at same place till it breaks. The specimen film is placed under a constant pressure in a folding endurance tester. It is then folded at a certain angle at a specific fold speed. It is the measure of folding of film without tearing. Moisture and plasticiser loss can decrease folding endurance [106].

5.8. Disintegration

Although no specific guidelines are available for testing disintegration of oral films. Disintegration by slide frame method, where films can be clamped into slide frames after putting a water droplet on film, is most frequently used. In another test protocol, film is kept in a petri dish and time for complete disintegration/dissolution is measured. In one other method, the film is placed on the surface of water in a petri dish and time to disintegrate/dissolve is measured. The disintegration time limit for FDOF is 30 s or less as per guidelines of US Centre for Drug Evaluation and Research. As per pharmacopoeia, fast releasing formulations have a disintegration time limit of 5-30 s and it can be performed in pharmacopoeial disintegration apparatus [107, 108].

5.9. Swelling Property

Swelling studies on FDOFs are conducted in simulated saliva. Procedure includes putting a film on a steel mesh and submerging into the medium. Increase in the film weight can be measured at set time intervals until film gains a constant weight. Degree of swelling can be calculated by using the formula w_t-w_0/w_0, where w_t and w_0 are weights of the film at time t and t_0 (initial time), respectively [107, 108]

5.10. Contact Angle

Contact angle can be measured with goniometer. Alternatively, a distilled water droplet may be kept on film surface and within 10 minutes, images can be recorded for water droplet by a digital camera. Later pictures can be analysed by using software for contact angle determination [107, 108].

5.11. Dissolution

For dissolution paddle or basket apparatus can be used and sink condition are essentially required to be maintained. Media can be selected as per standard requirements and dose of API. When films float in water or in a given media, a basket type apparatus is preferred. Recently Dow chemical company has explored specific dissolution methods for oral films *via* conductivity evaluation [108].

5.12. Assay and Content Uniformity

Assay method available for a particular API can be used for estimation of the labelled amount. Content uniformity can be determined by estimating API in each film. The limit for content uniformity is 85-115% for oral films [109].

5.13. Organoleptic Evaluation

FDOFs are supposed to disintegrate rapidly in the oral cavity so the film needs to have acceptable organoleptic properties. The film should have the desired sweetness and flavour, which must be acceptable to a large mass of population. Taste sensors/electronic tongues can be used as *in vitro* testing methods for organoleptic evaluation of FDOFs. *In vitro* taste assessment apparatus and methodologies are used for taste screening of oral pharmaceutical formulations. Electronic tongue measurements have also been reported for measuring the designed sweetness levels in the formulations [110, 111].

6. SOME RECENT STUDIES

Lots of research is going for developing FDOFs in recent years. Some of these important FDOFs published reports are summarised in Table **5**.

Table 5. Some recent FDOF formulation attempts and their advantages.

Authors	Preparation	Advantage	Ref.
Shimoda *et al.*, 2009	Dexamethasone FDOF for cancer induced vomiting and radiotherapy patients	Rapid disintegration, better patient compliance and rapid drug release	[2]
Valentina *et al.*, 2010	Ondansetron FDOF was compared with oral dispersible tablet for vomiting	Higher patient convenience	[3]
Saini *et al.*, 2011	FDOF using pullulan have been prepared and variable concentrations of pullulan have been used	Increased in disintegration and better dissolution profiles	[13]
Francesco Cilurzo *et al.*, 2008	Fast dissolving films made up of maltodextrin have been studied	Good flexibility, strength and better patient compliance	[22]
Francesco Cilurzo *et al.*, 2010	Authors have studied the effects of taste masking agent and nicotine on properties of nicotine film was studied	Different flavours were used for taste masking and milk flavour gave better taste masking effect	[23]
Kulkarni *et al.*, 2010	Comparison of different polymers in formulation of oral films	Pullulan and HPMCE-15 were found to be best film formers among all selected polymers	[24]
Mishra *et al.*, 2010	Rapid film of cetirizine dihydrochloride using pullulan as film forming agent has been developed	Better taste masking, strength and better patient compliance	[32]
Murata *et al.*, 2010	Dexamethasone and pilocarpine were used as API and pullulan was used as polymer in FDOFs	Result showed that pullulan in 2% concentration gave better drug release	[33]
Garg *et al.*, 2010	Oral film and microbicide gels have been studied	Novel technique has been developed for vaginal delivery to prevent HIV transmission	[34]
Reiner *et al.*, 2010	An innovative RapidFilm® have been developed for ondansetron	RapidFilm® and conventional oral dispersible dosages both were found bioequivalent	[87]
Joshi *et al.*, 2012	FDOFs of domperidone were developed	Better tensile strength and dissolution profiles	[112]
Rubia *et al.*, 2012	FDOFs of citalopram hydrobromide were developed	Good tensile strength and dissolution profiles	[113]
Minako *et al.*, 2012	FDOFs containing dexamethasone as an antiemetic medication were developed	Rapid disintegration, better patient compliance and better tensile strength	[114]
Shelke *et al.*, 2012	FDOFs of amlodipine besylate were developed	Rapid disintegration, dissolution, better patient compliance and better tensile strength	[115]

7. SOME PATENTS

Various US patents have been filed and issued for FDOFs out of which some are discussed below:

7.1. Patent 1

Bess *et al.* filed a patent application (11/429,547) on fast dissolving orally consumable films containing taste masking agents. Patent (7,648,712) was issued and assignee of this patent is McNeil-PPC, Inc. Physiologically acceptable edible oral films have been developed. Pullulan is used as film forming agent and API used is dextromethorphan. This invention is related to FDOFs containing an ion exchange resin as an agent to mask the taste of a pharmaceutically active agent incorporated therein.

7.2. Patent 2

Berry *et al.* filed a patent application (10,226,451) on development of a process for manufacturing of thin strip. Patent (6,824,829) was issued and assignee of this patent is Anupac Packaging, Inc. This manufacturing method for thin film strip includes coating of a liner substrate with wet slurry of film forming ingredients and subsequent drying in an oven to form a thin film. Further, moisture content of the film is measured after passing through drying oven and the film is rewound on itself. The rewound film is then stored in a closed environment to prevent moisture loss during further processing. The invention is related to the processing of thin films and in particular to the formation of coated oral film strips.

7.3. Patent 3

Spence *et al.* filed a patent application (09/836,474) on fast dissolving orally consumable films. Patent (7,025,983) was issued and assignee of this patent is Warner Lambert Company, LLC. Physiologically acceptable, edible films have been developed. The films consist of a water soluble film forming polymer such as pullulan. These edible films contain essential oils such as thymol, methyl salicylate, eucalyptol and menthol as antimicrobials in effective amounts. The edible films are very much effective in killing of the plaque-producing germs responsible for dental plaque, gingivitis and bad breath. The film can also incorporate with API, if desired. Methods for producing the films have also been described in the patent. The films can be used to deliver breath deodorising agents, antimicrobial agents and salivary stimulants to the oral cavity.

7.4. Patent 4

Zerbe *et al.* filed a patent application (08/904,607) on water soluble fast dissolving film for oral administration with instant wettability. Patent (5,948,430) was issued and assignee of this patent is LTS Lohman Therapie-Systeme GmbH. A composition consisting of APIs and/or breath/mouth freshening agents for oral cavity has been disclosed. Water soluble polymers have been used as carriers along with certain formulation ingredients to provide a therapeutic and/or cosmetic effect. The film is coated and dried utilising existing coating technology and exhibits instant wettability. These films show rapid dissolution/disintegration upon administration in the oral cavity. Invention is related to composition of oral films in which water soluble polymer with other ingredients have been used.

7.5. Patent 5

Fox filed a patent application (10/267,235) on water soluble sheet composition. Patent (6,800,295) was issued and assignee of this patent is The Dial Corporation. A composition in the form of a soluble sheet or thin film having a variety of uses, particularly in the personal care field, has been disclosed in the invention. A water soluble film forming polymer, polyvinyl alcohol, and a humectant such as propylene glycol have been used in formulating films. Surfactant may be added to generate foam when film comes in contact with water resulting in cleansing properties. Hydrocarbons can also be added to the liquid base composition to facilitate drying of the mass to form a flexible sheet product.

7.6. Patent 6

Horstmann *et al.* filed a patent application (10/314,549) on a method for producing film type dosage forms. Patent (6,800,329) was issued and assignee of this patent is LTS Lohman Therapie-Systeme AG. This process for the production of film for oral administration includes coating and drying with a solvent-containing spreadable mass on a substrate. Drying takes place in three stages. First drying stage is performed between 30-50°C followed by a second drying stage at 35-80°C and a third drying stage at 25-50°C.

7.7. Patent 7

Zerbe *et al.* filed a patent application (10/123,142) on flavoured film. Patent (7,132,113) was granted and assignee of patent is IntelGenx Corp. This patent discloses rapidly disintegrating flavoured film, containing HPC, modified starch and a flavour ingredient. The films of this invention completely disintegrate within 30 s in the oral cavity. The invention may be advantageously employed as breath freshening films and in food items to impart flavour. Overall invention relates generally to flavoured films particularly for foods and breath freshening purpose.

7.8. Patent 8

Berry *et al.* filed a patent application (10/922,502) on developing thin film strips. Patent (7,241,411) was granted and assignee of this patent is Acupac Packaging, Inc. A method of forming thin film strips by coating the substrate with a wet slurry of film forming ingredients have been disclosed. The process involves drying of wet slurry in drying apparatus to form a thin film. The moisture content is controlled upon exit from the drying apparatus, further storing the film in a minimal moisture loss environment during curing process.

7.9. Patent 9

Meathrel *et al.* filed a patent application (10/970,383) on FDOFs for diagnostic purpose. Patent (7,470,397) was granted and assignee of this patent is Adhesives Research, Inc. The invention provides FDOF compositions for use in diagnostics. Combination of component have been used which yield sufficient film strength and desired disintegration properties. The present invention contains a water soluble high molecular weight component, a water soluble low molecular weight component and one or more reagents for use in a diagnostic device.

7.10. Patent 10

Scott *et al.* filed a patent application (10/941,182) on pullulan film compositions. Patent (7,267,718) was granted and assignee of this patent is Warner Lambert Company, LLC. The invention is related to compositions based on pullulan and a system for the use in pharmaceutical, veterinary, food, cosmetics and capsules. The composition contains a surfactant also. By using aqueous solution of the inventive compositions, the hard pullulan capsules are produced by a conventional dipping moulding process under the same process condition range than conventional gelatin capsules.

7.11. Patent 11

Kumar *et al.* filed a patent application (10/423,398) on rapid dissolving orally consumable films containing sweeteners and other formulation additives. Patent (2003/0211136) was issued and assignee of this patent is Warner Lambert Company, LLC. Consumable film to adhere and dissolve in oral cavity of human consist of water soluble polymer, taste masking agent and bitter pharmaceutical active. Invention covers the use of a sweetener for taste masking of bitter APIs.

7.12. Patent 12

Friend *et al.* filed a patent application (10/744,479) on fast dissolving films for oral administration of drugs. Patent (2004/0208931) was issued and assignee of this patent is William Squire, Esq. The dosage unit consist of substrate having polymer, API and a layer consisting second polymer which is a graft co-polymer.

7.13. Patent 13

Fadden *et al.* filed a patent application (10/838,045) on fast dissolving orally consumable films which consists of modified starch for improved heat and moisture resistance. Patent (2004/0247648) was issued and assignee of this patent is Pfizer, Inc. Consumable film that adheres to and dissolve in oral cavity of humans and consisting of a modified starch with API and water soluble polymer are disclosed.

7.14. Patent 14

Ramesh filed a patent application (12/228702) on FDOFs for human erectile dysfunction containing bioactive agents, along with formulation additives and a patent (2009/0047330) was issued in 2009. The present invention consists of a film based on a novel edible polymer consisting of pharmaceutically acceptable polymers of natural and semi synthetic origins. Also includes emulsifying agents, suspending agents, colourants, *etc*. This film is used in various applications such as oral, mucosal and external environments.

7.15. Patent 15

Maibach filed a patent on film containing nitroglycerin and a patent (20100215774) was granted in 2006. This invention describes composition and methods of manufacture of orally-fast dissolvable films as a vehicle for administration of nitroglycerin. Apart from nitroglycerin film may contain other APIs which absorbs through the mucosal tissues of the oral cavity. The films include a water soluble film-forming polymer such as pullulan. This invention relates to the administration of nitroglycerin, and other active drugs, *via* consumable, edible films to be absorbed through mucosal tissue of oral cavity.

8. APPLICATIONS

FDOFs have found their applications in treating various ailments and some of these applications are as follows:

8.1. Vaccines

FDOFs can be given in the form of vaccines, which are stable at room temperature. This gives an advantage of freshening mouth and quick delivery from oral cavity. Rota virus vaccine has been prepared in form of oral film that gives better patient compliance with improved bioavailability [116].

8.2. Controlled and Sustained Release Drug Delivery

Various polymers like chitin, chitosan, *etc.* have a property of adhesion which makes them suitable for sustained release formulations. Oral film technology can be used for sustained action and provide minimum fluctuations in release of drug [117].

8.3. Fast Disintegrating Oral Films

With water soluble polymer faster disintegration can be obtained in FDOFs. FDOFs are preferred for treating almost any acute disease in paediatric, geriatric and psychotic patients. A number of marketed formulations are available for various applications [118].

8.4. Taste Masking

Taste masking is an important prerequisite for successful oral application of FDOFs. With the use of suitable polymers, adequate taste masking can be achieved in oral films. Taste masking can be done *via* encapsulation or coating of drug particle with suitable polymer [119].

CONCLUSIONS

FDOFs have become important delivery systems for several therapeutic applications. FDOFs are gaining popularity because of better patient compliance and quick action. API may be directly absorbed through sublingual or buccal route into the systemic circulation leading to faster onset and possible reduction in the dose. Oral films are consumer friendly and thus companies are trying to capture market with this new dosage form. Companies are using existing drug molecules for preparing oral films to deliver better therapeutic effect. Oral film technology has shown a new platform to companies for better growth and business potential in pharmaceuticals.

REFERENCES

[1] Ponchel G. Formulation of oral mucosal drug delivery systems for systemic delivery of bioactive materials. Adv Drug Deliv Rev 1993; 13: 75-87.

[http://dx.doi.org/10.1016/0169-409X(94)90027-2]

[2] Shimoda H, Taniguchi K, Nishimura M, *et al.* Preparation of a fast dissolving oral thin film containing dexamethasone: a possible application to antiemesis during cancer chemotherapy. Eur J Pharm Biopharm 2009; 73(3): 361-5.
[http://dx.doi.org/10.1016/j.ejpb.2009.08.010] [PMID: 19735731]

[3] Reiner V, Giarratana N, Monti NC, Breitenbach A, Klaffenbach P. Rapidfilm: an innovative pharmaceutical form designed to improve patient compliance. Int J Pharm 2010; 393(1-2): 55-60.
[http://dx.doi.org/10.1016/j.ijpharm.2010.03.055] [PMID: 20363308]

[4] Dixit RP, Puthli SP. Oral strip technology: overview and future potential. J Control Release 2009; 139(2): 94-107.
[http://dx.doi.org/10.1016/j.jconrel.2009.06.014] [PMID: 19559740]

[5] Corniello C. Quick dissolving strips: from concept to commercialization. Drug Del Technol 2006; 2: 68-71.

[6] Frankhauser C, Slominski G, Meyer S. Disintegrable oral films. US Patent 0202057, 2007.

[7] Fraser CG, Jennings HJ. A Glucan from tremella mesenterica NRRL-Y6158. Can J Chem 1971; 49: 1804-7.
[http://dx.doi.org/10.1139/v71-297]

[8] Corsaro MM, Castro DC, Evidente A, *et al.* Phytotoxic extracellular polysaccharide fractions from Cryphonectriaparasitica (Murr) Barr strains. Carbohydr Polym 1998; 37: 167-72.
[http://dx.doi.org/10.1016/S0144-8617(98)00050-2]

[9] Delben F, Forabosco A, Guerrini M, *et al.* Pullulans produced by strains of *Cryphonectria parasitica*-II Nuclear magnetic resonance evidence. Carbohydr Polym 1998; 37: 167-72.

[10] Chi Z, Zhao S. Optimization of medium and new cultivation conditions for pullulan production by a new pullulan-producing yeast strain. Enz Microb Tech 2003; 33: 206-11.
[http://dx.doi.org/10.1016/S0141-0229(03)00119-4]

[11] Scott R, Cade D, He X. Pullulan film compositions. US Patent 7267718, 2007.

[12] Yuen S. Pullulan and its applications. Process Biochem 1974; 9: 7-9.

[13] Saini S, Samta AC, Rana GS. Optimization of formulation of fast dissolving films made of pullulan polymer. Intl J Pharm Sc Rev Res 2011; 9: 127-31.

[14] Lydzinski S, Manegold T, Solarek D. Film containing starch. US Patent 0099692, 2003.

[15] Romero-Bastida CA, Bello-Perez LA, Gacia MA, *et al.* Physicochemical and micro structural characterization of films prepared by thermal and cold gelatinization from non-conventional sources of starches. Carbohydr Polym 2005; 60: 235-44.
[http://dx.doi.org/10.1016/j.carbpol.2005.01.004]

[16] Rindlav A, Hulleman SH, Gatenholm P. Formulation of starch films with varying crystallinity. Carbohydr Polym 1997; 34: 25-30.
[http://dx.doi.org/10.1016/S0144-8617(97)00093-3]

[17] Krogars K, Heinämäki J, Karjalainen M, Rantanen J, Luukkonen P, Yliruusi J. Development and characterization of aqueous amylose-rich maize starch dispersion for film formation. Eur J Pharm Biopharm 2003; 56(2): 215-21.
[http://dx.doi.org/10.1016/S0939-6411(03)00064-X] [PMID: 12957635]

[18] Mali S, Grossmann MV, Garcia MA, *et al.* Mechanical and thermal properties of yam starch films. Food Hydrocoll 2005; 19: 157-64.
[http://dx.doi.org/10.1016/j.foodhyd.2004.05.002]

[19] Gomez-Guillen MC, Turnay J. Structural and physical properties of gelatin extracted from different marine species: a comparative study. Food Hydrocoll 2002; 16: 25-34. [http://dx.doi.org/10.1016/S0268-005X(01)00035-2]

[20] Sobral PJ, Habitante AM. Phase transitions of pig skin gelatin. Food Hydrocoll 2001; 15: 377-82. [http://dx.doi.org/10.1016/S0268-005X(01)00060-1]

[21] Mac QR. Edible Dissolving Gelatin Strips. US Patent 7678397, 2010.

[22] Cilurzo F, Cupone IE, Minghetti P, Selmin F, Montanari L. Fast dissolving films made of maltodextrins. Eur J Pharm Biopharm 2008; 70(3): 895-900. [http://dx.doi.org/10.1016/j.ejpb.2008.06.032] [PMID: 18667164]

[23] Cilurzo F, Cupone IE, Minghetti P, *et al.* Nicotine fast dissolving films made of maltodextrins: a feasibility study. AAPS PharmSciTech 2010; 11(4): 1511-7. [http://dx.doi.org/10.1208/s12249-010-9525-6] [PMID: 20936440]

[24] Jagtap AR, Mitkare SS, Chalikwar RD, *et al.* Rosin: A novel film forming polymer for pharmaceuticals. Int J Pharm Res Dev 2010; 2(5): 210-2.

[25] Garsuch V, Breitkreutz J. Comparative investigations on different polymers for the preparation of fast-dissolving oral films. J Pharm Pharmacol 2010; 62(4): 539-45. [http://dx.doi.org/10.1211/jpp.62.04.0018] [PMID: 20604845]

[26] Fulzele SV, Satturwar PM, Dorle AK. Polymerised rosin: novel film forming polymer for drug delivery. Int J Pharm 2002; 249(1-2): 175-84. [http://dx.doi.org/10.1016/S0378-5173(02)00529-X] [PMID: 12433446]

[27] Elham B. Lycoat coating suits your plant extract tablets so well. Pharm Healthcare News 2008; 9: 1-10.

[28] Wu Y, Weller CL, Hamouz F, *et al.* Moisture loss and lipid oxidation for precooked ground-beef patties packaged in edible starch-alginate-based composite films. J Food Sci 2001; 66: 486-93. [http://dx.doi.org/10.1111/j.1365-2621.2001.tb16137.x]

[29] Manjanna KM, Shivakumar B, Pramod K. Formulation of oral sustained release aceclofenac sodium microbeads. Inter J Pharmtres 2009; 1: 940-52.

[30] Liu L, Fishman ML, Kost J, Hicks KB. Pectin-based systems for colon-specific drug delivery *via* oral route. Biomaterials 2003; 24(19): 3333-43. [http://dx.doi.org/10.1016/S0142-9612(03)00213-8] [PMID: 12763460]

[31] Varshosaz J, Emami J, Tavakoli N, *et al.* Pectin film coated pellets for colon-targeted delivery of budesonide: In-vitro/In-vivo valuation in induced ulcerative colitis in rat. Iran J Pharm Res 2012; 11(3): 733-45. [PMID: 24250500]

[32] Mishra R, Amin A. Formulation and characterization of rapidly dissolving films of cetrizine hydrochloride using pullulan as a film forming agent. J Pharm Ed Res 2011; 45: 71-7.

[33] Murta Y, Isobe T, Kofuji K, *et al.* Preparation of Fast dissolving films for oral dosage from natural polysaccharides. Materials (Basel) 2010; 3: 4291-9. [http://dx.doi.org/10.3390/ma3084291]

[34] Singh S, Gangwar S, Garg G, *et al.* Formulation and evaluation of rapidly disintegrating films of Levocetrizine Hydrochloride. Schol Res Lib 2010; 2: 434-9.

[35] Ghorwade V, Patil A, Patil S, *et al.* Formulation and evaluation of Montelukast sodium fast dissolving films by using gelatin as a film base. Res J Pharm Bio Chem Sci 2011; 2: 880-8.

[36] Shimoda H, Taniguchi K, Nishimura M, *et al.* Preparation of a fast dissolving oral thin film containing

dexamethasone: a possible application to antiemesis during cancer chemotherapy. Eur J Pharm Biopharm 2009; 73(3): 361-5.
[http://dx.doi.org/10.1016/j.ejpb.2009.08.010] [PMID: 19735731]

[37] Chambin O, Champion D, Debray C, Rochat-Gonthier MH, Le Meste M, Pourcelot Y. Effects of different cellulose derivatives on drug release mechanism studied at a preformulation stage. J Control Release 2004; 95(1): 101-8.
[http://dx.doi.org/10.1016/j.jconrel.2003.11.009] [PMID: 15013237]

[38] Grattard N, Pernin M, Marty B, Roudaut G, Champion D, Le Meste M. Study of release kinetics of small and high molecular weight substances dispersed into spray-dried ethylcellulose microspheres. J Control Release 2002; 84(3): 125-35.
[http://dx.doi.org/10.1016/S0168-3659(02)00260-2] [PMID: 12468216]

[39] Wesseling M, Kuppler F, Bodmeier R. Tackiness of acrylic and cellulosic polymer films used in the coating of solid dosage forms. Eur J Pharm Biopharm 1999; 47(1): 73-8.
[http://dx.doi.org/10.1016/S0939-6411(98)00091-5] [PMID: 10234529]

[40] de Moura MR, Avena-Bustillos RJ, McHugh TH, Krochta JM, Mattoso LH. Properties of novel hydroxypropyl methylcellulose films containing chitosan nanoparticles. J Food Sci 2008; 73(7): N31-7.
[http://dx.doi.org/10.1111/j.1750-3841.2008.00872.x] [PMID: 18803724]

[41] Podczeck F, Knight PE, Newton JM. The evaluation of modified microcrystalline cellulose for the preparation of pellets with high drug loading by extrusion/spheronization. Int J Pharm 2008; 350(1-2): 145-54.
[http://dx.doi.org/10.1016/j.ijpharm.2007.08.040] [PMID: 17905548]

[42] Wei L, Bingjie S, Peiyi W. Study on hydrogen bonds of carboxymethyl cellulose sodium film with two-dimensional correlation infrared spectroscopy. Carbohydr Polym 2009; 78: 454-61.
[http://dx.doi.org/10.1016/j.carbpol.2009.05.002]

[43] Bhatt NV, Nate MM, Bhatt RM, *et al.* Effect of gamma irriadiations on polyvinyl alcohol films doped with some dyes and their use in dosimetric studies. Ind J Pur Appl Phys 2007; 45: 545-8.

[44] Cristina DN, Catalina LC, Dana OD, *et al.* Polymeric films properties of poly vinyl alcohol and poly hydroxy urethane in different concentrations. UPB Sci Bull Ser 2009; 1: 71.

[45] Derek LH, Boualem H, Steven RK, *et al.* Unusual phase behaviour in mixtures of poly ethylene oxide and ethyl alcohol. J Polym Sci, B, Polym Phys 2006; 44: 557-64.
[http://dx.doi.org/10.1002/polb.20726]

[46] Wilson KE, Crossman E. The influence of tablet shape and pan speed on intra-tablet film coating uniformity. Drug Dev Ind Pharm 2007; 23: 1239-43.
[http://dx.doi.org/10.3109/03639049709146164]

[47] Haaf F, Sanner A, Straub F. Polymers of N-Vinylpyrrolidone: Synthesis, characterization and uses. Polym J 1985; 17(1): 143-52.
[http://dx.doi.org/10.1295/polymj.17.143]

[48] Prasanthi NL, Krishna CS, Gupta MS, *et al.* Design and development of sublingual fast dissolving films for an anti-asthmatic drug. Schol Res Lib 2011; 3(1): 382-95.

[49] Kunte S, Tandale P. Fast dissolving strips: A novel approach for the delivery of verapamil. J Pharm Bioallied Sci 2010; 2(4): 325-8.
[http://dx.doi.org/10.4103/0975-7406.72133] [PMID: 21180465]

[50] Nishimura M, Matsuura K, Tsukioka T, *et al.* *In vitro* and *in vivo* characteristics of prochlorperazine oral disintegrating film. Int J Pharm 2009; 368(1-2): 98-102.
[http://dx.doi.org/10.1016/j.ijpharm.2008.10.002] [PMID: 18992311]

[51] Patel R, Shardul N, Patel J, *et al.* Formulation development and evaluation of mouth melting film of Ondansetron. Arch Pharm Sci Res 2009; 1(2): 212-7.

[52] Kulkarni PK, Dixit M, Gunashekara K, *et al.* Formulation and evaluation of mouth dissolving film containing Rofecoxib. Int Res J Phar 2010; 2(3): 177-8.

[53] Rowe RC, Forse SF. The effect of polymer molecular weight on the incidence of film cracking and splitting on film coated tablets. J Pharm Pharmacol 1980; 32(8): 583-4. [http://dx.doi.org/10.1111/j.2042-7158.1980.tb13003.x] [PMID: 6106700]

[54] Rowe RC, Forse SF. The effect of plasticizer type and concentration on the incidence of bridging of intagliations on film-coated tablets. J Pharm Pharmacol 1981; 33(3): 174-5. [http://dx.doi.org/10.1111/j.2042-7158.1981.tb13744.x] [PMID: 6116761]

[55] Sheng JJ. Castor oil. In: Rowe RC, Sheskey PJ, Ovan SC, Eds. Handbook of pharmaceutical excipients. UK: Pharmaceutical press 2009; pp. 126-7.

[56] Guest RT. Dibutyl phthalate. In: Rowe RC, Sheskey PJ, Ovan SC, Eds. Handbook of pharmaceutical excipients. UK: Pharmaceutical press 2009; pp. 225-6.

[57] Farrell T. Dibutylsebacate. In: Rowe RC, Sheskey PJ, Owen SC, Eds. Handbook of pharmaceutical excipients. UK: Pharmaceutical press 2009; pp. 227-8.

[58] Quinn ME, Sheskey PJ. Tributyl Citrate. In: Rowe RC, Sheskey SC, Owen PJ, Eds. Handbook of pharmaceutical excipients. UK: Pharmaceutical press 2009; pp. 749-50.

[59] Teckoe J. Triethyl citrate. In: Rowe RC, Sheskey SC, Owen PJ, Eds. Handbook of pharmaceutical excipients. UK: Pharmaceutical press 2006; pp. 756-7.

[60] Browhn GL. Formation of films from polymer dispersions. J Polym Sci, Polym Phys Ed 1956; 22(102): 423-34.

[61] Sakellariou P, Rowe RC. Interactions in cellulose derivative films for oral drug delivery. Prog Polym Sci 1995; 20: 889-942. [http://dx.doi.org/10.1016/0079-6700(95)00008-4]

[62] Cao N, Yang X, Fu Y. Effects of various plasticizers on mechanical and water vapour barrier properties of gelatin films. Food Hydrocoll 2009; 23: 729-35. [http://dx.doi.org/10.1016/j.foodhyd.2008.07.017]

[63] Wu C, McGinity JW. Influence of ibuprofen as a solid-state plasticizer in Eudragit RS 30 D on the physicochemical properties of coated beads. AAPS PharmSciTech 2001; 2(4): 24. [http://dx.doi.org/10.1208/pt020424] [PMID: 14727861]

[64] Hariharan M, Bogue A. Orally dissolving film strips (ODFS): the final evolution of orally dissolving dosage forms. Drug Del Technol 2009; 9(2): 24-9.

[65] Ali S, Quadir A. High molecular weight povidone polymer-based films for fast dissolving drug delivery applications. Drug Del Technol 2007; 7(6): 36-43.

[66] Sohi H, Sultana Y, Khar RK. Taste masking technologies in oral pharmaceuticals: recent developments and approaches. Drug Dev Ind Pharm 2004; 30(5): 429-48. [http://dx.doi.org/10.1081/DDC-120037477] [PMID: 15244079]

[67] Szejtli J, Szente L. Elimination of bitter, disgusting tastes of drugs and foods by cyclodextrins. Eur J Pharm Biopharm 2005; 61(3): 115-25. [http://dx.doi.org/10.1016/j.ejpb.2005.05.006] [PMID: 16185857]

[68] Suzuki H, Onishi H, Takahashi Y, Iwata M, Machida Y. Development of oral acetaminophen chewable tablets with inhibited bitter taste. Int J Pharm 2003; 251(1-2): 123-32. [http://dx.doi.org/10.1016/S0378-5173(02)00595-1] [PMID: 12527182]

[69] Puri D, Bahelkar M. Evaluation of oral fast disintegrating tablets of taste masked famotidine in rat. Lat Amer J Pharm 2010; 29: 948-54.

[70] Sugao H, Yamazaki S, Shiozawa H, Yano K. Taste masking of bitter drug powder without loss of bioavailability by heat treatment of wax-coated microparticles. J Pharm Sci 1998; 87(1): 96-100. [http://dx.doi.org/10.1021/js970104g] [PMID: 9452976]

[71] Xu J, Bovet LL, Zhao K. Taste masking microspheres for orally disintegrating tablets. Int J Pharm 2008; 359(1-2): 63-9. [http://dx.doi.org/10.1016/j.ijpharm.2008.03.019] [PMID: 18455893]

[72] Mennella JA, Beauchamp GK. Optimising oral medications for children. Clin Ther 2008; 30(11): 2120-32. [http://dx.doi.org/10.1016/j.clinthera.2008.11.018] [PMID: 19108800]

[73] Hutteau F, Mathlouthi M, Portmann MO, *et al.* Physicochemical and psychophysical characteristics of binary mixtures of bulk and intense sweeteners. Food Chem 1998; 63(1): 9-16. [http://dx.doi.org/10.1016/S0308-8146(97)00243-4]

[74] Prakash I, Dubois GE, Clos JF, Wilkens KL, Fosdick LE. Development of rebiana, a natural, non-caloric sweetener. Food Chem Toxicol 2008; 46 (Suppl. 7): S75-82. [http://dx.doi.org/10.1016/j.fct.2008.05.004] [PMID: 18554769]

[75] Israel K, Leo V. Salivary stimulant. US Patent 4820506, 1989.

[76] McGregor R, Homan H, Gravina S. Fast dissolving film delivery of nucleotides that inhibit the unpleasant taste of bitter tasting medications. Patent Application WO 2004019885 A2, 2004.

[77] Hammon HK, Dean TJ. Colour and light. In: Sward GG, Ed. Paint Testing Manual-physical and chemical examination of paints varnishes lacquers, and colours. ASTM Special Technical Publication 1972; pp. 1-14.

[78] Kaur M, Rana AC, Seth N. Fast dissolving films: an innovative drug delivery system. Int J Pharm Res Allied Sci 2013; 2: 14-24.

[79] Sau-hung S, Robert S, Lori D. Fast dissolving orally consumable films. US Patent 6596298, 2003.

[80] Arya A, Chandra A, Sharma V, *et al.* Fast dissolving oral films: An innovative drug delivery system and dosage form. Int J Chem Tech Res 2010; 2(1): 576-83.

[81] Roumeliotis G. BioProgress uses films in drug delivery Accessed from: http://www.in-pharma-technologist.com/Ingredients/BioProgress-uses-films-in-drug-delivery Accessed on 10 Sep 2016.

[82] Wafertab: a revolutionary in pharmaceutical technology (Video) Accessed from: https://www.you-tube.com/watch?v=DZu9rYnKELE Accessed on 11 Sep 2016.

[83] Meldex International. Accessed from: http://ddm.staging01.azuragroup.com/@offers/dds/view/905/ Accessed on 11 Sep 2016.

[84] Borges AF. Development of novel pharmaceutical forms for oral administration of bioactive agents (Doctoral dissertation, University of Coimbra).

[85] RapidFilm® Oral film technology: an innovative form of oral medication. Accessed from: http://www.tesa-labtec.com/eng/RapidFilm/overview Accessed on 11 Sep 2016.

[86] Reiner V, Giarratana N, Monti NC, Breitenbach A, Klaffenbach P. Rapidfilm: an innovative pharmaceutical form designed to improve patient compliance. Int J Pharm 2010; 393(1-2): 55-60. [http://dx.doi.org/10.1016/j.ijpharm.2010.03.055] [PMID: 20363308]

[87] SciClone Pharmaceuticals Expands Portfolio by Licensing Ondansetron RapidFilm™ for Chinese Market. Accessed from: http://investor.sciclone.com/releasedetail.cfm?releaseid=454516 Accessed on 11 Sep 2016.

[88] List of approved drug from 01012010 TO 31122010 2010. Accessed from: http://cdsco.nic.in/writereaddata/LIST%20OF%20APPROVED%20DRUG%20FROM%2001.htm Accessed on 11 Sep 2016.

[89] VersaFilm™, Oral Film Technology. Accessed from: http://www.intelgenx.com/r-and-d-services/versafilm/default.aspx Accessed on 11 Sep 2016.

[90] Weintraub A. Drugs that melt in your mouth: Monosol Rx has its sights set on oral insulin 2011. Accessed from: http://www.monosolrx.com/news_11/news_051311.htm Accessed on 11 Sep 2016.

[91] Nehal SM, Garima G, Pramod KS. Short Review on A novel approach in oral fast dissolving drug delivery system and their patents. Adv Biol Res (Faisalabad) 2011; 5(6): 291-303.

[92] Ulrich S. Solvent cast technology. A versatile tool for thin film production. Prog Colloid Polym Sci 2005; 130: 1-14.

[93] Particle sciencs, Dissolving Films, Technical Brief. Drug Development Services 2010; 3: 1-2.

[94] Particle sciencs, Hot Melt Extrusion, Technical Brief. Drug Development Services 2011; 3: 1-2.

[95] Rina C, Hossein Z. Hot-Melt Extrusion Technique: A Review. Iran J Pharm Res 2004; 3: 3-16.

[96] Coppens KA, Hall MJ, Mitchell SA, *et al.* Hypromellose ethyl cellulose and polyethylene oxide used in hot melt extrusion. Pharm Technol 2006; 30(1): 1-6.

[97] Patil B, Mandore P, Sharma RK, *et al.* A Review: Novel Advances in semisolid dosage forms & patented technology in semisolid dosage forms. Int J Pharm Tech Res 2011; 3(1): 420-30.

[98] Dhirendra K, Lewis S, Udupa N, Atin K. Solid dispersions: a review. Pak J Pharm Sci 2009; 22(2): 234-46.
[PMID: 19339238]

[99] Golod SV, Prinz VY, Mashanov VI. Directional-rolling method for strained SiGe/Si films and its application to fabrication of hollow needles. Thin Solid Films 2005; 489: 169-76.
[http://dx.doi.org/10.1016/j.tsf.2005.05.013]

[100] Preis M, Breitkreutz J, Sandler N. Perspective: Concepts of printing technologies for oral film formulations. Int J Pharm 2015; 494(2): 578-84.
[http://dx.doi.org/10.1016/j.ijpharm.2015.02.032] [PMID: 25683143]

[101] Sward GG. Measurement of film thickness. In: Sward GG, Ed. Paint Testing Manual-physical and chemical examination of paints varnishes lacquers, and colours. ASTM Special technical Publication 1972; pp. 260-7.
[http://dx.doi.org/10.1520/STP37158S]

[102] Sward GG. Drying Time. In: Sward GG, Ed. Paint Testing Manual-physical and chemical examination of paints varnishes lacquers, and colours. ASTM Special technical Publication 1972; pp. 268-80.
[http://dx.doi.org/10.1520/STP37159S]

[103] Schurr GG. Tensile strength and elongation. In: Sward GG, Ed. Paint Testing Manual-physical and chemical examination of paints varnishes lacquers, and colours. ASTM Special Technical Publication 1972; pp. 338-40.
[http://dx.doi.org/10.1520/STP37164S]

[104] Sward GG. Abrasion Resistance. In: Sward GG, Ed. Paint Testing Manual-physical and chemical examination of paints varnishes lacquers and colours. ASTM Special Technical Publication 1972; pp. 31-313.

[105] Roberts AG. Dynamic mechanical and tensile properties. In: Sward GG, Ed. Paint Testing Manual-physical and chemical examination of paints varnishes lacquers, and colours. ASTM Special Technical Publication 2012; p. 624.

[106] Schurr GG. Flexibility. In: Sward GG, Ed. Paint Testing Manual-physical and chemical examination of paints varnishes lacquers and colours. ASTM Special Technical Publication 1972; pp. 333-7.

[107] Nagender KD, Keshavshetti GG, Mogale P, *et al.* Formulation and evaluation of fast dissolving oral films of metoprolol succinate. Int J Eng App Sci 2015; 6: 28-38.

[108] Barnhart S. Thin film oral dosage forms. In: Rathborne M, Hadgraft J, Roberts M, Eds. Modified release drug delivery technology. Drugs and the Pharmaceutical Sciences. Informa Healthcare 2008; pp. 209-16.

[109] Nishimura M, Matsuura K, Tsukioka T, *et al. In vitro* and *in vivo* characteristics of prochlorperazine oral disintegrating film. Int J Pharm 2009; 368(1-2): 98-102. [http://dx.doi.org/10.1016/j.ijpharm.2008.10.002] [PMID: 18992311]

[110] Anand V, Kataria M, Kukkar V, Saharan V, Choudhury PK. The latest trends in the taste assessment of pharmaceuticals. Drug Discov Today 2007; 12(5-6): 257-65. [http://dx.doi.org/10.1016/j.drudis.2007.01.010] [PMID: 17331891]

[111] Winquist F, Holmin S, Krantz-Rulcker C, *et al.* A hybrid electronic tongue. Anal Chim Acta 2006; 406: 147-57. [http://dx.doi.org/10.1016/S0003-2670(99)00767-9]

[112] Joshi P, Patel H, Patel V, Panchal R. Formulation development and evaluation of mouth dissolving film of domperidone. J Pharm Bioallied Sci 2012; 4(5) (Suppl. 1): S108-9. [http://dx.doi.org/10.4103/0975-7406.94159] [PMID: 23066181]

[113] Preparation and evaluation of oral fast dissolving films of citalopram hydrobromide. Intern J Biopharm 2012; 3(2): 103-6.

[114] Nishigaki M, Kawahara K, Nawa M, *et al.* Development of fast dissolving oral film containing dexamethasone as an antiemetic medication: clinical usefulness. Int J Pharm 2012; 424(1-2): 12-7. [http://dx.doi.org/10.1016/j.ijpharm.2011.12.057] [PMID: 22240389]

[115] Shelke PV, Dumbare AS, Gadhave MV, *et al.* Formulation and evaluation of rapidly disintegrating film of amlodipine besylate. J Drug Del Therapeut 2012; 2(2): 72-5.

[116] Malke S, Shidhaye S, Desai J, *et al.* Oral Films. Patient compliant dosage form for pediatrics. Internet J Pediatr Neonatol 2009; 11: 2.

[117] Kato Y, Onishi H, Machida Y. Application of chitin and chitosan derivatives in the pharmaceutical field. Curr Pharm Biotechnol 2003; 4(5): 303-9. [http://dx.doi.org/10.2174/1389201033489748] [PMID: 14529420]

[118] Habib W, Khankari R, Hontz J. Fast-dissolve drug delivery systems. Crit Rev Ther Drug Carrier Syst 2000; 17(1): 61-72. [http://dx.doi.org/10.1615/CritRevTherDrugCarrierSyst.v17.i1.20] [PMID: 10755211]

[119] Sohi H, Sultana Y, Khar RK. Taste masking technologies in oral pharmaceuticals: recent developments and approaches. Drug Dev Ind Pharm 2004; 30(5): 429-48. [http://dx.doi.org/10.1081/DDC-120037477] [PMID: 15244079]

CHAPTER 11

Novel Fast Dissolving/Disintegrating Dosage Forms

Vikas A. Saharan*

Department of Pharmaceutics, School of Pharmaceutical Sciences, Sardar Bhagwan Singh Post Graduate Institute of Biomedical Sciences and Research, Balawala, Dehradun 248161, Uttarakhand, India

Abstract: Fast disintegrating tablets (FDTs) were initially developed for immediate drug delivery, quicker onset of action and as age appropriate dosage form for special populations like geriatrics, paediatrics, psychotics, *etc*. Their quick dissolution/ disintegration in the oral cavity has made them suitable for incorporating microparticles/pellets for developing controlled drug delivery systems. Furthermore, advancement in manufacturing technologies and dosage forms have led to the introduction of newer dosage forms like oral disintegrating mini tablets (ODMTs), fast disintegrating capsules (FDCs), fast disintegrating pellets (FDPs) and orodispersible or to dissolve in oral powders. ODMTs are small size (2-3 mm in diameter) tablets prepared with characteristics of faster dissolution/disintegration. ODMTs have been found suitable and well acceptable in children. Perforation and vacuum drying methods have been used to convert traditional capsules into FDCs to overcome disadvantages of other FDDFs like expensive manufacturing, low payload, lengthy processes and insufficient masking of undesirable taste. Extrusion spheronisation and spray coating of drug with suitable excipients can led to FDPs, while orodispersible/effervescent powders can be filled in a unit dose packing. This chapter details about these novel FDDFs *vis a vis* to some novel advancements in their compositions.

Keywords: Capsules, Controlled release, Drug targeting, Granules, Mini tablets, Oral disintegration, Pellets, Powders.

1. INTRODUCTION

FDTs have been extensively explored for their advantages like ease of administration, wide acceptability, popularity and clinical advantages. Several new dosage forms in the family of FDDFs have emerged with time. Some of these have successfully reached to the market, while some others are in the final phases

* **Corresponding author Vikas A. Saharan:** Department of Pharmaceutics, School of Pharmaceutical Sciences, Sardar Bhagwan Singh Post Graduate Institute of Biomedical Sciences and Research (www.sbspgi.edu.in), Balawala, Dehradun 248161, Uttarakhand, India; Tel: +91-135-2686246; Mobile: +91-8439820796; Fax: +91-135-2686286; E-mail: vikas.pharmaceutics@gmail.com

of development. FDCs, ODMTs, FDPs and orodispersible/effervescent powders in a stick are some novel FDDFs. Table **1** provides some recent development attempts with some novel FDDFs.

Table 1. Recently developed novel FDDFs.

Drug	Important Excipients	Method/ Technology	FDDFs	Remarks	Ref.
—	Hard gelatin/HPMC capsules (size 1), microcrystalline cellulose (MCC) (Avicel PH101 and PH112), mannitol, lactose monohydrate, saccharose and maize starch	Vacuum-drying or perforating conventional hard capsules	FDCs	Disintegration time of perforated capsules (6–10 holes of diameter 25–50 mm) was 39 s. Vacuum-dried brittle capsules disintegrated orally in 7.1±4.8 s.	[1]
—	Hard gelatin capsules, PEG, HPMC capsules, gelatin (type B) granules with different bloom strengths (43, 80, 100, 180 and 260), polyethylene glycol (PEG) 400, 1500 and 4000, cross-linked sodium carboxymethyl cellulose (SCMC), Ac-Di-Sol®, Avicel® PH101, Tylopur® C600, Explotab®, sorbitol, xylitol, d(+)-lactose monohydrate, citric acid and saccharose	Optimised dipping process	Fastcaps (FDCs)	Decreasing bloom strength of gelatin and adding sugars or PEGs reduced disintegration time.	[2]
Hydrochlorothiazide	Parteck® ODT, Ludiflash®, Pearlitol® Flash, Prosolv® ODT, Pharmaburst® 500, magnesium stearate and Pruv®	Direct compression in tablet machine equipped with a mini-tableting tool (Euro-B 19-tip) and power feeder	ODMTs	Novel dosage forms for children with advantages of ease of administration, flexible dose measurement and use of safe excipients	[3]

(Table 1) contd.....

Drug	Important Excipients	Method/ Technology	FDDFs	Remarks	Ref.
Dextromethorphan HBr monohydrate	Amberlite® IRP69, ethylcellulose and Aquacoat® ECD, Surelease®, Kollicoat® SR30D, Mannogem™ EZ Spray and spray dried mannitol	IER drug complexes by batch process; polymer coating by Wurster process and high shear wet granulation process	Sustained release FDTs	Diffusion governed drug release; drug release followed Higuchi and Boyd model	[4]
Model bitter drug	Amberlite® IRP69, Eudragit® RS, Eudragit® RL, triethyl citrate, talc, mannitol, Ac-Di-Sol®, citric acid, sodium bicarbonate and magnesium stearate	Coated drug-resin complexes were compressed to tablets	Sustained release FDTs	Taste masking and sustained release properties of IER and fast disintegration/ dissolution of FDTs coupled in a single dosage form	[5]
Ibuprofen	Phospholipon® 80H, Lipoid® S75, Kollicoat® SR 30D, Kollidon® 90F, Amprac® 01, Eudragit® RD 100, Explotab®, Kollidon® CL, aspartame, Pearlitol® SD200 and magnesium stearate	Granulation; aqueous polymer pan coating; simple compression technology to prepare FDT	Fast dispersible slow releasing FDT	Reduction of gastric side effects	[6]
Nicorandil	Myristyl alcohol and stearyl alcohol		Dry emulsion loaded FDT	*In vitro* release of nicorandil sustained over 6 h from FDT	[7]
Ketoprofen	Eudragit® RS-30D, Starch 1500®, PEG 6000, lactose, mannitol and polyvinylpyrrolidone	Spray drying followed by direct compression	Sustained drug release FDTs	*In vivo* pharmacokinetic studies exhibited significant extended release profile	[8]
Paracetamol and theophylline, riboflavin	Pectinic acid and MCC Sanaq® 102 G	Extrusion spehronisation	FDPs	Pectinic acid (10% methoxylation) was used as an extrusion aiding excipient	[9]
Theophylline monohydrate	MCC II (MCC Sanaq® Burst)	Extrusion spehronisation	FDPs	A storage humidity of 55-80% was recommended to maintain faster disintegration/dissolution	[10]

(Table 1) contd.....

Drug	Important Excipients	Method/ Technology	FDDFs	Remarks	Ref.
Diphenhydramine HCl and griseofulvin	MCC II (MCC Sanaq® Burst)	Extrusion spehronisation	FDPs	MCC II was established as a pelletisation aid	[11]
Dexamethasone sodium phosphate	Sorbitol, xylitol, mannitol, sodium bicarbonate, citric acid and tartaric acid	Fluid bed rotary processing	Effervescent FDPs	Sequential experimental design to optimise formulation and processing parameters	[12]
Paracetamol	—	Filling orodispersible powder in Unistick®	Orodispersible Unistick®	Orodispersible powder in a stick developed as a new dosage form	

Fast disintegrating capsules (FDC) are prepared by either vacuum drying or perforating shells of conventional hard capsule. Conventional capsules are perforated by needle at laboratory scale and laser may be used at industrial level. Perforations in capsules enables quick uptake of water from saliva resulting in faster disintegration of capsules in the oral cavity. Vacuum drying is used to reduce the moisture content of conventional capsules shells rendering them more brittle. Brittle capsules easily break in the oral cavity by forces induced by movements of the tongue.

ODTs of small size (3 mm or lower) are generally referred as ODMTs. Directly compressible coprocessed excipient is blended with the drug and subsequently compressed in a tablet press equipped with a power feeder and a mini-tableting tool. ODMTs are easy to swallow due to their small size and faster dissolution/disintegration in mouth. ODMTs allow flexible dosing as these may be swallowed as such or as a dispersion or sprinkled on soft food or may be used to prepare oral solution/suspension for easy administration in children.

Pellets are generally prepared by extrusion spheronisation or by spray coating methods. If an adequate amount of disintegrant is added to the formulation, it may reduce disintegration/dissolution time of pellets. Unither Pharmaceuticals is developing powders in a stick called Unistick®. Unistick® are filled with orodispersible powders or powders meant to produce solution/suspension.

Sustained/controlled/targeted drug delivery of drugs requires use of polymers for their ability to modify or target drug release. In most instances microparticles or nanoparticles are fabricated and incorporated in conventional dosage forms. When sustained/controlled/targeted drug delivery is desired by oral route of administration, FDTs offers great potential in loading microparticles or nanoparticles. The advantages like minimum breakage and minimum structural losses, due to the use of low compression methodologies or non-compression methods in manufacturing FDTs, prevent burst release. Furthermore, sustained delivery of drug for 12/24 h is feasible with easy administration in special populations like paediatrics, geriatrics, psychotic patients and in situations where water is not available for swallowing tablets.

2. FAST DISINTEGRATING CAPSULES

Perforation and vacuum drying methodologies have been used to prepare FDCs from conventional hard capsules [1]. Fastcaps (hard capsule shells), for quick salivary disintegration and having adequate mechanical strength, were prepared from gelatin (low bloom strength) and other additives [2]. FDCs are able to overcome some disadvantages of other FDDFs, especially expensive manufacturing, low payload, lengthy processes and insufficient masking of the taste [1]. Advantages of FDCs are provided in Box **1** and their similarities to other FDDFs are provided in Table **2**.

Box 1: Advantages of FDCs

- Rapid disintegration in the saliva
- High drug loadings
- Possible solid and liquid fillings
- No compression steps required and thus suitable for coated taste masked or extended release drug particles/pellets/microspheres/microcapsules
- No need for large quantities of excipients
- Good mechanical properties
- Simple manufacturing
- Mechanical stability
- No requirement of special packaging (except for vacuum dried brittle capsules)
- Improved drug stability due to solid drug processing

Table 2. Comparison of FDCs and other FDDFs [1].

Attribute	FDCs	Zydis®	Tablets	Films
Disintegration rate	Fast	Fastest	Slow	Faster
Broad range of actives	Yes	No	Intermediate	No
Drug loading	Highest	Low	Higher	Low

(Table 2) contd.....

Attribute	FDCs	Zydis®	Tablets	Films
Modified release or taste masking	Yes	No	Yes	No
Stability Issues	Least	Moderate to high	Least	Moderate to high
Filling of liquid/semisolid formulations	No for perforated capsules /Yes for vacuum dried capsules	No	No	No
Requirement of special packaging	No for perforated capsules/Yes for vacuum dried capsules	Yes	Not Always	Yes

2.1. Perforation

On a laboratory scale, needle is used to perforate (2-10 holes of size 25-50 µm) empty or filled conventional hard capsules longitudinally or at top to reduce their disintegration time [1]. On a production scale, laser beam is used to create holes in hard gelatin capsule shells or filled capsules. The size of holes is critical as it is required to be smaller than the size of particles of powder/granule, so as to prevent the loss of contents. Alternatively, powders may be processed to granules having size greater than the size of perforations in the capsules.

Water soluble or water insoluble fillers are used in FDCs [1]. Perforated capsules (with 6 and 10 holes top/horizontal) filled with water insoluble or swellable fillers like Avicel PH101 disintegrate quickly in less than 60 s. *In vitro* disintegration time of perforated capsules, filled with water soluble excipients like lactose or saccharose, are higher than 60 s [1].

In one study, *in vitro* disintegration of perforated capsules was reduced to more than half (39 *vs.* 92 s for conventional capsules) [1]. Top or longitudinal location of holes did not significantly affect disintegration time. The content of perforated capsules spread rapidly in the oral cavity immediate after their oral disintegration. Oral disintegration time was even much lesser than *in vitro* disintegration time of perforated capsules due to the mechanical stresses induced by the movement of capsule in the oral cavity. Perforated and conventional hard gelatin capsules did not significantly differ when subjected to breakage at equal moisture content. A slight increase in breakage of the capsules was observed with the increase of number of holes. Breakage tests confirmed that FDCs prepared by perforation method are amenable to filling and packaging on automated machine.

2.2. Vacuum Drying

Vacuum drying of hard gelatin capsule shells removes moisture making them more brittle and faster disintegrating [1]. In one such method of preparing FDCs, accurately weighed hard gelatin capsules and HPMC capsules are kept in a desiccator at 51% relative humidity (RH) attained with the help of a saturated potassium carbonate. These empty or filled capsules are further dried in a vacuum oven at 30°C/40°C.

Moisture content of 4% or less is essential to obtain FDCs (Fastcaps). Moisture may migrate from the fillers to the capsule shell, which is a critical process to control. Fastcaps are, therefore, required to be filled with either pre-dried or non-hygroscopic excipients.

Fast disintegration requires the use of a low mechanical force in the oral cavity followed by a quick hydration and thereafter disintegration leading to a soft and pleasant mouth feel. Brittle capsules have been optimised for the fastest *in vivo* disintegration time of 7.1 s. The brittle capsules disintegrate/dissolve quickly in the mouth and release their content almost instantaneously. Moisture sensitivity and brittle nature of capsule demands special blister packaging from where dosage form can be readily removed by pulling a foil or layer. Over-wraps of aluminium foil over blisters or blister packs made from aluminium are also considered suitable for packaging of brittle capsules.

2.3. Fastcaps by Dipping Process

A dipping process, using stainless steel pins, has been developed to prepare Fastcaps at a small laboratory scale [2]. This process uses gelatin having bloom strength in range 43-260 at 35% w/w and viscosity of 500–600 cP to prepare a gelatin sol. Preservative, 0.15% w/w methylparaben, distilled water 64.85% w/w and 15% w/w other excipients (sorbitol or xylitol) or 5% w/w PEG are added to the gelatin sol. Stainless steel pins are immersed into a warm sol of gelatin, rotated and elevated in air to set a uniform film over pins. The pins are air dried at 25-30°C in a chamber for 0.5-1 h to achieve residual moisture of 15-18% in the capsule shells. Capsule shells are then removed from the chamber and trimmed to the required size. Critical processing factors affecting the quality of these capsule shells (Fastcaps) are steel pin withdrawing rate, viscosity and temperature of the gelatin sol.

Reduction in bloom strength from 260 to 40 decreases disintegration time of gelatin films to less than 60 s [2]. Mechanical properties of gelatin films were improved with the addition of 10% and 15% w/w of xylitol, which also reduced disintegration time. Hydrophilic additives like xylitol, sorbitol, PEG 1500 or 400 (5% w/w) enhanced dissolution of gelatin films resulting in shortening of their disintegration time.

The contents of the capsules also affect their disintegration/dissolution. Water-soluble contents like glucose, lactose, saccharides and/or disintegrants like sodium starch glycolate (SSG), MCC, crosslinked sodium carboxymethylcellulose (SCMC) were found effective in decreasing disintegration/dissolution times of capsules. Fastcaps, prepared from gelatin of bloom strength 43 and 80 and filled with MCC or lactose, disintegrated in just 28-36 s, which was just half the time required for conventional capsules filled with the same components [2]. No significant differences were found in mechanical properties of Fastcaps and conventional capsules. MCC and lactose are, therefore, considered best excipients for filling into Fastcaps. Fastcaps also offered quick *in vivo* disintegration in 9-13 s resulting in rapid spread of capsule contents in mouth. Addition of xylitol in the formulation provides a pleasant taste, cooling sensation and anticariogenic effect resulting in overall improvement in palatability.

3. ORALLY DISINTEGRATING MINI TABLETS

Mini-tablet and FDDF technologies have been coupled to develop ODMTs as a novel oral delivery system for paediatrics [3, 13]. ODMTs of diameter 3 mm or less, provides easy measuring abilities coupled with rapid disintegration of tablets in mouth, making them most appropriate dosage form for not only children but also for infants and toddlers [3]. ODMTs belong to the group of child-appropriate dosage form which are easy to administer, palatable and use clinically safe and stable excipients. A small dose like 1 mg drug per ODMT allows covering a broad dose range by simple counting of mini-tablets and thus avoiding the need to administer conventional tablets by breaking into halves or quarter tablets. This dose flexibility offered by ODMTs holds great potential for their paediatric use, recently and in future. Some advantages of ODMTs are presented in Box **2**.

Box 2: Advantages of ODMTs

- Easy to administer
- Palatable
- Use of safe, well-established and stable excipients
- Weight-based dosing , dose titration and individual dose adaption
- Good stability

Box 2 contd.....

- Low transport and storage costs
- Direct compression on conventional tableting machines
- Differentiation of the evaluated excipients could be made with regard to compressibility, friability and simulated wetting test-time

ODMTs with adequate crushing strength and short simulated wetting test (SWT) time have been obtained with the use of co-processed excipients like Ludiflash® (BASF), Pharmaburst® 500 (SPI Pharma), Parteck® ODT (Merck), Pearlitol® Flash (Roquette) and Prosolv® ODT (JRS Pharma) [13]. Narrow particle size distributions of coprocessed excipients have led to sufficient flow properties. Pharmaburst® 500 exhibited the narrowest particle size distribution and the highest median (d_{50}), resulting in good flowability as demonstrated by low Carr's Index. Best compressibility resulting in highest crushing strength (17.6 N after compression with 8 kN) in ODMTs was achieved with Parteck® ODT. Least compressibility was obtained with Pearlitol® Flash. Lowest SWT time (1.9-5.0 s) and best ratio of crushing strength to SWT-time (2.5 N/s) were achieved with Ludiflash®. All ODMTs indicated a sufficient friability below 1%, except ODMTs prepared with Prosolv® ODT and Pearlitol® Flash, compressed with 3 kN.

ODMTs containing 1 mg zinc sulphate per tablet have been developed as a child-appropriate dosage form for their use in developing countries [14]. The optimised formulation contained Pearlitol® Flash, 16.8% w/w sodium cyclamate, 1.6% w/w saccharin sodium and 9.8% w/w NaCl. The inexpensive and straight-forward approach of adding suitable sweeteners was sufficient to mask the taste of zinc sulphate.

ODMTs of enalapril maleate were prepared by rotary tablet press equipped with 2 mm punches [15]. ODMTs were easy to be swallowed and disintegrated within 5 s. ODMT formulation contained enalapril maleate, FlowLac®, Kollidon® CL-SF and Pruv® or magnesium stearate. Prepared ODMTs were superior in prolonging shelf life in comparison to suspension and dosing was more accurate when compared with halved tablets. ODMTs were, therefore, presented as a flexible dosing form for children suffering from hypertension.

3.1. Ideal Properties of Suitable Tableting Excipient

- Good flow properties for flawless and smooth tablet compression process
- Sufficient blend uniformity and content uniformity to formulate low dose

ODMTs
- Good compressibility for adequate crushing strength and low friability at low compression forces
- Short SWT time resulting in quick oral disintegration and suitability for use in paediatrics
- Low SWT and high crushing strength makes the excipient most appropriate
- Clinically tested safe in paediatric patients and acceptable by drug regulatory agency

3.2. Direct Compression of ODMTs

Powder mixture, containing drug and excipients, is subjected to direct compression to obtain biconvex mini-tablets with a compression force (maximum upper punch force) of 3-10 kN and speed of rotation 10 rpm on an instrumented rotary tablet press [3, 13]. Tablet press equipped with a power feeder and one mini-tableting tool (Euro-B 19-tip) is used in preparing ODMTs. ODMTs are dedusted for 1 min by an air jet sieve. The tableting and storage is generally performed in an air-conditioned room maintained at 45% RH and 21°C to prevent moisture uptake by hygroscopic coprocessed excipients.

3.3. Crushing Strength

Powder mixtures must possess good compressibility to obtain not only sufficient mechanical strength amenable to packaging and practical handling but also to prevent breakage of fragile tools used in compressing mini-tablets. Sensitivity of tablet hardness tester is not sufficient to differentiate hardness among ODMTs due to the use of low compression forces and small size of mini-tablets. Hence, the hardness testing is performed as measuring the force required to crush mini-tablets radially in a texture analyser [3]. One such model is TA-XT2i of Stable Micro Systems (Godalming, UK). During measurement of the crushing strength, the punch moves at the speed of 0.1 mm/s to a constant distance and the deformation is measured continuously to record a force-distance diagram. The maximum force required to break ODMTs is estimated.

3.4. Friability

Small size and low mass of ODMTs makes their appearance very similar to pellets, rather than to conventional tablets. Friability of ODMTs is, therefore, estimated by a modified method, which is very similar to the method used for measuring friability of spheroids/pellets/granules [16]. About 1 g of ODMTs are filled into a multi-dose container and subjected to shaking in a mechanical shaker at 200 vibrations/min [3]. Later, ODMTs are removed from the container and de-dusting is performed with the help of an air jet sieve for 1 min. Samples are weighed before and after the treatment and friability is calculated. Friability of less than 1% is considered acceptable for ODMTs.

3.5. Content Uniformity and Mass Variation

ODMTs are essentially low-dose dosage forms due to their small size and use of large amount of coprocessed excipients. Low dose of drug, direct compression and cohesive flow properties of drug make the uniformity of dosing a critical quality control attribute ODMTs are, thus, essentially examined to comply with the requirements of mass variation and content uniformity as per the pharmacopoeia [3].

3.6. Simulated Wetting Test Time (SWT Time)

SWT time is a modified procedure of estimating wetting time of ODTs [17, 18]. SWT time simulates the physiological environment of wet human tongue, without giving any regard to the movement of tongue. Due to the small size of ODMTs, a modified SWT time test is used [3]. In this modified method, 96-well plate is used. Each well contains a 5 mm diameter disc of Whatman® filter paper wetted with 20 μl of a 0.1% (w/w) Brilliant Blue 85E133 solution. A single ODMT is placed over the wet paper disc with the help of a forcep. SWT time is determined as the time required in which blue dye solution completely wets the tablet.

3.7. Acceptance and Compliance

In a double crossover random study involving 60 children of age 0.5 to 6 years, placebo ODMTs (size 2 mm, disintegration time <10 s) were administered orally with beverage or 15% glucose syrup [19]. ODMTs were well accepted by children and the level of acceptance was found higher or equal to the acceptance of the syrup. In age group 6-12 months, children find no difficulty in swallowing ODMTs and their acceptance was higher than sweet liquids. Children of age 2-4 years swallowed ODMTs after chewing and the acceptance was found still higher. It was also observed that acceptability of 1 × n(ODMT) >> 1 x 3 ml glucose syrup throughout all age categories. In another study, acceptability of placebo 3 mm diameter mini-tablets was assessed in 100 children of age 2-6 year [20]. The ability of swallowing in children increased with age and it was found that 46%, 53% and 85% children were able to swallow mini tablets in age 2 year, 3 year, 4 year or higher, respectively. Both studies concluded that mini tablets can be used as potential novel formulations for children.

Weight based dosing, taste masking and dissolution characteristics of ODMTs are important for improving acceptability and compliance. Taste masking is critical and challenging with respect to the size of ODMTs. Improvement in dissolution of poorly soluble drugs is very limited due to extremely small size of these tablets, which provides only a limited choice of excipients and drugs for drug product development. Studies are ongoing to characterise dissolution, bitterness suppression, weight based dosing, acceptability and compliance in children to establish ODMTs for their beneficial role in paediatrics.

3.8. Effect of Excipients on Quality of ODMTs

The type of coprocessing, composition and applied compression force could have a major influence on evaluation parameters of ODMTs. In most of the cases, superdisintegrants like maize starch and crospovidone have a beneficial effect on SWT time. The complex composition of coprocessed excipient Prosolv® ODT (comprised of crospovidone, fructose and MCC) shows SWT time dependency on compression force. ODMTs prepared with Ludiflash® have high compressibility, low friability and short SWT time.

Acceptable uniformity and small mass variations were achieved with all coprocessed excipients in 1 mg hydrochlorthiazide ODMTs [3]. Pearlitol® Flash showed best flowability. Parteck® ODT fulfilled good compatibility demands. Desired short SWT times were obtained with Ludiflash® and Pearlitol® Flash. Low SWT time and high crushing strength are highly desirable attributes in ODMTs. ODMTs, with and without drug, when prepared with Ludiflash® at compression force of 8 kN, exhibited SWT time of 5.0 s and hardness of 11.8 N. Incorporation of hydrochlorthiazide in Ludiflash® and compression at 8 kN resulted in adequate hardness of 8.1 N and acceptable SWT time of 4.9 s. Due to these favourable results, Ludiflash® was regarded as best excipient used in preparing ODMTs [3, 21].

4. TARGETED ORAL DRUG DELIVERY *VIA* MINI TABLETS

Rapidly disintegrating enteric coated mini-tablets have also been designed for a targeted oral delivery system [22]. Theophylline anhydrous (50% w/w), Prosolv® SMCC 90 (20% w/w), lactose monohydrate (q.s. 100% w/w) and disintegrant (0.5, 1.0, 2.0, 3.0, 4.0, 5.0% w/w) were sieved through a 600 μm sieve, blended for 15 min in a V blender, followed by the addition of magnesium stearate (0.5% w/w) and final mixing for 5 min. Mini tablets were prepared by direct compression using a rotary tablet press equipped with 5 mm diameter punches. Quick disintegration times of less than 60 s were achieved with 0.5–5.0% w/w of

CCS, 3.0–5.0%w/w of crospovidone, 0.5–5.0% w/w of Explotab® and 2.0–5.0% w/w of L-HPC. Use of 3% w/w of CCS gave superior drug dissolution compared to other disintegrants at same concentration. The rapidly disintegrating mini-tablet prepared using 0.5-5.0% w/w of CCS showed most uniform disintegration time. Coprocessed excipient Prosolv® SMCC 90 enhanced the compressibility of powder blend and allowed compression to hard tablets with low friability. An enteric coating over the prepared rapidly disintegrating mini tablets may be applied to design a targeted oral drug delivery system *via* mini tablets.

5. FAST DISINTEGRATING TABLETS WITH SUSTAINED/CONTROLLED RELEASE PROFILE

The advantages of both quick disintegration/dissolution and sustained/controlled release can be coupled in a single dosage form (Box **3**). FDTs have been programmed for quick oral dispersibility with sustained/controlled/delayed release characteristics, where dissolution/drug release starts from places away from the buccal region. The sustained/controlled delivery of drug for 12/24 h may be exploited with great ease of administration in paediatrics, geriatrics, psychotic patients and in situations of no or difficult access to water [4]. Sustained/controlled release FDTs reduce dosing frequency, provide better maintenance of therapeutic levels and improve patient compliance. Additionally such formulations offer great ease of administering medicines to patients experiencing difficulties in swallowing due to injuries of brain or spinal cord injury and diseases like multiple sclerosis, stroke, muscular dystrophy, GERD, Parkinson's disease, oesophageal cancer and oesophagitis [23]

Box 3: Advantages of FDT sustained/controlled release formulations

- Reducing dosing frequency
- Maintains therapeutic levels
- Improve patient compliance.
- Great ease of administering medicines to patients who suffer from dysphagia

5.1. Challenges for Sustained/Controlled Release FDT

- Adequate hardness to withstand transportation and handling
- Rapid disintegration of FDT into individual particles in the oral cavity
- Disintegrated particles must have a particle size less than 300 μm to prevent gritty feeling in mouth

- Polymer used shall not allow fusion of coated drug particles during compression of the tablet
- The process of tablet compression should not significantly alter drug release characteristics of coated drug particles. During tableting, polymer coated drug particles may deform but should not rupture or crack so as to maintain a constant and reproducible drug release rate

5.2. Highly Plastic Granules + IER Approach

Frosta® technology uses a conventional wet granulation method to prepare plastic granules which are subsequently compressed to FDTs [24, 25]. FDT formulations based on Frosta® technology and sustained release properties of ion-exchange resins (IERs) were combined to achieve sustained drug delivery of dextromethorphan *via* FDTs [4]. Linear *Bt–t* plots and application of Higuchi equation to drug release from resin complexes and coated resin complexes revealed diffusion of drug as the rate controlling step in the drug release from the matrix. Increase in thickness of coating reduced the diffusion of drug through coating. The disintegration time of prepared FDTs of coated dextromethorphan IER complex was very short (10-30 s). SEM studies showed that granules at the surface of tablet were compressed tightly, while granules present at the core of tablet were loose, separated by pores, which allows water to be absorbed quickly by capillary action leading to faster disintegration. As the tablet disintegrates into granules with saliva or water, it was followed by the release of the drug with a minimum effect of compaction pressures. Kollicoat® SR30D provided acceptable mechanical properties giving strong resistance to breaking or fracture of coating. Unlike to ethylcellulose, Kollicoat® SR30D prevented significant changes in drug release rates from tablets compressed at pressure 200-500 lbs, when compared to drug release rates from coated drug resin complexes [4].

Amberlite™ IRP69 (a strong cation exchange resin) was used to prepare resinates with a bitter model drug HCl salt [5]. The Amberlite™ IRP69-drug resinates were prepared by mixing hydrated IER particles and different concentrations of the model drug for 6 hours, so as to maximise drug loading onto IER particles. Resinates were dried in an oven followed by coating with a combination of methacrylate polymers to further control the release profile and reduce initial burst. Coated resinates were compressed to tablets using 11/32" round tooling into 250 mg tablets containing a dose of 25 mg of the drug. Mannitol, citric acid and sodium bicarbonate were used to mask the bitter taste as well as to enhance the disintegration time along with CCS (Ac-di-Sol®). The prepared formulations exemplified the dual advantage of taste-masking and sustained release characteristics of IERs by formulating FDTs.

5.3. Fast Disintegrating and Slow Releasing Ibuprofen Tablets

Kollidon CL as superdisintegrant was used to prepare FDTs of ibuprofen characterised by sustained drug release. Conventional wet granulation followed by compression was used to prepare FDTs of ibuprofen [6]. Gastric side effects and bitter taste of ibuprofen was reduced by preparing wet granules with a saturated lecithin (Phospholipon® 80H). Amprac® 01, Kollicoat® SR 30, Eudragit® RD 100 and Kollidon® 90F were used to provide a uniform film over granules by pan coating. Coated granules were mixed with aspartame, Peartlitol® SD 200 and Kollidon® CL and compressed to FDTs under low compression forces. Deaggregation time of tablets prepared with Kollidon CL was 32-70 s. Delay in drug release was the combined effect of the coating as well as the presence of lecithin in the granules. Prepared tablets were capable of quick oral disintegration and delayed release of drug to prevent gastric side effects of drug.

5.4. Sustained Release FDTs from Dry Emulsions

Nicorandil loaded dry emulsions were prepared with stearyl alcohol and myristyl alcohol followed by their compression to FDTs having fast disintegration time of 12-33 s [7]. The ratio of stearyl alcohol and myristyl alcohol was found critical in controlling the release of the drug from FDTs. FDTs were able to delay the release of the drug for more than 6 h. *In vivo* pharmacokinetic studies in beagle dogs showed similar AUC, a lower C_{max}, and delayed T_{max}, when results were compared to plain FDTs and commercial tablets.

5.5. Oral Disintegrating Tablets (ODTs) with Controlled Release Microparticulate Beads (Advatab®+ Diffucaps®)

Melperone permitting once-a-day controlled release ODTs, having disintegration time less than 30 s, were prepared in order to improve acceptance and compliance in patients suffering from schizophrenia and psychosis linked to Parkinson's disease [26]. Swallowing dysfunction is most common in early stages of Parkinson's disease. An ODT formulation is highly desirable to improve compliance and controlled release, in combination, will improve therapy in such patients.

Two technologies, Diffucaps® beads and Advatab® were used in preparing ODT controlled release tablets of melpreone HCl [26]. Coated controlled release beads were prepared by Diffucaps® technology and tableting was effected by Advatab® proprietary and patented technology. Diffucaps® involves the layering of drug on an inert core. Drug layered cores are coated with one or more layers of functional polymers in a fluidised bed apparatus. The composition and thickness of the coating polymers can be altered to achieve various drug release profiles. Advatab® technology utilises Advatab® base granules with other excipients and an external lubrication system in which the lubricant is only applied to the material contacting surfaces of punches and dies. The external lubrication system requires lower compression forces and minimum lubricant on tablet surface, which ensures rapid disintegration on contact with dissolution media or saliva in the oral cavity resulting in a successful ODT.

Melpreone is extremely water soluble drug at physiologically relevant pH range (1.2-6.8) with solubility of 700-800 mg/ml. Solubility decreases sharply below 100 mg/ml at pH 7.1 and above, especially above pH 8. Such high solubility is a great challenge in developing controlled release dosage form with minimum possibility of dose dumping. However, the advantage of poor solubility at higher pH can be exploited for controlled release once-daily ODT formulations by creating microenvironment of basic pH inside coated beads.

In the dissolution media or upon oral administration, water imbibed into controlled release bead creating an alkaline pH of 8 or higher, which makes drug release slower due to poor solubility of melperone in basic environment. Microparticles of size≥400 μm gave gritty feeling inside mouth. An ODT formulation was therefore targeted to have microparticles of size ≤400 μm for their successful incorporating in ODTs for good acceptability by patients. It was achieved by the use of inert cores of 45-60 mesh for the sustained release beads.

A core of 45-60 mesh sugar spheres was layered with melperone HCl (25% w/w) and a seal coat (2% w/w) of hydroxypropylcellulose (Klucel LF) was applied to prepare immediate release beads. An additional coating of an anhydrous dibasic sodium phosphate and one more coat of water-insoluble ethylcellulose (Ethocel Standard 10 Premium) with triethylcitrate or dibutyl sebacate as the plasticiser were applied to prepare Diffucaps® beads. These Diffucaps® beads were blended with rapidly dispersing microgranules (Advatab® base granules), MCC, sucralose, a flavour (peppermint or wintergreen) and compressed into ODT-CR tablets (50 mg dose weighing 1000 mg) on a rotary tablet machine equipped with an external lubrication system and 15 mm flat and round punches. The compression force (12-16 kN) was optimised to achieve hardness greater than 30 N and friability of 0.6% or less. ODT-CR formulations were optimised for an acceptable *in vitro* disintegration time of less than 30 s in a USP disintegration test and adequate controlled release characteristics for once-daily formulation.

5.6. Ketoprofen Orally Disintegrating Sustained Release Tablets

Orally disintegrating sustained release tablets of ketoprofen were prepared by a simple two-step process of spray drying and direct compression [8]. In the first step, sustained release ketoprofen granules were developed by spray drying the aqueous dispersion consisting Eudragit RS-30D, Starch 1500 and PEG 6000 at inlet temperature of 100°C and a feed rate of 1.5 mL/min. Obtained granules were mixed with lactose, mannitol and a cross-linked polyvinylpyrrolidone and subsequent direct compression. Prepared tablets quick disintegrated quickly within 30 s allowing to liberate coated granules for slow release of ketoprofen for 24 h. *In vivo* pharmacokinetic studies in beagle dogs also demonstrated significantly extended release profile, when compared to ketoprofen normal capsules.

6. FAST DISINTEGRATING PELLETS

Pellets are generally prepared by extrusion/spheronisation and can be made faster disintegrating by processing them with sufficient amounts of disintegrating agent. Apart from conventionally used MCC, pectinic acid and MCC II Sanaq® Burst have been exploited for preparing FDPs [9, 27]. FDPs provide the advantages of faster disintegration/dissolution and great flexibility of dosing similar to ODMTs.

Pectinic acid with 10% degree of methoxylation was a superior extrusion aid, when compared to MCC, in preparing FDPs by extrusion/spheronisation [9]. Mehoxylated pectinic acid was almost insoluble in water at pH values below 6-7 due to conformational changes in polymer resulting in prevention of hydration of the polymer. Irrespective of the drug or its dose, pectinic acid pellets released drug faster than MCC pellets. Quick fragmentation of pectinic acid pellets in test medium was found independent of pH. Cracks or holes on the surface of pectinic acid pellets played important role in drug release as water penetrates through the core much faster causing faster fragmentation and subsequent quick disintegration. However, MCC pellets released the drug by diffusion. Pellets prepared with pectinic acid were mechanically stable but more sensitive to the amount and type of the drug. Pectinic pellets also offered a high loading capacity (upto 80% loading) and faster disintegration giving an excellent avenue for fast release of a poorly water soluble drug like riboflavin.

MCC II was used for manufacturing FDPs by wet-extrusion/spheronisation [27]. MCC II is a different allomorph of MCC [11] MCC II exhibit superior pelletisation properties and results pellets having properties of faster disintegration and quick drug release. Theophylline pellets prepared with 20%

MCC II gave a disintegration time of 0.7 minute in a modified European Pharmacopoeia method [10]. MCC II based pellets had shown almost instantaneous diphenydramine HCl release profile comparable to that of Benadryl® and a faster griseofulvin release, when compared to pellets prepared with MCC I [11]. Pellets of MCC II were recommended to store at 55-80% RH at 20°C [10]. Lower humidity may convert the monohydrate to anhydrous form and higher humidities can affect disintegration properties irreversibly due to changes in MCC II. MCC II is a multifunctional excipient with filler, binder and disintegrant properties [28, 29]. It is pure MCC (100% w/w) with better taste than the other types of cellulose, directly compressible and offer faster disintegration in pellets and tablets. With all these properties, it has a great potential to become a diluents of choice in FDTs and fast disintegrating pellets [30]. It can avoid the use of a separate disintegrant in FDPs or FDTs.

Effervescent FDPs from dexamethasone sodium phosphate and water soluble excipients, *viz.* sorbitol, xylitol, mannitol, sodium bicarbonate, citric acid and tartaric acid, were prepared in a fluid bed rotary processor [12]. Ethanol and PEG 400 mixture was applied as binding liquid. Sequential experimental designs were applied to optimise both formulation and process variables. FDPs having disintegration time of 30 s and rate of drug release greater than 85% in 10 minutes were achieved. Effervescent FDPs were presented as a safe, efficacious and palatable dosage form. Effervescent FDPs seems to contribute enhanced patient compliance due to their direct dispersion in the oral cavity or dissolution in a small volume of water.

7. ORODISPERSIBLE OR TO DISSOLVE IN WATER POWDERS

Unither Pharmaceuticals has developed a stick-pack filling machine for filling powders in a single unit dose product referred to as Unistick® [31]. The machine can be used to three different sizes of stick-packs, *viz.* 120 mm, 80 mm and 60 mm. Powder in quantities 0.5 ml to 5 ml can be filled in these unit dosage forms. The proprietary process claims to fill hydrophobic (orodispersible or effervescent) besides the conventional powders. Unistick® is being offered as a life management solution to restore and revive pharmaceutical products in European markets. Effervescent paracetamol Unither 500 mg and 1000 mg, n-acetyl cysteine 200 mg powder stick and some other orodispersible or to dissolve in water powders are under development at Gannat R&D plant of Unither Pharmaceuticals. Carbocisteine Unistick® 750 mg/10 ml was approved by European Medicines Agency (EMA) and successfully entered in markets of France in 2013 [32].

CONCLUSIONS

FDC, prepared by perforation or vacuum drying, are useful in incorporating high dose of drugs and able to overcome poor taste masking abilities due to various filling volumes of capsules. Gelatin low bloom strength and use of suitable excipients have considerably improved the mechanical properties of the capsule shells so as to manufacture brittle capsules. Mechanical weaknesses in capsule shells make them vulnerable to easy and quick rupture in oral cavity resembling similar to other FDDFs. Moisture protection packaging, similar to freeze dried tablets, is also required for packaging of FDC.

Direct compression of drug with coprocessed excipients is a method of choice in preparing ODMTs. Availability of commercial coprocessed excipients has made ODMTs more affordable than standard liquid dosage forms. When compared to FDTs/ODTs, ODMTs have further improved the acceptability and compliance in children due to their small size and quick oral disintegration/dissolution. Characteristics of ODMTs like weight-based dosing, dose titration and individual dose adaption make them excellent dosage form avoiding measuring problems of liquid dosage forms. ODMTs may also be used as flexible dosage forms for preparing dispersion in water/syrup/juice/flavoured liquid, immediately before its oral administration. ODMTs may also be sprinkled on soft food and thereby provides an additional convenient approach for administering drug to children.

FDCs and ODMTs can be formulated for drugs that are used to treat diseases, like lower respiratory tract infections, diarrhoeal diseases, asthma, malaria *etc.*, which are the major causes of morbidity and mortality in children. FDPs have also been tried with water soluble excipients and by processing in fluid bed processor or extrusion/spheroniser. FDPs have also been looked as flexible dosage forms for paediatrics. Unistick® provides the advantages of convenient and cost-effective method of reducing processing steps by simply filling orodispersible powder in a packing.

Sustained/controlled/targeted drug delivery is also feasible with various FDDFs, as these dosage forms quickly disintegrate to disperse microcapsules/ microspheres without adversely affecting the intended release of the drug. Furthermore, some formulation approaches like freeze drying and moulding are more amenable to incorporate microcapsules/microspheres/coated micro-particulates in tablet forms with least breakage or fracture.

REFERENCES

[1] Ciper M, Bodmeier R. Modified conventional hard gelatin capsules as fast disintegrating dosage form

in the oral cavity. Eur J Pharm Biopharm 2006; 62(2): 178-84.
[http://dx.doi.org/10.1016/j.ejpb.2005.08.014] [PMID: 16260126]

[2] Ciper M, Bodmeier R. Preparation and characterization of novel fast disintegrating capsules (Fastcaps) for administration in the oral cavity. Int J Pharm 2005; 303(1-2): 62-71.
[http://dx.doi.org/10.1016/j.ijpharm.2005.07.004] [PMID: 16111845]

[3] Stoltenberg I, Breitkreutz J. Orally disintegrating mini-tablets (ODMTs)a novel solid oral dosage form for paediatric use. Eur J Pharm Biopharm 2011; 78(3): 462-9.
[http://dx.doi.org/10.1016/j.ejpb.2011.02.005] [PMID: 21324357]

[4] Jeong SH, Park K. Development of sustained release fast-disintegrating tablets using various polymer-coated ion-exchange resin complexes. Int J Pharm 2008; 353(1-2): 195-204.
[http://dx.doi.org/10.1016/j.ijpharm.2007.11.033] [PMID: 18164882]

[5] Gokhale A, Sundararajan P. Novel controlled release formulation for orally disintegrating tablets using ion exchange resins. Drug Des Deliv 2013; 13: 40-5.

[6] Fini A, Bergamante V, Ceschel GC, Ronchi C, de Moraes CA. Fast dispersible/slow releasing ibuprofen tablets. Eur J Pharm Biopharm 2008; 69(1): 335-41.
[http://dx.doi.org/10.1016/j.ejpb.2007.11.011] [PMID: 18182280]

[7] Jin Y, Ohkuma H, Wang H, Natsume H, Sugibayashi K, Morimoto Y. [Fast-disintegration oral tablets having sustained release property]. Yakugaku Zasshi 2002; 122(11): 989-94.
[http://dx.doi.org/10.1248/yakushi.122.989] [PMID: 12440156]

[8] Wei Q, Yang F, Luan L. Preparation and *in vitro/in vivo* evaluation of a ketoprofen orally disintegrating/sustained release tablet. Drug Dev Ind Pharm 2013; 39(6): 928-34.
[http://dx.doi.org/10.3109/03639045.2012.664146] [PMID: 22401710]

[9] Tho I, Sande SA, Kleinebudde P. Disintegrating pellets from a water-insoluble pectin derivative produced by extrusion/spheronisation. Eur J Pharm Biopharm 2003; 56(3): 371-80.
[http://dx.doi.org/10.1016/S0939-6411(03)00071-7] [PMID: 14602179]

[10] Krueger C, Thommes M, Kleinebudde P. Influence of storage condition on properties of MCC II-based pellets with theophylline-monohydrate. Eur J Pharm Biopharm 2014; 88(2): 483-91.
[http://dx.doi.org/10.1016/j.ejpb.2014.06.006] [PMID: 24950003]

[11] Rojas J, Kumar V. Evaluation of microcrystalline cellulose II (MCCII) as an alternative extrusion-spheronization aid. Pharmazie 2012; 67(7): 595-7.
[PMID: 22888514]

[12] Karatzas A, Politis S, Rekkas D. Application of DoE for the Development of Rapidly Dissolving Pellets Prepared by Direct Pelletization within the QbD Framework AAPS Annual Meeting and Exposition 2014.

[13] Stoltenberg I, Breitkreutz J. Suitability of ready-to-use excipients for preparation of orally disintegrating mini-tablets (ODMTs). FIP PSWC / AAPS Annual Meeting; New Orleans. 2010.

[14] Stoltenberg I, Breitkreutz J. ODMTs with taste-masked zinc sulphate as a child appropriate dosage form for developing countries 3rd European Paediatric Formulation Initiative (EuPFI) Meeting. Strasbourg, France. 2011.

[15] Hermes M, Breitkreutz J. Orodispersible minitablets as a child-appropriate dosage form with enalapril maleate: Avoiding the problems of extemporaneous formulations?. 3rd European Paediatric Formulation Initiative (EuPFI) Meeting; Strasbourg, France. 2011.

[16] Sucker H. Test methods for granulates. Pharm Ind 1982; 44: 312-6.

[17] Park J, Holman K, Bish G, *et al.* An Alternative to the USP Disintegration Test for Orally Disintegrating Tablets. Pharm Technol 2008; 32: 54-88.

[18] Bi Y, Sunada H, Yonezawa Y, Danjo K, Otsuka A, Iida K. Preparation and evaluation of a compressed tablet rapidly disintegrating in the oral cavity. Chem Pharm Bull (Tokyo) 1996; 44(11): 2121-7. [http://dx.doi.org/10.1248/cpb.44.2121] [PMID: 8945778]

[19] Spomer N, Klingmann V, Stoltenberg I, Lerch C, Meissner T, Breitkreutz J. Acceptance of uncoated mini-tablets in young children: results from a prospective exploratory cross-over study. Arch Dis Child 2012; 97(3): 283-6. [http://dx.doi.org/10.1136/archdischild-2011-300958] [PMID: 22253279]

[20] Thomson SA, Tuleu C, Wong IC, Keady S, Pitt KG, Sutcliffe AG. Minitablets: new modality to deliver medicines to preschool-aged children. Pediatrics 2009; 123(2): e235-8. [http://dx.doi.org/10.1542/peds.2008-2059] [PMID: 19171575]

[21] Heberstreit P, Osswald F, Widmaier R, *et al.* Ludiflash as excipient for paediatric use 2nd Conference of the European Paediatric Formulation Initiative (EUPFi). Berlin, Germany. 2010.

[22] Thitinan S, Jang S-F, McConville JT. A rapidly disintegrating mini-tablet for targeted oral delivery. AAPS Annual Meeting and Exposition Online Itinerary. 11/15/2008 - 11/20/2008; 2008.

[23] Birmachu W. Orally disintegrating extended release (ODT-ER) dosage forms. Drug Deliv 2010; (April): 33-4.

[24] Fu Y, Jeong SH, Park K. Fast-melting tablets based on highly plastic granules. J Control Release 2005; 109(1-3): 203-10. [http://dx.doi.org/10.1016/j.jconrel.2005.09.021] [PMID: 16260059]

[25] Jeong SH, Fu Y, Park K. Frosta: a new technology for making fast-melting tablets. Expert Opin Drug Deliv 2005; 2(6): 1107-16. [http://dx.doi.org/10.1517/17425247.2.6.1107] [PMID: 16296813]

[26] Venkatesh GM, Stevens PJ, Lai J-W. Development of orally disintegrating tablets comprising controlled-release multiparticulate beads. Drug Dev Ind Pharm 2012; 38(12): 1428-40. [http://dx.doi.org/10.3109/03639045.2011.653365] [PMID: 22356215]

[27] Krueger C, Thommes M, Kleinebudde P. MCC SANAQ burst: a new type of cellulose and its suitability to prepare fast disintegrating pellets. J Pharm Innov 2010; 5: 45-57. [http://dx.doi.org/10.1007/s12247-010-9080-4]

[28] Krueger C, Thommes M, Kleinebudde P. Influence of MCC II fraction and storage conditions on pellet properties. Eur J Pharm Biopharm 2013; 85(3 Pt B): 1039-45. [http://dx.doi.org/10.1016/j.ejpb.2013.07.001] [PMID: 23872176]

[29] Krueger C, Thommes M, Kleinebudde P. Spheronisation mechanism of MCC II-based pellets. Powder Technol 2013; 238: 176-87. [http://dx.doi.org/10.1016/j.powtec.2011.12.052]

[30] Leuenberger H, Leuenberger MN, Puchkov M. Right First Time: Computer-Aided Scale-up for manufacturing solid dosage forms with a shorter time to market. Swiss Pharma 2010; 32: 3-13.

[31] Powder Unistick®: New member to reinforce Unither's unit-dose family. 2015. Accessed from: http://www.unither-pharma.com/en/corporate-news/262-powder-unistick-new-member-to-reinforce-unither-s-sterile-unit-dose-family Accessed on 30th January 2015.

[32] Decrets, arretes, circulaires. Journal Officiel De La Republique Francaise 2013; 66.

CHAPTER 12

Approved and Marketed Fast Dissolving/ Disintegrating Drug Products

Vikas A. Saharan[1,*], **Anupama Singh**[1] and **Vandana Kharb**[2]

[1] *Department of Pharmaceutics, School of Pharmaceutical Sciences, Sardar Bhagwan Singh Post Graduate Institute of Biomedical Sciences and Research, Balawala, Dehradun 248161, Uttarakhand, India*

[2] *Sachdeva College of Pharmacy, Chandigarh-Ludhiana National Highway, Gharuan 140413, Punjab, India*

Abstract: Websites of various drug regulatory agencies like US FDA, EMA, MHRA, PMDA and CDSCO were visited and information about approval and market authorisations of FDDF drug products' was collected with an aim to provide updated lists. Additionally, information about marketed FDDF drug products was also retrieved from websites of pharmaceutical companies and other literature sources. This chapter comprehensively enlists various drug products approved and marketed in US, UK, Europe, Japan and India.

Keywords: Bioequivalence, Brand, CDSCO, Controlled release, EMA, FDA, Film, Generic, MDT, MHRA, Mouth dissolving, ODT, Orally disintegrating, Orange book, Orodispersible, Patent, PMDA, Proprietary, Tablet.

1. INTRODUCTION

From regulatory context, FDDF products are regarded as novel drug delivery systems, which require bioequivalence testing with their equivalent conventional dosage forms. Immediate release drug products shall be tested for bioequivalence with reference listed conventional drug products, if the FDDF product is first market entry. If any FDDF product is already available in the market, the new product (generic FDDF) shall be compared to the reference listed FDDF product. So, bioequivalence testing of a FDDF is an essential criterion for market entry of FDDF product of an approved drug. Bioequivalence of a FDDF product is

* **Corresponding author Vikas A. Saharan:** Department of Pharmaceutics, School of Pharmaceutical Sciences, Sardar Bhagwan Singh Post Graduate Institute of Biomedical Sciences and Research (www.sbspgi.edu.in), Balawala, Dehradun 248161, Uttarakhand, India; Tel: +91-135-2686246; Mobile: +91-8439820796; Fax: +91-135-2686246; E-mail: vikas.pharmaceutics@gmail.com

Vikas Anand Saharan (Ed.)

assessed by either pharmacokinetic or pharmacodynamic methods.

As per EMA guidelines, BCS biowaiver for FDDF product is considered only if the API is not absorbed in mouth [1]. However, there is an ongoing debate and several research reports have advocated use of *in vitro* testing of bioequivalence by performing dissolution studies in small volumes (*i.e.* 5 mL of volume) of dissolution studies, which can resemble the dissolution in mouth and thus suggested requirement to amend BCS solubility criterion for FDDFs like Orally Disintegrating Tablets (ODTs), Fast Disintegrating/Dissolving Tablets (FDTs), Fast Dissolving Oral Films (FDOFs), buccal and sublingual tablets [2]. A standardised bioequivalence protocol require FDDF products to be administered orally only after prior wetting of the mouth with 20 ml of water and a limitation of not taking water within 1 h of administration.

Various generic FDDF products have entered in the market to compete the success of patented FDDF products. FDDF Drug market is continuously expanding with the rise of regulatory requirements and increase in awareness of drug products for paediatrics, geriatrics and other special populations. Newer technologies are continuously emerging to shape a tablet or other dosage form meant for faster disintegration/dissolution. Pioneer technologies of manufacturing FDDF utilise process control to optimise disintegration/dissolution. New technologies have emerged, which controls crystal growth and porosity while utilising the conventional manufacturing processes in shaping tablets. The latest technological innovations involve the application of prescription design type approaches in formulating FDDF products. New fabrication method like 3-dimensional printing is also gaining access from research and development sections through pilot plant to manufacturing sections of pharmaceutical industries.

GlaxoSmithKline's Zofran® ODT (ondansetron) and Lilly's Zyprexa® Zydis® (olanzapine) are two commercially successful products, which have motivated the entry of generic FDTs [3]. However, Zyprexa® Zydis® formulation still enjoys marketing exclusivity till 7/26/2016 in US [4]. FDT market is expected to reach $12 billion globally by 2018 with the popularity and growth of FDTs in various developing countries. FDOF market is expected to reach $1 billion in 2015 [5]. FDDF market is also expanding with introduction of newer products like sustained/controlled release FDTs, which have been successfully launched. Development pipeline of FDDF products is also increasing parallel with other novel dosage forms like FDGs, FDPs, and ODMTs.

2. PROPRIETARY TECHNOLOGY BASED FDDF PRODUCTS

Various proprietary technologies for making FDTs are provided in Table **1** and successful marketed products based on these technologies are presented in Table **2** and Table **3**. Table **4** provides proprietary FDOF technologies and list of companies, which have successfully marketed their FDOF products. A list of marketed FDOF product is provided in Table **5**. Most of these FDDF technologies (Table **1** and Table **4**) are invented and patented in US, Europe and Japan. However, a few technologies have been developed in other countries but lack of aggressive marketing/licensing has resulted in only limited regional success.

Table 1. Various proprietary FDT technologies.

Proprietary FDT Technology	Company	Website	Technology Platform
Zydis®, Zydis® Ultra, Zydis® Nano, Zydis® Bio	Catalent	www.catalent.com	Lyophilisation
Lyoc®	Cima Labs	www.cimalabs.com	Lyophilisation
QuickSolv®	Jenssen	www.janssenpharmaceuticalsinc.com	Lyophilisation
Pharmafreeze®	SPI Pharmaceuticals	www.spipharma.com	Excipient system for lyophilisation
OraSolv®/DuraSolv®	Cima Labs	www.cimalabs.com	Compressed tablet
Flashtab®	Ethypharm	www.ethypharm.com	Compressed tablet
Wowtab®, Wowtab-Wet®, Wowtab-Dry®	Astellas (Yamanouchi)	www.astellas.com	Low pressure compression moulding
FlashDose®	Valeant (Biovail)	www.valeant.com	Sugar floss
OraQuick®	Perrigo	www.perrigo.com	Compressed tablets
Solblet®	Kyowa Hakko Kirin	www.kyowa-kirin.com	Compressed tablet, external lubrication
Advatab®/Ziplets	Aptalis (Eurand)	www.aptalispharma.com	Compressed tablet, external lubrication
Ziplets®	Aptalis (Eurand)	www.aptalispharma.com	Compressed tablet
Pharmaburst®	SPI Pharmaceuticals	www.spipharma.com	Excipient system for direct compression
SUITAB®, SUITAB-NEX®, SUITAB-MAX®, SATAB®, PEATAB®	Dainippon Sumitomo Pharma	http://www.ds-pharma.co.jp	Compressed tablet

(Table 1) contd.....

Proprietary FDT Technology	Company	Website	Technology Platform
RACTAB®	Towa Pharmaceutical	http://www.towayakuhin.co.jp	Low pressure compression of tablet followed by post-processing on the intensity of drying
IDTAB®	Otsuka Pharmaceutical	https://www.otsuka.co.jp	Identifiable tablet technology
EMP®	Eisai	www.eisai.com	Compression moulding followed by drying
Frosta®	Akina	http://akinainc.com	Conventional wet granulation process
ZipDose®	Aprecia	https://aprecia.com	Three dimensional printing of tablets
XR-ODT®, RDIM®	Neos Therapeutics Inc.	www.neostx.com	Controlled release ODT containing taste masked IER complex of drug
Orally Disintegrating Granules	Hermes Pharma	http://www.hermes-pharma.com	Orally disintegrating granules

Table 2. Marketed FDT products based on proprietary lyophilisation technologies.

Drug Product	Drug	Dose	Indication	Manufactured /Marketed by	FDT Technology
Abilify® OD Tablets	Aripiprazole	3 mg, 6 mg, 12 mg, 24 mg	Schizophrenia	Otsuka Pharmaceutical Co., Ltd.	Zydis®
Ativan®	Lorazepam	1 mg, 2.5 mg	Anxiety disorders	Pfizer, Wyeth, Valeant Pharmaceuticals	Zydis®
Claritin® RediTab	Loratadine	5 mg, 10 mg	Allergy	Bayer Schering Pharma, MSD K.K.	Zydis®
Feldene® melt	Piroxicam	20 mg	Pain relief	Pfizer	Zydis®
Grastek® Sublingual Tablet	Timothy Grass Pollen Allergen Extract (*Phleum pratense*)	2800 Bioequivalent Allergy Unit	Timothy and related grass pollen allergies	MSD, ALK-Abello	Zydis®
GRAZAX® 75,000 SQ-T oral lyophilisate	Grazax (*Phleum pratense*)	75,000 SQ-T (Standardised Quality units Tablet)	Grass pollen allergy (hay fever)	ALK-Abello	Zydis®

(Table 2) contd.....

Drug Product	Drug	Dose	Indication	Manufactured /Marketed by	FDT Technology
Klonopin® Wafers	Clonazepam	0.125 mg, 0.25 mg, 0.5 mg, 1 mg or 2 mg	Sedation	Roche	Zydis®
Imodium® Instant Melts, Imodium® Lingual, Imodium® Quick Dissolve	Loperamide	2 mg	Diarrhoea	Johnson & Johnson	Zydis®
Izofran® Zydis	Ondansetron HCl	4 mg, 8 mg	Nausea and vomiting induced by cytotoxic chemotherapy and radiotherapy	GlaxoSmithKline	Zydis®
Maxalt® MLT	Rizatriptan	10 mg	Headache	Merck & Co.	Zydis®
Metozolv® ODT	Metoclopramide HCl	10 mg, 15 mg	Gastroesophageal reflux disease (GERD) and recurrent diabetic gastroparesis	Salix Pharmaceuticals	Zydis®
Motilium®	Domperidone	5 mg, 10 mg	Nausea and vomiting	Johnson & Johnson	Zydis®
Ondansetron-RL Zydis Wafers	Ondansetron HCl	4 mg, 8 mg	Nausea and vomiting induced by cytotoxic chemotherapy and radiotherapy	GlaxoSmithKline	Zydis®
Ondaz® Zydis® Wafers	Ondansetron HCl	4 mg, 8 mg	Nausea and vomiting induced by cytotoxic chemotherapy and radiotherapy	Sandoz	Zydis®
Pepcid® RPD	Famotidine	10 mg, 20 mg	Peptic ulcer disease and GERD	Johnson & Johnson	Zydis®
Ragwitek® Sublingual Tablet	Short Ragweed Pollen Allergen Extract	12 Amb a 1-U	Ragweed pollen allergies	MSD, ALK-Abello	Zydis®
Zelapar®	Selegiline	2.5 mg	Parkinson's disease and depression	Valeant Pharmaceuticals	Zydis®
Seresta® Expidet	Oxazepam	10 mg	Tranquiliser	Wyeth	Zydis®
Zofran® Zydis®	Ondansetron HCl	4 mg, 8 mg	Nausea and vomiting induced by cytotoxic chemotherapy and radiotherapy	GlaxoSmithKline	Zydis®
Zyprexa® Zydis®	Olanzapine	2.5 mg, 5 mg, 10 mg	Schizophrenia and bipolar disorder	Eli Lilly	Zydis®

(Table 1) contd.....

Drug Product	Drug	Dose	Indication	Manufactured /Marketed by	FDT Technology
Proxalyoc®	Piroxicam	20 mg	Arthritis, rheumatoid arthritis and ankylosing spondylitis	Teva Sante	Lyoc®
Paralyoc®	Paracetamol	50 mg, 125 mg, 250 mg, 500 mg	Analgesic-antipyretic	Teva Sante	Lyoc®
Spasponlyoc®	Phloroglucinol hydrate	80 mg, 160 mg	Skin disorders, burns and wounds	Teva Sante	Lyoc®
Vogalene® Lyoc®	Metopimazine	7.5 mg	Vomiting and Nausea	Teva Sante	Lyoc®
Seglor® Lyoc®	Dihydroergotamine mesylate	5 mg, 10 mg	Migraine and orthostatic hypotension	UCB Pharma Sa	Lyoc®
Loperamide Lyoc®	Loperamide chlorhydrate	2 mg	Diarrhoea	Teva Sante	Lyoc®
Sermion® Lyoc®	Nicergoline	5 mg, 10 mg	Vasodilator and peripheral vascular disease	Pfizer, Sanofi-Aventis France	Lyoc®
Risperdal® M-tab/Quicklet®	Risperidone	0.5, 1, 2, 3, 4 mg	Schizophrenia and bipolar disorders	Jenssen (J and J)	QuickSolv®
Propulsid® Quicksolv®	Cisapride Monohydrate	20 mg	Nocturnal heartburn due to GERD	Janssen	QuickSolv®
Reminyl® OD Tablets	Galantamine hydrobromide	4 mg, 8 mg and 12 mg	Alzheimer's dementia	Janssen/Takeda	QuickSolv®

Table 3. Marketed FDTs based on compression technologies.

Drug Product	Drug	Dose	Indication	Marketed by	FDT Technology
Alavert®	Loratadine	10 mg	Allergy, sneezing, runny nose, itchy and watery eyes, itching of nose and throat	Wyeth Consumer Healthcare	DuraSolv®
Allegra®	Fexofenadine	30 mg	Seasonal allergy	Aventis Pharmaceuticals	OraSolv®
Aricept® ODT	Donepezil HCl	5 mg, 10 mg	Alzheimer's disease	Eisai	OraSolv®/ DuraSolv®
Clarinex® RediTabs	Desloratadine	2.5 mg, 5 mg	Allergic rhinitis and urticaria	Schering Plough	OraSolv®

(Table 3) contd.....

Drug Product	Drug	Dose	Indication	Marketed by	FDT Technology
Dimetapp® ND	Loratadine	10 mg	Hay fever or other upper respiratory allergies	Wyeth	DuraSolv®
FazaClo® LD and FazaClo® HD	Clozapine	12.5 mg, 25 mg, 50 mg, 100 mg, 150 mg, 200 mg	Schizophrenia	Alamo Pharmaceuticals/Azur Pharma	DuraSolv®
Fluxid®	Famotidine	20 mg, 49 mg	Duodenal ulcer and GERD	Azur Pharma	OraSolv®
Kamstro®	Baclofen	10 mg, 20 mg	Anti-spastic analgesic	UCB/Azur Pharma	DuraSolv®
Niravam®	Alprazolam	0.25, 0.5, 1 or 2 mg	Anxiety disorders	Azur Pharma	DuraSolv®
NuLev®	Hyoscyamine sulfate	0.125 mg	Peptic ulcer, spasm in stomach and bladder	UCB	DuraSolv®
NuLev®	Hyoscyamine	0.125 mg	Stomach, intestinal and bladder conditions including spasms	UCB	DuraSolv®
Orapred® ODT	Prednisolone sodium phosphate	10 mg, 15 mg, 30 mg	Asthma, atopic dermatitis, and seasonal and perennial allergic rhinitis	Concordia Pharmaceuticals	OraSolv®
Parcopa®	Levodopa and carbidopa)	25/100; 10/100; 25/250	Parkinson's disease	UCB/Azur Pharma	DuraSolv® /RapiTab®
Remeron® SolTab	Mirtazapine	15 mg, 30 mg, 45 mg	Depression	Organon Inc.	OraSolv®
Tempra® Quicklets / Tempra® Firs Tabs	Acetaminophen	80 mg, 160 mg	Pain and fever	Bristol-Myers Squibb / Mead Johnson	OraSolv®

(Table 3) contd.....

Drug Product	Drug	Dose	Indication	Marketed by	FDT Technology
Triaminic® Softchews	Pseudoephedrine HCl, dextromethorphan HBr monohydrate, chlorpheniramine maleate	15 mg; 5 mg; 1 mg	Cold and Cough	Novartis Consumer Health	OraSolv®
Triaminic® Softchews	Dextromethorphan HBr monohydrate	7.5 mg	Cough	Novartis Consumer Health	OraSolv®
Triaminic® Softchews	Pseudoephedrine HCl; acetaminophen	15 mg; 160 mg	Allergy sinus and headache	Novartis Consumer Health	OraSolv®
Triaminic® Softchews	Pseudoephedrine HCl	15 mg	Allergy and congestion	Novartis Consumer Health	OraSolv®
Triaminic® Softchews	Acetominophen, pseudoephedrine HCl, dextromethorphan HBr monohydrate	160 mg; 15 mg; 5 mg	Throat Pain and Cough	Novartis Consumer Health	OraSolv®
Triaminic® Softchews Cold and Allergy	Pseudoephedrine, chlorpheniramine maleate	15 mg; 1 mg	Cold and Allergy	Novartis Consumer Health	OraSolv®
Zomig® Rapimelt	Zolmitriptan	2.5 mg	Migraine	AstraZeneca	OraSolv®
Zomig® ZMT	Zolmitriptan	2.5 mg	Migraine	Oragnon Inc	DuraSolv®
Nasea® OD Tablet	Ramosetron HCl	0.1 mg	Nausea and vomiting	Astellas Pharma Inc.	Wowtab®
Benadryl® Fastmelt	Diphenhydramine citrate	12.5 mg	Allergy and sinus pressure relief	McNeil-PPC, Inc	Wowtab®
Children's Benadryl® Allergy & Cold Fastmelt	Diphenhydramine; pseudoephedrine	19 mg; 30 mg	Allergy, cold and sinus	McNeil-PPC, Inc	Wowtab®
Gaster® OD Tablet	Famotidine	10 mg, 20 mg	Peptic ulcers and gastritis	Astellas Pharma Inc.	Wowtab®
Harnal® D Tab	Tamsulosin HCl	0.1 mg, 0.2 mg	Benign prostatic hyperplasia	Astellas Pharma Inc.	Wowtab®
Irribow® OD Tablet	Ramosetron HCl	2.5 µg, 5 µg	Irritable bowel syndrome	Astellas Pharma Inc.	Wowtab®
Vesicare® OD Tab	Solifenacin Succinate	2.5 mg, 5 mg	Overactive bladder	Astellas Pharma Inc.	Wowtab®
Calpol® Six Plus Fastmelts	Paracetamol	250 mg	Pain and fever	Pfizer/McNeil Products Ltd	Flashtab®

(Table 3) contd.....

Drug Product	Drug	Dose	Indication	Marketed by	FDT Technology
Nurofen® Recovery (mint flavoured), Nurofen® Meltlets (lemon flavoured), Nurofen® Meltlets, Neurofen® tabs	Ibuprofen	100 mg, 200 mg	Pain, fever and inflammation	Boots/Reckitt Benckiser	Flashtab®
Oxynormoro®	Oxycodone	5 mg, 10 mg, 20 mg	Severe pain	Mundipharma	Flashtab®
Paracetamol Flashtab®	Paracetamol	500 mg	Pain and fever	Ranbaxy	Flashtab®
Solupred® Orodispersible	Prednisolone	20 mg	Asthma, atopic dermatitis, and seasonal and perennial allergic rhinitis	Sanofi-Aventis	Flashtab®
Tachipirina® Flashtab®	Paracetamol	250 mg, 500 mg	Pain and fever	Angelini	Flashtab®
Trambax® MD-tab	Tramadol HCl	50 mg	Moderate to severe pain	Ranbaxy	Flashtab®
Tramelene® Flashtab®	Tramadol HCl	50 mg	Moderate to severe pain	Ethypharm	Flashtab®
Zamadol® Melt / Travex®	Tramadol HCl	50 mg	Moderate to severe pain	MEDA Pharma	Flashtab®
Ondansetron Flashtab®	Ondansetron	4 mg, 8 mg	Emesis	UKPAR Teva	Flashtab®
Excedrin® Quicktabs	Acetaminophen; caffeine	500 mg; 65 mg	Pain and fever	Bristol-Myers Squibb	Flashtab®
Taglo® Flas	Acetaminophen	500 mg	Pain and fever	Laboratorios ERN, S.A	Flashtab®
Dolflash®	Acetaminophen	500 mg	Pain and fever	Sanofi-Synthelab	Flashtab®
Prevacid® Solutab (Delayed Release ODT)	Lansoprazole	15 mg, 30 mg	Duodenal and gastric ulcers, and the common symptoms GERD including heartburn and erosive oesophagitis	Takeda	Flashtab®
Tovalt® ODT	Zolpidem tartrate	5 mg, 10 mg	Insomnia	Biovail	FlashDose®

(Table 3) contd.....

Drug Product	Drug	Dose	Indication	Marketed by	FDT Technology
Relivia® Flashdose	Tramadol HCl	50 mg	Moderate to severe pain	Biovail	FlashDose®
Fluoxetine ODT	Fluoxetine	5 mg, 10 mg, 15 mg, 20 mg	Depression	Biovail	FlashDose®
Citalopram Hydrobromide ODT	Citalopram HBr	Eq. 10 mg base, Eq. 20 mg base, Eq. 40 mg base	Depression	Biovail	FlashDose®
Hyoscyamine Sulfate ODT	Hyoscyamine sulphate	0.125 mg	Ulcers	Perrigo (Previously KV Pharma)	OraQuick®
Nauzelin® OD	Domperidone	5 mg, 10 mg	Gastrointestinal prokinetic agent	Kyowa Hakko Kirin	Solblet®
Allelock® OD	Olopatadine HCl	2.5 mg, 5 mg	Allergy	Kyowa Hakko Kirin	Solblet®
Lamictal® ODT	Lamotrigine	25 mg, 50 mg, 100 mg, 200 mg	Bipolar disorders and epilepsy	Glaxosmithkline	Advatab®
Unisom® SleepMelt	Diphenhydramine HCl	25 mg	Night-time sleep aid	Chattem, Inc.	Advatab®
Cibalgina® Due Fast	Ibuprofen	100 mg, 200 mg	Inflammation and pain	Novartis Consumer Healthcare	Ziplets®
Caffé Magia®	Vitamin B and caffeine		To stay alert and awake	Akina	Frosta®
Ceto-Q®	Mannitol, calcium carbonate, xylitol, yucca extract, *etc.*		Toothpaste tablet	Akina	Frosta®
Pletaal® OD	Cilostazol	50 mg, 100 mg	Antiplatelet	Otsuka	IDTAB® technology
DOPS® OD Tablets	Droxidopa	100 mg, 200 mg	Parkinson's disease	Dainippon Sumitomo Pharma	SUITAB-MAX®
Amlodipine OD tablet	Amlodipine	2.5 mg, 5 mg, 10 mg	Hypertension	Towa	RACTAB®

Table 4. List of proprietary FDOF technologies and companies developing these technologies.

Proprietary FDOF Technology	Company	Website
PharmFilm®	MonoSol Rx, APR Pharma	http://www.monosolrx.com
Rapidfilm®	tesa Labtec	www.tesa-labtec.com
Rapidfilm®	APR Applied Pharma Research	http://www.apr.ch
Quick-Dis®	Lavipharm	http://www.lavipharm.gr
VersaFilm®	IntelGenx	http://www.intelgenx.com
Solves Strips®	Pace Wellness	http://pacewellness.com
	Biofilm	http://www.biofilm.co.uk
	ODF Technologies Inc.	http://www.odftechnologies.com
	FFT Medical	http://fftmedical.se
	Cynapsus Therapeutics	http://www.cynapsus.ca
	Biodelivery Science International	http://www.bdsi.com
	LTS Lohman	http://www.ltslohmann.de
	C L Pharma	http://www.clpharm.com
	Kyukyu Pharmaceutical	http://www.qqp.co.jp
	Sato	http://www.zentripsato.com
	NU Therapeutics	http://nutherapeutics.com
	Prestige Brands	http://prestigebrands.com/
	Umang Pharmaceuticals	http://www.umangpharmaceuticals.com

Table 5. Marketed FDOF products.

Drug Product	API and Dose	Indications	Companies Involved
Amlodipine Besilate OD Film	Amlodipine (2.5 mg)	Hypertension	Kyukyu Pharmaceutical and Biomedix
Antimal® ODF	Primaquine phosphate (26.3 mg)	Antiprotozoal	CL Pharm
Aspirin81	Aspirin (81 mg)	Arthritis, toothaches, and other pains aggravated by inflammation	Pace Wellness
BEMA® Buprenorphine	Buprenorphine	Therapeutic alternative for patients with incomplete pain relief or those unable to tolerate	Bio Delivery Sciences International
Benadryl® Allergy Quickdissolve	Diphenhydramine HCl (25 mg)	Common cold, hey fever and other respiratory allergies	McNeil
Breakyl®	Fentanyl (200 μg, 400 μg, 600 μg, 8000 μg, 1200 μg)	Breakthrough pain	Meda and LTS Lohmann Therapie- Systeme AG

(Table 5) contd.....

Drug Product	API and Dose	Indications	Companies Involved
Caffeine strips	Caffeine (40 mg)	Instant energey boost	Biofilm
Chloraceptic® Sore Throat Relief Strips	Benzocaine	Sore throat	Prestige Brands and Zengen
Confidence®	Sildenafil citrate (70.23 mg)	Erectile dysfunction	CL Pharm and YuYu Pharma, Inc.
Donepezil HCl OD film	Donepezil HCl (3 mg, 5 mg, 10 mg)	Alzheimer's disease	Kyukyu Pharmaceutical and Elmed Eisai Co., Ltd.
Donepzil HCl Orodispersible Film	Donepezil HCl (5 mg, 10 mg)	Dementia in Alzheimer	Hexal and Sandoz
EDForce® F	Sildenafil citrate (70.23 mg)	Erectile dysfunction	CL Pharm and YuHan corporation
Gas-X® Tongue Twisters® Thin Strips	Simethicone (40 mg, 62.5 mg, 125 mg)	Flatulence, hyperacidity, GERD and ulcers	Novartis
Ignis® Oral Disintegration Film	Sildenafil Citrate (70.23 mg)	Erectile dysfunction	CL Pharm
Jaigra®	Sildenafil citrate (70.23 mg)	Erectile dysfunction	CL Pharm and DongKoo Bio&Pharma
Loratadine OD Film	Loratadine (10 mg)	Hay fever or other upper respiratory allergies	Kyukyu Pharmaceutical and Mochida Pharmaceutical
Melatonin Strips	Melatonin	Insomnia	Pace Wellness
Nicabate®/Niquintin® Mint Oral Film	Nicotine (2.5 mg)	Tobacco dependence	Glaxosmithkline and LTS Lohmann Therapie-Systeme AG
Night Time Triaminic® Thin Strips Cold and Cough	Diphenhydramine HCl (12.5 mg) and phenlyephrine HCl (5 mg)	Anthihistaine/cough suppresant, nasal decongestant, itchy and runny nose	Novartis
Olanzapine Renatos® Orodispersible Film	Olanzapine (5 mg, 10 mg, 15 mg)	Schizophrenia, bipolar disorder	Renatos Pharmavertriebsges nbH and Labtec GmbH
Olopatadine HCl OD Film	Olopatadine HCl (2.5 mg, 5 mg)	Allergy	Kyukyu Pharmaceutical and Maruho
Ondansetron HCl Orally Disintegrating Strips	Ondansetron HCl (2 mg, 4 mg, 8 mg)	Chemotherapy induced nausea and vomiting	NU Therapeutics
Ondissolve® ODF	Ondansetron HCl (4 mg, 8 mg)	Chemotherapy and radiotherapy induced nausea and vomiting	Takeda Canada Inc. and tesa Labtec
Onsolis® (Buccal Soluble film)	Fentanyl (400 mcg)	Pain in opioid–tolerant patients	Bio Delivery Sciences International, Meda, Kunwha Pharmaceutical, TTY Biopharm) and LTS Lohmann Therapie-Systeme AG

(Table 5) contd.....

Drug Product	API and Dose	Indications	Companies Involved
Ramea® Oral Disintegration Film	Ramosetron HCl 0.1mg	Antiemetic	CL Pharm and KwangDong Pharmaceutical
Risperidone Hexal SF	Risperidone (0.5 mg, 1 mg)	Schizophrenia	Hexal, LabTec and Applied Pharma
Rizaport®	Rizatriptan	Migraine	IntelGenx and RedHill Biopharma
Setofilm®	Ondansetron HCl (4 mg, 8 mg)	Chemotherapy and radiotherapy induced nausea and vomiting	Norgine Ltd. and tesa Labtec
Sildenafil Citrate Orally Disintegrating Strips	Sildenafil Citrate (25 mg, 50 mg)	Erectile dysfunction	NU Therapeutics
Sildenafil Sandoz / Tornetis®/SlideHexal SF Orodispersible Film	Sildenfafil citrate (25 mg, 50 mg, 75 mg)	Erectile dysfunction	Hexal and Sandoz
Simethicone Orally Disintegrating Strips	Simethicone (62.5 mg)	Flatulence	NU Therapeutics
Simethicone Strips	Simethicone (40 mg)	Painful infant gas	Pace Wellness and Biofilm
Suboxone® Sublingual	Buprenorphine and naloxone (2 mg/0.5 mg, 1 mg/1 mg, 8 mg/2 mg, 12 mg/3 mg)	Opioid addiction	Indivior Inc. and MonoSol Rx
Subutex®	Buprenorphine (2 mg, 8 mg)	Opioid addiction	Reckitt Benkiser and MonoSol Rx
Tadalafil® Orally Disintegrating Strips	Tadalafil (10 mg, 20 mg)	Erectile dysfunction	NU Therapeutics
Tadalafil®	Taladafil	Erectile dysfunction	IntelGenx and RedHill Biopharma
Theraflu® Cold/Cough Nighttime strips	Phenylephrine (10 mg) and dextromethorphan HBr (25 mg)	Nasal congestion, runny nose, sneezing, itchy nose and throat	Novartis
Theraflu® Thin Strips Cough	Dextrometorphan HCl (5 mg)	Antitussive	Novartis
Theraflu® Thin Strips Daytime Cold and Cough	Dextromethorphan (3.67 mg) (equivalent to 5 mg Dextromethorphan HBr) and phenylephrine HCl (2.5 mg)	Nasal decongestant	Novartis
Theraflu® Thin Strips Multi Sympton	Diphenhydramine (25 mg)	Nasal and sinus congestion	Novartis
Traful® Direct	Triamcinolone acetonide	Stomatitis	Kyukyu Pharmaceutical and Daichi Sankyo Healthcare

(Table 5) contd.....

Drug Product	API and Dose	Indications	Companies Involved
Vinix®	Sildenafil citrate (70.23 mg)	Erectile dysfunction	CL Pharm
Voglibose OD Film	Voglibose (0.2 mg, 0.3 mg)	Diabetes	Kyukyu Pharmaceutical and Mochida Pharmaceutical
Zentrip®	Meclizine HCl (25 mg)	Motion sickness	Sato Pharmaceutical
Zolmitriptan Renatos	Zolmitriptan (2.5 mg)	Migraine	Renatos Pharmavertriebsges and Labtec gmbH
Zolpidem Tartrate OD Film	Zolpidem tartrate (5 mg, 10 mg)	Insomnia	Kyukyu Pharmaceutical and Mochida Pharmaceutical
Zuplenz® Oral Soluble Film	Ondansetron HCl (4 mg, 8 mg)	Chemotherapy and radiotherapy induced nausea and vomiting	Galena Biopharma, Vestiq Pharmaceuticals, Monosol Rx LLC and APR Applied Pharma

3. FDDF PRODUCTS IN UNITED STATES

Generic drug products or therapeutic equivalent products have same clinical effect and safety profile when administered to patients. US FDA approves therapeutic equivalent products in United States (US) as generic drug products, as per section 505 of the federal Food, Drug and Cosmetic Act (FDA), which is followed by their publication in the Orange Book.

Orange Book classifies therapeutic equivalent products on the basis of following general criterion:

- Products are approved as safe and effective
- Products are pharmaceutical equivalents in that they (a) contain identical amounts of the same active drug ingredient in the same dosage form and route of administration and (b) meet compendial or other applicable standards of strength, quality, purity and identity
- Products are bioequivalent in that (a) they do not present a known or potential bioequivalence problem, and they meet an acceptable *in vitro* standard or (b) if they do present such a known or potential problem, they are shown to meet an appropriate bioequivalence standard
- Products are adequately labelled
- Products are manufactured in compliance with Current Good Manufacturing Practice (cGMP) regulations.

Table **6** and Table **7** provide various prescription drug products and OTC drug products, respectively, approved by US FDA and enlisted in Orange Book. Table **8** provides a list of discontinued FDDF products.

Table 6. Fast dissolving/disintegrating prescription drug products approved by US FDA and listed in Orange Book.

Dosage Form, Type; Route of Administration, Drug/Drug Product	Manufacturer/ Distributor	Dosage Strengths	Approval Date
Tablet, Orally Disintegrating; Oral; Alprazolam	Actavis Elizabeth	0.25 mg, 0.5 mg, 1 mg, 2 mg	16 Mar 10
Tablet, Orally Disintegrating; Oral; Alprazolam	Par Pharm	0.25 mg, 0.5 mg, 1 mg, 2 mg	9 Jan 09
Tablet, Orally Disintegrating; Oral; Niravam® (Alprazolam)	UCB Inc	0.25 mg, 0.5 mg, 1 mg, 2 mg	19 Jan 05
Tablet, Orally Disintegrating; Oral; Abilify (Aripiprazole)	Otsuka	10 mg, 15 mg	7 Jun 06
Tablet, Orally Disintegrating; Oral; Carbidopa and Levodopa	Mylan	25 mg + 250 mg	18 Sep 08
Tablet, Orally Disintegrating; Oral; Carbidopa and Levodopa	Mylan	10 mg + 100 mg, 25 mg + 100 mg, 25 mg + 250 mg	18 Sep 08
Tablet, Orally Disintegrating; Oral; Carbidopa and Levodopa	Sun Pharm Inds	10 mg + 100 mg, 25 mg + 100 mg, 25 mg + 250 mg	31 Jul 09
Tablet, Orally Disintegrating; Oral; Clonazepam	Barr	0.12 mg, 0.25 mg, 0.5 mg, 1 mg, 2 mg	10 Aug 05
Tablet, Orally Disintegrating; Oral; Clonazepam	Par Pharm	0.12 mg, 0.25 mg, 0.5 mg, 1 mg, 2 mg	3 Aug 05
Tablet, Orally Disintegrating; Oral; Clonazepam	Sun Pharm Inds Inc	0.125 mg, 0.25 mg, 0.5 mg, 1 mg, 2 mg	27 Aug 14
Tablet, Orally Disintegrating; Oral; FazaClo® ODT (Clozapine)	Jazz Pharms III	12.5 mg	30 May 07
Tablet, Orally Disintegrating; Oral; FazaClo® ODT (Clozapine)	Jazz Pharms III	25 mg, 100 mg	10 Feb 04
Tablet, Orally Disintegrating; Oral; FazaClo® ODT (Clozapine)	Jazz Pharms III	150 mg, 200 mg	9 Jul 10
Tablet, Orally Disintegrating; Oral; Clarinex® (Desloratadine)	Merck Sharp Dohme	2.5 mg	14 Jul 05
Tablet, Orally Disintegrating; Oral; Clarinex® (Desloratadine)	Merck Sharp Dohme	5 mg	26 Jun 02
Tablet, Orally Disintegrating; Oral; Desloratadine	Reddys	2.5 mg, 5 mg	12 Jul 10
Tablet, Orally Disintegrating; Oral; Aricept® ODT (Donepezil HCl)	Eisai Inc	5 mg, 10 mg	18 Oct 04

(Table 6) contd.....

Dosage Form, Type; Route of Administration, Drug/Drug Product	Manufacturer/ Distributor	Dosage Strengths	Approval Date
Tablet, Orally Disintegrating; Oral; Donepezil HCl	Barr	5 mg, 10 mg	26 Nov 10
Tablet, Orally Disintegrating; Oral; Donepezil HCl	Macleods Pharms Ltd	5 mg, 10 mg	14 Dec 12
Tablet, Orally Disintegrating; Oral; Donepezil HCl	Sandoz	5 mg, 10 mg	14 Dec 12
Tablet, Orally Disintegrating; Oral; Donepezil HCl	Zydus Pharms Usa Inc	5 mg, 10 mg	10 May 11
Tablet, Orally Disintegrating; Oral; Lamictal® ODT (Lamotrigine)	Glaxosmithkline LLC	25 mg, 50 mg, 100 mg, 200 mg	8 May 09
Tablet, Orally Disintegrating; Oral; Lamotrigine	Impax Labs Inc	25 mg, 50 mg, 100 mg, 200 mg	15 Jul 13
Tablet, Delayed Release, Orally Disintegrating; Oral; Prevacid® (Lansoprazole)	Takeda Pharms USA	15 mg, 30 mg	30 Aug 02
Tablet, Delayed Release, Orally Disintegrating; Oral; Lansoprazole	Ani Pharms Inc	15 mg,30 mg	15 Oct 10
Tablet, Orally Disintegrating; Oral; Metozolv® ODT (Metoclopramide HCl)	Salix Pharms	Eq. 5 mg base	4 Sep 09
Tablet, Orally Disintegrating; Oral; Metozolv® ODT (Metoclopramide HCl)	Novel Labs Inc	Eq. 5 mg base, Eq. 10 mg base	15 Aug 14
Tablet, Orally Disintegrating; Oral; Mirtazapine	Actavis Elizabeth	15 mg, 30 mg, 45 mg	31 Aug 05
Tablet, Orally Disintegrating; Oral; Mirtazapine	Aurobindo Pharma Ltd	15 mg, 30 mg	8 Dec 05
Tablet, Orally Disintegrating; Oral; Mirtazapine	Aurobindo Pharma Ltd	45 mg	28 Feb 06
Tablet, Orally Disintegrating; Oral; Mirtazapine	Teva	15 mg, 30 mg	28 Jun 05
Tablet, Orally Disintegrating; Oral; Remeron® Soltab™ (Mirtazapine)	Organon Usa Inc	15 mg, 30 mg	12 Jan 01
Tablet, Orally Disintegrating; Oral; Olanzapine	Apotex Inc	5 mg, 10 mg, 15 mg, 20 mg	24 Oct 11
Tablet, Orally Disintegrating; Oral; Olanzapine	Aurobindo Pharma Ltd	5 mg, 10 mg, 15 mg, 20 mg	15 May 14
Tablet, Orally Disintegrating; Oral; Olanzapine	Barr Labs Inc	5 mg, 10 mg, 15 mg, 20 mg	30 Jan 12
Tablet, Orally Disintegrating; Oral; Olanzapine	Dr Reddys Labs Ltd	5 mg, 10 mg, 15 mg, 20 mg	24 Oct 11
Tablet, Orally Disintegrating; Oral; Olanzapine	Jubilant Generics	5 mg, 10 mg, 15 mg, 20 mg	12 Sep 12

(Table 6) contd.....

Dosage Form, Type; Route of Administration, Drug/Drug Product	Manufacturer/ Distributor	Dosage Strengths	Approval Date
Tablet, Orally Disintegrating; Oral; Olanzapine	Mylan Pharms Inc	7 mg, 10 mg, 15 mg, 20 mg	12 May 14
Tablet, Orally Disintegrating; Oral; Olanzapine	Par Pharm	5 mg, 10 mg, 15 mg, 20 mg	24 Oct 11
Tablet, Orally Disintegrating; Oral; Olanzapine	Sun Pharm Inds	5 mg, 10 mg, 15 mg, 20 mg	28 Feb 12
Tablet, Orally Disintegrating; Oral; Olanzapine	Torrent Pharms LLC	6 mg, 10 mg, 15 mg, 20 mg	25 Oct 11
Tablet, Orally Disintegrating; Oral; Zyprexa® Zydis® (Olanzapine)	Lilly	7 mg, 10 mg, 15 mg, 20 mg	6 Apr 00
Tablet, Orally Disintegrating; Oral; Oral Zofran® ODT (Ondansetron)	Glaxosmithkline	4 mg, 8 mg	27 Jan 99
Tablet, Orally Disintegrating; Oral; Ondansetron	Aurobindo Pharma	4 mg, 8 mg	12 Apr 10
Tablet, Orally Disintegrating; Oral; Ondansetron	Barr	4 mg, 8 mg	25 Jun 07
Tablet, Orally Disintegrating; Oral; Ondansetron	Glenmark Generics	4 mg, 8 mg	27 Jun 07
Tablet, Orally Disintegrating; Oral; Ondansetron	Mylan	4 mg, 8 mg	25 Jun 07
Tablet, Orally Disintegrating; Oral; Ondansetron	Ranbaxy	4 mg, 8 mg	24 Feb 11
Tablet, Orally Disintegrating; Oral; Ondansetron	Sandoz	4 mg, 8 mg	13 Aug 07
Tablet, Orally Disintegrating; Oral; Ondansetron	Sun Pharm Inds	4 mg, 8 mg	2 Aug 07
Tablet, Orally Disintegrating; Oral; Ondansetron	Teva	4 mg, 8 mg	25 Jun 07
Tablet, Orally Disintegrating; Oral; Zofran® ODT (Ondansetron)	Glaxosmithkline	4 mg, 8 mg	27 Jan 99
Film; Oral; Zuplenz®	Vestiq Pharms	4 mg, 8 mg	2 Jul 10
Tablet, Orally Disintegrating; Oral; Suprenza® (Phentermine Hydrochloride)	Citius Pharms	15 mg, 30 mg	13 Jun 11
Tablet, Orally Disintegrating; Oral; Suprenza® (Phentermine Hydrochloride)	Citius Pharms	37.5 mg	27 Mar 12
Tablet, Orally Disintegrating; Oral; Orapred® ODT (Prednisolone sodium phosphate)	Concordia Pharms Inc	Eq. 10 mg base, Eq. 15 mg base, Eq. 30 mg base	1 Jun 06
Tablet, Orally Disintegrating; Oral; Prednisolone Sodium Phosphate	Mylan Pharms Inc	Eq. 10 mg base, Eq. 15 mg base, Eq. 30 mg base	10 Apr 13

(Table 6) contd.....

Dosage Form, Type; Route of Administration, Drug/Drug Product	Manufacturer/ Distributor	Dosage Strengths	Approval Date
Tablet, Orally Disintegrating; Oral; Risperidone	Dr Reddys Labs Ltd	0.5 mg	24 Feb 09
Tablet, Orally Disintegrating; Oral; Risperidone	Dr Reddys Labs Ltd	1 mg	5 Oct 09
Tablet, Orally Disintegrating; Oral; Risperidone	Dr Reddys Labs Ltd	2 mg	24 Feb 09
Tablet, Orally Disintegrating; Oral; Risperidone	Jubilant Organosys	0.5 mg, 1 mg, 2 mg, 3 mg, 4 mg	4 Nov 11
Tablet, Orally Disintegrating; Oral; Risperidone	Mylan Pharms Inc	0.25 mg	12 Feb 13
Tablet, Orally Disintegrating; Oral; Risperidone	Mylan Pharms Inc	0.5 mg, 1 mg, 2 mg, 3 mg, 4 mg	30 Mar 11
Tablet, Orally Disintegrating; Oral; Risperidone	Par Pharm	0.25, 0.5 mg, 2 mg, 3 mg, 4 mg	30 Apr 09
Tablet, Orally Disintegrating; Oral; Risperidone	Par Pharm	1 mg	26 Oct 09
Tablet, Orally Disintegrating; Oral; Risperidone	Ranbaxy	0.5 mg, 1 mg, 2 mg, 3 mg, 4 mg	6 Aug 10
Tablet, Orally Disintegrating; Oral; Risperidone	Sandoz	0.5 mg, 1 mg, 2 mg, 3 mg, 4 mg	22 Dec 09
Tablet, Orally Disintegrating; Oral; Risperidone	Sun Pharm Ind ltd	0.5 mg, 1 mg, 2 mg, 3 mg, 4 mg	8 Apr 13
Tablet, Orally Disintegrating; Oral; Risperidone	Teva	0.5 mg, 1 mg, 2 mg	12 Mar 12
Tablet, Orally Disintegrating; Oral; Risperidone	Watson Labs Florida	0.5 mg, 1 mg, 2 mg, 3 mg, 4 mg	19 Apr 11
Tablet, Orally Disintegrating; Oral; Risperidone	Zydus Pharms USA	0.5 mg, 2 mg	1 May 09
Tablet, Orally Disintegrating; Oral; Risperdal (Risperidone)	Janssen Pharms	0.5 mg, 1 mg, 2 mg	2 Apr 03
Tablet, Orally Disintegrating; Oral; Risperdal (Risperidone)	Janssen Pharms	3 mg, 4 mg	23 Dec 04
Tablet, Orally Disintegrating; Oral; Maxalt-MLT® (Rizatriptan Benzoate)	Merck	Eq. 5 mg base, Eq. 10 mg base	29 Jun 98
Tablet, Orally Disintegrating; Oral; Rizatriptan Benzoate	Apotex Inc	Eq. 5 mg base, Eq. 10 mg base	1 Jul 13
Tablet, Orally Disintegrating; Oral; Rizatriptan Benzoate	Aurobindo Pharma Ltd	Eq. 5 mg base, Eq. 10 mg base	1 Jul 13
Tablet, Orally Disintegrating; Oral; Rizatriptan Benzoate	Glenmark Generics	Eq. 5 mg base, Eq. 10 mg base	1 Jul 13
Tablet, Orally Disintegrating; Oral; Rizatriptan Benzoate	Mylan Pharms Inc	Eq. 5 mg base, Eq. 10 mg base	31 Dec 12

(Table 6) contd.....

Dosage Form, Type; Route of Administration, Drug/Drug Product	Manufacturer/ Distributor	Dosage Strengths	Approval Date
Tablet, Orally Disintegrating; Oral; Rizatriptan Benzoate	Natco Pharma Ltd	Eq. 5 mg base, Eq. 10 mg base	1 Jul 13
Tablet, Orally Disintegrating; Oral; Rizatriptan Benzoate	Sandoz	Eq. 5 mg base, Eq. 10 mg base	1 Jul 13
Tablet, Orally Disintegrating; Oral; Zelapar® (Selegeline HCl)	Valeant Pharm Intl	1.25 mg	14 Jun 06
Tablet, Orally Disintegrating; Oral; Staxyn® (Vardenafil HCl)	Bayer Hlthcare	10 mg	17 Jun 10
Tablet, Orally Disintegrating; Oral; Zolmitriptan	Apotex Inc	2.5 mg, 5 mg	14 May 13
Tablet, Orally Disintegrating; Oral; Zolmitriptan	Glenmark Generics	2.5 mg, 5 mg	14 May 13
Tablet, Orally Disintegrating; Oral; Zolmitriptan	Zydus Pharms USA Inc	2.5 mg, 5 mg	15 May 13
Tablet, Orally Disintegrating; Oral; Zomig-ZMT® (Zolmitriptan)	Astrazeneca	2.5 mg, 5 mg	13 Feb 01

Table 7. Fast dissolving/disintegrating OTC drug products approved by US FDA and listed in Orange Book.

Dosage Form, Type; Route of Administration, Drug/Drug Product	Manufacturer/ Distributor	Dosage Strengths	Approval Date
Tablet, Orally Disintegrating; Oral; Children's Allegra® Allergy (Fexofenadine HCl)	Sanofi Aventis US	30 mg	24 Jan 11
Tablet, Orally Disintegrating; Oral; Children's Allegra® Hives	Sanofi Aventis US	30 mg	24 Jan 11
Tablet, Orally Disintegrating; Oral; Children's Fexofenadine HCl Allergy	Dr Reddys Labs Ltd	30 mg	18 Jan 13
Tablet, Orally Disintegrating; Oral; Children's Fexofenadine HCl Hives	Dr Reddys Labs Ltd	30 mg	18 Jan 13
Tablet, Orally Disintegrating; Oral; Alavert® (Loratadine)	Pfizer	10 mg	19 Dec 02
Tablet, Orally Disintegrating; Oral; Claritin® Hives Relief Reditab	Schering Plough	10 mg	19 Nov 03
Tablet, Orally Disintegrating; Oral; Claritin® Reditabs	Schering Plough	5 mg	12 Dec 06
Tablet, Orally Disintegrating; Oral; Claritin® Reditabs	Schering Plough	10 mg	27 Nov 02
Tablet, Orally Disintegrating; Oral; Loratadine	Impax Labs	10 mg	29 Sep 03
Tablet, Orally Disintegrating; Oral; Loratadine	Pfizer	10 mg	10 Feb 03
Tablet, Orally Disintegrating; Oral; Loratadine	Watson Labs Florida	10 mg	3 Nov 03

(Table 7) contd.....

Dosage Form, Type; Route of Administration, Drug/Drug Product	Manufacturer/ Distributor	Dosage Strengths	Approval Date
Tablet, Orally Disintegrating; Oral; Loratadine Redidose	Ranbaxy	10 mg	11 Apr 07
Tablet, Orally Disintegrating; Oral; Zyrtec® Allergy (Cetirizine HCl)	Mcneil Consumer	10 mg	3 Sep 10

Table 8. Fast dissolving/disintegrating drug products discontinued by US FDA and listed as discontinued in Orange Book.

Dosage Form, Type; Route of Administration, Drug/Drug Product	Manufacturer/ Distributor	Dosage Strengths	Approval Date
Film, Oral; Nexcede® (Ketoprofen)	Novartis	12.5 mg	25 Nov 09
Film; Buccal; Onsolis® (Fentanyl Citrate)	Meda Pharms	Eq. 0.2 mg base, 0.4 mg base, 0.6 mg base, 0.8 mg base, 1.2 mg base	16 Jul 09
Tablet, Orally Disintegrating; Oral Amlodipine Besylate	Synthon Pharms	Eq. 2.5 mg base, Eq. 5 mg base, Eq. 10 mg base	27 Sep 07
Tablet, Orally Disintegrating; Oral Abilify® (Aripiprazole)	Otsuka	20 mg, 30 mg	7 Jun 06
Tablet, Orally Disintegrating; Oral Kemstro® (Baclofen)	UCB Inc	10 mg, 20 mg	30 Oct 03
Tablet, Orally Disintegrating; Oral Propulsid® Quicksolv (Cisapride Monohydrate)	Janssen Pharma	Eq. 20 mg base	7 Nov 97
Tablet, Orally Disintegrating; Oral Citalopram HBr	Biovail Labs Intl	Eq. 10 mg base, Eq. 20 mg base, Eq. 40 mg base	20 Dec 05
Tablet, Orally Disintegrating; Oral Klonopin® Rapidly Disintegrating (Clonazepam)	Roche	0.125 mg, 0.25 mg, 0.5 mg, 1 mg, 2 mg	23 Dec 97
Tablet, Orally Disintegrating; Oral Fazaclo® ODT (Clozapine)	Jazz Pharms III	50 mg	3 Jun 05
Tablet, Orally Disintegrating; Oral Donepezil HCl	Mutual Pharm	5 mg, 10 mg	11 Dec 09
Tablet, Orally Disintegrating; Oral; Fluxid® (Famotidine)	UCB Inc	20 mg, 40 mg	24 Sep 04
Tablet, Orally Disintegrating; Oral; Pepsid® RPD (Famotidine)	Merck	20 mg, 40 mg	28 May 98
Tablet, Delayed Release, Orally Disintegrating; Oral Lansoprazole	Teva Pharms	15 mg, 30 mg	15 Oct 10
Tablet, Orally Disintegrating; Oral Metozolv® ODT (Metoclopramide HCl)	Salix Pharms	Eq. 10 mg base	4 Sep 09
Tablet, Orally Disintegrating; Oral Reglan® ODT (Metoclopramide HCl)	Meda Pharms	Eq. 5 mg base, Eq. 10 mg base	10 Jun 05

(Table 8) contd.....

Dosage Form, Type; Route of Administration, Drug/Drug Product	Manufacturer/ Distributor	Dosage Strengths	Approval Date
Tablet, Orally Disintegrating; Oral Mirtazapine	Actavis Elizabeth	15 mg, 30 mg, 45 mg	14 Feb 11
Tablet, Orally Disintegrating; Oral Mirtazapine	Actavis Totowa	15 mg, 30 mg, 45 mg	31 Aug 05
Tablet, Orally Disintegrating; Oral Ondansetron	Nesher Pharms	4 mg, 8 mg	25 Jun 07
Tablet, Orally Disintegrating; Oral Ondansetron	Par Pharm	4 mg, 8 mg, 16 mg, 24 mg	26 Dec 06
Tablet, Orally Disintegrating; Oral Simvastatin	Synthon Pharms	10 mg, 20 mg, 40 mg, 80 mg	9 Oct 07
Tablet, Orally Disintegrating; Oral Rybix® ODT (Tramadol HCl)	Shionogi Inc	50 mg	5 May 05
Tablet, Orally Disintegrating; Oral Tovalt ODT (Zolpidem Tartrate)	Biovail Labs Intl	5 mg, 10 mg	25 Apr 07
Tablet, Orally Disintegrating; Oral; Carbidopa and Levodopa	Impax Labs	10 mg + 100 mg, 25 mg + 100 mg, 25 mg + 250 mg	8 Jun 10
Tablet, Orally Disintegrating; Oral; Parcopa (Carbidopa and Levodopa)	UCB Inc	10 mg + 100 mg, 25 mg + 100 mg, 25 mg + 250 mg	27 Aug 04

4. FDDF PRODUCTS IN EUROPEAN UNION

European Medicines Agency (EMA) is the drug regulatory agency responsible for safety regulations of the food and drug products in European Union. FDDF products can be introduced in Europe market by a centralised procedure, decentralised procedure, national procedure or by mutual recognition procedure. Table **9** provides list of FDDF products approved by EMA. Products approved by MHRA (UK) are provided in Table **10**.

Table 9. Orodispersible tablets available in European market (Source http://www.ema.europa.eu/).

Brand	Drug	Dose	Indication	Manufacturer/ Distributor
Abilify®	Aripropazole	10 mg, 15 mg, 30 mg	Bipolar disorder and schizophrenia	Otsuka Pharmaceutical Europe Ltd
Aerius®	Desloratadine	2.5 mg, 5 mg	Urticaria, rhinitis, and allergy seasonal and perennial	Schering-Plough Europe
Agopton® Rapid	Lansoprazole	15 mg, 30 mg	Duodenal ulcer and gastric ulcer, reflux oesophagitis, symptomatic GERD, Zollinger-Ellison syndrome	Takeda Pharma GmbH

(Table 9) contd.....

Brand	Drug	Dose	Indication	Manufacturer/ Distributor
Alertin® Zydis®	Loratadine	10 mg	Allergic rhinitis and chronic idiopathic urticaria	Plough Farma, Lda
Azomyr®	Desloratadine	2.5, 5 mg	Urticaria, rhinitis, and allergy seasonal and perennial	Merck Sharp & Dohme Ltd.
Biperidys® Flash	Domperidone	20 mg	Nausea and vomiting	Pierre Fabre Médicament
Biperidys® Flash, comprimé orodispersible	Domperidone	20 mg	Nausea and vomiting	Pierre Fabre Médicament
Claritine® Zydis	Loratadine	10 mg	Allergic rhinitis and chronic idiopathic urticaria	Shering-Plough Farma, Lda
Domepridone Zentiva	Domperidone	10 mg	Nausea and vomiting	Sanofi-Aventis France
Domperidone Arrow	Domperidone	10 mg	Nausea and vomiting	Arrow Generiques
Domperidone Biogaran	Domperidone	10 mg	Nausea and vomiting	Biogaran
Domperidone Cristers	Domperidone	10 mg	Nausea and vomiting	Cristers
Domperidone EG	Domperidone	10 mg	Nausea and vomiting	EG Labo-Laboratoires Eurogenerics
Domperidone EG	Domperidone	10 mg	Nausea and vomiting	Eurogenerics SA
Domperidone instant EG	Domperidone	10 mg	Nausea and vomiting	Eurogenerics N.V.
Domperidone Mylan	Domperidone	10 mg	Nausea and vomiting	Mylan SAS
Domperidone Ratiopharm	Domperidone	10 mg	Nausea and vomiting	Rrtiopharm (Allemagne)
Domperidone Sandoz	Domperidone	10 mg	Nausea and vomiting	Sandoz
Domperidone Teva	Domperidone	10 mg	Nausea and vomiting	Teva Sante
Domperidone Pierre Fabre	Domperidone	10 mg	Nausea and vomiting	Pierre Fabre Médicament
Feldene® Dispersable Tablets, Feldene® Melt	Piroxicam	10 mg, 20 mg	Osteoarthritis, rheumatoid arthritis and ankylosing spondylitis	Pfizer Limited
Feldene® Lyotabs	Piroxicam	10 mg, 20 mg	Osteoarthritis, rheumatoid arthritis and ankylosing spondylitis	Aktuapharma N.V., Pfizer S.A, Pharmapartner N.V.

(Table 9) contd.....

Brand	Drug	Dose	Indication	Manufacturer/ Distributor
Fluoxetin Stada	Fluoxetine	20 mg	Depressive episode, obsessive-compulsive disorder and bulimia nervosa	Stada Arzneimittel AG
Fluoxetine Lilly	Fluoxetine	20 mg	Depressive episode, obsessive-compulsive disorder and bulimia nervosa	Lilly France
Fluoxetine Merck	Fluoxetine	20 mg	Depressive episode, obsessive-compulsive disorder and bulimia nervosa	Merck Generiques
Fluoxetine Qualimed	Fluoxetine	20 mg	Depressive episode, obsessive-compulsive disorder and bulimia nervosa	Qualimed
Lansox®	Lansoprazole	15 mg, 30 mg	Duodenal ulcer and gastric ulcer, reflux oesophagitis, symptomatic GERD and Zollinger-Ellison syndrome	Takeda Italia Farmaceutici S.p.A.
Lanzo®	Lansoprazole	15 mg, 30 mg	Duodenal ulcer and gastric ulcer, reflux oesophagitis, symptomatic GERD and Zollinger-Ellison syndrome	Wyeth AB
Laprazol® FasTab	Lansoprazole	15 mg, 30 mg	Duodenal ulcer and gastric ulcer, reflux oesophagitis, symptomatic GERD and Zollinger-Ellison syndrome	Vianex S.A.
Levitra®	Vardenafil	5 mg, 10 mg	Erectile dysfunction	Bayer Pharma AG
Limpidex®	Lansoprazole	15 mg, 30 mg	Duodenal ulcer and gastric ulcer, reflux oesophagitis, symptomatic GERD and Zollinger-Ellison syndrome	Sigma-Tau S.p.A.
Mirtatsapiini® Teva	Fluoxetine	15 mg, 30 mg, 45 mg	Depressive episode, obsessive-compulsive disorder and bulimia nervosa	Teva Pharma B.V
Motilium® Instant	Domperidone	10 mg	Nausea and vomiting	Johnson & Johnson Consumer N.V.
Motilium Instant 10 mg orodispersible tablet	Domperidone	10 mg	Nausea and vomiting	Johnson & Johnson Consumer N.V. / McNeil Products Limited
Muscoril®	Tiocolchicoside	8 mg	Muscle relaxant	Sanofi Aventis S.P.A.
Neoclarityn®	Desloratadine	2.5 mg, 5 mg	Urticaria, rhinitis, and allergy seasonal and perennial	Merck Sharp & Dohme Ltd.

(Table 9) contd.....

Brand	Drug	Dose	Indication	Manufacturer/ Distributor
Nimvastid®	Rivastigmine hydrogen tartrate	1.5 mg, 3 mg, 4.5 mg, 6 mg	Dementia, Parkinson disease and alzheimer disease	KRKA, d.d., Novo mesto, Slovenia
Norset®	Fluoxetine	15 mg, 30 mg, 45 mg	Depressive episode, obsessive-compulsive disorder and bulimia nervosa	Organon France
Ogasto®	Lansoprazole	15 mg, 30 mg	Duodenal ulcer and gastric ulcer, reflux oesophagitis, symptomatic GERD and Zollinger-Ellison syndrome	Seber Portuguesa Farmaceutica, SA
Olanzapine Apotex	Olanzapine	5 mg, 10 mg, 15 mg and 20 mg	Bipolar disorder and schizophrenia	Apotex Europe B.V.
Olanzapine Glenmark	Olanzapine	5 mg	Bipolar disorder and schizophrenia	Glenmark Europe
Olanzapine Teva	Olanzapine	5 mg, 10 mg, 15 mg, 20 mg	Bipolar disorder and schizophrenia	Teva Pharma B.V.
Olazax® Disperzi	Olanzapine	5 mg, 7.5 mg, 10 mg, 15 mg, 20 mg	Bipolar disorder and schizophrenia	Glenmark Pharmaceuticals s.r.o.
Opiren® Flas	Lansoprazole	15, 30 mg	Duodenal ulcer and gastric ulcer, reflux oesophagitis, symptomatic GERD and Zollinger-Ellison syndrome	Almirall Prodesfarma, S.A.
Oroperidys®	Domperidone	10 mg	Nausea and vomiting	Pierre Fabre Médicament
Prozac® Lilly	Fluoxetine	20 mg	Depressive episode, obsessive-compulsive disorder and bulimia nervosa	Lilly France
Raxar®	Domperidone	10 mg	Nausea and vomiting	Crinos S.P.A.
Relmus®	Tiocolchicoside	8 mg	Muscle relaxant	Sanofi - Produtos Farmacêuticos, Lda.
Remergil® Soltab™	Fluoxetine	15 mg, 30 mg, 45 mg	Depressive episode, obsessive-compulsive disorder and bulimia nervosa	Organon GmbH, Oberschleissheim
Remergon® Soltab™	Fluoxetine	15 mg, 30 mg, 45 mg	Depressive episode, obsessive-compulsive disorder and bulimia nervosa	Organon Europe B.V.

(Table 9) contd.....

Brand	Drug	Dose	Indication	Manufacturer/ Distributor
Remeron® Orodispersible Tablets	Fluoxetine	15 mg, 30 mg, 45 mg	Depressive episode, obsessive-compulsive disorder and bulimia nervosa	N. V. Organon, The Netherlands
Remeron® Smelt	Fluoxetine	15 mg, 30 mg, 45 mg	Depressive episode, obsessive-compulsive disorder and bulimia nervosa	NV. Organon, Holland
Remeron® Soltab™	Mirtazapine	15 mg, 30 mg	Depression	Organon Limited
Remeron® Soltab™	Fluoxetine	15 mg, 30 mg, 45 mg	Depressive episode, obsessive-compulsive disorder and bulimia nervosa	N.V. Organon
Remeron® Soltab™	Mirtazapine	15 mg, 30 mg, 45 mg	Depression	N.V. Organon
Risperdal® Quicklet®	Risperidone	0.5 mg, 1 mg, 2 mg, 3 mg, 4 mg	Schizophrenia and bipolar disorders	Janssen-Cilag Pharma GmbH, Janssen Farmacêutica, Johnson & Johnson
Risperidone J-C Instasolv	Risperidone	0.5 mg, 1 mg, 2 mg	Schizophrenia and bipolar disorders	Janssen Cilag N.V.
Rispolept® Quicklet®	Risperidone	2 mg	Schizophrenia and bipolar disorders	UAB, Johnson & Johnson
Rispolin® Quicklet®	Risperidone	0.5 mg, 1 mg, 2 mg, 3 mg, 4 mg	Schizophrenia and bipolar disorders	Janssen-Cilag Pharma GmbH
Sycrest®	Asenapine maleate	5 mg, 10 mg	Bipolar I disorder	N.V. Organon
Viagra®	Sildenafil	50 mg	Erectile dysfunction	Pfizer, Ltd.
Vivanza®	Vardenafil	5 mg, 10 mg, 20 mg	Erectile Dysfunction	Bayer Pharma AG
Vizarsin®	Sildenafil	25 mg	Erectile Dysfunction	Krka, d.d., Novo mesto, Slovenia
Zalasta®	Olanzapine	2.5 mg, 5 mg	Bipolar disorder and schizophrenia	KRKA, d.d., Novo mesto, Slovenia
Zispin® Soltab™	Fluoxetine	15 mg, 30 mg, 45 mg	Depressive episode, obsessive-compulsive disorder andulimia nervosa	Organon Laboratories Limited, Cambs

(Table 9) contd.....

Brand	Drug	Dose	Indication	Manufacturer/ Distributor
Zispin® SolTab™	Mirtazapine	15 mg, 30 mg, 45 mg	Depression	Organon (Ireland) Limited
Zonegram®	Zonisamide	25 mg, 50 mg, 100 mg, 300 mg	Epilepsies, Partial	Eisai Ltd
Zoton® FasTab™	Lansoprazole	15 mg, 30 mg	Duodenal ulcer and gastric ulcer, reflux oesophagitis, symptomatic GERD and Zollinger-Ellison syndrome	John Wyeth & Brother Limited, Wyeth Lederle S.p.A
Zyprexa® Zydis®, Zyprexa® Velotab™, Zypadhera®	Olanzapine	5 mg, 10 mg, 15 mg, 20 mg	Bipolar disorder and schizophrenia	Eli Lilly Netherland B.V

Table 10. Various fast dissolving/disintegrating drug products available in United Kingdom market (Source: http://www.medicines.org.uk/emc/).

Brand Name and Dosage Form	Drug	Dose	Manufacturer/ Distributor
Abilify® Orodispersible Tablets	Aripiprazole	10 mg, 15 mg, 30 mg	Otsuka Pharmaceuticals (UK) Ltd
Hayfever Relief Instant Melts® 10 mg	Loratadine	10 mg	The Boots Company PLC
Donepezil HCl Orodispersible Tablets	Donepezil HCl	5 mg	Sandoz Ltd
Donepezil HCl Orodispersible Tablets	Donepezil HCl Monohydrate	5 mg, 10 mg	Consilient Health Ltd
Donepezil HCl Orodispersible Tablets	Donepezil HCl	5 mg, 10 mg	Actavis UK Ltd
Levitra® Orodispersible Tablets	Vardenafil HCl	10 mg	Bayer PLC
Loratadine Orodispersible Tablets	Loratadine	10 mg	Sandoz Ltd
Mirtazapine Orodispersible Tablets	Mirtazapine	15 mg, 30 mg, 45 mg	Actavis UK Ltd
Mirtazapine Orodispersible Tablets	Mirtazapine	15 mg, 30 mg, 45 mg	Focus Pharmaceuticals Ltd
Olanzapine Orodispersible Tablets	Olanzapine	5 mg, 10 mg, 15 mg, 20 mg	Aurobindo Pharma-Milpharm Ltd.
Olanzapine Orodispersible Tablets	Olanzapine	10 mg, 15 mg	Zenvita
Olanzapine Orodispersible Tablets	Olanzapine	5 mg, 10 mg, 15 mg, 20 mg	Actavis UK Ltd
Olanzapine Orodispersible Tablets	Olanzapine	5 mg, 10 mg, 15 mg, 20 mg	Dr. Rdddy's Laboratories (UK) Ltd.

(Table 10) contd.....

Brand Name and Dosage Form	Drug	Dose	Manufacturer/ Distributor
Olanzapine Orodispersible Tablets	Olanzapine	10 mg, 15 mg, 20 mg	Sandoz Ltd
Setofilm® Orodispersible Film	Ondansetron	4 mg, 8 mg	Norgine Limited
Risperdal® Orodispersible Tablets	Risperidone	0.5 mg, 1 mg, 2 mg, 3 mg, 4 mg	Janssen-Cilag Ltd
Risperidone Orodispersible Tablets	Risperidone	0.5 mg, 1 mg, 2 mg, 3 mg, 4 mg	Consilient Health Ltd
Risperidone Orodispersible Tablets	Risperidone	2 mg	Sandoz Ltd
Rizatriptan Orodispersible Tablets	Rizatriptan benzoate	10 mg	Aurobindo Pharma-Milpharm Ltd.
Rizatriptan Orodispersible Tablets	Rizatriptan benzoate	10 mg	Sandoz Ltd
Rizatriptan Orodispersible Tablets	Rizatriptan benzoate	10 mg	Actavis UK Ltd
Zalasta® Orodispersible Tablets	Olanzapine	5 mg, 10 mg, 15 mg, 20 mg	Consilient Health Ltd
Zispin® Orodispersible Tablets	Zomitriptan	2.5 mg, 5 mg	Actavis UK Ltd
Zolmitriptan Orodispersible Tablets	Zomitriptan	2.5 mg, 5 mg	Zenvita
Zomig® Rapimelt Orodispersible Tablets	Zomitriptan	5 mg	AstraZeneca UK Ltd
Zyprexa® Velotab™ Orodispersible Tablets	Olanzapine	5 mg, 10 mg, 15 mg, 20	Eli Lilly and Company Ltd

5. FDDF PRODUCTS IN JAPAN

PMDA (Pharmaceuticals and Medical Devices Agency; www.pmda.go.jp) is drug regulatory agency of Japan, which works together with Ministry of Health, Labour and Welfare, Japan to protect the public health by assuring safety, efficacy and quality of pharmaceuticals and medical devices. PMDA approves market entry of new drug products in Japan. FDDF drug products, bioequivalent to their respective conventional drug products, are allowed to enter in Japanese drug market. Japanese Orange Book (http://www.jp-orangebook.gr.jp/english/) provides lists of products approved by PMDA. Additionally, bioequivalence data of FDDF products is also available in Japanese Orange Book. Table **11** provides a list of FDDF products, which have been approved from 2004-2012 in Japan. Table **12** provide details of various FDDF products enlisted in Orange Book of Japan.

Table 11. Fast dissolving/disintegrating drug products approved by PMDA Japan in duration 2004-2012.

Brand Name	Dose	Applicant Company	Drug	Approval Date	Approval/Partial/Change	Approval Notes and Indication
Abilify® OD Tablets	3 mg, 6 mg, 12 mg, 24 mg	Otsuka Pharmaceutical Co., Ltd.	Aripiprazole	Jan. 18, 2012	Approval	Drugs with a new additional indication and a new dosage in new dosage forms for the improvement of manic symptoms in patients with bipolar disorder.
Allelock® OD Tablets	2.5 mg, 5 mg	Kyowa Hakko Kirin Co., Ltd.	Olopatadine HCl	Jul. 23, 2010	Change	Drugs with a new additional paediatric dosage indicated for the treatment of allergic rhinitis, urticaria and itching associated with skin disease (eczema/dermatitis and pruritus cutaneous).
Amlodin® OD Tablets	2.5 mg, 5 mg	Dainippon Sumitomo Pharma Co., Ltd.	Amlodipine besilate	Feb. 23, 2009	Change	Drugs with a new dosage indicated for the treatment of hypertension and angina pectoris.
Amlodin® OD Tablets	2.5 mg, 5 mg	Dainippon Sumitomo Pharma Co., Ltd.	Amlodipine besilate	Jun.22, 2012	Change	Drugs with a new additional paediatric dosage indicated for the treatment of hypertension.
Amlodipine OD Tablets	2.5 mg, 5 mg	Towa	Amlodipine besilate	Jun.22, 2012	Change	Drugs with a new additional paediatric dosage indicated for the treatment of hypertension.

(Table 11) contd.....

Brand Name	Dose	Applicant Company	Drug	Approval Date	Approval/Partial/Change	Approval Notes and Indication
Basen® OD Tablets	0.2 mg	Takeda Pharmaceutical Company Limited	Voglibose	Oct. 16, 2009	Change	Drugs with a new additional indication and a new dosage for prevention of type 2 diabetes mellitus in patients with impaired glucose tolerance
Minirinmelt® OD Tablets	120 µg, 240 µg	Ferring Pharmaceuticals Co., Ltd.	Desmopressin acetate hydrate	Mar. 30, 2012	Approval	Drugs with a new route of administration indicated for the treatment of nocturnal enuresis associated with decreased urine osmolality or urinary specific gravity
Minirinmelt® OD Tablets	120 µg, 240 µg	Ferring Pharmaceuticals Co., Ltd.	Desmopressin acetate hydrate	Dec. 21, 2012	Change	Drugs with a new indication and a new dosage for the treatment of central diabetes insipidus.
Minirinmelt® OD Tablets	60 µg	Ferring Pharmaceuticals Co., Ltd.	Desmopressin acetate hydrate	Dec. 25, 2012	Approval	A drug with a new indication and a new dosage in an additional dosage form for the treatment of central diabetes insipidus.
Norvasc® OD Tablets	2.5 mg, 5 mg	Pfizer Japan Inc.	Amlodipine besilate	Feb. 23, 2009	Change	Drugs with a new dosage indicated for the treatment of hypertension and angina pectoris.
Norvasc® OD Tablets	2.5 mg, 5 mg	Pfizer Japan Inc.	Amlodipine besilate	Jun.22, 2012	Change	Drugs with a new additional paediatric dosage indicated for the treatment of hypertension.

(Table 11) contd.....

Brand Name	Dose	Applicant Company	Drug	Approval Date	Approval/Partial/Change	Approval Notes and Indication
Reminyl® OD Tablets	4 mg, 8 mg and 12 mg	Janssen Pharmaceutical K.K.	Galantamine HBr	Jan. 21, 2011	Approval	Drugs with a new active ingredient indicated for inhibition of progression of symptoms of dementia in mild and moderate Alzheimer's dementia.
Takepron® OD Tablets	15 mg, 30 mg	Takeda Pharmaceutical Co., Ltd.	Lansoprazole	Aug. 23,2007	Change	Drugs with a new indication and dosage for use as a secondary eradication therapy for infection with *Helicobacter pylori*
Takepron® OD Tablets	15 mg	Takeda Pharmaceutical Co., Ltd.	Lansoprazole	Jun. 15, 2006	Partial	Drugs with a new indication and dosage for treatment of non-erosive reflux disease.
Takepron® OD Tablets 15 mg, 30 mg	15 mg, 30 mg	Takeda Pharmaceutical Co., Ltd.	Lansoprazole	Jun. 18, 2010	Change	Drugs with a new additional indication for *H. pylori* eradication therapy for gastric MALT lymphoma, for the stomach after endoscopic treatment of early gastric cancer, and for idiopathic thrombocytopenic purpura, in *H. pylori* infection.
Takepron® OD Tablets	15 mg	Takeda Pharmaceutical Co., Ltd.	Lansoprazole	Jul. 23, 2010	Change	Drugs with a new additional indication and a new dosage for prevention of recurrence of gastric ulcer or duodenal ulcer in patients treated with low-dose aspirin

(Table 11) contd.....

Brand Name	Dose	Applicant Company	Drug	Approval Date	Approval/Partial/Change	Approval Notes and Indication
Takepron® OD Tablets	15 mg	Takeda Pharmaceutical Co., Ltd.	Lansoprazole	Aug. 20, 2010	Change	Drugs with a new additional indication and a new dosage for prevention of recurrence of gastric ulcer or duodenal ulcer in patients treated with NSAID.
Takepron® OD Tablets	15 mg, 30 mg	Takeda Pharmaceutical Co., Ltd.	Lansoprazole	Feb. 21, 2013	Change	Drugs with a new additional indication for the treatment of gastritis induced by *H. pylori* infection.

Table 12. FDDF products listed in Orange Book of Japan.

Brand Name	Drug	Dose	Therapeutic Category	Company
Glucobay® OD	Acarbose	50 mg	Antidiabetic agent	Bayer
Ambroxol Hydrochloride Sustained-Release OD Tablet	Ambroxol Hydrochloride	45 mg	Expectorants	Nipro Corporation
Ambroxol Hydrochloride L-OD Tab	Ambroxol Hydrochloride	45 mg	Expectorants	Sawai Pharmaceutical Co., Ltd.
Amlodipine OD Film	Amlodipine Besilate	2.5 mg, 5 mg	Vasodilators	Kyukyu-phama Co., Ltd
Amlodin® OD Tab	Amlodipine Besilate	2.5. mg, 5 mg, 10 mg	Vasodilators	Dainippon Sumitomo Pharma Co., Ltd.
Norvasc® OD Tablet	Amlodipine Besilate	2.5. mg, 5 mg, 10 mg	Vasodilators	Pfizer Japan Inc.
Amlodipine OD Tablet	Amlodipine Besilate	2.5. mg, 5 mg, 10 mg	Vasodilators	Choseido Pharmaceutical Co.,Ltd.
Amlodipine OD Tablet	Amlodipine Besilate	2.5. mg, 5 mg, 10 mg	Vasodilators	Kyorin Rimedio Co.,Ltd.
Amlodipine OD Tablet	Amlodipine Besilate	2.5. mg, 5 mg, 10 mg	Vasodilators	Nipro Corporation

(Table 12) contd.....

Brand Name	Drug	Dose	Therapeutic Category	Company
Amlodipine OD Tablet	Amlodipine Besilate	2.5. mg, 5 mg, 10 mg	Vasodilators	Tatsumi Kagaku co., Ltd.
Amlodipine OD Tablet	Amlodipine Besilate	2.5. mg, 5 mg, 10 mg	Vasodilators	Taisho Pharmaceutical Industries, Ltd.
Amlodipine OD Tablet	Amlodipine Besilate	2.5. mg, 5 mg, 10 mg	Vasodilators	Yoshindo Inc.
Amlodipine OD Tablet	Amlodipine Besilate	2.5. mg, 5 mg, 10 mg	Vasodilators	Zensei Pharmaceutical Industries Co., Ltd.
Amlodipine OD Tablet	Amlodipine Besilate	2.5. mg, 5 mg, 10 mg	Vasodilators	Sandoz K.K.
Amlodipine OD Tablet	Amlodipine Besilate	2.5. mg, 5 mg, 10 mg	Vasodilators	Takata Seiyaku Co.,Ltd.
Amlodipine OD Tablet	Amlodipine Besilate	2.5. mg, 5 mg, 10 mg	Vasodilators	Teva Pharma Japan Inc
Amlodipine OD Tablet	Amlodipine Besilate	2.5. mg, 5 mg, 10 mg	Vasodilators	Nichi-Iko Pharmaceutical Co.,Ltd.
Amlodipine OD Tablet	Amlodipine Besilate	2.5. mg, 5 mg, 10 mg	Vasodilators	Shiono Chemical Co.,Ltd.
Amlodipine OD Tablet	Amlodipine Besilate	2.5. mg, 5 mg, 10 mg	Vasodilators	Elmed Eisai Co.,Ltd.
Amlodipine OD Tablet	Amlodipine Besilate	2.5. mg, 5 mg, 10 mg	Vasodilators	Nihon Generi Co.,Ltd.
Amlodipine OD Tablet	Amlodipine Besilate	2.5. mg, 5 mg, 10 mg	Vasodilators	Kobayashi Kako Co.,Ltd.
Amlodipine OD Tablet	Amlodipine Besilate	2.5. mg, 5 mg, 10 mg	Vasodilators	Nissin Pharmaceutical Co.,Ltd.
Amlodipine OD Tablet	Amlodipine Besilate	2.5. mg, 5 mg, 10 mg	Vasodilators	Aska Pharmaceutical. Co., Ltd.
Amlodipine OD Tablet	Amlodipine Besilate	2.5. mg, 5 mg, 10 mg	Vasodilators	Kyowa Pharmaceutical Industry Co., Ltd.

(Table 12) contd.....

Brand Name	Drug	Dose	Therapeutic Category	Company
Amlodipine OD Tablet	Amlodipine Besilate	2.5. mg, 5 mg, 10 mg	Vasodilators	Isei-pharm Co.,Ltd
Amlodipine OD Tablet	Amlodipine Besilate	2.5. mg, 5 mg, 10 mg	Vasodilators	Nihon Pharmaceutical Industry Co.,Ltd.
Amlodipine OD Tablet	Amlodipine Besilate	2.5. mg, 5 mg, 10 mg	Vasodilators	Sawai Pharmaceutical Co.,Ltd
Amlodipine OD Tablet	Amlodipine Besilate	2.5. mg, 5 mg, 10 mg	Vasodilators	Towa Pharmaceutical Co., Ltd.
Amlodipine OD Tablet	Amlodipine Besilate	2.5. mg, 5 mg, 10 mg	Vasodilators	Taisho Pharmaceutical Industries, Ltd.
Amlodipine OD Tablet	Amlodipine Besilate	2.5. mg, 5 mg, 10 mg	Vasodilators	Meiji Seika Pharma Co., Ltd
Abilify® OD Tablet	Aripiprazole	3 mg, 6 mg, 12 mg, 24 mg	Psychotropic agent	Otsuka Pharmaceutical Co.,Ltd.
Atorvastatin OD Tablet	Atorvastatin Calcium Hydrate	5 mg, 10 mg	Agents for hyperlipidemias	Towa Pharmaceutical Co., Ltd.
Talion® OD Tablet	Bepotastine Besilate	5 mg, 10 mg	Other antiallergic agents	Mitsubishi Tanabe Pharma Corporation
Casodex® OD Tablet	Bicalutamide	80 mg	Other antitumor agents	AstraZeneca K.K.
Lendormin® D Tablet	Brotizolam	0.25 mg	Hypnotics and sedatives, antianxietics	Nippon Boehringer Ingelheim Co., Ltd.
Brotizolam OD Tablet	Brotizolam	0.25 mg	Hypnotics and sedatives, antianxietics	Daiko Pharmaceutical Co.,Ltd.
Brotizolam OD Tablet	Brotizolam	0.25 mg	Hypnotics and sedatives, antianxietics	Kyowa Pharmaceutical Industry Co., Ltd.
Brotizolam OD Tablet	Brotizolam	0.25 mg	Hypnotics and sedatives, antianxietics	Teva Pharma Japan Inc
Brotizolam OD Tablet	Brotizolam	0.25 mg	Hypnotics and sedatives, antianxietics	Medisa Shinyaku Inc.
Candesartan OD Tablet	Candesartan Cilexetil	2 mg, 4 mg, 8 mg, 12 mg	Antihypertensives	Elmed Eisai Co.,Ltd.

(Table 12) contd.....

Brand Name	Drug	Dose	Therapeutic Category	Company
Candesartan OD Tablet	Candesartan Cilexetil	2 mg, 4 mg, 8 mg, 12 mg	Antihypertensives	Kobayashi Kako Co.,Ltd.
Candesartan OD Tablet	Candesartan Cilexetil	2 mg, 4 mg, 8 mg, 12 mg	Antihypertensives	Sawai Pharmaceutical Co.,Ltd.
Cetirizine Hydrochloride OD Tablet	Cetirizine Hydrochloride	5 mg, 10 mg	Other antiallergic agents	Sawai Pharmaceutical Co.,Ltd.
Pletal® OD Tablet	Cilostazol	50 mg, 100 mg	Agents relating to blood and body fluids	Otsuka Pharmaceutical Co. Ltd.
Cilostazol OD Tablet	Cilostazol	50 mg, 100 mg	Agents relating to blood and body fluids	Daito Pharmaceutical Co.,Ltd.
Cilostazol OD Tablet	Cilostazol	50 mg, 100 mg	Agents relating to blood and body fluids	Sawai Pharmaceutical Co.,Ltd.
Cilostazol OD Tablet	Cilostazol	50 mg, 100 mg	Agents relating to blood and body fluids	Tsuruhara pharmaceutical Co.,Ltd.
Cilostazol OD Tablet	Cilostazol	50 mg, 100 mg	Agents relating to blood and body fluids	Towa Pharmaceutical Co., Ltd.
Cilostazol OD Tablet	Cilostazol	50 mg, 100 mg	Agents relating to blood and body fluids	Mylan Pharmaceutical Co.,Ltd
Cilostazol OD Tablet	Cilostazol	50 mg, 100 mg	Agents relating to blood and body fluids	Kotobuki pharmaceutical Co., Ltd.
Cilostazol OD Tablet	Cilostazol	50 mg, 100 mg	Agents relating to blood and body fluids	Nihon Pharmaceutical Industry Co.,Ltd.
Cilostazol OD Tablet	Cilostazol	50 mg, 100 mg	Agents relating to blood and body fluids	Takata Seiyaku Co.,Ltd.
Minirinmelt® OD Tablet	Desmopressin Acetate Hydrate	60 µg, 120 µg, 240 µg	Pituitary hormone preparations	Ferring Pharmaceuticals Co.Ltd.
Dinagest® OD Tablet	Dienogest	1 mg	Other hormone preparations (including antihormone preparations)	Mochida Pharmaceutical Co., Ltd.
Nauzelin® OD Tablet	Domperidone	5 mg, 10 mg	Other agents affecting digestive organs	Kyowa Hakko Kirn Co., Ltd.
Aricept® D Tablet	Donepezil HCl	3 mg, 5 mg, 10 mg	Other agents affecting central nervous system	Eisai Co., Ltd.

(Table 12) contd.....

Brand Name	Drug	Dose	Therapeutic Category	Company
Donepezil HCl OD Tablet	Donepezil HCl	3 mg, 5 mg, 10 mg	Other agents affecting central nervous system	Kotobuki pharmaceutical Co., Ltd.
Donepezil HCl OD Tablet	Donepezil HCl	3 mg, 5 mg, 10 mg	Other agents affecting central nervous system	Nipro Corporation
Donepezil HCl OD Tablet	Donepezil HCl	3 mg, 5 mg, 10 mg	Other agents affecting central nervous system	Taisho Pharmaceutical Industries, Ltd.
Donepezil HCl OD Tablet	Donepezil HCl	3 mg, 5 mg, 10 mg	Other agents affecting central nervous system	Kyowa Pharmaceutical Industry Co., Ltd.
Donepezil HCl OD Tablet	Donepezil HCl	3 mg, 5 mg, 10 mg	Other agents affecting central nervous system	Mitsubishi Tanabe Pharma Corporation
Donepezil HCl OD Tablet	Donepezil HCl	3 mg, 5 mg, 10 mg	Other agents affecting central nervous system	Teva Pharma Japan Inc
Donepezil HCl OD Tablet	Donepezil HCl	3 mg, 5 mg, 10 mg	Other agents affecting central nervous system	Daiichi Sankyo Espha Co., Ltd.
Donepezil HCl OD Tablet	Donepezil HCl	3 mg, 5 mg, 10 mg	Other agents affecting central nervous system	Dainippon Sumitomo Pharma Co., Ltd.
Donepezil HCl OD Tablet	Donepezil HCl	3 mg, 5 mg, 10 mg	Other agents affecting central nervous system	Fujifilm Pharma Co., Ltd
Donepezil HCl OD Tablet	Donepezil HCl	3 mg, 5 mg, 10 mg	Other agents affecting central nervous system	Nihon Generic Co.,Ltd.
Donepezil HCl OD Tablet	Donepezil HCl	3 mg, 5 mg, 10 mg	Other agents affecting central nervous system	Nihon Pharmaceutical Industry Co.,Ltd.
Donepezil HCl OD Tablet	Donepezil HCl	3 mg, 5 mg, 10 mg	Other agents affecting central nervous system	Tatsumi Kagaku co.,Ltd.
Donepezil HCl OD Tablet	Donepezil HCl	3 mg, 5 mg, 10 mg	Other agents affecting central nervous system	Yoshindo Inc.
Donepezil HCl OD Tablet	Donepezil HCl	3 mg, 5 mg, 10 mg	Other agents affecting central nervous system	Zensei Pharmaceutical Industries Co., Ltd.
Donepezil HCl OD Tablet	Donepezil HCl	3 mg, 5 mg, 10 mg	Other agents affecting central nervous system	Ohara Pharmaceutical Co.,Ltd.

(Table 12) contd.....

Brand Name	Drug	Dose	Therapeutic Category	Company
Donepezil HCl OD Tablet	Donepezil HCl	3 mg, 5 mg, 10 mg	Other agents affecting central nervous system	Shiono Chemical Co.,Ltd.
Donepezil HCl OD Tablet	Donepezil HCl	3 mg, 5 mg, 10 mg	Other agents affecting central nervous system	Kyorin Rimedio Co.,Ltd.
Donepezil HCl OD Tablet	Donepezil HCl	3 mg, 5 mg, 10 mg	Other agents affecting central nervous system	Nippon Chemiphar Co.,Ltd.
Donepezil HCl OD Tablet	Donepezil HCl	3 mg, 5 mg, 10 mg	Other agents affecting central nervous system	Sawai Pharmaceutical Co.,Ltd.
Donepezil HCl OD Tablet	Donepezil HCl	3 mg, 5 mg, 10 mg	Other agents affecting central nervous system	Sandoz K.K.
Donepezil HCl OD Tablet	Donepezil HCl	3 mg, 5 mg, 10 mg	Other agents affecting central nervous system	Takata Seiyaku Co.,Ltd.
Donepezil HCl OD Tablet	Donepezil HCl	3 mg, 5 mg, 10 mg	Other agents affecting central nervous system	Towa Pharmaceutical Co., Ltd.
Donepezil HCl OD Tablet	Donepezil HCl	3 mg, 5 mg, 10 mg	Other agents affecting central nervous system	Nichi-Iko Pharmaceutical Co.,Ltd.
Donepezil HCl OD Tablet	Donepezil HCl	3 mg, 5 mg, 10 mg	Other agents affecting central nervous system	Meiji Seika Pharma Co., Ltd
Donepezil HCl OD Tablet	Donepezil HCl	3 mg, 5 mg, 10 mg	Other agents affecting central nervous system	Daito Pharmaceutical Co.,Ltd.
Donepezil HCl OD Tablet	Donepezil HCl	3 mg, 5 mg, 10 mg	Other agents affecting central nervous system	Nissin Pharmaceutical Co.,Ltd.
Donepezil HCl OD Tablet	Donepezil HCl	3 mg, 5 mg, 10 mg	Other agents affecting central nervous system	Kyukyu-phama Co., Ltd.
Donepezil HCl OD film	Donepezil Hydrochlorthaizide	3 mg, 5 mg, 10 mg	Other agents affecting central nervous system	Kyukyu-phama Co., Ltd
Cardenalin OD	Doxazosin mesilate	0.5 mg, 1 mg, 2 mg, 4 mg	Antihypertensives	Pfizer Japan Inc.
Dops® OD	Droxidopa	200 mg	Antiparkinsonism agents	Dainippon Sumitomo Pharma Co., Ltd.

(Table 12) contd.....

Brand Name	Drug	Dose	Therapeutic Category	Company
Ebastel OD Tablet	Ebastine	5 mg, 10 mg	Antiallergic agent	Dainippon Sumitomo Pharma Co., Ltd.
Ebastine OD Tablet	Ebastine	5 mg, 10 mg	Antiallergic agent	Zensei Pharmaceutical Industries Co., Ltd.
Ebastine OD Tablet	Ebastine	5 mg, 10 mg	Antiallergic agent	Kyowa Pharmaceutical Industry Co., Ltd.
Ebastine OD Tablet	Ebastine	5 mg, 10 mg	Antiallergic agent	Pfizer Japan Inc.
Ebastine OD Tablet	Ebastine	5 mg, 10 mg	Antiallergic agent	Daiko Pharmaceutical Co.,Ltd.
Ebastine OD Tablet	Ebastine	5 mg, 10 mg	Antiallergic agent	Medisa Shinyaku Inc.
Ebastine OD Tablet	Ebastine	5 mg, 10 mg	Antiallergic agent	Nipro Corporation
Ebastine OD Tablet	Ebastine	5 mg, 10 mg	Antiallergic agent	Nissin Pharmaceutical Co.,Ltd.
Ebastine OD Tablet	Ebastine	5 mg, 10 mg	Antiallergic agent	Shiono Chemical Co.,Ltd.
Ebastine OD Tablet	Ebastine	5 mg, 10 mg	Antiallergic agent	Yoshindo Inc.
Ebastine OD Tablet	Ebastine	5 mg, 10 mg	Antiallergic agent	Daito Pharmaceutical Co.,Ltd.
Ebastine OD Tablet	Ebastine	5 mg, 10 mg	Antiallergic agent	Nippon Chemiphar Co.,Ltd.
Ebastine OD Tablet	Ebastine	5 mg, 10 mg	Antiallergic agent	Sawai Pharmaceutical Co.,Ltd.
Ebastine OD Tablet	Ebastine	5 mg, 10 mg	Antiallergic agent	Teva Pharma Japan Inc
Ebastine OD Tablet	Ebastine	5 mg, 10 mg	Antiallergic agent	Takata Seiyaku Co.,Ltd.
Ebastine OD Tablet	Ebastine	5 mg, 10 mg	Antiallergic agent	Nichi-Iko Pharmaceutical Co.,Ltd.
Gaster® OD Tablet	Famotidine	10 mg, 20 mg	Agents for peptic ulcer	Astellas Pharma Inc.
Stomarcon D Tablet	Famotidine	10 mg, 20 mg	Agents for peptic ulcer	Taisho Pharmaceutical Industries, Ltd.
Famotidine OD Tablet	Famotidine	10 mg, 20 mg	Agents for peptic ulcer	Teva Pharma Japan Inc
Famotidine D Tablet	Famotidine	10 mg, 20 mg	Agents for peptic ulcer	Nihon Generic Co.,Ltd.

(Table 12) contd.....

Brand Name	Drug	Dose	Therapeutic Category	Company
Famotidine OD Tablet	Famotidine	10 mg, 20 mg	Agents for peptic ulcer	Tobishi Pharmaceutical Co., Ltd.
Gasric D Tablet	Famotidine	10 mg, 20 mg	Agents for peptic ulcer	Nissin Pharmaceutical Co.,Ltd.
Climagen®-OD Tablet	Famotidine	10 mg, 20 mg	Agents for peptic ulcer	Mylan Pharmaceutical Co.,Ltd
Famotidine D Tablet	Famotidine	10 mg, 20 mg	Agents for peptic ulcer	Sannova Co., Ltd.
Famotidine D Tablet	Famotidine	10 mg, 20 mg	Agents for peptic ulcer	Sawai Pharmaceutical Co.,Ltd.
Famotidine D Tablet	Famotidine	10 mg, 20 mg	Agents for peptic ulcer	Tobishi Pharmaceutical Co., Ltd.
Famotidine OD Tablet	Famotidine	10 mg, 20 mg	Agents for peptic ulcer	Yoshindo Inc.
Famotidine OD Tablet	Famotidine	10 mg, 20 mg	Agents for peptic ulcer	Oara Pharmaceutical Co.,Ltd.
Famotidine OD Tablet	Famotidine	10 mg, 20 mg	Agents for peptic ulcer	Shiono Chemical Co.,Ltd.
Famotidine OD Tablet	Famotidine	10 mg, 20 mg	Agents for peptic ulcer	Towa Pharmaceutical Co., Ltd.
Famotidine D Tablet	Famotidine	10 mg, 20 mg	Agents for peptic ulcer	Medisa Shinyaku Inc.
Famotidine D Tablet	Famotidine	10 mg, 20 mg	Agents for peptic ulcer	Nichi-Iko Pharmaceutical Co.,Ltd.
Fexofenadine HCl OD Tablet	Fexofenadine HCl	30 mg, 60 mg	Antiallergic agents	Nipro Corporation
Fexofenadine HCl OD Tablet	Fexofenadine HCl	30 mg, 60 mg	Antiallergic agents	Ceolia Pharma Co., Ltd.
Fexofenadine HCl OD Tablet	Fexofenadine HCl	30 mg, 60 mg	Antiallergic agents	Sawai Pharmaceutical Co.,Ltd.
Fexofenadine HCl OD Tablet	Fexofenadine HCl	30 mg, 60 mg	Antiallergic agents	Elmed Eisai Co.,Ltd
Fexofenadine HCl OD Tablet	Fexofenadine HCl	30 mg, 60 mg	Antiallergic agents	Kobayashi Kako Co.,Ltd.
Fexofenadine HCl OD Tablet	Fexofenadine HCl	30 mg, 60 mg	Antiallergic agents	Towa Pharmaceutical Co., Ltd.
Fexofenadine HCl OD Tablet	Fexofenadine HCl	30 mg, 60 mg	Antiallergic agents	Pfizer Japan Inc.
Allegra® OD Tablet	Fexofenadine HCl	60 mg	Antiallergic agents	Sanofi K.K.

(Table 12) contd.....

Brand Name	Drug	Dose	Therapeutic Category	Company
Fexofenadine HCl OD Tablet	Fexofenadine HCl	60 mg	Antiallergic agents	Fujifilm Pharma Co., Ltd
Fexofenadine HCl OD Tablet	Fexofenadine HCl	60 mg	Antiallergic agents	Yoshindo Inc.
Reminyl® OD Tablet	Galantamine HBr	4 mg, 8 mg, 12 mg	Other agents affecting central nervous system	Janssen Pharmaceutical K.K.
Amaryl® OD Tablet	Glimepiride	0.5 mg, 1 mg, 3 mg	Antidiabetic agents	Sanofi K.K.
Glimepiride OD Tablet	Glimepiride	0.5 mg, 1 mg, 3 mg	Antidiabetic agents	Elmed Eisai Co.,Ltd.
Glimepiride OD Tablet	Glimepiride	0.5 mg, 1 mg, 3 mg	Antidiabetic agents	Kobayashi Kako Co.,Ltd.
Glimepiride OD Tablet	Glimepiride	0.5 mg, 1 mg, 3 mg	Antidiabetic agents	Shiono Chemical Co.,Ltd.
Glimepiride OD Tablet	Glimepiride	0.5 mg, 1 mg, 3 mg	Antidiabetic agents	Teva Pharma Japan Inc
Glimepiride OD Tablet	Glimepiride	0.5 mg, 1 mg, 3 mg	Antidiabetic agents	Towa Pharmaceutical Co., Ltd.
Glimepiride OD Tablet	Glimepiride	0.5 mg, 1 mg, 3 mg	Antidiabetic agents	Nichi-Iko Pharmaceutical Co.,Ltd.
Glimepiride OD Tablet	Glimepiride	0.5 mg, 1 mg, 3 mg	Antidiabetic agents	Daiko Pharmaceutical Co.,Ltd.
Hydrochlorthiazide OD Tablet	Hydrochlorthiazide	12.5 mg	Diuretics	Towa Pharmaceutical Co., Ltd.
Uritos® OD Tablet 0.1mg	Imidafenacin	0.1 mg	Other agents for urogenital and anal organ	Kyorin Pharmaceutical Co.,Ltd.
Staybla® OD Tablet 0.1mg	Imidafenacin	0.1 mg	Other agents for urogenital and anal organ	Ono Pharmaceutical Co., Ltd.
Gaslon® N OD Tablet	Irsogladine Maleate	2 mg, 4 mg	Agents for peptic ulcer	Nippon Shinyaku Co., Ltd.
Protecadin® OD Tablet	Lafutidine	5 mg, 10 mg	Agents for peptic ulcer	Taiho Pharmaceutical Co., Ltd.

(Table 12) contd.....

Brand Name	Drug	Dose	Therapeutic Category	Company
Takepron® OD	Lansoprazole	15 mg, 30 mg	Agents for peptic ulcer	Takeda Pharmaceutical Co., Ltd.
Lansoprazole OD Tablet	Lansoprazole	15 mg, 30 mg	Agents for peptic ulcer	Shiono Chemical Co.,Ltd.
Lansoprazole OD Tablet	Lansoprazole	15 mg, 30 mg	Agents for peptic ulcer	Teva Pharma Japan Inc
Lansoprazole OD Tablet	Lansoprazole	15 mg, 30 mg	Agents for peptic ulcer	Nichi-Iko Pharmaceutical Co.,Ltd.
Lansoprazole OD Tablet	Lansoprazole	15 mg, 30 mg	Agents for peptic ulcer	Sawai Pharmaceutical Co.,Ltd
Lansoprazole OD Tablet	Lansoprazole	15 mg, 30 mg	Agents for peptic ulcer	Towa Pharmaceutical Co., Ltd.
Lansoprazole OD Tablet	Lansoprazole	15 mg, 30 mg	Agents for peptic ulcer	Daiko Pharmaceutical Co.,Ltd.
Lansoprazole OD Tablet	Lansoprazole	15 mg, 30 mg	Agents for peptic ulcer	Nihon Generic Co.,Ltd.
Levofloxacin OD Tablet	Levofloxacin Hydrate	250 mg, 500 mg	Synthetic antibacterials	Towa Pharmaceutical Co., Ltd.
Claritin® Reditabs® Tablet	Loratadine	10 mg	Other antiallergic agents	Msd K.K.
Loratadine OD Tablet	Loratadine	10 mg	Other antiallergic agents	Aska Pharmaceutical. Co., Ltd.
Loratadine OD Tablet	Loratadine	10 mg	Other antiallergic agents	Choseido Pharmaceutical Co.,Ltd.
Loratadine OD Tablet	Loratadine	10 mg	Other antiallergic agents	Daiko Pharmaceutical Co.,Ltd.
Loratadine OD Tablet	Loratadine	10 mg	Other antiallergic agents	Elmed Eisai Co.,Ltd.
Loratadine OD Tablet	Loratadine	10 mg	Other antiallergic agents	Fujifilm Pharma Co., Ltd
Loratadine OD Tablet	Loratadine	10 mg	Other antiallergic agents	Nihon Generic Co.,Ltd.
Loratadine OD Tablet	Loratadine	10 mg	Other antiallergic agents	Nipro Corporation
Loratadine OD Tablet	Loratadine	10 mg	Other antiallergic agents	Taisho Pharmaceutical Industries, Ltd.
Loratadine OD Tablet	Loratadine	10 mg	Other antiallergic agents	Yoshindo Inc.
Loratadine OD Tablet	Loratadine	10 mg	Other antiallergic agents	Kyowa Pharmaceutical Industry Co., Ltd.

(Table 12) contd.....

Brand Name	Drug	Dose	Therapeutic Category	Company
Loratadine OD Tablet	Loratadine	10 mg	Other antiallergic agents	Daito Pharmaceutical Co.,Ltd.
Loratadine OD Tablet	Loratadine	10 mg	Other antiallergic agents	Sawai Pharmaceutical Co.,Ltd.
Loratadine OD Tablet	Loratadine	10 mg	Other antiallergic agents	Towa Pharmaceutical Co., Ltd.
Loratadine OD Tablet	Loratadine	10 mg	Other antiallergic agents	Pfizer Japan Inc.
Loratadine OD Tablet	Loratadine	10 mg	Other antiallergic agents	Mylan Pharmaceutical Co.,Ltd
Loratadine OD Tablet	Loratadine	10 mg	Other antiallergic agents	Kyorin Rimedio Co.,Ltd.
Loratadine OD Tablet	Loratadine	10 mg	Other antiallergic agents	Nichi-Iko Pharmaceutical Co.,Ltd.
Loratadine OD Tablet	Loratadine	10 mg	Other antiallergic agents	Nissin Pharmaceutical Co.,Ltd.
Loratadine OD Tablet	Loratadine	10 mg	Other antiallergic agents	Kobayashi Kako Co.,Ltd.
Loratadine OD Filme	Loratadine	10 mg	Other antiallergic agents	Kyukyu-phama Co., Ltd.
Memary® OD Tab	Memantine HCl	5 mg, 10 mg, 20 mg	Other agents affecting central nervous system	Daiichi Sankyo Co., Ltd.
Metligine® D Tablet	Midodrine HCl	2 mg	Vasoconstrictors	Taisho Pharmaceutical Co., Ltd.
Flivas® OD Tablets	Naftopidil	25 mg, 50 mg, 75 mg	Other agents for urogenital and anal organ	Asahi Kasei Pharma Co.,Ltd.
Nitropen® Tablet	Nitroglycerin	0.3 mg	Vasodilators	Nippon Kayaku Co., Ltd.
Zyprexa® Zydis® Tablet	Olanzapine	2.5 mg, 5 mg, 10 mg	Psychotropic agents	Eli Lilly Japan K.K.
Olopatadine HCl OD Film	Olopatadine	2.5 mg, 5 mg	Antiallergic agents	Kyukyu-phama Co., Ltd
Allelock® OD Tab	Olopatadine HCl	2.5 mg, 5 mg	Antiallergic agents	Kyowa Hakko Kirn Co., Ltd.
Olopatadine HCl OD Tablet	Olopatadine HCl	2.5 mg, 5 mg	Antiallergic agents	Kobayashi Kako Co.,Ltd.
Olopatadine HCl OD Tablet	Olopatadine HCl	2.5 mg, 5 mg	Antiallergic agents	Sawai Pharmaceutical Co.,Ltd.

(Table 12) contd.....

Brand Name	Drug	Dose	Therapeutic Category	Company
Olopatadine HCl OD Tablet	Olopatadine HCl	2.5 mg, 5 mg	Antiallergic agents	Takata Seiyaku Co.,Ltd.
Olopatadine HCl OD Tablet	Olopatadine HCl	2.5 mg, 5 mg	Antiallergic agents	Taisho Pharmaceutical Industries, Ltd.
Olopatadine HCl OD Tablet	Olopatadine HCl	2.5 mg, 5 mg	Antiallergic agents	Nichi-Iko Pharmaceutical Co.,Ltd.
Olopatadine HCl OD Tablet	Olopatadine HCl	2.5 mg, 5 mg	Antiallergic agents	Daito Pharmaceutical Co.,Ltd.
Olopatadine HCl OD Tablet	Olopatadine HCl	2.5 mg, 5 mg	Antiallergic agents	Kyowa Pharmaceutical Industry Co., Ltd.
Olopatadine HCl OD Tablet	Olopatadine HCl	2.5 mg, 5 mg	Antiallergic agents	Iwaki Seiyaku Co.,Ltd
Olopatadine HCl OD Tablet	Olopatadine HCl	2.5 mg, 5 mg	Antiallergic agents	Nippon Chemiphar Co.,Ltd.
Olopatadine HCl OD Tablet	Olopatadine HCl	2.5 mg, 5 mg	Antiallergic agents	Towa Pharmaceutical Co., Ltd.
Olopatadine HCl OD Tablet	Olopatadine HCl	2.5 mg, 5 mg	Antiallergic agents	Pfizer Japan Inc.
Olopatadine HCl OD Tablet	Olopatadine HCl	2.5 mg, 5 mg	Antiallergic agents	Meiji Seika Pharma Co., Ltd
Olopatadine HCl OD Tablet	Olopatadine HCl	2.5 mg, 5 mg	Antiallergic agents	Kyukyu-phama Co., Ltd.
Zofran® Zydis® 4	Ondansetron	4 mg	Other agents affecting digestive organs	Glaxo Smithkline K.K.
Paroxetine OD Tablet	Paroxetine Hydrochloride Hydrate	5 mg, 10 mg, 20 mg	Psychotropic agents	Towa Pharmaceutical Co., Ltd.
Actos® OD Tablet	Pioglitazone HCl	15 mg, 30 mg	Antidiabetic agents	Takeda Pharmaceutical Co., Ltd.
Pioglitazone OD Tablet	Pioglitazone HCl	15 mg, 30 mg	Antidiabetic agents	Nihon Pharmaceutical Industry Co.,Ltd.
Pioglitazone OD Tablet	Pioglitazone HCl	15 mg, 30 mg	Antidiabetic agents	Kyowa Pharmaceutical Industry Co., Ltd.
Pioglitazone OD Tablet	Pioglitazone HCl	15 mg, 30 mg	Antidiabetic agents	Kyorin Rimedio Co.,Ltd.
Pioglitazone OD Tablet	Pioglitazone HCl	15 mg, 30 mg	Antidiabetic agents	Nippon Chemiphar Co.,Ltd.

(Table 12) contd.....

Brand Name	Drug	Dose	Therapeutic Category	Company
Pioglitazone OD Tablet	Pioglitazone HCl	15 mg, 30 mg	Antidiabetic agents	Taisho Pharmaceutical Industries, Ltd.
Pioglitazone OD Tablet	Pioglitazone HCl	15 mg, 30 mg	Antidiabetic agents	Nichi-Iko Pharmaceutical Co.,Ltd.
Pioglitazone OD Tablet	Pioglitazone HCl	15 mg, 30 mg	Antidiabetic agents	Pfizer Japan Inc.
Pioglitazone OD Tablet	Pioglitazone HCl	15 mg, 30 mg	Antidiabetic agents	Daiichi Sankyo Espha Co., Ltd.
Pioglitazone OD Tablet	Pioglitazone HCl	15 mg, 30 mg	Antidiabetic agents	Fujifilm Pharma Co., Ltd
Pioglitazone OD Tablet	Pioglitazone HCl	15 mg, 30 mg	Antidiabetic agents	Kobayashi Kako Co.,Ltd.
Pioglitazone OD Tablet	Pioglitazone HCl	15 mg, 30 mg	Antidiabetic agents	Nissin Pharmaceutical Co.,Ltd.
Pioglitazone OD Tablet	Pioglitazone HCl	15 mg, 30 mg	Antidiabetic agents	Tatsumi Kagaku co.,Ltd.
Pioglitazone OD Tablet	Pioglitazone HCl	15 mg, 30 mg	Antidiabetic agents	Takata Seiyaku Co.,Ltd.
Pioglitazone OD Tablet	Pioglitazone HCl	15 mg, 30 mg	Antidiabetic agents	Towa Pharmaceutical Co., Ltd.
Livalo® OD Tab	Pitavastatin Calcium	1 mg, 2 mg	Agents for hyperlipidemias	Kowa Company, Ltd.
Pitavastatin Ca OD Tablet	Pitavastatin Calcium	1 mg, 2 mg, 4 mg	Agents for hyperlipidemias	Towa Pharmaceutical Co., Ltd.
Promac® D Tablet	Polaprezinc	75 mg	Agents for peptic ulcer	Zeria Pharmaceutical Co., Ltd.
Polaprezic OD Tablet	Polaprezinc	75 mg	Agents for peptic ulcer	Sawai Pharmaceutical Co.,Ltd.
Pramipexole Hydrochloride OD Tablet	Pramipexole HCl Hydrate	0.125 mg, 0.5 mg	Antiparkinsonism agents	Towa Pharmaceutical Co., Ltd.
Caltan-OD® Tab	Precipitated Calcium Carbonate	250 mg, 500 mg	Other cardiovascular agents	Mylan Pharmaceutical Co.,Ltd
Nasea® OD Tablet	Ramosetron HCl	0.1 mg	Other agents affecting digestive organs	Astellas Pharma Inc.
Irribow® OD Tablet	Ramosetron HCl	2.5 µg, 5 µg	Other agents affecting digestive organs	Astellas Pharma Inc.
Rebamipide OD Tablet	Rebamipide	100 mg	Agents for peptic ulcer	Nissin Pharmaceutical Co.,Ltd.
Rebamipide OD Tablet	Rebamipide	100 mg	Agents for peptic ulcer	Yoshindo Inc.

(Table 12) contd.....

Brand Name	Drug	Dose	Therapeutic Category	Company
Rebamipide OD Tablet	Rebamipide	100 mg	Agents for peptic ulcer	Meiji Seika Pharma Co., Ltd
Risperdal® OD Tablet	Risperidone	0.5 mg, 1 mg, 2 mg, 3 mg	Psychotropic agents	Janssen Pharmaceutical K.K.
Risperidone OD Tab	Risperidone	0.5 mg, 1 mg, 2 mg, 3 mg	Psychotropic agents	Kyowa Pharmaceutical Industry Co., Ltd.
Risperidone OD Tab	Risperidone	0.5 mg, 1 mg, 2 mg, 3 mg	Psychotropic agents	Takata Seiyaku Co.,Ltd.
Risperidone OD Tab	Risperidone	0.5 mg, 1 mg, 2 mg, 3 mg	Psychotropic agents	Sawai Pharmaceutical Co.,Ltd.
Risperidone OD Tab	Risperidone	0.5 mg, 1 mg, 2 mg, 3 mg	Psychotropic agents	Towa Pharmaceutical Co., Ltd.
Risperidone OD Tab	Risperidone	0.5 mg, 1 mg, 2 mg, 3 mg	Psychotropic agents	Zensei Pharmaceutical Industries Co., Ltd.
Maxalt® RPD Tablet 10mg	Rizatriptan Benzoate	10 mg	Vasoconstrictors	Kyorin Pharmaceutical Co.,Ltd.
Selegiline FP OD Tab	Selegiline HCl	2.5 mg	Antiparkinsonism agents	FP Pharmaceutical Corporation
Vesicare® OD Tab	Solifenacin Succinate	2.5 mg, 5 mg	Other agents for urogenital and anal organ	Astellas Pharma Inc.
Ceredist® OD Tablet	Taltirelin Hydrate	5 mg	Other agents affecting central nervous system	Mitsubishi Tanabe Pharma Corporation
Taltirelin-OD	Taltirelin Hydrate	5 mg	Other agents affecting central nervous system	Nihon Generic Co.,Ltd.
Taltirelin-OD	Taltirelin Hydrate	5 mg	Other agents affecting central nervous system	Kyowa Pharmaceutical Industry Co., Ltd.
Taltirelin-OD	Taltirelin Hydrate	5 mg	Other agents affecting central nervous system	Nichi-Iko Pharmaceutical Co.,Ltd.

(Table 12) contd.....

Brand Name	Drug	Dose	Therapeutic Category	Company
Harnal® D Tab	Tamsulosin HCl	0.1 mg, 0.2 mg	Other agents for urogenital and anal organ	Astellas Pharma Inc.
Tamsulosin HCl OD Tablet	Tamsulosin HCl	0.1 mg, 0.2 mg	Other agents for urogenital and anal organ	Pfizer Japan Inc.
Tamsulosin HCl OD Tablet	Tamsulosin HCl	0.1 mg, 0.2 mg	Other agents for urogenital and anal organ	Taisho Pharmaceutical Industries, Ltd.
Tamsulosin HCl OD Tablet	Tamsulosin HCl	0.1 mg, 0.2 mg	Other agents for urogenital and anal organ	Kyowa Pharmaceutical Industry Co., Ltd.
Tamsulosin HCl OD Tablet	Tamsulosin HCl	0.1 mg, 0.2 mg	Other agents for urogenital and anal organ	Nihon Pharmaceutical Industry Co.,Ltd.
Tamsulosin HCl OD Tablet	Tamsulosin HCl	0.1 mg, 0.2 mg	Other agents for urogenital and anal organ	Sawai Pharmaceutical Co.,Ltd.
Tamsulosin HCl OD Tablet	Tamsulosin HCl	0.1 mg, 0.2 mg	Other agents for urogenital and anal organ	Nichi-Iko Pharmaceutical Co.,Ltd.
Tamsulosin HCl OD Tablet	Tamsulosin HCl	0.1 mg, 0.2 mg	Other agents for urogenital and anal organ	Nissin Pharmaceutical Co.,Ltd.
Tamsulosin HCl OD Tablet	Tamsulosin HCl	0.1 mg, 0.2 mg	Other agents for urogenital and anal organ	Meiji Seika Pharma Co., Ltd
Tamsulosin HCl OD Tablet	Tamsulosin HCl	0.1 mg, 0.2 mg	Other agents for urogenital and anal organ	Choseido Pharmaceutical Co.,Ltd.
Tamsulosin HCl OD Tablet	Tamsulosin HCl	0.1 mg, 0.2 mg	Other agents for urogenital and anal organ	Towa Pharmaceutical Co., Ltd.
Restream® OD Tablet 0.1mg	Tamsulosin HCl	0.1 mg, 0.2 mg	Other agents for urogenital and anal organ	Aska Pharmaceutical. Co., Ltd.
TS-1® Combination OD Tablet	Tegafur, Gimeracil, Oteracil Potassium	20 mg, 25 mg	Antimetabolic agents	Taiho Pharmaceutical Co., Ltd.
Tramal® OD Tablet	Tramadol HCl	25 mg, 50 mg	Antipyretics, analgesics and anti-inflammatory agents	Nippon Shinyaku Co., Ltd.
Diovan® OD Tab	Valsartan	20 mg, 40 mg, 80 mg, 160 mg	Antihypertensives	Novartis Pharma K.K.

(Table 12) contd.....

Brand Name	Drug	Dose	Therapeutic Category	Company
Valsartan OD Tablet	Valsartan	20 mg, 40 mg, 80 mg, 160 mg	Antihypertensives	Towa Pharmaceutical Co., Ltd.
Hemolingual Tablet	Venous Plexus Extract	0.18 mg	Antihemorrhoidals	Tobishi Pharmaceutical Co., Ltd.
Voglibose OD Film	Voglibose	0.2 mg, 0.3 mg	Antidiabetic agents	Kyukyu-phama Co., Ltd
Basen® OD Tablet	Voglibose	0.2 mg, 0.3 mg	Antidiabetic agents	Takeda Pharmaceutical Co., Ltd.
Beglilat® OD Tablet	Voglibose	0.2 mg, 0.3 mg	Antidiabetic agents	Taisho Pharmaceutical Industries, Ltd.
Voglibose OD Tablet	Voglibose	0.2 mg, 0.3 mg	Antidiabetic agents	Shiono Chemical Co.,Ltd.
Voglibose OD Tablet	Voglibose	0.2 mg, 0.3 mg	Antidiabetic agents	Sawai Pharmaceutical Co.,Ltd.
Voglibose OD Tablet	Voglibose	0.2 mg, 0.3 mg	Antidiabetic agents	Teva Pharma Japan Inc
Voglibose OD Tablet	Voglibose	0.2 mg, 0.3 mg	Antidiabetic agents	Takata Seiyaku Co.,Ltd.
Voglibose OD Tablet	Voglibose	0.2 mg, 0.3 mg	Antidiabetic agents	Nichi-Iko Pharmaceutical Co.,Ltd.
Voglibose OD Tablet	Voglibose	0.2 mg, 0.3 mg	Antidiabetic agents	Mylan Pharmaceutical Co.,Ltd
Voglibose OD Tablet	Voglibose	0.2 mg, 0.3 mg	Antidiabetic agents	Medisa Shinyaku Inc.
Voglibose OD Tablet	Voglibose	0.2 mg, 0.3 mg	Antidiabetic agents	Kobayashi Kako Co.,Ltd.
Voglibose OD Tablet	Voglibose	0.2 mg, 0.3 mg	Antidiabetic agents	Towa Pharmaceutical Co., Ltd.
Zomig® RM Tablet	Zolmitriptan	2.5 mg	Vasoconstrictors	AstraZeneca K.K.
Zolpidem Tartrate OD Film	Zolpidem Tartrate	5 mg, 10 mg	Hypnotics and sedatives, antianxietics	Kyukyu-phama Co., Ltd
Zolpidem Tartrate OD Tablet	Zolpidem Tartrate	5 mg, 10 mg	Hypnotics and sedatives, antianxietics	Elmed Eisai Co.,Ltd.
Zolpidem Tartrate OD Tablet	Zolpidem Tartrate	5 mg, 10 mg	Hypnotics and sedatives, antianxietics	Kobayashi Kako Co.,Ltd.
Zolpidem Tartrate OD Tablet	Zolpidem Tartrate	5 mg, 10 mg	Hypnotics and sedatives, antianxietics	Sawai Pharmaceutical Co.,Ltd.

(Table 12) contd.....

Brand Name	Drug	Dose	Therapeutic Category	Company
Zolpidem Tartrate OD Tablet	Zolpidem Tartrate	5 mg, 10 mg	Hypnotics and sedatives, antianxietics	Towa Pharmaceutical Co., Ltd.
Zolpidem Tartrate OD Tablet	Zolpidem Tartrate	5 mg, 10 mg	Hypnotics and sedatives, antianxietics	Nichi-Iko Pharmaceutical Co.,Ltd.
Trerief® OD Tablet	Zonisamide	25 mg	Antiparkinsonism agents	Dainippon Sumitomo Pharma Co., Ltd.

6. FDDF PRODUCTS IN INDIA

CDSCO (Central Drug Standards and Control Organisation, www.cdsco.nic.in) is central drug regulatory agency of India, which regulates and approves the entry of new drugs and drug products. In past seven years various fast disintegrating/dissolving drug products have been approved by CDSCO (Table **13**). Table **14** provides list of available drug products in Indian drug market. In Indian market, FDDF products are most commonly refereed to as Mouth Dissolving (MD) products.

Table 13. FDDF products approved by CDSCO India in duration 2007-2014 (Source www.cdsco.nic.in).

Description of FDDF Product	Indication	Date of Approval
Escitalopram Oxalate IP Eq to Escitalopram 10 mg + Clonazepam IP 0.5 mg Mouth dissolving tablet	Comorbid depression and anxiety disorder	04.04.14
Celecoxib Mouth Dissolving Tablet, 50 mg, 100 mg, 200 mg	Osteoarthritis and rheumatoid arthritis	25.02.2010
Dextromethorphan Orodispersible Strip, 5.5mg, 11 mg	Persistent dry irritating cough in adults	28.01.08
Donepezil HCl Orodispersible Tablet, 5 mg, 10 mg	Mild to moderate severe Alzheimer's dementia	15.10.2009
Lamotrigine Orodispersible Tablet, 12.5 mg	Anticonvulsant	20.03.2010
Levocetirizine Di-HCl Mouth Dissolving Tablets, 5 mg	Allergic rhinitis and chronic urticaria	25.07.2007
Levodopa 100/100/250 mg + Carbidopa10/25/25 mg, Mouth Dissolving Tablet	Idiopathic Parkinson's disease	04.03.09
Ondansetron Fast Dissolving Strips, 4 mg, 8 mg	Chemotherapy induced nausea and vomiting and post-operative nausea and vomiting	22.11.2011
Ondansetron Hydrochloride Mouth Melting Strips, 4 mg	Chemotherapeutic induced nausea and vomiting	29.3.12

(Table 13) contd.....

Description of FDDF Product	Indication	Date of Approval
Ondansetron Orally Disintegrating Tablet, 4 mg, 8mg	Chemotherapy induced nausea and vomiting	28.09.2007
Ondansetron Rapid Film Oral Strip, 4 mg, 8 mg	For chemotherapeutic induced nausea and vomiting.	16.11.10
Pantoprazole Mouth Dissolving Tablet, 20 mg, 40 mg	For the treatment of gastric ulcer, duodenal ulcer and GERD.	30.03.2010
Prednisolone Sodium Phosphate Orally Disintegrating Tablet, 10 mg, 15 mg, 30 mg	Glucocorticoids activity including collagen disease, allergic disease and hypersensitive reaction	26.11.2009
Rizatriptan Benzoate Orally Disintegrating Tablet, 10 mg	Migraine	24.05.2010
Sildenafil Citrate Orally Disintegrating Strips, 25mg/50mg	Erectile dysfunction	05.07.2013
Simethicone Orally Disintegrating Strip, 62.5 mg	Flatulance and as adjuvant in hyperacidity	14.11.2010
Tadalafil® Orally Disintegrating Strip, 10 mg, 20 mg	Erectile dysfunction	30.07.2014
Tolperisone HCl Mouth Dissolving tablet 50 mg, 100 mg	Muscle weakness and muscular hypertension	04.11.10
Voglibose tablet (Mouth dissolving), 0.2 mg/0.3 mg	Parantial hyperphemia in diabetes mellitus only	28.12.07

Table 14. Various fast dissolving/disintegrating drug products available in Indian market (Source: Drug Today and www.drugupdate.com).

Brand Name	Drug	Dose	Therapeutic Category	Company
Aripat® MD	Aripiprazole	10 mg, 15 mg, 20 mg, 30 mg	Antimaniac	Gentech H. Care
Sulpitac® MD	Amisulpiride	50 mg, 100 mg	Schizophrenia	Sun Pharma
Cetracare® MD	Cetirizine Dihydrochloride	10 mg	Antiallergic	Royal Lab
E-Cet® MD	Cetirizine Dihydrochloride	10 mg	Antiallergic	Marline Bio-Care
Rincet® MD	Cetirizine Dihydrochloride	10 mg	Antiallergic	Springer Bio-Tech
Varcet® MD	Cetirizine Dihydrochloride	10 mg	Antiallergic	Zota Healthcare
Zotacet® MD	Cetirizine HCl	10 mg	Antiallergic	Zota Pharma
Clodep® MD	Clonazepam	0.25 mg, 0.5 mg, 1 mg	Anticonvulsant	Parasol

(Table 14) contd.....

Brand Name	Drug	Dose	Therapeutic Category	Company
Clonapax® MD	Clonazepam	0.25 mg, 0.5 mg, 1 mg, 2 mg	Anticonvulsant	Reliance
Gemclo® MD	Clonazepam	0.25 mg, 0.5 mg, 1 mg, 2 mg	Anticonvulsant	Psychogem
Hope® MD	Clonazepam	0.25 mg	Anticonvulsant	RKG Pharma
Lonazep® MD	Clonazepam	0.25 mg, 0.5 mg, 1 mg, 2 mg	Anticonvulsant	Sun Pharma
Domaray® MD	Domperidone	10 mg	Antiemetics and antinauseants	Ray Remedies
Domit® MD	Domperidone	10 mg	Antiemetics and antinauseants	Shinto Biotec
Maridom® MD	Domperidone	10 mg	Antiemetics and antinauseants	Marc H. Care
Velrid® MD	Domperidone	10 mg	Antiemetics and antinauseants	Shreyam Health Care
Vomidon® MD	Domperidone	10 mg	Antiemetics and antinauseants	Olcare Lab
5HT3A® -MD	Ondansetron HCl	4 mg	Antiemetics and antinauseants	Baltic Pharma
Astadon® MD	Ondansetron HCl	4 mg	Antiemetics and antinauseants	Astalon Pharma
Estil® MD	Ondansetron HCl	4 mg	Antiemetics and antinauseants	Gladcare
Ondiphar® MD	Ondansetron HCl	4 mg	Antiemetics and antinauseants	Biophar L. Sciences
Onrid® MD	Ondansetron HCl	4 mg	Antiemetics and antinauseants	Kapeetus Medicorp
On-Zen-MD	Ondansetron HCl	4 mg	Antiemetics and antinauseants	Zenik Pharma
Vomirax® MD Tab	Ondansetron HCl	4 mg	Antiemetics and antinauseants	Rax H. Care
Vomitron® MD Tab	Ondansetron HCl	4 mg	Antiemetics and antinauseants	Marc Lab
Vomitix® MD	Ondansetron HCl	4 mg	Antiemetics and antinauseants	Saphnyx
Zofer® MD	Ondansetron HCl	4 mg, 8 mg	Antiemetics and antinauseants	Sun Pharma
Zomitron® MD	Ondansetron HCl	4 mg	Antiemetics and antinauseants	Healer's Lab

(Table 14) contd.....

Brand Name	Drug	Dose	Therapeutic Category	Company
Navtil® MD	Perochlorperazine maleate	5 mg	Antiemetics and antinauseants	RKG Pharma
Bigvin-1500 MD	Mecobalamin	1500 mcg	Peripheral neuropathy	Bestochem
Cobamet® OD	Mecobalamin	1500 mcg	Peripheral neuropathy	
Mecozen® MD	Mecobalamin	1500 mcg	Peripheral neuropathy	Sain Medicaments
Admenta® MD	Memantine HCl	5 mg, 10 mg	Dementia of the Alzheimers type	Sun Pharma
Mosid® MT	Mosapride citrate	2.5 mg, 5 mg	Chronic gastritis	Torrent
Romilast® MD Tab	Montelukast	4, 5 mg	Asthma	Ranbaxy Pharma
Mel-OD	Meloxicam	7.5 mg and 15 mg	NSAID	Zydus (Cadila)
Abinim® MD	Nimesulide	100 mg	NSAID	Alpic Biotech
Amonim® MD	Nimesulide	100 mg	NSAID	Mak Pharma
Crusid®MD	Nimesulide	100 mg	NSAID	Events Pharma
Imosan-100 MD	Nimesulide	100 mg	NSAID	Arvincare
Insure® MD	Nimesulide	100 mg	NSAID	Suzen Pharma
Melide® MD	Nimesulide	100 mg	NSAID	Milimax H. Care
Neme® MD	Nimesulide	100 mg	NSAID	Wel'N'Drugs
Nexus® MD	Nimesulide	100 mg	NSAID	Lexus
Nimed-MD	Nimesulide	100 mg	NSAID	Taurus Laboratories
Nime-MD	Nimesulide	100 mg	NSAID	Archise Life Science
Nimex® MD	Nimesulide	100 mg	NSAID	Mexon Health Care
Nimez® MD	Nimesulide	100 mg	NSAID	Zota Pharma
Nimlyn-MD	Nimesulide	100 mg	NSAID	Shade-Lynn
Nimovon® MD	Nimesulide	100 mg	NSAID	Ajanta
Nimude® MD	Nimesulide	100 mg	NSAID	Merril Pharma
Nimulid® MD	Nimesulide	100 mg	NSAID	Panacea Biotec
Nimvar® MD	Nimesulide	100 mg	NSAID	Zota Healthcare
Olnim® MD	Nimesulide	100 mg	NSAID	Olcare Lab
Softel® MD	Nimesulide	100 mg	NSAID	Symbiosis Labs
Sulbid® MD	Nimesulide	100 mg	NSAID	Alpic Remedies
Topmide®	Nimesulide	100 mg	NSAID	Antigen Health Care
Jolyon® MD	Olanzapine	5, 10, 15 mg	Antimaniac	Lupin
Lezapin® MD	Olanzapine	5, 10 mg	Antimaniac	Dycine
Manza® RDT	Olanzapine	5, 10 mg	Antimaniac	Mano Pharma (Orchid)

(Table 14) contd.....

Brand Name	Drug	Dose	Therapeutic Category	Company
Olanex® Instab	Olanzapine	2.5, 5, 7.5, 10 mg	Antimaniac	Ranbaxy (Solus)
Oleanx® RT (Oleanz RapiTab)	Olanzapine	2.5, 5, 7.5, 10, 15, 20 mg	Antimaniac	Sun Pharma
Olimelt®	Olanzapine	2.5, 5, 7.5, 10, 15, 20 mg	Antimaniac	Intas
Ozapin® MD	Olanzapine	2.5, 5, 7.5, 10, 15, 20 mg	Antimaniac	IPCA (Innova)
Schizol® MD	Olanzapine	5, 7.5, 10, 15, 20 mg	Antimaniac	Gentech HC
Tolaz® MD	Olanzapine	2.5, 5, 7.5, 10 mg	Antimaniac	Torrent (Mind)
Genrest® MD	Risperidone	0.5 mg, 1 mg	Psychotic disorders, schizophrenia and acute mania	4Life
Sizodon® MD	Risperidone	0.5 mg, 1 mg, 2mg	Psychotic disorders, schizophrenia and acute mania	Sun Pharma
Zisper® MD	Risperidone	1 mg, 2 mg, 3 mg	Psychotic disorders, schizophrenia and acute mania	Neu Foreva
TRD-MD	Tramadol HCl	50 mg	Opioid analgesics	Modi Mundi Pharma
Vogin® MD	Voglibose	0.2 mg, 0.3 mg	Antidiabetic	Divine Savior
Vosemet® MD	Voglibose	0.2 mg, 0.3 mg	Antidiabetic	Medihealth Lifesciences
Vogem® MD	Voglibose	0.2 mg, 0.3 mg	Antidiabetic	CeeDee Lifecare

CONCLUSIONS

Drug market in US, EU, Japan and Asian countries like India is continuously expanding with fast disintegrating/dissolving drug products. However, patent based FDDF products mostly belong to US, EU and Japan. Pharmaceutical companies like Catalent, Cima Labs and Ethypharm are aggressively marketing their proprietary technologies and expanding their market with the presence of newer FDDFs products through their alliance companies or by granting licenses to other companies. Among various FDDF products, FDTs have been exploited extensively for drug delivery. FDOF prescription products are recently introduced and in some markets they are yet to enter and expand. Controlled release FDTs are latest entrants in FDDF market with only a few (one or two products) in each geographic region. Other novel FDDF products like FDGs, ODMTs and FDPs are continuously developing and thus they may require more time for their successful market launches.

WEBSITES OF VARIOUS DRUG REGULATORY AGENCIES AND OTHER DRUG PRODUCT DATABASES

Central Drug Standards and Contral Organisation, India	www.cdsco.nic.in
DailyMed, US National Library of Medicine	http://dailymed.nlm.nih.gov
Drug Today	www.drugtodayonline.com
Drug Update	www.drugupdate.com
Drugs	www.drugs.com
Electronic Medicines Compendium (eMC), Datapharm.	http://www.ukmi.nhs.uk/default.asp
Electronic Medicines Compendium (eMC). Datapharm. Products.	http://www.medicines.org.uk/emc/
European Medicines Agency, UK	http://www.ema.europa.eu/
Food and Drug Administration, United States. US FDA	www.fda.gov
Medicines and Healthcare Regulatory Agency, United Kingdom.	https://www.gov.uk/government/organisations/medicines-and-healthcare-products-regulatory-agency
Orange Book (United States): Approved Drug Products with Therapeutic Equivalence	www.accessdata.fda.gov/scripts/cder/ob/
Orange Book, Japan	http://www.jp-orangebook.gr.jp/english/
Pharmaceutical and Medical Devices Agency, Japan	www.pmda.go.jp

WEBSITES OF VARIOUS COMPANIES VISITED DURING FEB-MARCH 2015

Akina	http://akinainc.com
APR Applied Pharma Research	http://www.apr.ch
Aprecia	https://aprecia.com
Aptalis	www.aptalispharma.com
Astellas	www.astellas.com
Biodelivery Science International	http://www.bdsi.com
Biofilm	http://www.biofilm.co.uk
C L Pharma	http://www.clpharm.com
Catalent	www.catalent.com
Cima Labs	www.cimalabs.com

Cima Labs	www.cimalabs.com
Cynapsus Therapeutics	http://www.cynapsus.ca
Dainippon Sumitomo Pharma	http://www.ds-pharma.co.jp
Eisai	www.eisai.com
Ethypharm	www.ethypharm.com
FFT Medical	http://fftmedical.se
Hermes Pharma	http://www.hermes-pharma.com
IntelGenx	http://www.intelgenx.com
Jenssen	www.janssenpharmaceuticalsinc.com
Kyowa Hakko Kirn	www.kyowa-kirin.com
Kyukyu Pharmaceutical	http://www.qqp.co.jp
Lavipharm	http://www.lavipharm.gr
LTS Lohman	http://www.ltslohmann.de
MonoSol Rx	http://www.monosolrx.com
Neos Therapeutics Inc.	www.neostx.com
NU Therapeutics	http://nutherapeutics.com
ODF Technolologies Inc.	http://www.odftechnologies.com
Otsuka Pharmaceutical	https://www.otsuka.co.jp
Pace Wellness	http://pacewellness.com
Perrigo	www.perrigo.com
Prestige Brands	http://prestigebrands.com/
Sato	http://www.zentripsato.com
SPI Pharmaceuticals	www.spipharma.com
tesa Latec	www.tesa-labtec.com
Towa Pharmaceutical	http://www.towayakuhin.co.jp
Umang Pharmaceuticals	http://www.umangpharmaceuticals.com
Valeant	www.valeant.com

REFERENCES

[1] EMA Guideline on the Investigation of bioequivalence. London: Committee for Medicinal Products for Human Use (CHMP). European Medicines Agency (EMA); 2010.

[2] García-Arieta A, Gordon J. Bioequivalence requirements in the European Union: critical discussion. AAPS J 2012; 14(4): 738-48. [http://dx.doi.org/10.1208/s12248-012-9382-1] [PMID: 22826032]

[3] Harmon TM. Orally disintegrating tablets: A valuable life cycle management strategy 2007. Accessed from: www.pharmaceuticalcommerce.com. Accessed on 3rd March 2015.

[4] FDA. Approved Drug Products with Therapeutic Equivalence Evaluations (Orange Book). US Department of Health and Human Services, Food And Drug Administration, Center For Drug Evaluation And Research, Office Of Medical Products And Tobacco Office Of Generic Drugs. 34th ed., 2014.

[5] Orally Disintegrating Tablet and Film Technologies. Technologies, Products, & Market Analysis. 7th ed., 2013. Accessed from: http://www.technology-catalysts.com/pdf/ODT7_brochure.pdf. Accessed on 3rd March 2015.

SUBJECT INDEX

W

X

Y

Z

www.ingramcontent.com/pod-product-compliance
Lightning Source LLC
LaVergne TN
LVHW072314210926
848482LV00021B/229